HEALTH ECONOMICS OF
Dementia

HEALTH ECONOMICS OF
Dementia

Edited by

ANDERS WIMO
Department of Family Medicine, Umeå University, Sweden and
Division of Clinical Neuroscience and Family Medicine, Karolinska Institute, Stockholm, Sweden

BENGT JÖNSSON
Department of Health Economics, Stockholm School of Economics, Stockholm, Sweden

GÖRAN KARLSSON
Department of Health Economics, Stockholm School of Economics, Stockholm, Sweden

BENGT WINBLAD
Division of Geriatric Medicine, Karolinska Institute, Stockholm, Sweden

JOHN WILEY & SONS

Chichester • New York • Weinheim • Brisbane • Singapore • Toronto

Other Wiley Editorial Offices

John Wiley & Sons, Inc., 605 Third Avenue,
New York, NY 10158-0012, USA

WILEY-VCH Verlag GmbH, Pappelallee 3,
D-69469 Weinheim, Germany

Jacaranda Wiley Ltd, 33 Park Road, Milton,
Queensland 4064, Australia

John Wiley & Sons (Asia) Pte Ltd, 2 Clementi Loop #02-01,
Jin Xing Distripark, Singapore 129809

John Wiley & Sons (Canada) Ltd, 22 Worcester Road,
Rexdale, Ontario M9W 1L1, Canada

Library of Congress Cataloging-in-Publication Data

Health economics of dementia / edited by Anders Wimo . . . [et al.].
    p. cm.
  Includes bibliographical references and index.
  ISBN 0-471-98376-4 (cased)
  1. Dementia—Economic aspects. 2. Medical economics.
 I. Wimo, Anders.
 RC521.H43 1998
 362.1'9683—dc21   98–16101
                                                        CIP

British Library Cataloguing in Publication Data

A catalogue record for this book is available from the British Library

ISBN 0-471-98376-4

Contents

Contributors

Ove Almkvist, Division of Geriatric Medicine B84, Huddinge Hospital, S-14186 Huddinge, Sweden

Yumiko Arai, Head of Research Unit for Nursing, Caring Sciences and Psychology, National Institute for Longevity Sciences, 36-3 Gengo, Obu-shi, Aichi, 474-8522, Japan

Stefanie Auer, New York University Medical Center, Education and Resources Program, 550 First Avenue, New York, NY 10016, USA

Thomas Bernhardt, Bayer Vital GmbH & Co. KG, Leverkusen, Germany

Luc Bonneux, Erasmus University Rotterdam, Institute for Medical Technology Assessment, Department of Public Health, PO Box 1738, 3000 DR Rotterdam, The Netherlands

Henry Brodaty, Professor, Academic Department of Psychogeriatrics, University of New South Wales, Prince Henry Hospital, Little Bay, Sydney, NSW 2036, Australia

Werner B. F. Brouwer, Erasmus University Rotterdam, Institute for Medical Technology Assessment, Department of Public Health, PO Box 1738, 3000 DR Rotterdam, The Netherlands

Rachelle Smith Doody, Baylor College of Medicine, Department of Neurology, 6550 Fannin, Suite 1801, Houston, TX 77030, USA

Michael F. Drummond, Professor, Centre for Health Economics, University of York, Heslington, York, YO1 5DD, UK

Sture Eriksson, Professor, Division of Geriatric Medicine, Umeå University, 901 87 Umeå, Sweden

Johan Fastbom, Dept. of Clinical Neuroscience and Family Medicine, Division of Geriatric Medicine, KFC Novum, S-141 86, Huddinge, Sweden

Howard Feldman, Professor, Division of Neurology, University of British Columbia, S192-2211 Wesbrook Mall, Vancouver, B.C. V6T 2B5, Canada

Emile Franssen, New York University Medical Center, Education and Resources Program, 550 First Avenue, New York, NY 10016, USA

Laura Fratiglioni, Olivecronas väg 4, Aldrecentrum, PO Box 6401, 113 82 Stockholm, Sweden

Serge Gauthier, Professor, Centre for Studies in Aging, McGill University, Montreal, Quebec H4M IR3, Canada

Maria Stella T. Giron, Stockholm Gerontology Research Centre & Department of Clinical Neuroscience and Family Medicine, Division of Geriatric Medicine, Karolinska Institute, Stockholm, Sweden

Steven Gracon, Warner-Lambert Company, Parke-Davis Pharmaceutical Research, 2800 Plymouth Road, Ann Arbor, Michigan 48105, USA

Margareta Grafström, Olivecronas väg 4, Aldrecentrum, PO Box 6401, 113 82 Stockholm, Sweden

Andreas Grass, Bayer Vital GmbH & Co., KG, Leverkusen, Germany

Stefan Håkansson, Professor, Department of Health Economics, The Swedish Institute for Health Service Development, Spri, P.O. Box 70487, S-107 26 Stockholm, Sweden

Richard C. Hermann, Harvard School of Public Health, Department of Health Policy and Management, 718 Huntington Avenue, Boston, MA 02115, USA

Suzanne Hill, Faculty of Medicine and Health Sciences, University of Newcastle, Callaghan, Newcastle, New South Wales, Australia

Rolf Horn, Bad Honnef

Naoki Ikegami, Professor, Department of Health Policy and Management, School of Medicine, Keio University, 35 Shinanomachi, Shinjuku-Ku, Tokyo, 160, Japan

Bernard Ineichen, Imperial College School of Medicine, Department of Public Health, Chelsea and Westminster Hospital, 369 Fulham Rd., London, SW10 9NH, UK

Lennarth Johansson, Socialtjanstgruppen, Socialstyrelsen, 106 30 Stockholm, Sweden

Bengt Jönsson, Professor, Department of Health Economics, Stockholm School of Economics, Stockholm, Sweden

Göran Karlsson, Department of Health Economics, Stockholm School of Economics, Stockholm, Sweden

Sunnie Kenowski, New York University Medical Center, Education and Resources Program, 550 First Avenue, New York, NY 10016, USA

Martin Knapp, Personal Social Services Research Unit, London School of Economics and Political Science, Houghton Street, London WC2A 2AE, UK

Marc A. Koopmanschap, Erasmus University Rotterdam, Institute for Medical Technology Assessment, Department of Public Health, PO Box 1738, 3000 DR Rotterdam, The Netherlands

Elaine A. Leventhal, UMDNJ, Robert Wood Johnson Medical School, University Medical Group, Clinical Academic Building, 125 Paterson Street, New Brunswick, NJ 08903, USA

David Lie, Academic Department of Psychogeriatrics, University of New South Wales, Prince Henry Hospital, Little Bay, Sydney, NSW 2036, Australia

Gunnar Ljunggren, Department of Clinical Neuroscience, Division of Geriatric Medicine, Karolinska Institute, S-141 86 Stockholm, Sweden

Paul J. van der Maas, Erasmus University Rotterdam, Institute for Medical Technology Assessment, Department of Public Health, PO Box 1738, 3000 DR Rotterdam, The Netherlands

Oliver Mast, Bayer Vital GmbH & Co., KG, Leverkusen, Germany

Vera Mastey, Pfizer Pharmaceuticals Group, Pfizer Inc., 235 East 42nd Street, New York, NY 10017-5755, USA

Wendy Max, Professor, Institute for Health & Aging, University of California, 3333 California Street, Room 340, San Francisco, CA 94143-0646, USA

Patricia McGettigan, Faculty of Medicine and Health Sciences, University of Newcastle, Callaghan, Newcastle, New South Wales, Australia

Willem J. Meerding, Erasmus University Rotterdam, Institute for Medical Technology Assessment, Department of Public Health, PO Box 1738, 3000 DR Rotterdam, The Netherlands

Hans-Jürgen Möller, Munich University

John N. Morris, Hebrew Rehabilitation Center for Aged, HRCA Research and Training Institute, Boston, Massachusetts, USA

Peter J. Neumann, Harvard School of Public Health, Department of Health Policy and Management, 718 Huntington Avenue, Boston, MA 02115, USA

Astrid Norberg, Professor, Department of Advanced Nursing, Umeå University, 901 87 Umeå, Sweden

Louise Nygård, Department of Geriatric Medicine, Huddinge University Hospital, 141 86 Huddinge, Sweden

Johan J. Polder, Erasmus University Rotterdam, Institute for Medical Technology Assessment, Department of Public Health, PO Box 1738, 3000 DR Rotterdam, The Netherlands

Stephen G. Post, School of Medicine, Center for Biomedical Ethics, Case Western Reserve University, Cleveland OH 44106, USA

Bernard M. Prigent, Associate Medical Director, Research and Development, Pfizer Canada Inc, Kirkland, Canada

Barry Reisberg, New York University Medical Center, Education and Resources Program, 550 First Avenue, New York, NY 10016, USA

P. O. Sandman, Department of Geriatric Medicine, University of Umeå, 901 87 Umeå, Sweden

Lon S. Schneider, Professor, University of Southern California, School of Medicine, 1975 Zonal Avenue, KAM-400 Los Angeles, CA 90033, USA

J.-M. Graf v.d. Schulenburg, North German Centre for Health Services Research HSR, Hanover University, 30167 Hanover, Germany

Ines Schulenburg, North German Centre for Health Services Research HSR, Hanover University, 30167 Hanover, Germany

F. Smith, Warner-Lambert Company, Parke-Davis Pharmaceutical Research, 2800 Plymouth Road, Ann Arbor, Michigan 48105, USA

Frank A. Sonnenberg, UMDNJ, Robert Wood Johnson Medical School, University Medical Group, Clinical Academic Building, 125 Paterson Street, New Brunswick, NJ 08903, USA

Liduin Souren, New York University Medical Center, Education and Resources Program, 550 First Avenue, New York, NY 10016, USA

Milton C. Weinstein, Harvard School of Public Health, Department of Health Policy and Management, 718 Huntington Avenue, Boston, MA 02115, USA

A.-L. Wetterholm, Department of Clinical Neuroscience & Family Medicine, Karolinska Institute, Division of Geriatric Medicine, Huddinge Hospital, S-141 86, Sweden

Peter Whitehouse, Professor, University Alzheimer Center, 11100 Euclid Avenue, Case Western Reserve University, Cleveland, OH 44106, USA

Carol J. Whitlatch, Professor, The Margaret Blenkner Research Center, The Benjamin Rose Institute, 850 Euclid Ave., Cleveland, OH 44114-3301, USA

Rachel Wigglesworth, Personal Social Services Research Unit, London School of Economics and Political Science, Houghton Street, London WC2A 2AE, UK

Anders Wimo, Professor, HC Bergsjo, Box 16, S-820 70 Bergsjo, Sweden

Bengt Winblad, Professor, Department of Clinical Neuroscience & Family Medicine, Karolinska Institute, Division of Geriatric Medicine, Huddinge Hospital, S-141 86, Sweden

Elke Witthaus, Department of Clinical Development, Hoechst Marion Roussel GmbH, HMR Entwicklung, H 840 D-659 26 Frankfurt am Main, Germany

Preface

The expanding number of people worldwide suffering from different dementia disorders presents an enormous challenge for the health care and social support systems, irrespective of how they are organized and financed. There is also a great ethical challenge in dementia care since the diseases themselves influence the patients' capacity to advocate for their own interests. Dementia disorders also considerably influence the situation of the caregivers. Care of dementia is costly and in these days of determining priorities, the combination of expensive care and a highly prevalent group of chronic diseases where patients have great problems in looking after their interests, makes us focus on the fundamental issues in all health economics analyses.

Health economics of dementia is in its infancy with a small scientific base, and the purpose of this book is mainly methodological: to present and discuss the methodological issues in this field. We have invited contributions from those whom we consider to be among the most prominent scientists in the areas that we regard as important for health economics of dementia. Although health economics focuses on the costs and outcome of care, it is also necessary to have a broad background for such analyses and therefore we have included a section in this book that presents some basic prerequisites for dementia care.

However, we do not claim to present a complete picture of all problems related to the health economics of dementia and we do not guarantee that the contributions are in perfect harmony as regards content or theoretical approach. Some of the contributions partly overlap and some controversies are also highlighted. However, this illustrates the current development of the health economics of dementia.

This is the first comprehensive book on the health economics of dementia and we hope that it will contribute to the discussions of how future research in this field should be designed and performed. The editors are grateful to all the contributors to this volume, and to the publisher for support during its production.

Stockholm, 1998
Anders Wimo
Bengt Jönsson
Göran Karlsson
Bengt Winblad

1 General Aspects

1.1 Classification and Diagnostics

LAURA FRATIGLIONI

Division of Geriatric Medicine, Karolinska Institute, Stockholm and Neurologic Clinic, Careggi University Hospital, Florence

The term 'dementia' describes a syndrome characterised by a wide range of symptoms due to brain dysfunction. It can be defined as the acquired and sustained deterioration of intellectual functions in an alert patient (Morris, 1996). The essential features are losses of cognitive and emotional abilities severe enough to interfere with daily functioning and quality of life. Because dementia can be produced by many different underlying diseases, the order of onset and relative prominence of the cognitive disturbances and associated symptoms vary with different dementing disorders (American Psychiatric Association, 1997; Geldmacher and Whitehouse, 1996). However, uniform diagnostic criteria have been developed and are commonly implemented for the identification of dementia.

DIAGNOSTIC CRITERIA FOR DEMENTIA

The most frequently used criteria are provided by the American Psychiatric Association in the third version of *Diagnostic and Statistical Manual* (DSM-III-R, 1987) or in the recently published new edition (DSM-IV, 1994), and by the diagnostic guidelines described in the International Classification of Disease (ICD-10, 1992). The definition of dementia according to these three systems is reported in Table 1.1.1.

According to these classification criteria, memory disturbances alone are not sufficient for the diagnosis of dementia. Moreover, other disorders causing cognitive impairment, such as delirium, amnestic disorder, mental retardation, and major depression, need to be excluded. The DSM-IV criteria introduce the disturbances of executive functioning (the ability to think abstractly and to plan, initiate, sequence, monitor, and stop complex behaviour) instead of personality changes required by DSM-III-R. Cognitive decline from previous level is also newly introduced in DSM-IV. Similarly to DSM-IV, ICD-10 guidelines specify that memory disturbances alone are not sufficient for the diagnosis, and that cognitive disturbances are based on evidence of a decline. Differently from

Health Economics of Dementia. Edited by Anders Wimo, Bengt Jönsson, Göran Karlsson and Bengt Winblad.
© 1998 John Wiley & Sons Ltd.

Table 1.1.1. Definition of dementia according to different diagnostic criteria

DSM-III-R (1987)	ICD-10 (1992)	DSM-IV (1994)
Impairment in memory	Decline in both memory	Impairment in memory
and	and	and
at least one of the following: abstract thinking, judgement impairment, aphasia, agnosia, or personality change	thinking, of a degree sufficient	at least one of the following: agnosia, apraxia, aphasia, or executive functioning impairment
Cognitive deficits interfere with work or social activities or relationships with others	to impair functioning in daily living	Cognitive deficits are severe enough to interfere with occupational/social activities
		and
		represent a decline from previous level

DSM-IV, the ICD-10 guidelines consider dementia as a chronic or progressive disorder, and require a duration of symptomatology of at least 6 months.

The validity of dementia diagnosis is problematic, especially in the early stages of the disease when mild cognitive impairment must be differentiated from cognitive changes resulting from normal ageing. It has been stressed that the essence of dementia diagnosis and different dementia disorders, too, depends on the knowledge and skills of a physician in eliciting a valid history, documenting the impairment and characteristic findings during the examination, and carrying out appropriate differential diagnosis (Berg and Morris, 1994). Thus, this process is especially difficult in community surveys carried out for epidemiological and public health purposes, due to a more limited contact with the subject and his/her family, and a higher proportion of mild cases in the population than in the clinical setting. The distinction between dementia and normal ageing becomes more difficult with increasing age (Fratiglioni et al, 1992). Old subjects decrease social and work activities in a variable way depending more on family situation, personality, physical health status, and type of society than on their degree of cognitive impairment. Multimorbidity is more common in old age, and can interfere in some way with cognitive functioning during the examination.

The validity of dementia diagnosis has been investigated in terms of agreement between different clinicians, and diagnostic confirmation at follow-up (Schofield et al, 1995; Agüero Torres et al, 1998). The agreements, expressed as kappa index, range from 0.59 to 0.86 in different studies where DSM-III-R criteria were used (Fratiglioni et al, 1992; Baldereschi et al, 1994; O'Connor et al, 1996). Because kappa index measures the agreement beyond chance (MacLure and Willet, 1987), this agreement is regarded as good.

CLASSIFICATION OF DEMENTING DISORDERS

Neurological diseases display a limited repertoire of cognitive, behavioural, and neurological symptoms and signs, so it is not surprising that conditions with distinctively different aetiology and neuropathology may share clinical features. Different classifications have been proposed, either based on clinical (Cummings and Benson, 1992), or aetiopathological (Morris, 1996), or clinicopathological (Pryse-Phillips and Galasko, 1996) aspects. We suggest a subdivision of the most common dementing disorders into four groups according to the frequency of dementia in the core symptomatology of each specific disease (Table 1.1.2).

Several diagnostic criteria have been developed, especially for the most common dementing disorders, Alzheimer's disease (AD) and Vascular dementia (VaD), but operational criteria for frontotemporal lobe dementia (The Lund and Manchester Groups, 1994) and for senile dementia of Lewy body type (McKeith et al, 1996) have been published, too.

DIAGNOSTIC CRITERIA FOR ALZHEIMER'S DISEASE

As no specific biological markers have been identified, the diagnosis is essentially a clinical one. Both DSM and ICD include specific criteria for AD. A third leading set of diagnostic criteria is that suggested in a consensus document by a working group organised by the National Institute of Neurological Disorders and Stroke, and the Alzheimer's Disease and Related Disorders Association (NINCDS–ADRDA criteria; McKhann et al, 1984) (Table 1.1.3).

Not surprisingly, the three sets of criteria share many common features. In order to make a diagnosis of AD, all three require (1) an insidious onset of dementia, (2) a gradually progressive deteriorating course, and (3) the exclusion of all other specific causes of dementia. In ICD-10, absence of apoplectic onset or focal neurological signs early in the illness are exclusion criteria. The NINCDS–ADRDA criteria take a somewhat different approach by grading the level of diagnostic certainty. Differences between definite, probable and possible AD diagnosis reflect the available information and how closely the patient's syndrome resembles 'classic' AD. A definite diagnosis can be reached when pathological evidence of AD is added to a diagnosis of clinical probable AD. Probable AD is characterised by deficits in two or more areas of cognition, and possible AD is diagnosed when only one cognitive area is affected in the absence of any other identifiable cause, or when the clinical course is atypical, or when a second disease potentially related to dementia is present but it is not considered to be the cause of dementia.

Table 1.1.2. Disorders known to cause dementia

Group	Specific diseases
Dementia as the core symptomatology	
Degenerative disorders	Alzheimer's disease
	Frontal lobe dementias
	Diffuse Lewy Body disease
	Alcoholic dementia
Vascular disorders	Multi-infarct dementias
	Biswanger's disease
	Amyloid angiopathy
	Rare vasculopathies
Prion and infectious disorders	Subacute spongiform encephalopathies (Creutzfeldt–Jakob)
	AIDS-dementia
	Chronic meningoencephalopathies (neurosyphilis)
Dementia as a part of the core symptomatology	Huntington's disease
	Parkinson with dementia
	ALS–Parkinson–Dementia complex
	Progressive supranuclear palsy
	Hydrocephalus
	Metabolic disorders (B12 deficiency, renal dialysis, hypothyroidism)
Dementia as a rare symptom in common disorders	Multiple Sclerosis
	Head trauma
	Primary and metastatic brain tumours
	Subdural haematoma
Dementia as a symptom in rare disorders	Mostly metabolic diseases (see review in Morris, 1996, and Coker, 1991)

Table 1.1.3. Definition and diagnostic criteria of Alzheimer's disease

Definition	Diagnostic criteria
Dementia characterised by insidious onset and progressive deterioration. Other dementing disorders need to be excluded	DSM-III-R (1987)
	DSM-IV (1994)
	ICD-10 (1992)
	NINCDS–ADRDA (1984)

The validity of AD diagnosis has been studied in terms of reproducibility and confirmation at autopsy. The agreement, expressed as kappa index, between different clinicians in making AD diagnosis was 0.49 (Lopez et al, 1990), 0.72 (Baldereschi et al, 1994), and 0.63 (Farrer et al, 1995) when NINCDS–ADRDA criteria were used. The reproducibility of DSM-III-R resulted in a kappa value of 0.55 (Kukull et al, 1990), and 0.67 (Fratiglioni et

Table 1.1.4. Definition and diagnostic criteria of Vascular dementia

Short definition	Diagnostic criteria
Post-stroke dementia or Multi-infarct dementia	DSM-III-R (1987) ICD-10 (1992) Hachinski score (1975) and modified forms[a]
Dementia due to cerebrovascular disorders	DSM-IV (1994) Erkinjuntti et al (1988) ADDTC, Chui et al (1992) NINDS–AIREN Román et al (1993)
Vascular Cognitive Impairment	Hachinski and Bowler (1993) (Operational criteria not yet defined)

[a] Rosen et al (1979); Portera-Sanchez et al (1982); Loeb and Gandolfo (1983); Katzman and Kawas (1986); Fischer et al (1991).

al, 1992). The accuracy rate of clinically based diagnosis when compared with pathological findings varies from 0.62 to 0.92 (Klatka et al, 1996).

DIAGNOSTIC CRITERIA FOR VASCULAR DEMENTIA

After the initial definition of 'multi-infarct dementia' as a post-stroke dementia, the broader term 'Vascular dementia' has been suggested to identify the acquired intellectual impairment resulting from brain injury due to a cerebrovascular disorder (Tatemichi et al, 1994). This definition properly includes both haemorrhagic and ischemic cerebrovascular diseases, although it is generally agreed that ischemic damage is the predominant cause of VaD. The term cerebrovascular disorder includes both conventional mechanisms such as thromboembolic disease and also hypoxic-ischemic brain insults from circulatory failure related to cardiac arrest and systemic hypotension. Finally, Hachinski and Bowler, 1993, and Bowler and Hachinski, 1995, propose a new concept, 'Vascular cognitive impairment', in which all cognitive disturbances related to cerebrovascular disorders are included, disregarding degree of severity and primary focus on memory.

Following these definitions, different sets of criteria have been proposed (Table 1.1.4). Despite all the efforts, VaD is still difficult to diagnose and remains a controversial topic (Hachinski, 1992). One of the main reasons is the emerging evidence from pathological and aetiologic studies, of overlap between degenerative and vascular dementing disorders. At autopsy, vascular lesions are frequently associated with AD, and maybe they affect presence and severity of the symptoms (Snowdon et al, 1997; Pasquier and Leys, 1997); cognitive impairment and dementia increase the risk of stroke (Ferrucci et al, 1996; Moroney et al, 1997); and vascular risk factors have been found to be associated with increased risk of AD (Skoog et al, 1996).

Traditional methods such as DSM diagnostic criteria or Hachinski ischemic score (Hachinski et al, 1975) have been strongly criticised (O'Brien, 1988). Two major diagnostic criteria systems have been proposed (Chui et al, 1992; Román et al, 1993), both of which attempted to include all aspects of vascular dementia in operational criteria. All require three essential features to diagnose VaD: defining dementia, identifying the presence of cerebrovascular dementia, and establishing a causal link between the two disorders. Differently from DSM-III or IV, and from ICD-10, dementia here is defined by impairment in memory, and in at least two other cognitive domains. The presence of cerebrovascular disease can be derived from clinical history, examination or brain imaging. The aetiologic relevance is left to clinical judgement in DSM-III and IV, whereas in NINCDS–AIREN causality is based on a temporal relationship, abrupt or stepwise deterioration or fluctuating course, or specific brain imaging findings. Because important gaps in knowledge concerning vascular dementia still exist, no single system of diagnostic criteria can be considered definitive (Drachman, 1993).

REFERENCES

Agüero Torres, H., Fratiglioni, L., Guo, Z., Viitanen, M., and Winblad, B. (1998). Prognostic factors in very old demented adults: a seven-year follow-up from a population-based survey in Stockholm, *J. Am. Ger. Soc.*, in press.

American Psychiatric Association (1997). Practice guideline for the treatment of patients with Alzheimer's disease and other dementias of late life, *Am. J. Psychiatry*, Suppl 154, 1–39.

American Psychiatric Association (1987). *Diagnostic and Statistical Manual of Mental Disorders, 3rd edn revised* (DSM-III-R), pp. 97–163, American Psychiatric Association, Washington, DC.

American Psychiatric Association (1994). *Diagnostic and Statistical Manual of Mental Disorders, 4th edn* (DSM-IV), pp. 133–155, American Psychiatric Association, Washington, DC.

Baldereschi, M., Amato, M. P., Nencini, P., Pracucci, G., Lippi, A., Amaducci, L., Gauthier, S., Beatty, L., Quiroga, P., Klassen, G., Galea, A., Muscat, P., Osuntokun, B., Ogunniyi, A., Portera-Sanchez, A., Bermejo, F., Hendrie, H., Burdine, V., Brashear, A., Farlow, M., Maggi, S., and Katzman, R. (1994). Cross-national interrater agreement on the clinical diagnostic criteria for dementia, *Neurology*, **44**, 239–242.

Berg, L., and Morris, J. C. (1994). Diagnosis, in R. D. Terry, R. Katzman, and K. L. Bick (Eds), *Alzheimer Disease*, pp. 9–25, Raven Press, New York.

Bowler, J. V., and Hachinski, V. (1995). Vascular cognitive impairment: a new approach to vascular dementia, in V. Hachinski (Ed.), *Cerebrovascular Disease*, pp. 357–376, Baillière Tindall, London.

Chui, H. C., Victoroff, J. I., Margolin, D., Jagust, W., Shankle, R., and Katzman, R. (1992). Criteria for the diagnosis of Ischemic Vascular Dementia proposed by the State of California Alzheimer's Disease Diagnostic and Treatment Centers, *Neurology*, **42**, 473–480.

Coker, S. B. (1991). The diagnosis of childhood degenerative disorders presenting as dementia in adults, *Neurology*, **41**, 794–798.

Cummings, J. L., and Benson, D. F. (1992). *Dementia. A Clinical Approach*, Butterworth-Heinemann, Boston.

Drachman, D. A. (1993). New criteria for the diagnosis of vascular dementia: do we know enough yet? *Neurology*, **43**, 246–249.

Erkinjuntti, T., Haltia, M., Palo, J., Sulkava, R., and Paetau, A. (1988). Accuracy of the clinical diagnosis of vascular dementia: a prospective clinical and post-mortem neuropathological study, *J. Neurol. Neurosurg. Psychiatry*, **51**, 1037–1044.

Farrer, L. A., Cupples, L. A., Blackburn, S., Kiely, D. K., Auerbach, S., Growdon, J. H., Connor-Lacke, L., Karlinsky, H., Thibert, A., Burke, J. R., Utley, C., Chui, H., Ireland, A., Duara, R., Lopez-Alberola, R., Larson, E. B., O'Connell, S., and Kukull, W. A. (1995). Consistency of clinical diagnosis in a community-based longitudinal study of dementia and Alzheimer's disease, *Neurology*, **45**, 2159–2164.

Ferrucci, L., Guralnik, J. M., Salive, M. E., Pahor, M., Corti, M.-C., Baroni, A., and Havlik, R.J. (1996). Cognitive impairment and risk of stroke in the older population, *J. Am. Ger. Soc.*, **44**, 237–241.

Fischer, P., Jellinger, K., Gatterer, G. et al (1991). Prospective neuropathological validation of Hachinski's Ischemic Score in dementia, *J. Neurol. Neurosurg. Psychiatry*, **54**, 580–583.

Fratiglioni, L., Grut, M., Forsell, Y., Viitanen, M., and Winblad, B. (1992). Clinical diagnosis of Alzheimer's disease and other dementias in a population survey. Agreement and causes of disagreement in applying DSM-III-R criteria, *Arch. Neurol.*, **49**, 227–232.

Geldmacher, D. S., and Whitehouse, P. J. (1996). Evaluation of Dementia, *New Engl. J. of Medn*, **335**, 330–335.

Hachinski, V. (1992). Preventable senility: a call for action against the vascular dementias, *Lancet*, **340**, 645–647.

Hachinski, V. C., and Bowler, J. V. (1993). Vascular dementia, *Neurology*, **43**, 2159–2160.

Hachinski, V. C., Iliff, L. D., Zilhka, E., Du Boulay, G. H., McAllister, V. L., Marshall, J., Russel, R. W. R., and Symon, L. (1975). Cerebral blood flow in dementia, *Arch. Neurol.*, **32**, 632–637.

Katzman, R., and Kawas, C. (1986). The evolution of the diagnosis of dementia: past, present, and future, in *Neurology*. Proceedings of the XIIIth World Congress of Neurology, Hamburg (Eds K. Poeck, H-J. Freund, and H. Ganshirt), pp. 43–49, Springer-Verlag, New York.

Kertesz, A., Davidson, W., and Fox, H. (1997). Frontal behavioral inventory: diagnostic criteria for frontal lobe dementia, *Can. J. Neurol. Sciences*, **24**, 29–36.

Klatka, L. A., Schiffer, R. B., Powers, J. M., and Kazee, A. M. (1996). Incorrect diagnosis of Alzheimer's disease, *Arch. Neurol.*, **53**, 35–42.

Kukull, W. A., Larson, E. B., Reifler, B. V., Lampe, T. H., Yerby, M., and Hughes, J. (1990). Interrater reliability of Alzheimer's disease diagnosis, *Neurology*, **40**, 257–260.

Loeb, C., and Gandolfo, C. (1983). Diagnostic evaluation of degenerative and vascular dementia, *Stroke*, **14**, 399–401.

Lopez, O. L., Swihart, A. A., Becker, J. T., Reinmuth, O. M., Reynolds, C. F., Rezek, D. L., and Daly, F. L. (1990). Reliability of NINCDS–ADRDA criteria for the diagnosis of Alzheimer's disease, *Neurology*, **40**, 1517–1522.

MacLure, M., and Willett, W. (1987). Misinterpretation and misuse of the Kappa statistic, *Am. J. Epidemiol.*, **126**, 161–169.

McKeith, I. G., Galasko, D., Kosaka, K., Perry, E. K., Dickson, D. W., Hansen, L. A., Salmon, D. P., Lowe, J., Mirra, S. S., Byrne, E. J., Lennox, G., Quinn, N. P.,

Edwardson, J. A., Ince, P. G., Bergeron, C., Burns, A., Miller, B. L., Lovestone, S., Collerton, D., Jansen, E. N. H., Ballard, C., de Vos, R. A. I., Wilcock, G. K., Jellinger, K. A., and Perry, R. H. (1996). Consensus guidelines for the clinical and pathologic diagnosis of dementia with Lewy bodies (DLB): Report of the consortium on DLB international workshop, *Neurology*, **47**, 1113–1124.

McKhann, G., Drachman, D., Folstein, M., Katzman, R., Price, D., and Stadlan, M. (1984). Clinical diagnosis of Alzheimer's disease: Report of the NINCDS–ADRDA Work Group under the auspices of Department of Health and Human Services Task Force on Alzheimer's Disease, *Neurology*, **34**, 939–944.

Moroney, J. T., Bagiella, E., Tatemichi, T. K., Paik, M. C., Stern, Y., and Desmond, D. W. (1997). Dementia after stroke increases the risk of long-term stroke recurrence, *Neurology*, **48**, 1317–1325.

Morris, J. C. (1996). Classification of dementia and Alzheimer's disease, *Acta. Neurol. Scand.*, Suppl 165, 41–50.

O'Brien, M. D. (1988). Vascular dementia is underdiagnosed, *Arch. Neurol.*, **45**, 797–798.

O'Connor, D. W., Blessed, G., Cooper, B., Jonker, C., Morris, J. C., Presnell, I. B., Ames, D., Kay, D. W. K., Bickel, H., Schäufele, M., Wind, A., Coats, M., and Berg, L. (1996). Cross-national interrater reliability of dementia diagnosis in the elderly and factors associated with disagreement, *Neurology*, **47**, 1194–1199.

Pasquier, F., and Leys, D. (1997). Why are stroke patients prone to develop dementia? *J. Neurol.*, **244**, 135–142.

Portera-Sanchez, A., del Ser, T., Bermejo, F. et al (1982). Clinical diagnosis of senile dementia of Alzheimer type and vascular dementia, in *Neural Aging and its Implications in Human Neurological Pathology* (Eds R. D. Terry, C. L. Bilis, and G. Toffano), pp. 169–188, Raven Press, New York.

Pryse-Phillips, W., and Galasko, D. (1996). Non-Alzheimer dementias, in *Clinical Diagnosis and Management of Alzheimer's Disease* (Ed. S. Gauthier), pp. 51–66, Martin Dunitz, Canada.

Román, G. C., Tatemichi, T. K., Erkinjuntti, T., Cummings, J. L., Masdeu, J. C., Garcia, J. H., Amaducci, L., Orgogozo, J.-M., Brun, A., Hofman, A., Moody, D. M., O'Brien, M. D., Yamaguchi, T., Grafman, J., Drayer, B. P., Bennett, D. A., Fisher, M., Ogata, J., Kokmen, E., Bermejo, F., Wolf, P. A., Gorelick, P. B., Bick, K. L., Pajeau, A. K., Bell, M. A., DeCarli, C., Culebras, A., Korczyn, A. D., Bogousslavsky, J., Hartmann, A., and Scheinberg, P. (1993). Vascular dementia: diagnostic criteria for research studies. Report of the NINDS–AIREN International Work Group, *Neurology*, **43**, 250–260.

Rosen, W. G., Terry, R. D., Fuld, P. et al (1979). Pathological Verification of Ischemic Score in Differentiation of Dementias, *Ann. Neurol.*, **7**, 486–488.

Schofield, P. W., Tang, M., Marder, K., Bell, K., Dooneief, G., Lantigua, R., Wilder, D., Gurland, B., Stern, Y., and Mayeux, R. (1995). Consistency of clinical diagnosis in a community-based longitudinal study of dementia and Alzheimer's disease, *Neurology*, **45**, 2159–2164.

Skoog, I., Lernfelt, B., Landahl, S. et al (1996). 15-year longitudinal study of blood pressure and dementia, *Lancet*, **347**, 1141–1145.

Snowdon, D. A., Greiner, L. H., Mortimer, J. A., Riley, K. P., Greiner, P. A., and Markesbery, W. R. (1997). Brain infarction and the clinical expression of Alzheimer disease. The Nun Study, *JAMA*, **277**, 813–817.

Tatemichi, T. K., Sacktor, N., and Mayeux, R. (1994). Dementia associated with cerebrovascular disease, other degenerative diseases, and metabolic disorders, in *Alzheimer Disease* (Eds R. D. Terry, R. Katzman, and K. L. Bick), pp. 123–166, Raven Press, New York.

The Lund and Manchester Groups (1994). Clinical and neuropathological criteria for frontotemporal dementia, *J. Neurol. Neurosurg. Psychiatry*, **57**, 416–418.
World Health Organisation (1992). *International statistical classification of diseases and related health problems*, 10th revision (ICD-10). Chapter V, categories F00–F99. Mental, behavioural and developmental disorders, clinical description and diagnostic guidelines. World Health Organisation, Geneva.

1.2 Epidemiology

LAURA FRATIGLIONI
Division of Geriatric Medicine, Karolinska Institute, Stockholm and Neurologic Clinic, Careggi University Hospital, Florence

The first epidemiological studies concerning dementia and different types of dementia were carried out during the 1960s in the Scandinavian countries; however, it was during the 1980s that epidemiological methods first began to be widely used in the field of dementia. They were used to describe the occurrence and frequency patterns of the dementias, and to identify risk factors for different dementing disorders. Finally, in the 1990s, follow-up studies regarding both the aetiology and natural history of the dementias have been initiated. The contribution of epidemiological research to understanding the dementias, up to the present time, can be summarised in the following three points:

1. The distribution pattern of the dementing disorders has been described in sufficient detail to be utilised for planning medical and social services, at least in all Western countries.
2. Some risk factors have been clearly identified, and interesting working hypotheses in the field of aetiopathogenesis have been suggested, giving the impression (and hope) that we are not far away from the time when preventive interventions can be implemented.
3. Although longitudinal data on the natural history of the dementias are still limited, some aspects of disease progression, as well as impact on survival and quality of life, are sufficiently outlined to be useful at the community level for allocating medical and social resources, and at the individual level for counselling patients and relatives.

OCCURRENCE

The occurrence of a disease can be measured as the proportion of subjects affected by the disease in a defined population at a specific instant (prevalence), or as the number of new cases that develop in a population of individuals at risk during a specific time interval (incidence). Whereas the prevalence provides

Health Economics of Dementia. Edited by Anders Wimo, Bengt Jönsson, Göran Karlsson and Bengt Winblad.
© 1998 John Wiley & Sons Ltd.

Table 1.2.1. Age-specific prevalence, per 100, of all dementias in different countries. Values are expressed as ranges derived from different studies

Age groups	Europe[a]	North America[b]	Asia[c]	Africa[d]
60–64	0.4–1.0	0.2–0.3	0.3	
65–69	0.9–1.4	0.8–0.9	1.0–2.4	
70–74	2.1–4.1	1.3–2.0	1.5–7.0	0.9
75–79	4.6–14.6	3.6–6.3	10.8–15.1	
80–84	9.6–27	8.9–12.7	16.3–38.9	0.7
85–89	20.4–38.3	16.3–29.7		
90–94	28.3–57.3	40.4–74.3		9.6
95+	42.3–55.8	58.6		

[a] Hofman et al (1991); Juva et al (1993); Engedal and Haugen (1993); Wernicke and Reischies (1994); Fichter et al (1995); Ott et al (1995); Johansson and Zarit (1995); Prencipe et al (1996); Gip et al (1997); De Ronchi et al (1998).
[b] Kokmen et al (1989); Bachman et al (1992); Ebly et al (1994); Graves et al (1997).
[c] Ueda et al (1992); Hasegawa et al (1986); Zhang et al (1990); Park et al (1994); Shaji et al (1996).
[d] Hendrie et al (1995).

an estimate of the risk that an individual will be ill at a certain point in time, the incidence estimates the risk of becoming ill. The prevalence is determined both by incidence and disease survival.

PREVALENCE OF DEMENTIA AND DIFFERENT DEMENTING DISORDERS

Dementia prevalence depends greatly on the age structure of the population, as the disease prevalence doubles almost every 5 years (Jorm, 1991; Hofman et al, 1991). Prevalence is low in subjects under the age of 60, and increases even in the most advanced ages (Gip et al, 1997). Approximately one out of every 100 people age 60–69 is demented, but the corresponding value reaches 50% in 90+ year old adults. Some prevalence figures from different countries are presented in Table 1.2.1. Variation among countries seems to reflect methodological differences among studies rather than real differences (Corrada et al, 1995). However, some authors have reported possible ethnic variation, as higher prevalence has been found among black Americans (Schoenberg et al, 1985; Perkins et al, 1997) and American Hispanics (Perkins et al, 1997), and lower values have been observed among Nigerian Africans (Hendrie et al, 1995).

Despite similar overall prevalence for dementia in North America, Europe, and Asia, the relative proportions attributed to Alzheimer's disease (AD) and Vascular dementia (VaD) differ markedly. In most Western countries, 50–70% of the total dementia prevalence is attributed to AD, and 20–30% to VaD. In most Asian studies, higher percentages are found for VaD. Only few reports differ from this pattern (Skoog et al, 1993; Park et al, 1994). It seems that most

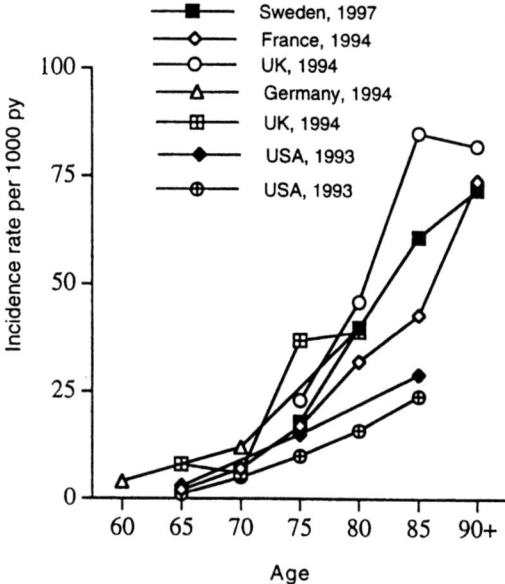

Figure 1.2.1. Age-specific incidence rates for dementia per 1000 person-years in different countries (Kokmen et al, 1993; Bachman et al, 1993; Letenneur et al, 1994; Paykel et al, 1994; Bickel and Cooper, 1994; Boothby et al, 1994; Fratiglioni et al, 1997)

of the inconsistency is due to the estimate of VaD figures, rather than AD. The interpretation of these geographical differences needs to take into account (1) variation in diagnostic criteria and procedure, (2) differential survival, and (3) differential geographical distribution of vascular risk factors and stroke.

INCIDENCE OF DEMENTIA AND DIFFERENT DEMENTING DISORDERS

Most of our knowledge concerning the occurrence of the dementias is based on prevalence rather than incidence figures. A limited number of incidence studies are present in the literature, especially regarding different dementing disorders. In Figures 1.2.1–1.2.3, the findings from some of these studies are summarised. All figures are surprisingly similar, when methodological differences among different studies are taken into account. During one year, there are two persons per 1000 people ages 65–69 who become demented; when the population is older than 90 years, this number increases to 70–80 new cases in one year per 1000 people. AD is the most frequent dementing disorder, accounting for 80% in the oldest age group. Both dementia and AD incidence increase steeply with age, while the relationship between VaD and age is not so clear.

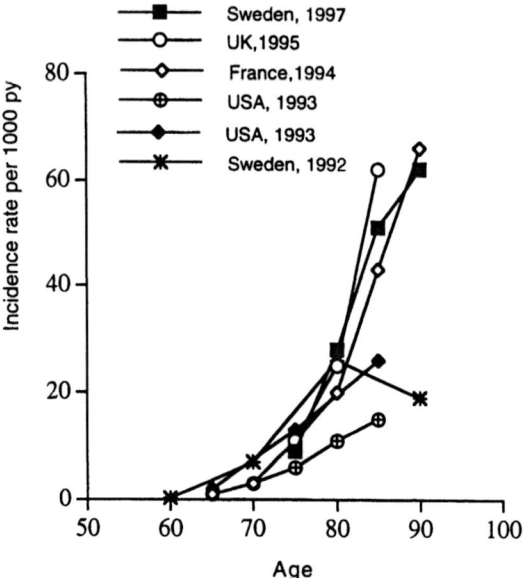

Figure 1.2.2. Age-specific incidence rates for Alzheimer's disease per 1000 person-years in different countries (Hagnell et al, 1992; Kokmen et al, 1993; Bachman et al, 1993; Letenneur et al, 1994; Brayne et al, 1995; Fratiglioni et al, 1997)

RISK FACTORS

Numerous aetiologic studies have been carried out with the aim of identifying risk factors for different dementing disorders. Most of these studies focus on AD; data concerning vascular dementia and other dementia types are limited. In the last few years, a new research area has been developed in which the outcome is any type of dementia, rather than a specific dementing disorder.

RISK FACTORS FOR ALZHEIMER'S DISEASE

Most studies use the case-control approach with prevalent cases, rather than incident cases, and a retrospective assessment of the exposure. Some studies have collected information on risk factors directly from the subjects before dementia onset, most have used an informant as a surrogate for the demented person who could not be interviewed due to the nature of the disease. All of these limitations and methodological differences need to be kept in mind when considering the inconsistent findings reported in the literature. Comprehensive reviews have recently been published, in which aetiologic hypotheses are described in detail (van Duijn, 1996; Fratiglioni, 1996). These two papers

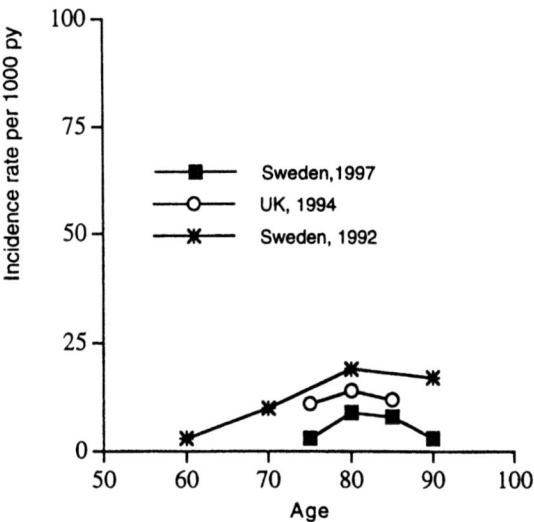

Figure 1.2.3. Age-specific incidence rates for Vascular dementia per 1000 person-years in different countries (Hagnell et al, 1992; Brayne et al, 1995; Fratiglioni et al, 1997)

Table 1.2.2. Risk and protective factors for Alzheimer's disease

| Definitively accepted | Putative | | Putative protective factors |
	Recently suggested	Older hypotheses	
Age	Female gender	Previous diseases, e.g. depression	NSAID use
ApoE e4 allele	Low education	Head trauma	Postmenopausal oestrogen therapy
Familial aggregation	Hypertension	Alcohol intake	
	Specific occupational exposures	Smoking (protective?)	
		Aluminium in drinking water	

provide references where not otherwise specified. A summary of the current knowledge on risk factors for AD is presented in Table 1.2.2.

Definite risk factors

Age, apolipoprotein E (ApoE) polymorphism, and family history of dementia have been extensively investigated, and all studies consistently show that increasing age, ApoE e4 allele, and familial aggregation increase the risk of

AD. AD occurrence rises with increasing age, as shown by all available incidence studies (Figure 1.2.2). However, whether AD is an age-dependent or ageing-dependent disease is an ongoing debate (Ritchie and Kildea, 1996), as data from very old subjects (over 90) are limited. Prevalence figures in the very old are controversial and difficult to interpret due to the possible differential survival (Drachman, 1994). In the Kungsholmen Project, when a 90+ year-old population was added to the initial cohort, we found that prevalence figures increased from 38% in 90–94 year-old subjects to 56% in 95+ year-old persons (Gip et al, 1997), a finding similar to that reported in the Canadian Study of Health and Aging (Ebly et al, 1994).

Familial aggregation of dementia has been found to be associated with both early- and late-onset AD. It is likely that the familial aggregation is the result of the combined effect of genetic and environmental factors. Twin studies can address this question in a unique way (Breitner, 1994). In a Finnish study, the incidence of AD was significantly higher in monozygotic twins than in dizygotic (Räihä et al, 1996). In the Study of Dementia in Swedish Twins, heritability of AD liability was estimated to be 0.74, the other variance being attributable to environmental factors (Gatz et al, 1997).

ApoE is an important transport protein in lipid metabolism, with three major isoforms coded by alleles e2, e3 and e4 at a single locus on chromosome 19. The e4 allele has been consistently found associated with increased risk of AD, with a decreasing effect in old age (Farrer et al, 1997). In the Kungsholmen Project, the risk for 75+ year-old subjects with ApoE e4 allele is approximately threefold that of persons without the e4 allele (Winblad et al, 1997). The proportion of cases due to ApoE e4 allele was estimated in this study as 17%, only slightly higher than the value of 14% reported in the East Boston Study (Evans et al, 1997).

Putative risk factors, suggested in recent studies

Several prevalence studies suggest a higher risk for AD among women, but results from incidence studies are controversial. In the Kungsholmen Project (Fratiglioni et al, 1997) and the Rotterdam Study (Ott et al, 1997b), a higher incidence of dementia and AD among women has been found, confirming a previous report on presenile dementia (McGonigal et al, 1993). Other studies have not found any statistically significant difference between the genders (Hagnell et al, 1992; Kokmen et al, 1993; Bachman et al, 1993; Letenneur et al, 1994; Brayne et al, 1995).

Higher dementia prevalence among poorly educated persons has been reported by most surveys, although the evidence is not so strong for AD (Fratiglioni et al, 1991). Some incidence studies have confirmed an inverse relationship between dementia and educational attainment (Stern et al, 1994), but others have failed to find such a linkage (Beard et al, 1992; Paykel et al, 1994; Cobb et al, 1995). Katzman (1993) hypothesises that education may increase brain reserve by increasing synaptic density in the neocortical association cortex. Other authors have expanded the reserve hypothesis by taking into account the possible beneficial influence of mental activity throughout the entire life span (Stern et al, 1994; Orrell and Sahakian, 1995). Still other observers suggest that education and occupation are likely surrogates for intelligence, which could be the real factor inversely related to increased AD risk (Plassman et al, 1995; Svedberg et al, 1996). In addition, the association between education and dementia may be due to confounders such as occupational exposure, social status, life habits, and previous comorbidity. A recent study in an Italian population of middle to high socio-economic status reported an association between no education and dementia or AD that was independent of gender, occupation, life habits, and hypertension. These findings suggest that the first decade of life is a critical period related to developing dementia later in life (De Ronchi et al, 1998).

In 1993, an association between manual work and increased risk of late-onset AD was reported from the Kungsholmen Project, suggesting the possible implication of one or more occupational exposures (Fratiglioni et al, 1993). Similar findings were reported successively from other studies, whereas previous investigations had been negative. Recently, exposure to organic solvents (Kukull et al, 1995), and occupational magnetic fields (Sobel et al, 1995 and 1996) have been found to be associated with an increased risk of AD.

Hypertension, which is the most powerful risk factor for cerebrovascular disease, is believed also to be an important risk factor for vascular dementia. However, relatively few data pertaining to the direct relationship between blood pressure and dementia are available. Mid-life hypertension has been found to predict late-life cognitive impairment (Elias et al, 1993; Launer et al, 1995), and an increase of 1 standard deviation in systolic blood pressure has been shown to be related to a 60% increased risk of vascular dementia, but not of AD (Yoshitake et al, 1995). Recently, a study of 382 subjects showed that individuals who developed dementia later in life had higher systolic and diastolic pressure, suggesting that elevated blood pressure may increase the risk of dementia, including AD (Skoog et al, 1996). In the Kungsholmen Project, low blood pressure (systolic ≤ 140 mm Hg or diastolic ≤ 75 mm Hg) was associated with higher prevalence of AD (Guo et al, 1996), and blood pressure reduction was associated with increased incidence of dementia and AD (Guo et al, 1998).

Putative risk factors—older hypotheses

After the first reports, the association between dementia and previous thyroid diseases/previous depressive episodes has not been further studied. In contrast, further data support the hypothesis regarding previous head trauma as a risk factor for AD (Mayeux et al, 1993). It has been suggested that head injury may play a role in the aetiology of AD through a synergistic relationship with the ApoE e4 allele (Mayeux et al, 1995), probably interacting in determining the deposition of amyloid b-protein (Nicoll et al, 1995).

It is known that alcohol may lead to many physical and mental problems in individuals of any age. Alcohol is a recognised cause of a specific form of dementia, 'alcoholic dementia'. In addition, use of alcohol has been reported to increase the risk of vascular dementia (Yoshitake et al, 1995). Most of the studies concerning the role of alcohol consumption in the aetiology of AD have shown no association. In the Kungsholmen Project, alcohol abuse has been found to be associated with increased AD prevalence (Fratiglioni et al, 1993). However, a recent French study in the Bordeaux area reported an inverse relationship between moderate wine drinking and incident dementia, leading to the hypothesis that moderate doses of alcohol may protect against dementia (Orgogozo et al, 1997).

In some studies, smoking has been found to be inversely associated to AD, even with a significant dose-dependent relation (van Duijn and Hofman, 1991), but most investigations have not found any association, and two studies have reported a positive relationship (Lee, 1994). Moreover, analysis of prospective data from the Rotterdam Study did not confirm the previously reported protective effect; on the contrary, a twofold increased risk of AD in smokers was detected (Ott et al, 1997b).

Finally, there is still insufficient evidence that aluminium in drinking water is a risk factor for AD. Negative reports have recently been published (Forster et al, 1995; Jacqmin-Gadda et al, 1996).

Possible protective factors

Recently, attention has been drawn to possible protective effects against AD of two different types of drugs: non-steroidal anti-inflammatory drugs (NSAID) and postmenopausal oestrogen therapy.

A number of epidemiological studies have reported an inverse association between the use of NSAIDs and AD. These drugs might inhibit the immunological mechanisms that have been reported to be involved in the AD process. Most of these studies included prevalent cases, and some of them were cross-sectional with a contemporary assessment of disease and exposure (McGeer et al, 1997). More recently, three longitudinal studies have been performed, with inconsistent results, one supporting (Stewart et al, 1997) and two failing to support (Fourrier et al, 1996; Henderson et al, 1997) the hypothesis of a protective effect of NSAIDs against AD. More data are necessary in order to be able either to accept or to rule out this hypothesis.

Four recent studies in which information on oestrogen replacement therapy was collected before dementia onset have reported a decreased risk of AD in subjects with postmenopausal oestrogen use, confirming previous cross-sectional observations (Henderson, 1997). Clinical studies of postmenopausal women suggested beneficial oestrogen effects on specific cognitive skills.

Preliminary results of trials of oestrogen in women with AD have shown similar results (Birge, 1997). At the moment, however, the effect of potential confounders cannot be excluded; thus, the hypothesis regarding the efficacy of oestrogen in lowering AD risk in women needs further testing.

RISK FACTORS FOR VASCULAR DEMENTIA

Epidemiological studies designed to detect risk factors for vascular dementia are still limited; they are hampered by lack of general consensus on disease definition and diagnostic criteria. Moreover, some risk factors are included in the definition or in operational criteria. Interesting reviews have recently been published (Hébert and Brayne, 1995; Amar and Wilcock, 1996; Gorelick, 1997; Pasquier and Leys, 1997) and all have concluded that further studies with sound methodological design are needed.

Age is the only consistent risk factor for VaD, with all other potential risk factors still requiring further investigation. Clear examples of the latter are gender and race. Men are thought to be at a higher risk of VaD, but evidence from epidemiological studies is lacking. It has been shown that Orientals and probably Blacks are at higher risk of VaD than Caucasian populations (Jorm, 1991). However, high prevalence figures similar to those reported in Japan have been found in a study in Gothenburg in 85 year old subjects (Skoog et al, 1993).

Most studies have examined whether stroke-related factors, such as number, location and size, modify the risk of VaD. These studies have led to some consistent findings: greater tissue loss, number of infarcts and strategic locations are associated with a high risk of developing dementia (Gorelick, 1997). Atherogenic factors may be involved in the aetiopathogenesis of VaD, but it is not well known if risk factors for developing VaD differ from those found in stroke. Some factors seem to be directly associated with VaD (hypertension, diabetes), while others (smoking, cholesterol, heart disease) are indirect (Hébert and Brayne, 1995). Finally, genetic factors have rarely been studied, despite the existence of hereditary VaD such as 'autosomal dominant hereditary cerebral haemorrhage with amyloidosis-Dutch type', and CADA-SIL (Joutel et al, 1997).

RISK FACTORS FOR DEMENTIA

Studying risk factors for dementia constitutes a new approach that reflects an orientation towards intervention. The detection of any risk factor that can be prevented/modified can help in decreasing the occurrence of dementia syndrome. If we are able to decrease the occurrence of the dementia through treatment or elimination of these hypothetical risk factors, an important goal has been achieved. In addition, this approach to dementia as a whole avoids all misclassification bias due to the difficulties in differentiating AD and VaD.

Until now the main finding from this approach is the detection of a group of 'vascular risk factors' that have emerged as being strongly associated with dementia. Apart from stroke, which has been found to increase the risk of dementia ninefold in the first year and to double the risk each year thereafter (Tatemichi et al, 1992; Kokmen et al, 1996), several other factors seem to increase the risk of dementia sometimes even if no clinical strokes have occurred: diabetes mellitus (Ott et al, 1996; Leibson et al, 1997b), atrial fibrillation (Ott et al, 1997a), atherosclerosis (Hofman et al, 1997), ECG ischemia (Prince et al, 1994), alcohol (Saunders et al, 1991; Smith and Atkinson, 1995), severe systolic hypertension (Guo et al, 1998), and high saturated fat and cholesterol intake (Kalmijn et al, 1997).

NATURAL HISTORY OF DEMENTIA

Current knowledge of the natural history of dementia is still limited. In general, studies have focused on AD patients, have sampled relatively young older adults in the hospital, or have selected from nursing home populations, and have used a variety of follow-up intervals, outcomes and putative predictors. Briefly, we discuss data concerning the evolution of dementia in terms of dementia severity and progression (functional decline, institutionalisation) and mortality.

DEMENTIA SEVERITY AND PROGRESSION

As opposed to people with mild physical handicaps, a subject affected by even a mild form of dementia needs assistance and some surveillance. Moreover, those suffering from severe disease require high-level, specialised care. For these reasons, prevalence figures disaggregated for disease severity are relevant. Population surveys from different countries report average proportions of 30%, 40% and 30% for mild, moderate and severe dementia, respectively (Rocca et al, 1991; O'Connor et al, 1989; Skoog et al, 1993; Ebly et al, 1994; Fratiglioni et al, 1994; Fichter et al, 1995; Juva et al, 1993).

The disease progresses dramatically. In three years, 54% of demented cases enrolled in the CERAD study reached the severe stage as according to the Clinical Dementia Rating scale (Galasko et al, 1995). In the Kungsholmen Project, the proportion of severe forms among prevalent cases increased from 19% at baseline, to 48% after three years, and to 67% after seven years (Agüero Torres, 1998). This progression is due to both cognitive and functional decline.

Cognitive decline

The annual average rate of cognitive decline as measured by the Mini-Mental Status Examination varies from −4.0 to −2.4 points in different studies

(Agüero Torres, 1998). In the Kungsholmen Project, the decline was constant during the two follow-up periods, -2.4 points during the first three years and -2.9 in the following three years (Agüero Torres et al, 1998a).

Many different predictors of more rapid cognitive decline have been reported in the literature. Although differences in methodological aspects are numerous and substantial, the length of follow-up is both the most relevant and most neglected one. Several studies recognise higher cognitive function and functional disability as the strongest predictors of a worse prognosis (Agüero Torres et al, 1998a).

Functional decline

Complete functional dependence in activities of daily living (ADL) was found in 14% of demented cases at entry in the CERAD study; this reached a proportion of 54% after three years (Galasko et al, 1995). In the Swedish study, 30% of demented persons were totally dependent at entry, and 50% of the survivors needed complete assistance with ADL after seven years. Of demented subjects, 78% needed assistance with at least one ADL item, versus 26% of the non-demented. Main factors associated with functional dependence were age, dementia, cerebrovascular disease, heart disease and hip fracture (Agüero Torres et al, 1998b).

Functional dependence in one or more activities of daily living afflicted 32% of the population at baseline; 9% of those who were initially functionally independent developed dependence within three years. Dementia was associated with functional dependence in the entire population, and with low MMSE performance in non-demented subjects. These factors were also the major determinants of the development of dependence and decline over three years. Diseases associated with functional dependence at baseline did not emerge as significant determinants of functional dependence at follow-up, apart from hip fracture. Half of the functional dependence developed during three years was attributable to dementia (Agüero Torres et al, 1998b).

Institutionalisation

In industrialised countries, the most prevalent disorders among elderly adults in nursing homes or other institutions are mental disease and cognitive impairment (Sandman et al, 1988; Ineichen, 1990). Moreover, it has been constantly reported that mental problems and dysfunction in daily activities are some of the best predictors of institutionalisation (Shapiro and Tate, 1988; Woo et al, 1994).

Institutionalisation in dementia cases seems to vary depending on age structure, urban or rural residence, and culture of the investigated populations. In northern Europe and North America, approximately 50% of the demented cases are in nursing homes (Sulkava et al, 1985; Skoog et al, 1993; Engedal and Haugen, 1993; Juva et al, 1993; Ebly et al, 1994; Fratiglioni et al, 1994; Fichter et al, 1995), whereas in southern Europe this value seems much lower (Rocca et al, 1990). In general, more severe cases and higher institutionalisation rates have been found among VaD than AD cases (Sulkava et al, 1985; Skoog et al, 1993; Fratiglioni et al, 1994).

Studies on predictors of institutionalisation have detected three main categories of relevant factors: (1) social-related variables such as marital status or presence of a caregiver; (2) caregiver burden; and (3) disease severity, expressed both as functional and cognitive dysfunction (Lieberman and Kramer, 1991; Cohen et al, 1993; Haupt and Kurz, 1993; Severson et al, 1994; Scott et al, 1997; Heyman et al, 1997).

MORTALITY

Death certificates grossly under-report dementia, even when underlying causes of death are taken into account. For that reason mortality data are scanty. In the Kungsholmen Project, which studies a 75+ year-old population, 70% of incident dementia cases died during the five years following the diagnosis, with a mortality rate specific for dementia of 2.4 per 100 person-years (Agüero Torres, 1998).

Several community-based studies have found an increased risk of death in demented persons compared to non-demented subjects, reporting a relative risk of death ranging between 1.4 and 4.4 (Agüero Torres, 1998). In the Swedish study, the risk of death among demented subjects was twice that among non-demented people, after controlling for sociodemographic variables and comorbidity. Of all deaths, 14% could be attributed to dementia. However, the main impact both at the individual and community levels was on the youngest old group and on women. After the age of 85, dementia still shortens life, especially among women, but much less than in younger old subjects (Agüero Torres, 1998).

Older age, male gender, low education, comorbidity and functional disability are the most frequent reported indicators of shorter survival in dementia (Agüero Torres, 1998).

CONCLUSIONS

At the moment we can conclude that dementia is a long and progressive process and one of the major causes of functional dependence, and that it shortens life even in the very old. In spite of methodological difficulties, it is possible to identify demented subjects with a worse prognosis by using clinical and demographic data. Clinicians and health care planners should be aware of the potential usefulness of such a readily available prognostic indicator as functional dependence, which is a good predictor of both shorter survival and disability.

REFERENCES

Agüero Torres, H. (1998). Natural history of Alzheimer's disease and other dementias. Data from a population survey. *Thesis*, Karolinska Institute, Stockholm.

Agüero Torres, H., Fratiglioni, L., Guo, Z., Viitanen, M., and Winblad, B. (1998a). Prognostic factors in very old demented adults: a seven-year follow-up from a population-based survey in Stockholm, *J. Am. Ger. Soc.*, in press.

Agüero Torres, H., Fratiglioni, L., Guo, Z., Viitanen, M., von Strauss, E., and Winblad, B. (1998b). Dementia is the major cause of functional dependence in the elderly. Three-year follow-up data from a population-based study, *Am. J. Public Health.*, in press.

Amar, K., and Wilcock, G. (1996). Vascular dementia, *BMJ*, **312**, 227–231.

Bachman, D. L., Wolf, P. A., Linn, R., Knoefel, J. E., Cobb, J., Belanger, A., D'Agostino, R. B., and White, L. R. (1992). Prevalence of dementia and probable senile dementia of the Alzheimer type in the Framingham Study, *Neurology*, **42**, 115–119.

Bachman, D. L., Wolf, P. A., Linn, R. T., Knoefel, J. E., Cobb, J. L., Belanger, A. J., White, L. R., and D'Agostino, R. B. (1993). Incidence of dementia and probable Alzheimer's disease in a general population: the Framingham Study, *Neurology*, **43**, 515–519.

Beard, C. M., Kokmen, E., Offord, K. P., and Kurland, L. T. (1992). Lack of association between Alzheimer's disease and education, occupation, marital status, or living arrangement, *Neurology*, **42**, 2063–2068.

Bickel, H., and Cooper, B. (1994). Incidence and relative risk of dementia in an urban elderly population: findings of a prospective field study, *Psychol. Med.*, **24**, 179–192.

Birge, S. J. (1997). The role of oestrogen in the treatment of Alzheimer's disease, *Neurology*, **48** (Suppl 7), S36–S41.

Boothby, H., Blizard, R., Livingston, G., and Mann, A. H. (1994). The Gospel Oak Study stage III: the incidence of dementia, *Psychol. Med.*, **24**, 89–95.

Brayne, C., Gill, C., Huppert, F. A., Barkley, C., Gehlhaar, E., Girling, D. M., O'Connor, D. W., and Paykel, E. S. (1995). Incidence of clinically diagnosed subtypes of dementia in an elderly population. Cambridge Project for later life, *Br. J. Psychiatry*, **167**, 255–262.

Breitner, J. C. S. (1994). New epidemiologic strategies in Alzheimer's disease may provide clues to prevention and cause, *Neurobiol. Aging*, **15** (Suppl 2), 175–177.

Callahan, C. M., Hall, K. S., Hui, S. L., Musick, B. S., Unverzagt, F. W., and Hendrie, H. C. (1996). Relationship of age, education, and occupation with dementia among a community-based sample of African Americans, *Arch. Neurol.*, **53**, 134–140.

Cobb, J. L., Wolf, P. A., White, R., and D'Agostino, R. B. (1995). The effect of education on the incidence of dementia and Alzheimer's disease in the Framingham Study, *Neurology*, **45**, 1707–1712.

Cohen, C. A., Gold, D. P., Shulman, K. I., Wortley, J. T., McDonald, G., and Wargon, M. (1993). Factors determining the decision to institutionalize dementing individuals: a prospective study, *Gerontologist*, **33**, 714–720.

Corrada, M., Brookmeyer, R., and Kawas, C. (1995). Sources of variability in prevalence rates of Alzheimer's disease, *Int. J. Epidemiol.*, **24**, 1000–1004.

De Ronchi, D., Fratiglioni, L., Rucci, P., Paternicò, A., Graziani, S., and Dalmonte, E. (1998). The effect of education on dementia occurrence in an Italian population with middle to high socio-economic status, *Neurology*, in press.

Drachman, D. A. (1994). If we live long enough, will we all be demented? *Neurology*, **144**, 1563–1565.

Ebly, E. M., Parhad, I. M., Hogan, D. B., and Fung, T. S. (1994). Prevalence and types of dementia in the very old: results from the Canadian Study of Health and Aging, *Neurology*, **44**, 1593–1600.

Elias, M. F., Wolf, P. A., D'Agostino, R. B., Cobb, J., and White, L. R. (1993). Untreated blood pressure level is inversely related to cognitive functioning: the Framingham Study, *Am. J. Epidemiol.*, **138**, 353–364.

Engedal, K., and Haugen, P. K. (1993). The prevalence of dementia in a sample of elderly Norwegians, *Int. J. Geriatr. Psychiat.*, **8**, 565–570.

Evans, D. A., Beckett, L. A., Field, T. S., Feng, L., Albert, M. S., Bennett, D. A., Tycko, B., and Mayeux, R. (1997). Apolipoprotein E e4 and incidence of Alzheimer's disease in a community population of older persons, *JAMA*, **277**, 822–824.

Farrer, L. A., Cupples, L. A., Haines, J. L., Hyman, B., Kukull, W. A., Mayeux, R., Myers, R. H., Pericak-Vance, M. A., Risch, N., and van Duijn, C. M. (1997). Effects of age, sex, and ethnicity on the association between Apolipoprotein E Genotype and Alzheimer's disease, *JAMA*, **278**, 1349–1356.

Fichter, M. M., Meller, I., Schröppel, H., and Steinkirchner, R. (1995). Dementia and cognitive impairment in the oldest old in the community. Prevalence and comorbidity, *Br. J. Psychiatry*, **166**, 621–629.

Forster, D. P., Newens, A. J., Kay, D. W. K., and Edwardson, J. A. (1995). Risk factors in clinically diagnosed presenile dementia of the Alzheimer type: a case-control study in northern England, *J. Epidemiol. Com. Health*, **49**, 253–258.

Fourrier, A., Letenneur, L., Bégaud, B., and Dartigues, J. F. (1996). Nonsteroidal antiiflammatory drug use and cognitive function in the elderly: inconclusive results from a population-based cohort study, *J. Clin. Epidemiol.*, **49**, 1201.

Fratiglioni, L. (1996). Epidemiology of Alzheimer's disease and current possibilities for prevention, *Acta Neurol. Scand.*, **165** (Suppl), 33–40.

Fratiglioni, L., Ahlbom, A., Viitanen, M., and Winblad, B. (1993). Risk factors for late-onset Alzheimer's disease: a population-based case-control study, *Ann. Neurol.*, **33**, 258–266.

Fratiglioni, L., Forsell, Y., Agüero Torres, H., and Winblad, B. (1994). Severity of dementia and institutionalization in the elderly: Prevalence data from an urban area in Sweden, *Neuroepidemiology*, **13**, 79–88.

Fratiglioni, L., Grut, M., Forsell, Y., Viitanen, M., Grafström, M., Holmén, K., Ericsson, K., Bäckman, L., Ahlbom, A., and Winblad, B. (1991). Prevalence of Alzheimer's disease and other dementias in an elderly urban population: relationship with age, sex, and education, *Neurology*, **41**, 1886–1892.

Fratiglioni, L., Viitanen, M., von Strauss, E., Tontodonati, V., Herlitz, A., and Winblad, B. (1997). Very old women at highest risk of dementia and Alzheimer's disease: incidence data from the Kungsholmen Project, Stockholm, *Neurology*, **48**, 132–138.

Galasko, D., Edland, S. D., Morris, J. C., Clark, C., Mohs, R., and Koss, E. (1995). The Consortium to Establish a Registry for Alzheimer's Disease (CERAD). Part XI. Clinical milestones in patients with Alzheimer's disease followed over 3 years, *Neurology*, **45**, 1451–1455.

Gatz, M., Pedersen, N., Berg, S., Johansson, B., Johansson, K., Mortimer, J. A.,

Posner, S. F., Viitanen, M., Winblad, B., and Ahlbom, A. (1997). Heritability for Alzheimer's disease: The study of dementia in Swedish twins, *Journal of Gerontology*, **52A**, M117–M125.

Gip, K., Viitanen, M., von Strauss, E., Winblad, B., and Fratiglioni, L. (1997). Prevalence of dementia in Nonagerians, in *Alzheimer's Disease: Biology, Diagnosis and Therapeutics*, K. Iqbal, B. Winblad, and H. M. Wisniewski (Eds), pp. 45–48, John Wiley, Chichester.

Gorelick, P. B. (1997). Status of risk factors for dementia associated with stroke, *Stroke*, **28**, 459–463.

Graves, A. B., Larson, E. B., Edland, S. D., Bowen, J. D., McCormick, W. C., McCurry, S. M., Rice, M. M., Wenzlow, A., and Uomoto, J. M. (1997). Prevalence of dementia and subtypes in the Japanese American population of King County, Washington State, *Am. J. Epidemiol.*, **144**, 760–771.

Guo, Z., Viitanen, M., Fratiglioni, L., and Winblad, B. (1996). Low blood pressure and dementia in elderly people: the Kungsholmen Project, *BMJ*, **312**, 805–808.

Guo, Z., Fratiglioni, L., Viitanen, M., Fastborn, J., and Winblad, B. (1998). Blood pressure and dementia in persons over 75 years old: follow-up results from the Kungsholmen Project, *Neurology*, submitted.

Hagnell, O., Öjesjö, L., and Rorsman, B. (1992). Incidence of dementia in the Lundby study, *Neuroepidemiology*, **11** (Suppl 1), 61–66.

Hasegawa, K., Homma, A., and Imai, Y. (1986). An epidemiological study of age-related dementia in the community, *Int. J. Geriatr. Psychiat.*, **1**, 45–55.

Haupt, M., and Kurz, A. (1993). Predictors of nursing home placement in patients with Alzheimer's disease, *Int. J. Geriatr. Psychiat.* **8**, 741–746.

Hébert, R., and Brayne, C. (1995). Epidemiology of vascular dementia, *Neuroepidemiology*, **14**, 240–257.

Henderson, A. S., Jorm, A. F., Christensen, H., Jacomb, P. A., and Korten, A. E. (1997). Aspirin, anti-inflammatory drugs and risk of dementia, *Int. J. Geriatr. Psychiat.*, **12**, 926–930.

Henderson, V. W. (1997). The epidemiology of estrogen replacement therapy and Alzheimer's disease, *Neurology*, **48** (Suppl 7), S27–S35.

Hendrie, H. C., Osuntokun, B. O., Hall, K. S. et al (1995). Prevalence of Alzheimer's disease and dementia in two communities: Nigerian Africans and African Americans, *Am. J. Psychiatry*, **152**, 1485–1492.

Heyman, A., Peterson, B., Fillenbaum, G., and Pieper, C. (1997). Predictors of time to institutionalization of patients with Alzheimer's disease: The CERAD experience, Part XVII, *Neurology*, **48**, 1304–1309.

Hofman, A., Rocca, W. A., Brayne, C., Breteler, M. M. B., Clarke, M., Cooper, B., Copeland, J. R. M., Dartigues, J. F., Da Silva Droux, A., Hagnell, O., Heeren, T. J., Engedal, K., Jonker, C., Lindesay, J., Lobo, A., Mann, A. H., Mölsä, P. K., Morgan, K., O'Connor, D. W., Sulkava, R., Kay, D. W. K., and Amaducci, L. (1991). The prevalence of dementia in Europe: a collaborative study of 1980–1990 findings, *Int. J. Epidemiol.*, **20**, 736–748.

Hofman, A., Ott, A., Breteler, M. M. B., Bots, M. L., Slooter, A. J. C., van Harskamp, F., van Duijn, C. N., Van Broeckhoven, C., and Grobbee, D. E. (1997). Atherosclerosis, apolipoprotein E, and prevalence of dementia and Alzheimer's disease in the Rotterdam Study, *Lancet*, **349**, 151–154.

Ineichen, B. (1990). The extent of dementia among old people in residential care, *Int. J. Geriatr. Psychiat.*, **5**, 327–335.

Jacqmin-Gadda, H., Commenges, D., Letenneur, L., and Dartigues, J.-F. (1996). Silica and aluminum in drinking water and cognitive impairment in the elderly, *Epidemiology*, **7**, 281–285.

Johansson, B., and Zarit, S. H. (1995). Prevalence and incidence of dementia in the oldest old: a longitudinal study of a population-based sample of 84–90-year olds in Sweden, *Int. J .Geriatr. Psychiat.*, **10**, 359–366.

Jorm, A. F. (1991). Cross-national comparison of the occurrence of Alzheimer's disease and vascular dementias, *Eur. Arch. Psychiatry Clin. Neurosci.*, **240**, 218–222.

Jorm, A. F., Korten, A. E., and Henderson, A. S. (1987). The prevalence of dementia: a quantitative integration of the literature, *Acta Psychiatr. Scand.*, **76**, 465–479.

Joutel et al (1997). CADASIL: cerebral autosomal dominant arteriopathy with subcortical infarcts and leukoencephalopathy, *Lancet*, **350**, 1511–1515.

Juva, K., Sulkava, R., Erkinjuntti, T., Valvanne, J., and Tilvis, R. (1993). Prevalence of dementia in the city of Helsinki, *Acta Neurol. Scand.*, **87**, 106–110.

Kalmijn, S., Launer, L. J., Ott, A., Witteman, J. C. M., Hofman, A., and Breteler, M. M. B. (1997). Dietary fat intake and the risk of incident dementia in the Rotterdam Study, *Ann. Neurol.*, **42**, 776–782.

Katzman, R. (1993). Education and the prevalence of dementia and Alzheimer's disease, *Neurology*, **43**, 13–20.

Kokmen, E., Beard, C. M., Offord, K. P., and Kurland, L. T. (1989). Prevalence of medically diagnosed dementia in a defined United States population: Rochester, Minnesota, January 1, 1975, *Neurology*, **39**, 773–776.

Kokmen, E., Beard, C. M., O'Brien, P. C., Offord, K. P., and Kurland, L. T. (1993). Is the incidence of dementing illness changing? A 25-year time trend study in Rochester, Minnesota (1960–1984), *Neurology*, **43**, 1887–1892.

Kokmen, E., Whisnant, J. P., O'Fallon, W. M., Chu, C.-P., and Beard, C. M. (1996). Dementia after ischemic stroke: a population-based study in Rochester, Minnesota (1960–1984), *Neurology*, **46**, 154–159.

Kukull, W. A., Larson, E. B., Bowen, J. D., McCormick, W. C., Teri, L., Pfanschmidt, M. L., Thompson, J. D., OMeara, E. S., Brenner, D. E., and van Belle, G. (1995). Solvent exposure as a risk factor for Alzheimer's disease: a case-control study, *Am. J. Epidemiol.*, **141**, 1059–1071.

Launer, L. J., Masaki, K., Petrovitch, H., Foley, D., and Havlik, R. J. (1995) The association between midlife blood pressure levels and late-life cognitive function: the Honolulu-Asia Aging Study, *JAMA*, **274**, 1846–1851.

Lee, P. N. (1994). Smoking and Alzheimer's disease: a review of the epidemiological evidence, *Neuroepidemiology*, **13**, 131–144.

Leibson, C. L., Rocca, W. A., Hanson, V. A., Cha, R., Kokmen, E., O'Brien, P. C., and Palumbo, P. J. (1997). Risk of dementia among persons with diabetes mellitus: a population-based cohort study, *Am. J. Epidemiol.*, **145**, 301–308.

Letenneur, L., Commenges, D., Dartigues, J. F., and Barbeger-Gateau, P. (1994). Incidence of dementia and Alzheimer's disease in elderly community residents of South-Western France, *Int. J. Epidemiol.*, **23**, 1256–1261.

Liebermann, M. A., and Kramer, J. H. (1991). Factors affecting decisions to institutionalize demented elderly, *Gerontologist*, **31**, 371–374.

McGeer, P. L., Schulzer, M., and McGeer, E. G. (1997). Arthritis and anti-inflammatory agents as possible factors for Alzheimer's disease: a review of 17 epidemiological studies, *Neurology*, **47**, 425–432.

Mayeux, R., Ottman, R., Tang, M. X., Noboa-Bauza, L., Marder, K., Gurland, B., and Stern, Y. (1993). Genetic susceptibility and head injury as risk factors for Alzheimer's disease among community-dwelling elderly persons and their first-degree relatives, *Ann. Neurol.*, **33**, 494–501.

Mayeux, R., Ottman, R., Maestre, G., Ngai, C., Tang, M.-X., Ginsberg, H., Chun, M., Tycko, B., and Shelanski, M. (1995). Synergistic effects of traumatic head injury and apolipoprotein-e4 in patients with Alzheimer's disease, *Neurology*, **45**, 555–557.

McGonigal, G., Thomas, B., McQuade, C., Starr, J. M., MacLennan, W. J., and Whalley, L. J. (1993). Epidemiology of Alzheimer's presenile dementia in Scotland, 1974–88, *BMJ*, **306**, 680–683.

Nicoll, J. A. R., Roberts, G. W., and Graham, D. I. (1995). Apolipoprotein E e4 allele is associated with deposition of amyloid b-protein following head injury, *Nature Medicine*, **1**, 135–137.

O'Connor, D. W., Pollitt, P. A., Hyde, J. B., Fellows, J. L., Miller, N. D., Brook, C. P. B., Reiss, B. B., and Roth, M. (1989). The prevalence of dementia as measured by the Cambridge Mental Disorders of the Elderly Examination, *Acta Psychiatr. Scand.*, **79**, 190–198.

Orgogozo, J.-M., Dartigues, J.-F., Lafont, S., Letenneur, L., Commenges, D., Salamon, R., Renaud, S., and Breteler, M. (1997). Wine consumption and dementia in the elderly: a prospective community study in the Bordeaux area, *Rev. Neurol. (Paris)*, **153**(2), 1–8.

Orrell, M., and Sahakian, B. (1995). Education and dementia. Research evidence supports the concept 'use it or lose it', *BMJ*, **310**, 951–952.

Ott, A., Breteler, M. M., van Harskamp, F., Grobbee, D. E., and Hofman, A. (1995). Prevalence of Alzheimer's disease and vascular dementia: association with education. The Rotterdam Study, *BMJ*, **310**, 970–973.

Ott, A., Breteler, M. M. B., de Bruyne, M. C., van Harskamp, F., Grobbee, D. E., and Hofman, A. (1997a). Atrial fibrillation and dementia in a population-based study. The Rotterdam Study, *Stroke*, **28**, 316–321.

Ott, A., Breteler, M. M. B., van Harskamp, F., Grobbee, D. E., and Hofman, A. (1997b). The incidence of dementia in the Rotterdam Study, in *Alzheimer's Disease: Biology, Diagnosis and Therapeutics*, K. Iqbal, B. Winblad, T. Nishimura, M. Takeda, H. M. Wisniewski (Eds), pp. 3–10, John Wiley, Chichester.

Ott, A., Stolk, R. P., Hofman, A., van Harskamp, F., Grobbee, D. E., and Breteler, M. M. B. (1996). Association of diabetes mellitus and dementia: The Rotterdam Study, *Diabetologia*, **39**, 1392–1397.

Paganini-Hill, A., and Henderson, V. W. (1996). Estrogen replacement therapy and risk of Alzheimer's disease, *Arch. Intern. Med.*, **156**, 2213–2217.

Park, J., Ko, H. J., Park, Y. N., and Jung, C.-H. (1994). Dementia among the elderly in a rural Korean population, *Br. J. Psychiatry*, **164**, 796–801.

Pasquier, F., and Leys, D. (1997). Why are stroke patients prone to develop dementia? *J. Neurol.*, **244**, 135–142.

Paykel, E. S., Brayne, C., Huppert, F. A., Gill, C., Barkley, C., Gehlhaar, E., Beardsall, L., Girling, D. M., Pollitt, P., and O'Connor, D. (1994). Incidence of dementia in a population older than 75 years in the United Kingdom, *Arch. Gen. Psychiatry*, **51**, 325–332.

Perkins, P., Annergers, J. F., Doody, R. S., Cooke, N., Aday, L., and Vernon, S. W. (1997). Incidence and prevalence of dementia in a multiethnic cohort of municipal retirees, *Neurology*, **49**, 44–50.

Plassman, B. L., Welsh, K. A., Helms, M., Brandt, J., Page, W. F., and Breitner, J. C. S. (1995). Intelligence and education as predictors of cognitive state in late life: a 50-year follow-up, *Neurology*, **45**, 1446–1450.

Prencipe, M., Casini, A. R., Ferretti, C., Lattanzio, M. T., Fiorelli, M., and Culasso, F. (1996). Prevalence of dementia in an elderly rural population: effects of age, sex and education, *J. Neurol. Neurosurg. Psychiatry*, **60**, 628–633.

Prince, M., Cullen, M., and Mann, A. (1994). Risk factors for Alzheimer's disease and dementia: a case-control study based on the MRC elderly hypertension trial, *Neurology*, **44**, 97–104.

Ritchie, K., and Kildea, D. (1996). Is senile dementia age-related or ageing-related?—

Evidence from meta-analysis of dementia prevalence in the oldest old, *Lancet*, **346**, 931–934.

Rocca, W. A., Bonaiuto, S., Lippi, A., Luciani, P., Turtù, F., Cavarzeran, F., and Amaducci, L. (1990). Prevalence of clinically diagnosed Alzheimer's disease and other dementing disorders: a door-to-door survey in Appignano, Macerata province, Italy, *Neurology*, **40**, 626–631.

Rocca, W. A., Hofman, A., Brayne, C., Breteler, M. M. B., Clarke, M., Copeland, J. R. M., Dartigues, J.-F., Engedal, K. et al (1991). Frequency and distribution of Alzheimer's disease in Europe: a collaborative study of 1980–1990 prevalence findings, *Ann. Neurol.*, **30**, 381–390.

Räihä, I., Kaprio, J., Koskenvuo, M., Rajala, T., and Sourander, L. (1996). Alzheimer's disease in Finnish twins, *Lancet*, **347**, 573–578.

Sandman, P. O., Adolfsson, R., Norberg, A., Nyström, L., and Winblad, B. (1988). Long-term care of the elderly. A descriptive study of 3600 institutionalized patients in the county of Västerbotten, Sweden, *Compr. Gerontol. A.*, **2**, 120–133.

Saunders, P. A., Copeland, J. R. M., Dewey, M. E., Davidson, I. A., McWilliam, C., Sharma, V., and Sullivan, C. (1991). Heavy drinking as a risk factor for depression and dementia in elderly men, *Br. J. Psychiatry*, **159**, 213–216.

Schoenberg, B. S., Anderson, D. W., and Haerer, A. F. (1985). Severe dementia. Prevalence and clinical features in a biracial US population, *Arch. Neurol.*, **42**, 740–743.

Scott, W. K., Edwards, K. B., Davis, D. R., Cornman, C. B., and Macera, C. A. (1997). Risk of institutionalization among community long-term care clients with dementia, *Gerontologist*, **37**, 46–51.

Severson, M. A., Smith, G. E., Tangalos, E. G., Petersen, R. C., Kokmen, E., Ivnik, R. J., Atkinson, E. J., and Kurland, L. T. (1994). Patterns and predictors of institutionalization in community-based dementia patients, *J. Am. Ger. Soc.*, **42**, 181–185.

Shaji, S., Promodu, K., Abraham, T., Roy, K. J., and Verghese, A. (1996). An epidemiological study of dementia in a rural community in Kerala, India, *Br. J. Psychiatry*, **168**, 745–749.

Shapiro, E., and Tate, R. (1988). Who is really at risk of institutionalization? *Gerontologist*, **28**, 237–245.

Skoog, I., Lernfelt, B., Landahl, S. et al (1996). 15-year longitudinal study of blood pressure and dementia, *Lancet*, **347**, 1141–1145.

Skoog, I., Nilsson, L., Palmertz, B., Andreasson, L. A., and Svanborg, A. (1993). A population-based study of dementia in 85-year olds, *N. Engl. J. Med.*, **328**, 153–158.

Smith, D. M., and Atkinson, R. M. (1995). Alcoholism and dementia, *Int. J. Addict.*, **30** (13–14), 1843–1869.

Sobel, E., Davanipour, Z., Sulkava, R., Erkinjuntti, T., Wikström, J., Henderson, V. W., Buckwalter, G., Bowman, J. D., and Lee, P.-J. (1995). Occupations with exposure to electromagnetic fields: a possible risk factor for Alzheimer's disease, *Am. J. Epidemiol.*, **142**, 515–524.

Sobel, E., Dunn, M., Davanipour, Z., Qian, Z., and Chui, H. C. (1996). Elevated risk of Alzheimer's disease among workers with likely electromagnetic field exposure, *Neurology*, **47**, 1477–1481.

Stern, Y., Gurland, B., Tatemichi, T. K., Tang, M. X., Wilder, D., and Mayeux, R. (1994). Influence of education and occupation in the incidence of Alzheimer's disease, *JAMA*, **271**, 1004–1010.

Stewart, W. F., Kawas, C., Corrada, M., and Metter, E. J. (1997). Risk of Alzheimer's disease and duration of NSAID use, *Neurology*, **48**, 626–632.

Sulkava, R., Wikström, J., Aromaa, A., Raitasalo, R., Lehtinen, V., Lahtela, K., and Palo, J. (1985). Prevalence of severe dementia in Finland, *Neurology*, **35**, 1025–1029.

Svedberg, P., Gatz, M., and Pedersen, N. L. (1996). Reconsidering education as a risk factor for Alzheimer's disease, *Gerontologist*, **36**, 251–252.

Tang, M-X., Jacobs, D., Stern, Y., Marder, K., Schofield, P., Gurland, B., and Andrews, H. (1996). Effect of oestrogen during menopause on risk and age at onset of Alzheimer's disease, *Lancet*, **348**, 429–432.

Tatemichi, T. K., Desmond, D. W., Mayeux, R., Paik, M., Stern, Y., Sano, M., Remien, R. H., Williams, J. B. W., Mohr, J. P., Hauser, W. A., and Figueroa, M. (1992). Dementia after stroke: baseline frequency, risks, and clinical features in a hospitalized cohort, *Neurology*, **42**, 1185–1193.

The Canadian Study of Health and Aging (1994). Risk factors for Alzheimer's disease in Canada, *Neurology*, **44**, 2073–2080.

Ueda, K., Kawano, K., Hasuo, Y., and Fujishima, M. (1992). Prevalence and aetiology of dementia in a Japanese community, *Stroke*, **23**, 798–803.

van Duijn, C. M. (1996). Epidemiology of the dementias: recent developments and new approaches, *J. Neurol., Neurosurg., Psychiatry*, **60**, 478–488.

van Duijn, C. M., Clayton, D. G., Chandra, V., Fratiglioni, L., Graves, A. B., Heyman, A., Jorm, A. F., Kokmen, E., Kondo, K., Mortimer, J. A., Rocca, W. A., Shalat, S. L., Soininen, H., and Hofman, A. (1994). Interaction between genetic and environmental risk factors for Alzheimer's disease: a reanalysis of case-control studies, *Genetic. Epidemiol.*, **11**, 539–551.

van Duijn, C. M., Havekes, L. M., Van Broeckhoven, C., de Kniiff, P., and Hofman, A. (1995). Apolipoprotein E genotype and association between smoking and early onset Alzheimer's disease, *BMJ*, **310**, 627–631.

van Duijn, C. M., and Hofman, A. (1991). Relation between nicotine intake and Alzheimer's disease, *BMJ*, **302**, 1491–1494.

van Duijn, C. M., de Knijff, P., Cruts, M., Wehnert, A., Havekes, L. M., Hofman, A., and Broeckhoven, C. V. (1994). Apolipoprotein e4 allele in a population-based study of early-onset Alzheimer's disease, *Nat. Genet.*, **7**, 74–77.

Wernicke, T. F., and Reischies, F. M. (1994). Prevalence of dementia in old age: clinical diagnoses in subjects aged 95 years and older, *Neurology*, **44**, 250–253.

White, L., Petrovitch, H., Ross, G. W., Masaki, K. H., Abbott, R. D., Teng, E. L., Rodriguez, B. L., Blanchette, P. L., Havlik, R. J., Wergowske, G., Chiu, D., Foley, D. J., Murdaugh, C., and Curb, J. D. (1996). Prevalence of dementia in older Japanese-American men in Hawaii. The Honolulu-Asia Aging Study, *JAMA*, **276**, 955–960.

Winblad, B., Corder, E., Fratiglioni, L., Basun, H., Lannfelt, L., and Viitanen, M. (1997). The prevalence of clinical dementia diagnosis varies with Apolipoprotein E polymorphism in a population sample of very old adults, in *Alzheimer's Disease: Biology, Diagnosis and Therapeutics*, K. Iqbal, B. Winblad, T. Nishimura, M. Takeda, H. M. Wisniewski (Eds), pp. 39–44, John Wiley, Chichester.

Woo, J., Ho, S. C., Lau, J., and Yuen, Y. K. (1994). Age and marital status are major factors associated with institutionalization in elderly Hong Kong Chinese, *J. Epidemiol Com. Health*, **48**, 306–309.

Yoshitake, T., Kiyohara, Y., Kato, I., Ohmura, T., Iwamoto, H., Nakayama, K., Ohmori, S., Nomiyama, K., Kawano, H., Ueda, K., Sueishi, K., Tsuneyoshi, M., and Fujishima, M. (1995). Incidence and risk factors of vascular dementia and Alzheimer's disease in a defined elderly Japanese population: the Hisayama Study, *Neurology*, **45**, 1161–1168.

Zhang, M., Katzman, R., Salmon, D., Jin, H., Cai, G., Wang, Z., Qu, G., Grant, I., Yu, E., Levy, P., Klauber, M. R., and Liu, W. T. (1990). The prevalence of dementia and Alzheimer's disease in Shanghai, China: Impact of age, gender, and education, *Ann. Neurol.*, **27**, 428–437.

1.3 Symptomatology: Functional Capacity and Behaviour

HENRY BRODATY and DAVID LIE

Department of Psychogeriatrics, Prince Henry Hospital, Sydney, Australia

INTRODUCTION

There are many types of dementia each of which can become manifest in a multitude of ways, influenced by the person, the environment, the disease pathology and the stage of disease progression. This chapter focuses on the clinical features of dementia, the common behavioural and psychological signs and symptoms (BPSSD) that complicate dementia, and the rate of decline including discussion of nursing home admission (NHA) and mortality.

While Alzheimer's disease (AD) will be used as the prototype in discussing the clinical aspects of dementia, there are limitations in using this paradigm. For example, in cases of dementia where frontal lobe damage predominates (such as in fronto-temporal dementias and as often arises in severe head injury), changes in personality and loss of judgement may be more prominent and occur earlier than gross memory disturbance and result in far greater disability. In addition, a variety of pathologies may be present in the one person leading to mixed clinical pictures rather than classical textbook cases. Alcohol dependence may lead to brain damage from head injury, from nutritional deprivation as well as from the direct toxic effects of alcohol itself. Alzheimer-type dementia is often complicated by cerebrovascular disease.

The framework for the chapter is to examine the cognitive, functional and behavioural changes that accompany AD, its effects on caregivers (CGs), and the requirements for services across the stages of dementia that characterise its decline. We pay particular attention to the emotional and behavioural disturbances of dementia as it is often these, rather than cognitive impairments *per se*, which tend to bring patients to the attention of medical services, place unbearable demands upon CGs and ultimately lead to the need for institutional care. Finally, we discuss differences observable in some of the other common dementias, namely vascular dementia (VaD), fronto-temporal dementia, diffuse Lewy body disease, Parkinson's disease, alcohol-related dementia and head injury.

Health Economics of Dementia. Edited by Anders Wimo, Bengt Jönsson, Göran Karlsson and Bengt Winblad.
© 1998 John Wiley & Sons Ltd.

SYMPTOMATOLOGY AND THE TIME COURSE OF DEMENTIA

Although dementia is an acquired syndrome of multiple cognitive impairments, losses may arise in a predictable sequence and in the case of some progressive conditions, especially AD, typical stages of illness may be described.

PRE-DIAGNOSIS

Before diagnosis symptoms are often vague and difficult to pin-point. Typically there is loss of short-term memory reported as misplacing objects, forgetting familiar names or inability to recall recent incidents or conversations. Subtle personality changes, clearer to others in retrospect, include irritability, depression, narrowing of interests and loss of emotional expressivity. Other cognitive deficits, if they occur at all, may include word-finding and conceptual difficulties. It is often hard to distinguish the features of early dementia from benign age-associated memory impairment. Indeed there is debate as to whether such abnormalities occur on a continuum with dementia or are part of a separate process of 'benign senescent forgetfulness' (Huppert and Brayne, 1994). Deficits in a number of cognitive areas, such as evidence of word-finding difficulties or difficulty in following a story, memory difficulties despite effort, and progression of cognitive decline augur poorly. Assessment may be hampered by sensory impairment, physical discomfort, side-effects of medication, concurrent emotional reactions to losses or test-related anxiety.

DIAGNOSIS

On average, people with AD or their families date the onset of symptoms about two to three years before the diagnosis is made. A family member rather than the person with AD is more likely to instigate assessment. The first point of contact for assessment, which will vary according to the severity and prominence of particular symptoms, may be the primary care physician, aged care and community service or hospital staff.

Dementia may appear to have an abrupt onset if suddenly unmasked. Spouses sometimes hide the dementing person's problems from other family members until they themselves fall ill or are no longer able to cope with caring. The patient who lives alone may not be suspected of dementia until she wanders away and becomes lost in her own neighbourhood. Others with dementia may be found living in squalor. In hospitals, cognitive assessment may occur for the first time when a patient develops delirium or because the patient becomes agitated or disorientated in an unfamiliar environment.

Dementia or memory clinics may receive referrals from relatives, family physicians or occasionally from patients themselves, especially where a strong family history of dementia is present. Memory loss or personality changes may lead to neurological consultation and psychiatrists may be consulted in particular where depression or psychosis are complicating features or where frontal lobe features predominate.

In this very early stage there is usually no functional decline or behavioural abnormality. Perhaps more complex or demanding activities are not performed to the usual standard. For example, the competition bridge player who notices that his declining memory is handicapping his game, or the architect who is having difficulty conceptualising her next design. Behavioural changes are usually negligible or subtle although spouses may report lack of usual verve. Workmates may be more aware of problems while CGs may have vague, often unvoiced concerns during this period. We know of no empirical data on the impact of dementia on CGs pre-diagnosis. The only requirement for services is for counselling and provision of information.

EARLY STAGE OF DEMENTIA

Cognitive deficits, which are the most prominent presenting features of AD, are mostly cortical in nature. Of the four (+4) As—amnesia, aphasia, apraxia and agnosia (plus acalculia, alexia, agraphia and associated features—loss of executive functions), the first two are generally evident early in the disease course. Memory abnormalities are mild but impair new learning, while language abnormalities are limited to word-finding difficulty and poor naming for low frequency items, visuospatial problems are revealed only by complex visuospatial tasks, such as navigating through unfamiliar neighbourhoods or copying complex figures (Cummings and Benson, 1992; Absher and Cummings, 1994).

Insight is often held to be poor but our experience from a Memory Disorders Clinic was that a third of patients being assessed retained insight into their condition, a third had partial insight and a third lacked insight (Brodaty, 1990). As expected insight was better preserved earlier in the disease.

Decline in cognitive, occupational or social function is required for the diagnosis of dementia (American Psychiatric Association, 1994). However, such decline may be subtle: differences may be only apparent to co-habitants, family or workmates. For example, one man was reported to lack his usual quickness with repartee, and a woman who for years had organised the mailing of Christmas cards found she became muddled and frustrated. Finances may suffer and driving may become hazardous.

Personality alterations are the rule. In the St Louis longitudinal study 80% of persons with mild AD exhibited personality changes compared to 10% of a control population of non-demented older persons (Rubin, Morris and Berg, 1987). Two patterns of personality change are apparent: a flattening of the landscape—disengagement, apathy, lack of interest; and a heightening of the peaks and deepening of the valleys—caricaturing of personality traits, disinhibition and exaggerated emotional responses.

Depression occurring in early dementia is more likely to be a reaction to the diagnosis, while depression occurring later is more likely to be part of the degenerative process (Brodaty and Luscombe, 1996; Reisberg et al, 1987). In AD behavioural aberrations are uncommon in this early stage.

As a general rule, the consequences of deficits at all stages are dependent on contextual factors such as pre-morbid personality and attainments, social and financial resources, concurrent physical problems (including sensory deficits), and the physical and cultural environment.

While mild impairment may bring loss of employment for some, those engaged in repetitive tasks or receiving adequate supervision may continue to work. Similarly, planning of household tasks may suffer but most are able to continue with routine home-making activities. Some higher level instrumental activities of daily living (IADLs) (use of money, medicines, telephone and transport) may be compromised or taken over by other family members.

Major changes in marital and family relationships may arise with a variety of consequences. On the one hand the increased burden on spouses may result in closer involvement of family. In other cases new demands may lead to physical or emotional abuse of the dementing person or illness in the carer.

The progressive changes in personality may be especially traumatic to the spouse. Thus, poor motivation and flat facial appearance may be perceived as loss of commitment to the marital relationship or at the least lead to loss of companionship.

Lastly, mild dementia may complicate the logistics of the management of other illnesses, particularly those relying on timed, consistent administration of medication or attendance for appointments.

MIDDLE STAGE OF DEMENTIA

As memory problems become more pronounced other cognitive deficits are apparent. Deficits in conceptualisation, judgement, planning, organisation, abstract thinking and language as well as parietal lobe signs such as ideomotor apraxia, agnosia and acalculia can be elicited. Auditory and written comprehension, especially for semantically complex material, and visuospatial abilities decline. Verbal output is fluent but relatively impoverished, repetition is preserved but nominal aphasia and paraphasias are apparent.

The earlier personality changes become more obvious and are compounded by frontal apathy and amotivation. Hygiene and personal grooming decline. Behavioural and psychological signs and symptoms of dementia (BPSSD) develop (see below), notably delusions, hallucinations and depression. Aggressiveness, loss of normal sleep rhythm and wandering are particular problems. Extrapyramidal motor abnormalities begin to appear on physical examination including slowed movements and gait (bradykinesia) and increased muscular tone.

Reliance on others for IADLs is almost total save for the most basic or over-learned routines. One woman could no longer cook except for the traditional weekly roast dinner, nor clean except for folding clothes and linen, an act which she performed repeatedly and purposelessly.

Even basic activities of daily living (ADLs) require assistance or prompting. Almost continuous supervision is required as independent living is no longer feasible. The capacity to give Power of Attorney or write a Will becomes tenuous and financial management generally falls to others.

The emotional, physical and social impact on caregivers is profound. Caregiver psychological morbidity is likely to be high, especially if BPSSD occur. Increased isolation, financial strain and forsaken employment often follow.

LATE STAGE OF DEMENTIA

In the late stage of dementia there is no short-term memory although occasional lucid moments may give families the false impression of preserved abilities. Verbal output is spare and may be characterised by palilalia or echolalia. Motor changes are more obvious with extrapyramidal features, primitive reflexes and motor retardation often apparent. Gait deteriorates to chair-fast and eventually bed-fast states. Independence is further lost until a functional stage of complete dependence is reached. Eventually the affected person is doubly incontinent and must be fed, toileted and washed by others.

Abnormal behaviours and psychiatric phenomena usually abate, though sometimes very regressed behaviours, such as constant screaming, may signal otherwise uncommunicable distress.

Paradoxically, CGs may find this last stage easier, as BPSSD ease and as care becomes more routine and task-orientated but less interactive. Even so, physical demands on CGs can be telling and assistance is required. While the decision to institutionalise is filled with guilt and angst, CGs whose dependants are in nursing homes have lower levels and rates of psychological morbidity than those still caring at home. Death re-ignites the grief of 'the funeral that never ends'. Bereavement is often felt doubly keenly as the centre of the CG's world disappears.

Services required are practical help such as home nursing and personal care assistance, periodic residential respite care, and emotional support in dealing with nursing home placement and later with bereavement.

BEHAVIOURAL AND PSYCHOLOGICAL SIGNS AND SYMPTOMS OF DEMENTIA (BPSSD)

These features are diverse and common in AD. Their importance lies in their influence on diagnosis, management, prognosis, institutionalisation, family

CGs and societal costs. For example, behavioural disturbances consistently account for about 25% of the variance in caregiver distress and are proven risk factors for institutionalisation (Brodaty, 1996). Further, BPSSD may provide a window into the pathogenesis of psychiatric phenomena in cognitively intact persons. For example, elucidation of a distinctive pathology in persons with AD and delusions compared to those with AD and no delusions may be instructive in understanding the pathogenesis of delusions.

BPSSD can often be cured or at least ameliorated. Successful treatment improves the quality of life of the affected person and those around him or her. Management follows the rule of correcting any underlying causes that can be identified, use of behavioural techniques building on analysis of abnormal behaviours, manipulation of the environment rather than the person, and judicious use of pharmacotherapy which must be carefully and legally (bearing in mind the need for informed consent) prescribed and periodically reviewed in order to ensure their continued need. All therapies, not only pharmaco-therapeutic, should be prescribed with rigour, but use of drugs requires special care because of the susceptibility of the dementing person to side-effects.

PSYCHOLOGICAL SIGNS AND SYMPTOMS

Depression

Depression is usually defined according to DSM-IV criteria, that is at least five symptoms of depression for at least two weeks interfering with normal function. Such definitions are difficult to apply in persons with dementia as clinical features of the two conditions overlap, for example loss of interest, agitation, retardation. Furthermore, it can be impossible to obtain a two-week history in the context of loss of memory.

Such diagnostic difficulties may explain the greatly divergent prevalence rates of clinical depression reported in AD—from 0–86%! The modal rate is around 20–25% but more recent studies estimate prevalences of 5–10% (Brodaty and Luscombe, 1996).

Aetiology is diverse. Psychological reaction and concern about the future are significant contributors to depression, particularly early in the disease process or soon after diagnosis. The AD pathology itself appears to be aetiological by way of reduction in brain amines and loss of cells in the locus coeruleus. The prevalence of depression and the severity of depressive symptoms appear to increase with increasing dementia severity, though this relationship may not hold in the late stage of the disease when there may be insufficient brain tissue to maintain a pervasive depression.

Management requires attention to aetiological factors. Antidepressants have a role, though little empirical data have accumulated on their efficacy. In general, avoidance of drugs with anticholinergic side-effects is recommended given the cholinergic hypothesis of memory impairment in AD. As such the selective serotonin reuptake inhibitors (SSRIs) or a more recently developed selective noradrenalin reuptake inhibitor or reversible monoamine oxidase inhibitor are preferred (Carrier and Brodaty, 1996).

Delusions

Persistent fixed false beliefs are relatively common in AD. Estimated prevalence rates are that about 30% of persons with AD will experience delusions or paranoid ideation at some time during their dementia, and about half of them in the previous 12 months (Burns et al, 1990a). The clinical picture is usually of simple delusions of theft or infidelity; more complex, elaborate delusions are less common.

   Biological and psychological aetiologies operate here too. There is some evidence that the basal ganglia are more likely to show pathology. Psychologically, it is understandable that a person will feel less secure as faculties fade. Personal valuables, which can impart a sense of confidence, may be secreted in soon forgotten places and then not found, leading the affected person to accuse others of stealing. Management requires attention to environmental factors, working with the family and prudent use of antipsychotic medication.

Hallucinations

Hallucinations, which are perceptions in the absence of a stimulus, can occur in any of the sensory modalities, though auditory and visual hallucinations are commonest. About 16% of people with AD will have hallucinations at some time during their dementia (Burns et al, 1990b; Rubin et al, 1988). The peak periods for hallucinations are the middle and later phases of the dementing process. There may be an association between sensory impairment and hallucinations. Hallucinations may portend a more rapid decline of the dementia. Management includes correction of sensory deficits and, if the hallucinations are distressing, use of antipsychotics.

Misidentification syndromes

These syndromes include misidentifications of a familiar person, often the spouse, as a stranger—so-called Capgras phenomenon; of oneself in a mirror as a stranger; of non-existent people as being in the house—the phantom boarder phenomenon; and, of the images on television as being real. They can be very distressing to the patient and family, and are very common, occurring in about one in three persons with AD during the course of their dementia (Burns et al, 1990b; Rubin et al, 1988).

Creative management methods attempt to cue perceptions differently, for example by asking the spouse to groom or dress differently, or by obscuring all but a small central part of the mirror. Anti-psychotic medications have a place.

BEHAVIOURAL DISTURBANCES

Aggression

Significant physically aggressive behaviour occurs commonly, perhaps in over one fifth of AD patients, more so as the disease progresses, though not in end-stage dementia, and more often in men.

Socio-environmental and behavioural management strategies are preferred; often a trigger may be identified and appropriate methods devised for avoiding the precipitant. For example, a behavioural diary identified that one man's aggressive outbursts followed morning showers by a female nursing assistant. Alteration of bathing patterns to his previous custom of evening baths, now supervised by the resident's wife, led to his behaviour settling. Pharmacological treatments have had less success but remain useful, especially in conjunction with behavioural methods. Antipsychotics are generally the first line of treatment; sedatives, anticonvulsants and antidepressants are sometimes effective.

Wandering

This is another common and difficult behaviour, which may be more complex than it seems at first glance. Wandering may be aimless, goal directed as in seeking a lost partner, part of a general anxiety state, a manifestation of akathisia resulting from the very medication used to treat the agitation, or even a sign of an agitated melancholic depression.

Management depends on the type of wandering. For the most common type, aimless wandering, good residential design is critical. Use of diversional therapy, such as music and creative activities, may help too. Pharmacotherapy has a limited role.

Screaming

Vocal disruptive behaviour can be a nightmare for everyone around the resident. Sometimes it reflects an underlying depression, physical pain, or a yearning for attention. Management is directed to rectification of the under-lying condition if this can be identified and employment of behavioural techniques such as providing attention or other rewards when the person is quiet, and ignoring the person or using time out for prolonged episodes of screaming.

Sleep disturbance

Persons with AD usually sleep sufficient hours but the architecture of the sleep cycle is disrupted so that they may be awake in the middle of the night when they can create havoc for others. Pain, physical disease and depression may also be causes of insomnia. Hypnotics may help sleep but compromise cognitive function the next day.

Agitation

This is a vague term often used to connote aggression, vocal disruption or wandering. Strictly defined it means a motor restlessness reflecting inner mental perturbation and may indicate a clinical depression or anxiety disorder. Management is behavioural, socio-environmental and pharmacotherapeutic.

Apathy and indifference

These are very common but under-reported behaviours as apathetic patients are often easier to manage and less demanding especially in residential facilities. On the other hand, spouse carers become extremely frustrated by their partner's lack of initiative, communicativeness, affection and general interest. Sometimes called abulia, these behaviours are associated with frontal lobe pathology, especially medially.

Sexual disinhibition

Disinhibited behaviours are not as common as apathetic ones but are frequent enough to pose a serious problem in the care of people with AD. They are also typically associated with frontal lobe pathology, especially in the orbito-basal region. In addition to the management principles enunciated previously, anti-androgen or feminising hormones are sometimes used as a last resort in men with very troublesome sexually aggressive behaviours.

Eating disturbances

These may be a loss of the ability to manipulate cutlery, loss of discrimination in what is eaten, indiscriminate eating, overeating (analogous to the Kluver–Bucy syndrome), stereotyped patterns of food intake (e.g. always eating the same food every time) or compulsive eating. Eventually the patient 'forgets' how to eat or even swallow. Spoon-feeding may give way to nasogastric or percutaneous enterogastric feeding. Most patients with AD ultimately lose weight despite adequate food intake and normal bowel motions.

DECLINE, NURSING HOME ADMISSION (NHA) AND DEATH

RATES OF DECLINE

Rates of decline are usually measured by annual rates of change in cognition. Decline, however, is not uniform: it may be interrupted by plateaux and monitoring of cognitive abilities usually indicates a trilinear pattern probably reflecting the limitations of measures such as the Mini-Mental State Examination (MMSE) (Yesavage et al, 1988). Thus there is slower decline in the early phase (possibly indicating a ceiling effect of the instrument) and in the late phase (floor effect) and a more rapid change in the middle phase. Broader estimates of staging and decline are provided by the Clinical Dementia Rating Scale (Berg, 1988) and the FAST (Reisberg, 1988).

This variability in cognitive decline also reflects the 'noise' of variables, such as the patient's mood, motivation, intercurrent illnesses, medications, practice effects and tester inconsistencies (Corey-Bloom et al, 1994). Education, age and psychiatric comorbidity may also influence rates of progression. Reported annual rates of change on the MMSE have averaged about 2.8–3.5 points with wide variability (range = 1.8–4.2, SD = approx 4.5) (Yesavage et al, 1988; Salmon et al, 1990; Teri et al, 1990; Burns et al, 1991; Corey-Bloom et al, 1994). On the Blessed Information, Memory and Concentration scale (Blessed et al, 1968), the mean annual rate of change was reported to be 3.2–4.5 with SD = 3.0–3.6 (Katzman et al, 1988; Thal et al, 1988; Ortof and Crystal, 1989; Salmon et al, 1990). Subjects with milder degrees of dementia declined less rapidly in these studies.

DEMENTIA AND NURSING HOMES (NHs)

Admission to an institution is a major milestone in the progress of the disease and is commonly used as an endpoint in dementia research. Significantly, NHA is usually very stressful for patient, CG and extended family. An understanding of what determines NHA may be helpful in ensuring that this is not arranged prematurely but only when appropriate.

Both dementia and CG variables are important predictors of NHA. The level of severity of the dementia, the degree of dependence and the rate of progression have all been linked to NHA (Drachman et al, 1990; Brodaty et al,

1993). In particular, the development of incontinence, the failure of patients to recognise the family member who is the principal CG, the nature and severity of BPSSD and CG stress levels appear to be potent influences on the decision to institutionalise. Many studies have documented the correlation between BPSSD and NHA, with aggression, insomnia, wandering and psychosis being important predictors of institutionalisation. Type of dementia may be important too, probably because it influences the rate of progression and the development of BPSSD. Thus persons with vascular dementia (VaD) have a more rapid rate of decline and enter NHs earlier than those with AD (Brodaty et al, 1993). Those with fronto-temporal dementias may be admitted earlier too, mainly because of their increased propensity to develop behavioural complications. Caregivers who are not spouses are more likely to institutionalise persons with dementia, as are CGs who are stressed, have fewer social supports or who have indicated a desire to institutionalise. Care 'managers', those who organise others to provide care, tend to institutionalise earlier than care 'providers', those who provide hands-on care themselves (Gilleard, 1984).

DEMENTIA AND DEATH

Persons with dementia die sooner than age-matched population controls, an effect more striking in younger persons. The average life-span from onset to death is difficult to judge because the onset of degenerative dementias is usually insidious. Over the last century there has been an increase in survival time for persons with AD (Christie, 1994). VaD consistently has a greater mortality rate compared to AD. In a sample of patients with predominantly mild dementia followed up over five years almost double the proportion of patients with VaD (63.6%) had died compared to those with AD (38.4%) (Brodaty et al, 1993), which was comparable to reports from others (Barclay et al, 1985; Drachman et al, 1990).

Other factors said to predict decreased survival are age, poor physical health, hallucinations, primitive reflexes, parietal lobe signs, incontinence, more rapid rate of decline, severity of decline, neuroleptic treatment and white matter changes on neuroimaging (Christie, 1994; Panisset and Stern, 1996; Scheltens et al, 1995). The influence of apolipoprotein E ϵ4 on rate of decline remains unclear with contradictory findings reported (Panisset and Stern, 1996).

The causes of death of persons with dementia are poorly specified. Bronchopneumonia is the most common accounting for over 50% of AD cases (Sulkava et al, 1983; Molsa et al, 1986), nearly 70% of VaD cases (Molsa et al, 1986) and 80% of other dementias (Sulkava et al, 1983). In one study, patients with dementia were three times as likely to die of bronchopneumonia as non-demented subjects (Kay, 1962). Another cause over-represented in dementia subjects is pulmonary embolism (Burns, 1992).

OTHER DEMENTIAS

VASCULAR DEMENTIA

The replacement of the term multi-infarct dementia (MID) with VaD emphasises the growing understanding of the complexity and multiplicity of causes that may result in dementia from cerebrovascular pathologies. Criteria for the classification of VaD have been proposed (Chui et al, 1992; Román et al, 1993). Unlike AD, the prevalence of VaD is higher in men than women. Also VaD tends to present earlier than AD.

Autopsy-based studies have reported that VaD accounts for up to 20% of cases of dementia and that mixed AD and VaD account for another 10–20%. VaD is thus the second most common type of dementia in the world, though the VaD/AD ratio is reversed in Japan and Russia (Jorm et al, 1987) for reasons which are incompletely understood.

The pathogenetic mechanisms for vascular disease are infarction which may be single or multiple and occur in arterial territory, in watershed areas or as lacunes; non-infarction ischaemia; and haemorrhage (Peisah et al, 1993). Infarctions may present as clinical or 'silent' strokes. Small strokes may have an additive or multiplicative effect and a critical threshold (about 100 ml) may need to be reached in order to overcome the brain's compensatory mechanisms and present the clinical picture of dementia (Hachinski et al, 1974; Tomlinson et al, 1970). Single small infarcts can, by themselves, cause VaD if they occur in certain strategic locations such as the angular gyrus, posterior cerebral artery territory, anterior cerebral artery territory, parietal lobe, thalamus and basal forebrain (Román et al, 1993). Binswanger's disease is a subcortical leukoencephalopathy in which chronic hypertension plays a major role.

The clinical presentation may be abrupt after a stroke and thereafter static, remitting or progressive or gradual with slow or stepwise progression. In general, clinical features suggestive of a subcortical process such as gait disorder, frequent falls, urinary frequency and incontinence early in the course of the dementing illness favour a diagnosis of VaD. Psychiatric symptoms such as depression and mood changes are common in VaD (Cummings, 1992). Common focal findings are hemiparesis or local facial weakness, sensory loss, pseudobulbar syndrome and extrapyramidal signs such as rigidity and akinesia (Román et al, 1993). As well as symptoms and signs of focal neurological deficits, neuroimaging with CT and MRI assists in diagnosis. Radiological criteria have been proposed for making the diagnosis of VaD (Chui et al, 1992; Román et al, 1993).

Clinical features held to differentiate VaD from AD include abrupt onset, stepwise deterioration, fluctuating course, nocturnal confusion, relative preservation of personality, emotional incontinence, history of hypertension, history of strokes, associated atherosclerosis, focal neurological symptoms and focal neurological signs (Hachinski et al, 1975).

In general, the effects on family caregivers, the impact of the disease on family and others and the need for services are much the same as for AD. Depression may be more common but other psychiatric complications less so (the rate of deterioration is faster and with earlier NHA and death [see above]).

LEWY BODY DISEASE

Lewy body disease or diffuse Lewy body disease is a type of dementia with characteristic pathological and clinical features. It is said to be the second or third most common form of dementia after AD and possibly after VaD. Lewy body disease affects primarily middle age to older individuals although an early onset form similar to juvenile Parkinson's disease has been described (Doody and Massman, 1994).

McKeith et al (1992) proposed clinical criteria for the diagnosis of Lewy body disease, namely dementia of at least three months duration, fluctuating confusion, visual hallucinations, extrapyramidal features and/or extreme sensitivity to neuroleptics, frequent falls and Parkinsonian features. The frequent presence of hallucinations combined with the exquisite sensitivity to anti-psychotic medications makes the management of such patients even more difficult than usual. Fortunately, patients with Lewy body disease may be more responsive to cholinergic enhancement strategies such as donepezil which are now being used in AD and may reduce the frequency and severity of some BPSSD (Cummings, 1997).

FRONTO-TEMPORAL DEMENTIAS (FTD)

Several pathological processes may result in the presentation of a fronto-temporal dementia. Pick's disease was the first recognised and is characterised by frontal and/or temporal atrophy with preservation of the parietal and occipital regions. The hippocampus is usually atrophic but not invariably and subcortical structures are often affected. The histological hallmark is the Pick body, an intracellular inclusion found in neocortical and hippocampal neurones (Knopman, 1994). Other pathological types of FTD, also called Pick Syndrome, are dementia lacking distinctive histological features, progressive subcortical gliosis and focal lobar atrophy.

Clinically, patients with fronto-temporal dementia present as apathetic, disinhibited or eccentric. Their social skills deteriorate much earlier than those of patients with AD and they may show signs of Kluver–Bucy syndrome early. Their language output is decreased, sometimes markedly, and they have evidence of semantic anomia whereas those with AD are more likely to have a lexical anomia. On the other hand parietal lobe functions such as construction, calculation, reading and writing are relatively spared. Memory loss, an early feature in AD, is variably affected and deficits may not be noted until later in the disease.

The early manifestation and frequency of personality and behavioural changes that occur in these dementias pose particular strains on caregivers. Patients present earlier than those with AD and are more likely to have a family history, both of which may impose additional burdens on patients and their families.

DEMENTIA RELATED TO ALCOHOLIC BRAIN DAMAGE

The aetiological role of alcohol itself in the dementia associated with prolonged heavy alcohol consumption is controversial. Impairments may result from the toxic effects of alcohol as well as other aspects of the 'alcoholic lifestyle'—poor nutrition (especially thiamine deficiency leading to Wernicke–Korsakoff's syndrome) and head injury (Renner and Morris, 1994). Joyce (1994) considered that most organic brain syndromes in alcoholic patients are variants of Wernicke–Korsakoff syndrome. Korsakoff's syndrome (see Kopelman, 1995) is considered an amnestic disorder, that is it produces memory loss with relative sparing of other cognitive functions. Yet abnormalities of abstract thinking and visuospatial function are found so commonly that Lishman (1990) argued for the existence of a true dementia secondary to chronic alcoholism. Psychiatric complications of heavy alcohol use, such as hallucinosis, depression, anxiety and excessive use of other substances, are additional considerations.

The dementia is said to be mild and following abstinence does not progress; abstinence may result in significant improvement although full recovery is rare (Brandt et al, 1983; Cummings and Benson, 1992; Renner and Morris, 1994). Patients typically display forgetfulness, psychomotor retardation, disorientation, vague thinking, perseveration, loss of abstract thinking and diminished attentiveness. There is often preservation of personality and retained social skills. Concurrent physical problems are frequent and include gait abnormalities, subdural haematoma, falls, alcoholic peripheral neuropathy, cerebellar degeneration, hypertension, cardiomyopathy and liver disease as well as respiratory conditions related to heavy cigarette consumption. Our impression is that behavioural and psychological complications are more common in men with alcoholic dementia than those with AD especially if there is continuing intake of alcohol or other substances.

For whatever reasons, a subgroup of people with a history of heavy drinking suffer from permanent, disabling cognitive disturbance and create specific challenges for caregivers and health services. Relatives may be ambivalent about providing support to maintain community living where substance dependence has been complicated by longstanding abuse.

The need for institutionalisation of alcoholics usually results from a combination of severe impairment in short-term memory, loss of planning ability and progressive alienation of supportive relationships due to previous behavioural and interpersonal problems. Autonomy versus beneficence debates are frequent and centre on compelling a person to abstain from alcohol and move to secure residential placement versus independent but unsafe living arrangements.

DEMENTIA ARISING FROM TRAUMATIC BRAIN INJURY

Motor vehicle accidents are the most frequent cause of head trauma in industrialised nations. Improvements in acute care have increased the numbers of survivors from severe traumatic brain injury. Dementia complicating traumatic brain injury often occurs in males aged 15–24, older people who have fallen and sustained head injuries, for example subdural haematoma, and alcohol-dependent persons who have fallen or been assaulted. Aside from direct injury to brain tissue itself, neurological damage may also arise from intracranial complications such as haematoma and from injury to other body areas, for example hypoxia secondary to chest trauma. The clinical picture that develops is determined by the site and nature of injuries with damage to frontal and temporal poles a frequent sequel.

In the aftermath of injury, the patient cannot remember what has occurred while comatose and for some period after emerging from unconsciousness. Anterograde post-traumatic amnesia describes ongoing difficulties with acquisition of new material in this period whilst retrograde post-traumatic amnesia is an inability to remember events for up to several months prior to the accident. This is followed by a period of more rapid recovery for up to 6 to 12 months and progression to a plateau phase over 12 to 24 months following the time of injury.

Prognosis is difficult to judge. Severe memory deficits are generally associated with prolonged post-traumatic amnesia, but permanent cognitive impairment may arise from relatively short periods of unconsciousness and continuing recovery may occur over months. Additional cognitive changes commonly include aphasia, disorganisation, rigidity, slowness of thinking, poor concentration and difficulty with abstract ideas. Mood, personality and motor abnormalities such as ataxia are common.

Impact

The functional consequences for the individual suffering traumatic brain injury relate to the summated effects of the traumatic event, including other physical injuries, psychological sequelae, for example post-traumatic stress syndromes, and social factors such as legal complications and occupational and relationship changes, and the degree of recovery achieved.

Features of frontal lobe injury present significant barriers to social and occupational recovery. Personality changes are difficult for family and friends to accept and may include apathy and withdrawal, irritability, aggressiveness, social disinhibition and lack of insight. These changes are often severe enough to cause loss of peer support and sometimes marriage breakup.

Patients who are otherwise physically well may be stigmatised when poor concentration and continuing difficulties with memory, planning and organisation lead to repeated job failures (loss of ability to drive or other life goals). Young men ordinarily achieving independence often become frustrated if they have to rely on parental carers who in turn can become exhausted with the physical and psychological demands of caring for a disabled adult child, especially where aggression is a feature.

Behavioural disturbance and other psychiatric problems may lead to institutional care, often in ill-suited aged care facilities. Diversional programmes and environment are often unsuitable and staff often become apprehensive of the threat of violence. Psychiatric facilities sometimes house those who are particularly assaultative. The use of psychotropic medication for behavioural and psychological sequelae is made problematic by an increased incidence of adverse reactions and a paucity of good outcome studies to guide best practice.

CONCLUSION

The manifestations of dementia are diverse. However by considering the typical pattern of AD, and understanding the differences from other dementias, the clinician and family can usefully though approximately predict the course of the disease and know what to expect.

ACKNOWLEDGEMENTS

Jennifer Grice prepared the manuscript. Georgina Luscombe assisted with proof reading. The section in this chapter on BPSSD is taken from: Behavioural and pyschological signs and symptoms of dementia, *The News*, Dementia Issue 2/97. Reprinted with permission from Counsellor.

REFERENCES

Absher, J. R., and Cummings, J. L. (1994). Cognitive and non-cognitive aspects of dementia syndromes, an overview, in A. Burns and R. Levy (Eds), *Dementia*, pp. 59–76, Chapman & Hall Medical, London.

American Psychiatric Association (1994). *Diagnostic and Statistical Manual of Mental Disorders* (4th edn, American Psychiatric Association), Washington, DC.

Barclay, L. L., Zemcov, A., Bless, J. P., and Jansone, J. (1985). Survival in Alzheimer's disease and vascular dementias, *Neurology*, **35**, 834–480.

Berg, L. (1988). Clinical dementia rating (CDR), *Psychopharmacol. Bull.*, **24**, 637–639.

Blessed, G., Tomlinson, B. E., and Roth, M. (1968). The association between quantitative measures of dementia and senile change in the cerebral grey matter of elderly
subjects, *Br. J. Psychiatr.*, **114**, 797–811.

Brandt, J., Butters, N., Ryan, C., and Bayog, R. (1983). Cognitive loss and recovery in
long-term alcohol abusers, *Arch. Gen. Psychiatr.*, **40**, 435–442.

Brodaty, H. (1990). Low diagnostic yield in a memory disorders clinic, *Int.
Psychogeriatr.*, **2**(2), 149–159.

Brodaty, H. (1996). Caregivers and behavioral disturbances: effects and interventions,
Int. Psychogeriatr., **8**(3), 455–458.

Brodaty, H., and Luscombe, G. (1996). Depression in persons with dementia, *Int.
Psychogeriatr.*, **8**(4), 609–622.

Brodaty, H., McGilchrist, C., Harris, L., and Peters, K. (1993). Time until
institutionalization and death in patients with dementia, *Arch. Neurol.*, **50**, 643–650.

Burns, A. (1992). Cause of death in dementia, *Int. J. Geriatr. Psychiatr.*, **7**, 461–464.

Burns, A., Jacoby, R., and Levy, R. (1990a). Psychiatric phenomena in Alzheimer's
disease II I: disorders of thought content, *Br. J. Psychiatry*, **157**, 72–76.

Burns, A., Jacoby, R., and Levy, R. (1990b). Psychiatric phenomena in Alzheimer's
disease II: disorders of perception, *Br. J. Psychiatr.*, 157, 76–81.

Burns, A., Jacoby, R., and Levy, R. (1991). Progression of cognitive impairment in
Alzheimer's disease, *J. Am. Geriatr. Soc.*, **39**, 34–45.

Carrier, L., and Brodaty, H. (1996). Mood and behaviour management, in S. Gauthier
(Ed.), *Clinical Diagnosis and Management of Alzheimer's Disease*, pp. 205–220,
Martin Dunitz, London.

Christie, A. B. (1994). Survival in Alzheimer's disease, in A. Burns and R. Levy (Eds),
Dementia, pp. 89–100, Chapman & Hall, London.

Chui, H. C., Victoroff, J. I., Margolin, M. D., Jagust, M. D., Shankle, R., and
Katzman, M. D. (1992). Criteria for the diagnosis of ischaemic vascular dementia
proposed by the State of California Alzheimer's Disease Diagnostic and Treatment
Centers, *Neurology*, **42**, 473–480.

Coorey-Bloom, J., Galasko, D., and Thal, L. J. (1994). Longitudinal changes in
cognition, in A. Burns and R. Levy (Eds), *Dementia*, pp. 79–88, Chapman & Hall,
London.

Cummings, J. L. (1992). Neuropsychiatric aspects of Alzheimer's disease and other
dementing illnesses, in S. C. Yudofsky and R. E. Hales (Eds), *The American
Psychiatric Textbook of Neuropsychiatry*, pp. 605–621, American Psychiatric Press,
Washington DC.

Cummings, J. L. (1997). Cholinergic treatment of non-cognitive symptoms of
Alzheimer's disease, *Alzheimer's Disease International Conference*, Helsinki, 1st
October 1997.

Cummings, J. L., and Benson, D. F. (1992). *Dementia: A Clinical Approach* (2nd edn),
Butterworths, New York.

Doody, R. S., and Massman, P. J. (1994). Other extrapyramidal dementias, in J. C.
Morris (Ed.), *Handbook of Dementing Illnesses*, pp. 323–326, Marcel Dekker, New
York.

Drachman, D. A., O'Donnell, B. F., Lew, R. A., and Swearer, J. M. (1990). The
prognosis in Alzheimer's disease, *Arch. Neurol.*, **47**, 851–856.

Gilleard, C. J. (1984). *Living with Dementia: Community Care of the Elderly Mentally
Infirm*, Croom Helm, London.

Hachinski, V. C., Iliff, L. D., Zilhka, E., Du Boulay, G. H., McAllister, V. L.,
Marshall, J. et al (1975). Cerebral blood flow in dementia, *Arch. Neurol.*, **32**, 632–
637.

Hachinski, V. C., Lassen, N. A., and Marshall, J. (1974). Multi-infarct dementia: a cause of mental deterioration in the elderly, *Lancet*, **2**, 207–210.

Huppert, F. A., and Brayne, C. (1994). What is the relationship between dementia and normal aging? in F. A. Huppert, C. Brayne and D. W. O'Connor (Eds), *Dementia and Normal Ageing*, Cambridge, Cambridge University Press.

Jorm, A. S., Korten, A. E., and Henderson, A. S. (1987). The prevalence of dementia: a quantitative integration of the literature, *Acta Psychiatr. Scand.*, **76**, 465–479.

Joyce, E. M. (1994). Aetiology of alcoholic brain damage: alcohol neurotoxicity or thiamine malnutrition? *Brit. Med. Bull.*, **50**, 99–114.

Katzman, R., Brown, T., Thal, L. J., Fuld, P. A., Aronson, M., Butters, N., Klauber, M. R., Wiederholt, W., Pay, M., Xiong, R. B. et al (1988). Comparison of rate of annual change of mental status score in four independent studies of patients with Alzheimer's disease, *Ann. Neurol.*, **24**, 384–389.

Kay, D. W. K. (1962). Outcome and cause of death in mental disorders of old age: a long-term follow-up of functional and organic psychoses, *Acta Psychiatr. Scand.*, **39**, 249–276.

Knopman, D. (1994). The non-Alzheimer degenerative dementias, in J. C. Morris (Ed.), *Handbook of Dementing Illnesses*, pp. 265–281, Marcel Dekker, New York.

Kopelman, M. D. (1995). The Korsakoff syndrome, *Brit. J. Psych.*, **166**, 154–173.

Lishman, W. A. (1990). Alcohol and the brain, *Brit. J. Psych.*, **157**, 635–644.

McKeith, I. G., Perry, R. H., Fairbairn, A. F., Jabeen, S., and Perry, E. K. (1992). Operational criteria for senile dementia of Lewy body type (SDLT), *Psychol. Med.*, **22**, 911–922.

Molsa, P. K., Martilla, R. J., and Rinne, U. K. (1986). Survival and cause of death in Alzheimer's disease and multi-infarct dementia, *Acta Neurol. Scand.*, **74**, 103–127.

Ortof, E., and Crystal, H. A. (1989). Rate of progression of Alzheimer's disease, *J. Am. Geriatr. Soc.*, **37**, 511–514.

Panisset, M., and Stern, Y. (1996). Prognostic factors in Alzheimer's disease, in S. Gauthier (Ed.), *Clinical Diagnosis and Management of Alzheimer's Disease*, pp. 129–135, Martin Dunitz, London.

Peisah, C., Sachdev, P., and Brodaty, H. (1993). Vascular dementia, *Int. Review Psychiatr.*, **5**, 381–395.

Reisberg, B. (1988). Functional assessment staging (FAST), *Psychopharmacol. Bull.*, **24**, 653–659.

Reisberg, B., Bornstein, J., Salob, S. P., Ferris, S. H., Franssen, E., and Geongotas, A. (1987). Behavioural symptoms in Alzheimer's disease: phenomenology and treatment, *J. Clin. Psychiatr.*, **48**, 9–15.

Renner, J. A., and Morris, J. C. (1994). Alcohol-associated dementia, in J. C. Morris (Ed.), *Handbook of Dementing Illnesses*, pp. 403–406, Marcel Dekker, New York.

Román, J. C., Tatemichi, T. K., Erkinjuntti, T., Cummings, J. L., Masdeu, J. C., Garcia, J. H., Amaducci, L., Orgogozo, J. M., Brun, A., Hofman, A. et al (1993). Vascular dementia: diagnostic criteria for research studies, *Neurology*, **43**, 250–260.

Rubin, E. H., Morris, J. C., and Berg, L. (1987). Progression of personality changes in patients with mild senile dementia of the Alzheimer's type, *J. Am. Geriat. Soc.*, **35**, 721–725.

Rubin, E. H., Drevets, W. C., and Burke, W. J. (1988). The nature of psychotic symptoms on senile dementia of the Alzheimer type, *J. Geriatr. Psychiatr. Neurol.*, **1**, 16–20.

Salmon, D. P., Thal, L. J., Butters, N., and Heindel, W. C. (1990). Longitudinal evaluation of dementia of the Alzheimer type: a comparison of 3 standardized mental status examinations, *Neurology*, **40**, 1225–1230.

Saunders, P. A., Dewey, M. E., and Copeland, J. R. M. (1991). Heavy drinking as a risk factor for depression and dementia in elderly men, *Brit. J. Psych.*, **159**, 213–216.

Scheltens, P., Barkhof, F., Leys, D., Wolters, E. C., Ravid, R., and Kamphorst, W. (1995). Histopathologic correlates of white matter changes on MRI on Alzheimer's disease and normal aging, *Neurology*, **45**(5), 883–888.

Sulkava, R., Haltia, M., Paetau, A., Wikstrom, J., and Palo, J. (1983). Accuracy of clinical diagnosis in primary degenerative dementia: correlation with neuropathological findings, *J. Neurol. Neurosurg. Psychiatr.*, **46**, 9–13.

Teri, L., Hughes, S. P., and Larson, E. B. (1990). Cognitive deterioration in Alzheimer's disease: behavioural and health factors, *J. Gerontol.*, **45**, 58–63.

Thal, L. J., Grundman, M., and Klauber, M. R. (1988). Dementia: characteristics of a referral population and factors associated with progression, *Neurology*, **38**, 1083–1090.

Tomlinson, V. E., Blessed, S., and Roth, M. (1970). Observations on the brains of demented old people, *J. Neurological Science*, **11**, 205–242.

Yesavage, J. A., Poulsen, S. L., Sheikh, J., and Tanke, E. (1988). Rates of change of common measures of impairment in senile dementia of the Alzheimer type, *Psychopharmacol. Bull.*, **24**, 531–534.

1.4 Care Options and Service Innovations in Dementia Care

LENNARTH JOHANSSON
The National Board of Health and Welfare, Stockholm, Sweden

CARE OPTIONS FOR DEPENDENT ELDERLY

In most Western countries, 'ageing-in-place' has become the guiding social policy principle in elderly welfare (OECD, 1994). Aged people should remain as long as possible in their own homes and services and care should be 'brought to' the elderly instead of 'moving' the elderly to the services and the care. In practice, this has implied a rapid development of supportive services for the elderly. Besides these home-based personal care services, a range of housing options have been developed in order to offer even very dependent older people the opportunity to age with dignity.

The strengthening of home-based care is a common goal in almost all industrial countries in order to ensure elderly people an autonomous living for as long as possible. However, a common difficulty is the continuously widening gap between care demands on the one hand and care supply and scarce resources on the other hand. In many countries profound changes in the development of the population can be detected, implying a socio-political challenge of the first rank. The 'oldest old' age group is of particular significance because of its sharp increase in the number as well as in the severity of illnesses and, consequently, in the need of care and shelter. When the rise in costs in the health and care sector remains unchanged, the need for lowering at least a further increase of costs will constitute the driving force behind the debates for reforms in care for the elderly.

Despite common goals in ageing policy, there are marked differences in the strategies and the implementation of measures that have been undertaken to achieve the objective of an autonomous living. For instance, as regards the development of home care, the Scandinavian countries have always been the precursors of a well-organised and flexible provision of home care to a low cost for the individual user (Daatland, 1996). However, due to the economic recession municipalities are now cutting down on services. In the last decade emphasis was also laid on the run-down of, or at least on no further

Health Economics of Dementia. Edited by Anders Wimo, Bengt Jönsson, Göran Karlsson and Bengt Winblad.
© 1998 John Wiley & Sons Ltd.

stockpiling of, institutional beds. In those countries, as for example in Scandinavia and in the Netherlands, initiatives have been taken in order to convert buildings for institutionalised care into dwellings which provide housing and care in a more 'home-like' setting. In addition to living comfort and access to service and care around the clock, the feeling of security plays a prominent role in the decision of the elderly whether or not to move to special dwellings or residential care.

Economic, demographic and political influences are reflected in the principles and assumptions on which policies have been developed during the 1990s. These policies advocate greater flexibility in housing, service and care options for older people. There are three main types of options: those based on ordinary housing, including ways of helping people to stay in this housing; options for moving into various types of grouped housing for independent living with some support; and institutional long-term care. Distinctions between types of provision are becoming blurred and innovative forms combine different types. For example, older people's housing situations vary considerably—both between and within countries—differences that tend to increase.

This ambiguity in terms of definitions and concepts sometimes creates challenging problems in cross-national comparisons and research. As definitions and concepts are strongly influenced by culture and context, their comparability is often reduced. Another problem of a more practical nature is how to find comparable data, when statistics are often compiled for different purposes, using varying definitions. However, what could be looked upon as a problem in cross-national comparative research could on the other hand be viewed as an interesting model for service provision; a continuum of care. Users, carers and service providers in many countries are in favour of a seamless system of service provision; options which stand for security and continuity in elder care.

However, there are many elderly people living at home, suffering from dementia, whose mental condition is poor and who are not well supported in the community. There are several explanations for this; either they lack closely involved relatives, their condition and circumstances are not regularly monitored or they reject formal services. Other reasons could be that those services are ill-coordinated, unavailable or only occasionally available. These people either remain at home, often in very adverse conditions, or they are admitted to institutions when they might be sustained at home. In either case enhanced care would be beneficial to them.

Then, whilst some research pursues the cause or causes and, ultimately, the cure for the various types of dementia, other studies investigate ways of managing the course of the disease other than by hospitalisation. Dementia has been defined more and more as a 'social disease' with responsibility for the long-term support of patients viewed as more appropriately undertaken by local authorities within the context of community care. Whether the various models of care management being developed by social work/services departments are able to support older people with dementia at home effectively and adequately will depend largely on the willingness of family carers to continue their involvement. That continued willingness of carers may depend on the flexibility and sufficiency of support services and of skilled care managers aware of the physical and mental costs which such commitment to people with dementia can impose (Aneshensel et al, 1995).

Traditionally, the dependent elderly have mostly faced a choice between two extremes of care: home care by their families and institutional care, often provided by the public system. This bipolar system is breaking or has broken down. Under demographic and, mostly, financial pressures, but also in order to cater for the changing needs and demands of the elderly, there is a search— in some countries more advanced than in others—for alternative forms of care and new arrangements between these two extremes of care.

According to Hugman (1994), the range of services from domiciliary care to hospital care can be viewed as two interrelated continua structured around the elements of residence and care. On the residence dimension there is the distinction between the older person's own home (in which they may have lived for many years as a younger adult) at one extreme, and at the other extreme an institution where older people live communally and to which they move late in life solely because they need care. On the care dimension the opposite ends can be defined in terms of the extent to which the support takes the form of an occasional social visit, through direct assistance with specific daily living tasks, such as the provision of meals, to full, around the clock, nursing care.

At their most extreme these two dimensions 'overlap' so that residence and degree of care appear to be closely related. For example, older people who receive meals-on-wheels in their own homes once or twice a week, when compared to those who reside in long-stay hospital wards, are illustrative of opposite ends of both continua. Mid-range examples, however, may appear more complex in their variations. For instance, intensive domiciliary care in the older person's own home when compared with sheltered housing that does not include direct assistance: the former combines low levels of communality with a high level of care, while the latter can be typified as involving moderate communality combined with a low level of care. As Hugman concludes, the degree of communality in living arrangements is not necessarily directly related to the extent of care provided, although in practice there are a number of connections (Hugman, 1994). The increasing range of services could improve the opportunities to address and tailor services to individual needs, but it could also create increasing problems in identifying the target population (Dooghe and Vanden Boer, 1993).

The settings in which services could be offered, and ways of defining differences between types of care, have also been examined by Higgins (1989), who argues that there is no clear distinction between institution and community and that many care settings have elements of both. Institutional care can take place in the community, for example in hostels for people with mental illness who have moved from a large institution to a smaller one. Much community care takes place in institutions, for example day hospital or respite care, but most care takes place in the home, provided by the family. Higgins suggests that services may be divided into those available *in a home*, for example an institution such as a hospital, or a home in the community such as a hostel or nursing home; *from home*, for example day care or respite care; or *at home*, such as domiciliary care by agencies or family. In this model there is no need for the concept community, which Higgins finds unhelpful (Higgins, 1989).

The imprecisely defined 'community' element of community care, based mainly on rhetoric, is of little use in comparative analysis. However, Higgins' distinction between 'institution' and 'home' is also problematic. The place where people usually sleep at night is their home, whether or not it is considered to be an institution. If a distinction is to be made between institution and home, the concept 'institution' must also be clearly defined. To categorise settings in which help is provided, a twofold typology, based on Higgins' 'from home' and 'at home', will be more useful. The type of home, such as ordinary housing, group home, nursing home, may then be specified where relevant. The main distinction between settings in which care is provided will thus be whether the service is received in the home where the person usually lives, or whether they leave that home to receive it, for example in a day care setting.

SERVICE INNOVATIONS

When establishing a system of service provision as well as individual care packages, it is of crucial importance to adopt a policy with a multipurposed approach for several reasons (Aneshensel et al, 1995). First, the needs and resources of the impaired elderly and their caregivers are diverse; even those at the same stage of their illnesses and their caregiving careers differ considerably in their requirements for assistance and support systems. Thus, a wide range of service alternatives are necessary. Second, concerns change over time, and new challenges arise and remain in one's multiple domains of functioning. The mix of services, therefore, must be able to evolve over time in response to changes in the patient's condition and the family's ability to provide appropriate care. Third, policy initiatives also ought to consider the interconnection of the multiple parties affected by dementia. It is not sufficient to address patient needs in isolation from the primary caregiver, or those of the primary caregiver in isolation from the patient or the rest of the family. Given the heterogeneity of needs, resources, and structural composition of families, a variety of services should be flexibly and selectively available. These services should provide treatment and stimulating activities for patients, respite and relief from caregiving for the care provider, and support and counselling to families as they build their resources for the long haul. Although not ignoring medical aspects of dementia and economic implications, policy must primarily address the social and behavioural consequences of dementia.

In recent decades, a number of interesting service innovations have emerged in the field of dementia care in different countries. These innovations and programmes have often started as local initiatives, as a response to needs not being met by formal services. Others could be characterised as an extension of present services or as an alternative mode of providing service and care to the demented elderly and the carer. In some countries these innovations have been incorporated in the regular services, a process that sometimes has been supported by national/federal funding. The local foci of the programmes often stand for a strong voluntary and community involvement and a mixture of private and public efforts. Many of these programmes have not been evaluated, but there is a growing body of knowledge building up. The range of innovations span from home-based services to rethinking institutional dementia care.

HOME-BASED CARE

CARERS' INFORMATION, COUNSELLING AND TRAINING

Replicated evidence from well-designed cohort- or case-controlled studies and multiple time-series designs has shown that providing information, education and/or counselling helps to alleviate care stress when specifically aimed at reducing uncertainty and developing effective coping mechanisms (Morris et al, 1989; Toseland et al, 1989; Braithwaite, 1990).

Both educational (Chiverton and Caine, 1989) and group interventions (Whitlatch et al, 1991) are effective in improving carers' knowledge, decreasing family burden, improving coping skills and promoting emotional well-being. Toseland and Smith (1990), in a comparative study, found that, if provided under specialist supervision, counselling by other carers was as effective as that provided by professionals. Supervision should be given by a practitioner with knowledge and skills in the patient group.

Appropriately designed leaflets and written guides have good evidence of success with informal carers, both in use and practicality (Toner, 1987).

Brodaty and Gresham (1989) report a comparative study of carers and patients who had 10 days' residential training together in a special hospital unit. There was a substantial reduction of psychological stress and of hospital admissions, and an increase in the time patients remained in the community compared to an equivalent respite care stay.

Sutcliffe and Larner (1988), in a small but carefully controlled study, taught carers to use anxiety management and anger control methods. This intervention led to a greater reduction in strain than the provision of information regarding dementia. Gendron et al (1986) provided training sessions in relaxation and assertiveness and report increased problem-solving skills and stress reduction in trained carers compared to controls at six months follow-up. In an intervention study, Mittelman et al (1993) randomly assigned spouse-caregivers of AD patients to either a treatment group (individual counselling and support group participation) or a control group (routine support). The results show that the treatment group had less than half as many nursing home placements as the control group.

SERVICES AND PRACTICAL SUPPORT AT HOME

The evidence for health gain in carers and sufferers through the provision of services which substitute for aspects of their care and which help the sufferer with everyday tasks at home is clear (Gilleard, 1984; Levin et al, 1989). There is little published work on the effectiveness of each service in isolation, mainly because of the overwhelming evidence that users and carers prefer and benefit most when these services are provided as part of an overall package of care (Zarit et al, 1998).

Levin et al (1989) examined the impact of services on the psychological health, as measured by the General Health Questionnaire, of the informal carers of elderly people with dementia living in the community. Home helps, community nursing and day services reduced the adverse effects for relatives continuing to care at home and these services were particularly effective in combination.

Outcomes for carers were improved by early identification, achieved by actively working with GPs, and by providing comprehensive medical and social assessments, continuing back-up and review, collaborative working with other agencies and active medical and nursing treatments.

In Sweden, a new programme in dementia care has been developed in recent years—the 'Dementia Nurse'. The dementia nurse functions as a care manager for the demented patient and the carers. The task is to provide outreach activities, make home visits to inform families about service and care oppor-tunities and to offer counselling. The dementia nurse is the hub for communi-cation between different service providers and she often is the 'glue' between different professionals and levels of care. In 1997, about 20% of the Swedish municipalities have established this kind of nursing function and it appears that interest is growing among others to do the same. So far, this programme has not been evaluated, but the practical experiences are overwhelmingly positive.

DAY SERVICES

The evidence, including well-designed controlled trials, shows that day services decrease carer stress (Montgomery, 1995; Zarit et al, 1998). There is little evidence as to what form day care should take, although there are patients with dementia who, because of their behaviour problems or medical needs, are not suited to day services without specialist health staff. Also, the form of day care offered ranges from programmes of age-appropriate activities to custodial care.

Care attendant and sitting schemes are interesting alternatives to day care but fuller evaluations are needed and the extent to which they might substitute for day hospitals has not been examined. Voluntary schemes run by the Alzheimer's Disease Society and other voluntary organisations exist in many countries, although provision is patchy and inconsistent in a national perspective. Studies are rare but there is no indication from any of the literature in this field that voluntary sector services can substitute totally for local and flexible day hospital support in meeting needs for specialist treatment and care during the day.

Small dementia-specific day centres in domestic settings with empathic, trained staff and using a normalising approach appear best placed to provide good quality day care for many people with dementia (Wimo et al, 1990). Wimo et al (1993) found in a prospective control study that day care could postpone institutionalisation, probably by offering the caregivers relief. Wells et al (1990) did not find that day care reduced caregivers' stress, but its major benefit was that caregivers were given more time on their own. Day care does not require a specific centre but can be provided in private homes and could therefore be developed on a wide scale in rural as well as urban areas. Generic day centres can also cater for people with dementia, either on separate days, or by addressing their particular needs on days of mixed attendance through the organisation of separate groups or the provision of high levels of suitably trained staff. As the needs of people with dementia and their informal caregivers are so varied it is important to have a range of services to choose from, although services ought to be defined by the characteristics of the locality and will inevitably be limited by financial constraints.

RESPITE CARE

Reviewing current literature on short breaks or respite care for people with dementia, terminology is not the only difficulty to emerge. There are also paradoxes with regard to the role of respite in community care. It was set up originally to help carers continue to care. While the literature tends to be inconclusive regarding this particular outcome, most studies point to respite as being a pertinent and positive factor in the care process, yet it is a diminishing resource. The closure of long-stay wards where traditionally many people with dementia received respite care, the varying cost of many local authority respite beds, and the lack and cost of provision in the private sector are all having an impact. Both underprovision and lack of service uptake are reported.

The evidence, including well-designed controlled trials, without randomisation, shows respite care to relieve carer stress (Harper et al, 1988; Lawton et al,

1989; Montgomery, 1995; Zarit et al, 1998). Levin et al (1989) found respite care facilitated permanent admissions into residential care on a planned basis, and reduced crisis admissions. As crisis admissions are highly associated with care breakdown, this probably indicates health gain for carers.

In combination with other community services, however, well-organised respite care is effective in helping carers to manage sufferers at home for longer. However, the degree of confusion and dependency of some patients is increased by respite care. Apart from the effects on sufferers, this also affects the morale of carers. Careful individual assessment of the patient's suitability and a high degree of flexibility in respite provision should overcome such difficulties (Levin and Moriarty, 1990).

INTERMEDIATE CARE

During the 1980s, new housing and care alternatives for demented patients were developed in many countries. For example, in Sweden *Group living care* became an important model (Johansson, 1990; Wimo et al, 1991; Annerstedt, 1993; Malmberg and Zarit, 1993) in the mid 1980s. During recent years, group livings have become an alternative to institutions for people with great need of care and supervision. They include co-operative housing arrangements for, among others, those with physical handicaps or psychiatric problems. Most common, however, is group living for cognitively impaired persons. 'Group living' has no standard definition, but it usually means a small housing collective for 6–8 persons, in which each resident has his own room, shares communal areas and has access to service and care provided by resident staff around the clock.

A primary impetus for its creation was the belief that the medical emphasis in nursing homes does not provide sufficient social and physical stimulation for dementia patients. Group homes consist of individual apartments for each resident, which are linked to common areas and secured to the outside. The staff-to-patient ratio is quite high by international standards (1:1 during the daytime), and staff undergo extensive formal training. Programmes emphasise engaging in everyday activities, such as assisting with cooking, cleaning, and laundry. A distinctive feature is that residents have considerable autonomy. Patients lease and furnish their apartments, and can go inside or outside when they like, locking the door behind them. This autonomy is integrated with security features that enable group homes to serve moderately to moderately severe dementia patients.

The overall Swedish group living concept consists of small, home-like units in flats or houses, staffed around the clock. Here, small groups of 6–9 demented patients will live together like an extended family, each renting their private area and part of the common living area (living room, kitchen and laundry). They are usually activated and socially trained in the daily, common housekeeping activities, which are performed together with the staff. A patient will be moved to group living care when home care is assessed to be inadequate. It is assumed that the residents have medical diagnoses of dementia. The inclusion criteria, however, may vary between municipalities as does the praxis of how severely demented a patient may be permitted to become and still be cared for in group living. Often group living provides care for patients in the last stages of dementia. In consequence, the patients' status will then be similar to those in the nursing homes. The level of competence among staff may vary between different municipalities.

According to Annerstedt's evaluation (1995), group living can act therapeutically in reducing secondary symptoms and preserving independence, during a limited period of dementia. Subsequently, group living can fill an important gap in dementia care, intermediate between home care and traditional institutional care.

In Canada the approach in changing the philosophy of care of the demented is, as in Sweden, a decision made by government authorities, based on empirical studies, extrapolations from related research and from basic principles, goals, concepts and values and the knowledge of accumulated practice. Prescriptions and recommendations for good quality highlight the progressive nature of the illness, the variations of symptoms, functional capacities and characteristics within the group, the trade-offs implicit in virtually every design decision and the need for creativity and flexibility in adapting the environment to changing needs (Lips, 1992).

There are usually five features generally cited in literature as the criteria for designating a unit as specialised for care of persons with dementia:

- The unit is physically separated from the facility (nursing home, hospital) of which it is a part
- It has a client population consisting mainly of persons with dementia
- It has special design features
- It has staff with specialised training
- It has special activity and/or therapeutic programmes

In Britain the 'Domus philosophy' for residential care of demented elderly has been developed as part of the psychogeriatric services. It is an attempt to improve the quality of care by specifically addressing the staff anxieties and attitudes that lead to institutional maintenance and poor quality of life for residents.

The programme is based on four assumptions:

- The domus is the resident's home for life
- The needs of the staff are as important as those of the residents
- The domus should aim to correct the avoidable consequences of dementia and accommodate those that are unavoidable

- The residents' individual psychological needs may take precedence over the physical aspects of their care

Further prospective studies are, however, needed to establish this model of residential care (Lindesay et al, 1991).

In France an innovative form of communal non-medical care, so-called 'cantous', appeared as long ago as 1968 and these are now widespread. In cantous the physical environment is adapted especially to the demented individual's needs. Promoters of the cantou concept initially defined nine criteria:

- Community living in a separate enclosed area
- Permanent residents
- 12–15 rooms organised around a common living area
- Residents suffer from senile dementia
- Non-medical institutions
- Activities principally centred around tasks of daily living
- Stable, multipurpose staff
- Administrative autonomy
- Participation of families in institutional life

The question of which type of structure of care is most beneficial for which type of pathology and at which stage of its evolution has been raised (Ritchie et al, 1992).

INSTITUTIONAL CARE

THE DEVELOPMENT OF SPECIALISED UNITS

The management of cognitively impaired nursing home residents can be challenging. Studies conducted in nursing homes have described problems in the care of residents with dementia, including: untrained staff, negative staff attitudes, little to no treatment offered, frequent use of physical restraints and psychoactive medications, and so on.

Nursing homes provide care for different types and mixes of patients. More rarely, there are special units in nursing homes designed only for demented patients. Care is seldom differentiated according to the patient's level of dementia. The physical setting in a nursing home may vary from small, intimate caring units to big wards for 50–60 patients. The organisation of care may also vary. From the 1980s the trend was to make wards, designed for permanent nursing home care, into more home-like settings, 'local nursing homes', separating them physically from the big hospitals. The privacy in the patient's housing is stressed. The concept of nursing home care in Sweden today is not unambiguous. There are medically well-equipped units, providing staff with high competence available around the clock. There are also units, designed for housing and basic care, with medical attendance available on request, from which patients have to be remitted to emergency wards in case of more severe intercurrent diseases. In some places there are special wards for severely vocally disruptive and/or socially disturbing patients. More often, however, these patients are mingled with the other demented or non-demented patients on the wards.

One popular response in the US to these problems—also illustrated by experiences from Sweden—has been the development of special units, termed special care units, for Alzheimer's residents in nursing homes. These units, which are referred to as dementia units, represent separate living quarters in the form of a hallway or other closed-off portion of the nursing home. They often differ from the rest of the home in terms of physical design and the provision of activities and programming tailored to the needs of residents with dementing illnesses. The dementia unit movement has received public and government support and in 1996 some 15% of nursing homes had SCU or specialised programmes for people with dementia.

However, opinions of health professionals about this are divided. Rabins (1986) identified the following advantages of dementia units: specially designed environments, trained and recruited staff, concentrated resources, ability to develop formal behavioural management policies and practices for all residents, alleviation of families' anxiety, and separation of cognitively impaired persons from those who are more intact. Their disadvantages include higher financial costs, difficulty in determining admission criteria, resistance to placement by residents or families, difficulty in recruitment of staff, negative effect of labelling the unit, higher staff turnover rates, and lowered staff expectations. Rabins states that research is needed to determine the effectiveness of these units. He cautions that more experience and knowledge are needed before nursing homes launch a widespread effort to establish dementia units.

Thus, the limited number of studies to date leave several questions unanswered. Nevertheless, family members and health care providers must still decide on the course of treatment for Alzheimer's disease victims. Often the choices are few and can offer only palliative relief. Dementia units of nursing homes may now provide new hope. The number and diversity of these programmes offer settings in which many questions can begin to be answered.

More data are needed on the outcomes of specialised dementia care to justify costs in time and effort presently going into the units, to justify more widely available government assistance, to determine which therapies are effective, to determine which populations can be helped, to help establish standards of care for the industry, and to guide families in their struggle to find appropriate care for the afflicted. Sloane and Mathew (1991) conclude their review of special care units with 'support this concept because of its potential both for providing a continuum of care and for exploring new treatments' (p. 256).

CONCLUSIONS

In the end, in confronting the dementing illnesses one could conclude that, so far, current procedures are more the result of unplanned responses to a series of changes and developments in medicine and society, rather than a thoughtful strategy for addressing the consequences of degenerative diseases in later life. Because modern medicine can keep people alive longer, even in the face of chronic degenerative conditions like dementia, should we passively allow this to happen? If so, should we not provide adequate support to the families and to the institutions caring for these patients? We need to remember that providing medical care in these circumstances represents a choice over withholding it. We need to consider if it is a choice we want to make and accept the consequences of that decision.

In the face of the protracted and terrible demeaning diseases, the real heroes are the family caregivers, whose exhaustive efforts go a long way to preserving dignity and honour. In a situation in which there is no good solution, where the disease is relentlessly debilitating and ultimately terminal, caregivers struggle to give meaning to their efforts and to the lives of their loved ones. They deserve an increased involvement from national and local governments that leads to a compassionate system of support—a partnership—for caregivers and patients.

REFERENCES

Aneshensel, C. A., Pearlin, L. I., Mullan, J. T., Zarit, S. H., and Whitlatch, C. J. (1995). *Profiles In Caregiving. The Unexpected Career*, San Diego, CA, Academic Press.

Annerstedt, L. (1993). Development and consequences of group living in Sweden. A new mode of care for the demented elderly, *Social Science and Medicine*, **37**(12), 1529–1538.

Annerstedt, L. (1995). On group-living care for the demented elderly. Experiences from the Malmö model, Lund: Lund University (Dissertation).

Braithwaite, V. A. (1990). *Bound to Care*, Sydney, Allen & Unwin.

Brodaty, H., and Gresham, M. (1989). Effects of a training programme to reduce stress in carers of patients with dementia, *British Medical Journal*, **299**, 1375–1379.

Chiverton, P., and Caine, E. D. (1989). Education to assist spouses in coping with Alzheimer's disease: a controlled trial, *Journal of American Geriatric Society*, **37**, 593–598.

Daatland, S. O. (1996). Adapting the Scandinavian model care for the elderly. In *Caring for frail elderly people. Policies in evolution*. Paris, OECD, Social Policy Studies, no. 19.

Dooghe, G., and Vanden Boer, L. (1993). *Sheltered Accommodation for Elderly People in an International Perspective*, Amsterdam, Swets & Zeitlinger.

Gendron, C. E., Poitras, L. R., and Engels, M. L. (1986). Skills training with supporters of the demented, *Journal of American Geriatric Society*, **34**, 875–880.

Gilleard, C. J. (1984). *Living with Dementia: Community Care of the Elderly Mentally Infirm*, London, Croom Helm.

Harper, N., McDowell, D. I. C., Turner, J. J., and Sharma, A. I. C. (1988). Planned admission to a geriatric unit: one aspect of respite care, *Age and Ageing*, **17**, 199–204.

Higgins, J. (1989). Defining community care: realities and myths, *Social Policy and Administration*, **23**(1), 3–15.

Hugman, R. (1994). *Aging and the Care of Older People in Europe*, New York, St Martin's Press.

Johansson, L. (1990). Group dwellings for dementia patients. A new care alternative. *Ageing International*, **16**(1), 35–37.

Lawton, M. P., Brody, E. M., and Saperstein, A. R. (1989). A controlled study of respite services for caregivers of Alzheimer's patients. *Gerontologist*, **29**, 8–16.

Levin, E., and Moriarty, J. (1990). Ready to cope again: breaks for the carers of confused elderly people, National Institute of Social Work Report to the Dept of Health.

Levin, E., Sinclair, I., and Gorbach, P. (1989). *Families, Services and Confusion in Old Age*, Aldershot, Avebury.

Lindesay, J., Briggs, K., Lawes, M., Macdonald, A., and Herzberg, J. (1991). The Domus philosophy, a comparative evaluation of a new approach to residential care for the demented elderly, *Journal of Geriatric Psychiatry*, **6**, 727–736.

Lips, T. J. (1992). Designing facilities for people with dementia, a new resource for planners and caregivers, in G. Gutman (Ed.), *Shelter and Care for Persons with Dementia*, Vancouver, Simon Fraser University.

Malmberg, B., and Zarit, S. H. (1993). Group homes for people with dementia, *Gerontologist*, **31**, 682–686.

Mittelman, M. S., Ferris, S. H., Steinberg, G., Schulman, E., Mackell, J. A., Ambinder, A., and Cohen, J. (1993). An intervention that delays institutionalization of Alzheimer's disease patients: treatment of spouse-caregivers, *Gerontologist*, **33**(6), 730–740.

Montgomery, R. I. V. (1995). Examining respite care, promises and limitations, in R. A. Kane and I. D. Penrod (Eds), *Family Caregiving in an Aging Society*, Thousand Oaks, CA, Sage.

Morris, L. W., Morris, R. G., and Britton, P. G. (1989). Cognitive style and perceived control in spouse caregivers of dementia sufferers, *British Journal of Medical Psychology*, **62**, 1973–1979.

OECD (1994). *New orientations for social policy*, Paris, OECD, Social Policy Studies, no 12.

Rabins, P. V. (1986). Establishing Alzheimer's disease units in nursing homes, pros and cons, *Hospital and Community Psychiatry*, **37**, 120–121.

Ritchie, I., Colvez, A., Ankri, I., Ledesert, B., Gardent, H., and Fontaine, A. (1992). The evolution of long-term care for demented elderly: a comparative study of hospital and collective non-medical care in France, *International Journal of Geriatric Psychiatry*, **7**, 549–577.

Sloane, P. D., and Mathew, L. J. (1991). The future role of specialized dementia care, in P. D. Sloane and L. J. Mathew (Eds), *Dementia Units in Long-Term Care*, Baltimore, Johns Hopkins University Press.

Sutcliffe, C., and Larner, S. (1988). Counselling carers of the elderly at home, a preliminary study, *British Journal of Clinical Psychology*, **27**, 177–178.

Toner, H. L. (1987). Effectiveness of a written guide for carers of dementia sufferers, *British Journal of Clinical and Social Psychology*, **5**(1), 24–26.

Toseland, R. W., Rossiter, C. M., and Labreque, M. S. (1989). The effectiveness of peer-led and professionally led groups to support family caregivers, *Gerontologist*, **29**, 465–471.

Toseland, R. W., and Smith, G. C. (1990). Effectiveness of individual counselling by professional and peer helpers for family caregivers of the elderly, *Psychology and Aging*, **5**, 256–263.

Wells, Y. D., Jorm, A. F., Jordan, F., and Lefroy, R. (1990). Effects on care-givers of special day care programmes for dementia sufferers, *Australian and New Zealand Journal of Psychiatry*, **24**, 82–90.

Whitlach, C. I., Zarit, S. H., Goodwin, P. E., and von Eye, A. (1995). Influence of psychoeducational interventions on the course of family care, *Clinical Gerontologist*, **16**, 117–130.

Wimo, A., Mattsson, B., Adolfsson, R., Eriksson, T., and Nelvig, A. (1993). Dementia day care and its effect on symptoms and institutionalisation—a controlled Swedish study, *Scandinavian Journal of Primary Health Care*, **11**, 117–123.

Wimo, A., Wallin, J. O., Lundgren, K., Rönnbeck, E., Asplund, K., Mattson, B., and Krakau, I. (1990). Impact of day care on dementia patients—costs, well-being and relatives' view, *Family Practice*, **7**, 279–287.

Wimo, A., Wallin, J. O., Lundgren, K., Rönnbeck, E., Asplund, K., Mattson, B., and Krakau, I. (1991). Group living, an alternative for dementia patients. A cost analysis, *International Journal of Geriatric Psychiatry*, **6**, 21–30.

Zarit, S. H., Johansson, L., and Jarrott, S. E. (1998). Family caregiving: stresses, social programs and clinical interventions, in I. H. Nordhus, S. Berg, G. Vanden Bos and P. Fromholt (Eds), *Clinical Gerontology* (to be published).

1.5 Different Ways of Organizing and Financing Health Care

STEFAN HÅKANSSON

University of Stockholm and Swedish Institute for Health Service Development (Spri), Stockholm

For many years there has been a gap between the increasing demand for health care caused by the introduction of new technologies, the ageing population, and rising patient expectations on the one hand, and what countries consider they can afford on the other. In Europe especially, the member states of the European Union (EU) are cutting back public spending in order to reduce their budget deficits to the target set by the Maastricht Treaty for joining the proposed European Monetary Union (EMU). Coupled with an economic recession this financial pruning has led to increased unemployment, while social welfare costs have strained local government budgets. Arguments have been put forward that, for western European countries to remain competitive in a globalizing world economy, their public sector spending levels must be reduced in order to free capital for private investment.

In western Europe the aggregate health care expenditure during the *1960s and 1970s* rose at a relatively rapid pace, both in absolute terms and compared to percentage growth of GDP generally. In the *1980s* the health care spending in most countries was broadly stable because of macro-level expenditure controls in response to the economic consequences of the oil crises of 1973 and 1978, and the consequent 'stagflation' of the early 1980s. In 1991 a severe recession began across Europe and a small but significant upturn in aggregate expenditures. The cost of pharmaceuticals was one factor contributing to this increase, and this has in turn become the subject of considerable cost-containment initiatives of late (Saltman and Figueras, 1997).

During the period 1971–1992 the total employment in the United States increased by almost 50%, in Japan by 25%, but in the European Union only by 13%. Both in the USA and Japan the vast majority of new jobs were in the private sector, whereas in Europe only 50% were in the private sector.

In some countries, the overall percentage increase was as much statistical as real, partly reflecting a fall in overall GDP and thus in the denominator of the ratio that expresses the percentage of GDP given over to health. Finland

Health Economics of Dementia. Edited by Anders Wimo, Bengt Jönsson, Göran Karlsson and Bengt Winblad.

provides an extreme example of this pattern: aggregate health spending grew from 7.4% in 1989 to 9.3% in 1992, largely as a result of a 16% reduction in total GDP over those three years due to the collapse of the former Soviet Union which was a big market for Finland's exports (Saltman and Figueras, 1997).

THE CORRELATION BETWEEN HEALTH CARE SPENDING AND GROSS DOMESTIC PRODUCT (GDP)

In Table 1.5.1 the OECD countries have been ranked according to health care expenditure per capita, expressed in purchasing power parities (PPP). The table also shows the GDP per capita and the health care expenditure as percentage of GDP. The percentage devoted to health care varied from 4.0% of GDP in Poland to 14.2% in the United States. In 1995 the United States spent $3644 per capita, which is two and a half times the OECD average, which was $1414 (8.1% of GDP). However, rather dramatic changes in the position in health care spending from 1970 to 1995 are shown in Appendix 1.5.1. Sweden's position is especially worth noting: from second place in 1970 and 1980 to seventeenth place in 1995, which is a reflection of the country's decline in economic growth.

In order to get a concrete example of what 'potential' for cost saving there is when using international comparison, we shall take the US as a case. If the United States spent the same amount per capita as Canada (US$2069), it would have spent $400 billion less, which is a reduction of 40% of its health care spending of $988.5 billion in 1995.

A study by the OECD of health care spending during 1980–1992 showed the United States had the greatest difference between growth in nominal per capita health spending (9.3%) and growth in nominal per capita GDP (5.8%), which means that for a 1% increase in GDP there is a 1.5% increase in health care spending. When taking account of the general inflation (GDP deflator) and medical price inflation the real volume and intensity growth in health spending was 2.4% annually, whereas the consumption and investment opportunities forgone in other sectors because of growth in health spending was 4.6% annually. Excess health care inflation appears to be a far more serious problem in the pluralistic US health system than it is in the more uniform systems of other countries (Schieber et al, 1994).

Despite the fact that the validity of the OECD data is continually being discussed and improved (Waldo and Sonefeld, 1991; Rublee and Schneider, 1991) this database is easily accessible and is the most widely used in international comparisons. The real problem is that there are no standardized, internationally accepted definitions of health care components (Schieber and Poullier, 1991).

Table 1.5.1. GDP, total expenditure on health per capita (PPP in US$) and total expenditure on health *as percentage of GDP 1995* (percentage of OECD average in parentheses)

	GDP per capita	Total expenditure on health per capita	Total health expenditure as percentage of GDP
United States	25 635 (146)	3 644 (258)	14.2 (176)
Switzerland	24 523 (140)	2 378 (168)	9.7 (120)
Luxembourg	31 537 (180)	2 206 (156)	7.0 (87)
Germany	20 470 (117)	2 134 (151)	10.4 (129)
Canada	21 252 (121)	2 069 (146)	9.7 (120)
France	19 919 (113)	1 972 (140)	9.9 (123)
Norway	22 810 (130)	1 821 (129)	8.0 (99)
Iceland	21 761 (124)	1 774 (125)	8.2 (102)
Australia	20 152 (115)	1 741 (123)	8.6 (107)
Netherlands	19 751 (113)	1 731 (122)	8.8 (109)
Belgium	20 814 (119)	1 665 (118)	8.0 (99)
Austria	20 782 (118)	1 634 (116)	7.9 (98)
Japan	21 912 (125)	1 581 (112)	7.2 (89)
Italy	19 487 (111)	1 507 (107)	7.7 (96)
Finland	17 781 (101)	1 373 (97)	7.7 (96)
Denmark	21 537 (123)	1 368 (97)	6.4 (79)
Sweden	18 671 (106)	1 353 (96)	7.2 (89)
United Kingdom	17 923 (102)	1 246 (88)	6.9 (86)
New Zealand	16 932 (96)	1 203 (85)	7.1 (88)
Ireland	17 413 (99)	1 106 (78)	6.4 (79)
Spain	14 076 (80)	1 075 (76)	7.6 (94)
Portugal	12 586 (72)	1 035 (73)	8.2 (102)
Czech Republic	9 459 (54)	749 (53)	7.9 (98)
Greece	12 174 (69)	703 (50)	5.8 (72)
Hungary	7 948 (45)	562 (40)	7.1 (88)
Korea	12 571 (72)	487 (34)	3.9 (48)
Mexico	7 876 (45)	386 (27)	4.9 (61)
Turkey	5 766 (33)	272[a] (19)	4.7 (59)
Poland	5 495 (31)	219[a] (15)	4.0 (49)
EU average	18 995 (108)	1 474 (104)	7.8 (96)
Non EU average	16 007 (91)	1 349 (95)	8.4 (105)
OECD average	17 552 (100)	1 414 (100)	8.1 (100)

[a] 1994 figures.

Source: OECD Health Data 97. Update 29 July 1997.

It has been known for decades that there is a strong correlation between health care expenditure and GDP: the richer a country is, the more is spent on health care (Newhouse, 1977; Leu, 1986; Parkin et al, 1992; Gerdtham, 1992).

As can be seen from Figure 1.5.1 the correlation is rather high. In the OECD countries 76% of the difference in health care expenditure can be explained by GDP. There are two 'outliers' in the figure. One is the US which

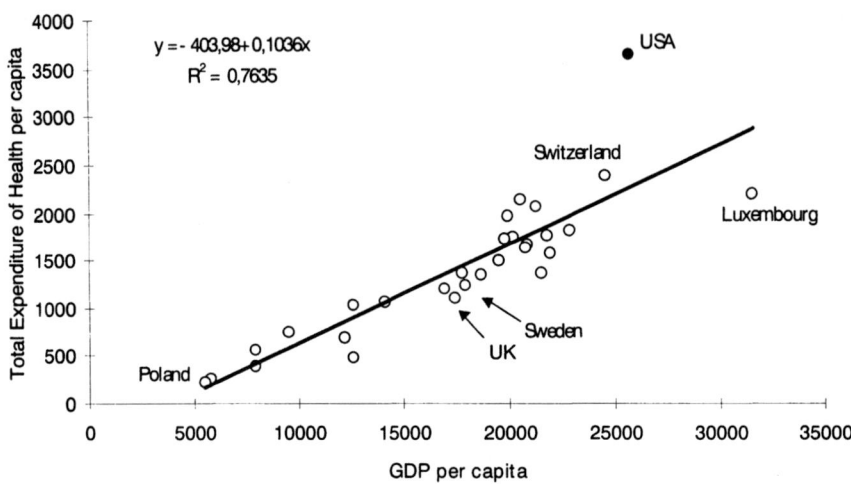

Figure 1.5.1. The relation in 1995 between GDP and total expenditure on health for OECD countries (PPP in US$). *Source*: OECD Health Data 97, 1994 Health Expenditures for Poland and Turkey

spent far more than could be expected from its GDP. Another is Luxembourg, which spent less than could be expected from its high GDP. If these countries were excluded the explanatory power would increase to about 90%.

When analyzing the causes for the increased health spending, both the age structure and public spending have been found to be factors that can explain variations in cost between the OECD countries. Earlier studies of the relation between health spending and GDP 'showed' a positive income elasticity of about 1.3, meaning that when GDP increased by 1%, health spending increased by 1.3%. This means that health care is a 'luxury' good by an economic definition. However, in later studies (Blomqvist and Carter, 1997; O'Connell, 1996) these results have been questioned. The result of the O'Connell study suggests that country-specific factors play an important role in determining per capita health spending when controlling for national income and the public sector financing of health services. The income coefficient, which may be interpreted as an income elasticity, is estimated to be less than one. The age structure of the population significantly affects health spending in some countries, with the magnitude of the effect varying among countries. For other countries, age structure does not appear to influence health spending. Seven countries have positive and significant country-specific age coefficients. For 8 of the 21 countries included in the analysis the age coefficients are negative and for 6 countries the age coefficients are not significant (O'Connell, 1996).

Regarding the percentage of public spending it seems that there has been a movement towards convergence between tax-based and insurance-based systems (see Appendix 1.5.2).

In a study of productivity growth in health care in the OECD countries Färe et al (1997) found that little productivity growth had occurred over the period 1974 to 1989. The two countries which have had the highest cumulative growth were Denmark (+15%) and the United States (+5%). In both countries the growth was due solely to technical change over this period.

TRENDS IN HEALTH CARE SPENDING BETWEEN DIFFERENT HEALTH CARE SYSTEMS

There are four key sources of funds for health care: taxation, contribution to social insurance schemes, voluntary subscriptions to private insurance schemes and out-of-pocket payments. These four sources can be classified as compulsory or statutory systems (social health insurance and taxation) or as voluntary systems (voluntary insurance and out-of-pocket payments).

Many health care systems in European countries rely on a mix of all four sources. There is no 'pure' system: tax-based financing systems typically also include elements of social insurance, and insurance-based systems often include strong elements of tax-based financing. Moreover, whether tax-based or insurance-based, virtually all health care systems in the region either include, or have plans to include, some elements of the two types of voluntary financing (Saltman and Figueras, 1997).

In Table 1.5.2 the development of total expenditure on health as a percentage of GDP during the period 1970–1995 is shown. The percentage has increased in all systems and there is also a tendency among 'well-established' systems for the figure for tax-based systems in 1995 (7.4%) to be lower than that for insurance-based systems (8.7%).

WHAT DO WE GET FROM THE HEALTH CARE SYSTEM?

It is a very cumbersome undertaking to measure the outcomes of different health care systems. Two indicators very often used are life expectancy and infant mortality. In 1995 the life expectancy at birth for females was highest in Japan (82.8 years) and lowest in Turkey (70.3 years) among the OECD countries. For men the highest figure was in Iceland (76.5 years) and the lowest in Hungary (65.3 years). When it comes to infant mortality the figures vary from about 4% in Finland, Norway, Sweden and Japan to 11.0% in Greece, 13.5% in Poland, 16.5% in Mexico and 44.4% in Turkey (see Appendix 1.5.3).

Another common indicator used in international comparisons is the percentage of low-weight deliveries at hospitals. As can be seen from Appendix 1.5.3 the variations in the OECD countries are from 3.2% in Iceland to 8.6%

Table 1.5.2. Total expenditure on health as percentage of GDP 1970, 1980, 1990 and 1995

	1970	1980	1990	1995
Well-established tax-based system	*5.6*	*7.1*	*7.5*	*7.5*
Australia	5.7	7.3	8.2	8.6
Denmark	6.1	6.8	6.5	6.4
Finland	5.7	6.5	8.0	7.7
Iceland	5	6.2	8.0	8.2
Ireland	5.3	8.8	6.6	6.4
Norway	4.6	7	7.8	8.0
Sweden	7.1	9.4	8.8	7.2
UK	4.5	5.6	6.0	6.9
Well-established insurance-based system	*5.2*	*7.5*	*7.8*	*8.5*
Austria	5.4	7.9	7.1	7.9
Belgium	4.1	6.6	7.6	8.0
France	5.8	7.6	8.9	9.9
Germany	6.4	9.0	8.9	10.4
Luxembourg	3.7	6.2	6.6	7.0
Netherlands	5.9	7.9	8.3	8.8
In transition to tax-based system	*4.0*	*5.7*	*6.7*	*7.4*
Greece	3.3	3.6	4.2	5.8
Italy	5.2	7	8.1	7.7
Portugal	2.8	5.8	6.5	8.2
Spain	3.7	5.7	6.9	7.6
In transition to insurance-based system	*2.4*	*3.3*	*2.5*	*4.7*
Turkey	2.4	3.3	2.5	4.7[a]
USA	7.2	9.1	12.7	14.2
OECD average	5.3	7.0	7.6	8.1

[a] 1994 figures.
Source: OECD Health Data 97. Update 29 July 1997.

in Hungary. It is a matter of debate how much the above variations are due to the health care systems and how much has to do with other factors, for example the economic standard and its distribution among citizens.

SATISFACTION FROM HEALTH SYSTEMS

In the late 1980s some public opinion surveys were conducted, especially in the United States, regarding citizens' satisfaction with their health care system (Blendon et al, 1990, 1995).

THE UNITED STATES, CANADA AND WESTERN GERMANY

Blendon et al (1995) have made some interesting comparisons between citizens in the United States, Canada and Western Germany between the years 1988,

Table 1.5.3. Ratings of health care systems in the United States, Canada, and Western Germany in 1988, 1990, and 1994 (%)

	United States		Canada		Western Germany	
	1988	1994	1988	1994	1988	1994
Only minor changes are necessary	10	18	56	29	41	30
Fundamental changes are needed	60	53	38	59	35	55
We need to completely rebuild it	29	28	5	12	13	11
Not sure	1	2	1	–	11	4

Source: Blendon, R. J., Benson, J., Donelan, K. et al (1995). Who has the best health system? A second look. *Health Affairs*, **14**(4), 220–230. Copyright © 1995 The People-to-People Health Foundation, Inc. All Rights Reserved. Reproduced with permission.

1990 and 1994. The survey was conducted during June–September 1994. The sample was about 1200 Americans, about 1500 Canadians and about 1210 Germans. From Table 1.5.3 it is evident that the Americans were more dissatisfied with their health care systems than people in the other countries. But the gap in satisfaction between the United States and the other two countries narrowed dramatically during that period. One of the reasons for the drop in satisfaction with the health care system in Canada and Germany could be that prior to 1994 these countries were experiencing strong cost-containment efforts.

In the study there was a remarkable difference between the countries regarding attitudes towards health care spending. In spite of the fact that the United States is the country which spends by far the most on health care (about 14% of GDP), 48% of the respondents thought that the country was spending too little on health care. Only 29% of Americans see the United States as an overspending nation. On the question: 'Can modern medicine cure any illness with access to advanced technology?' 33% of the Americans, 27% of the Canadians but only 11% of the Western Germans answered yes. But the most dramatic difference is the Americans' antipathy to government. According to the poll only 29% of the Americans had confidence in leaders of major health institutions. For the federal health care agencies the figure was as low as 7%. In Canada the figure was 45% and in Western Germany 53%.

EUROPEAN UNION

In early spring 1996 a Eurobarometer survey was conducted in the 15 European Union member states on citizens' views on health care systems and spending (Mossialos, 1977). Satisfaction was highest in Denmark (90.5%) and Finland (86.9%) and lowest in Italy (16.5%), Greece (18.5%) and Portugal (20.2%). The average for the European Union was 51.0%. It appears that satisfaction was highest in northern Europe and lowest in southern Europe. For more details, see Appendix 1.5.4. When a regression analysis is made

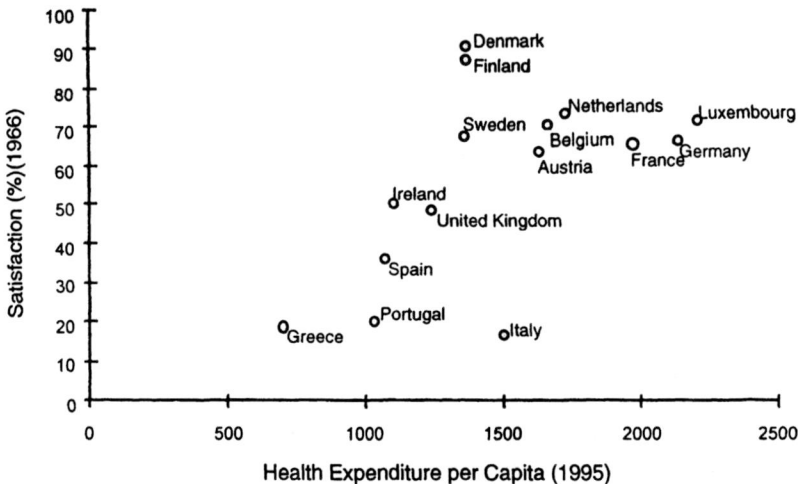

Figure 1.5.2. Satisfaction from health care systems in the 15 EU member states and per total expenditures on health per capita (PPP in US$). *Source*: Mossialos (1997), OECD Health Data 97

between health spending and satisfaction the result is a positive correlation which can be seen in Figure 1.5.2. The figure differs from Mossialos' in that GDP data from 1995 are used instead of 1993.

MANAGED CARE

The concept of managed care is hardly new. The Kaiser plans began in the American West in the 1930s (Ellwood and Lundberg, 1996). The term 'health maintenance organization' did not enter the lexicon until Paul Ellwood, a Minnesota physician and big thinker, coined it in his push to get the government to support prepaid health care. The result was the HMO Act of 1973, which in part extended government grants to start up HMOs (Green, 1997).

During the last few years there has been a dramatic focus in the health care debate both inside and outside the US concerning the concept of 'managed care'. A *managed care plan* is traditionally an insurance company working in partnership with hospitals, doctors, and other health care professionals to provide a comprehensive, planned, and coordinated program of health care (Health Care Financing Review/1996 Statistical Supplement). The growth of managed care in the US became rapid only after large corporations decided that they had to bring their steeply rising costs for health benefits under control. By the beginning of 1997, two thirds of all Americans working for medium-sized and large firms belonged to a managed-care plan, usually to one of several plans offered by their employers. The plans determine most of the kinds of treatment available—ambulatory services, consultations with specialist, and inpatient care (Ginzberg and Ostow, 1997).

Managed care was a response to pressure from private and public purchasers to slow the expenditure explosion. Between 1960 and 1990, spending on health care grew at almost 6% per annum (adjusted for inflation)—more than double the growth rate of the rest of the economy. Such a disparity, if left unchecked for another 30 years, would have resulted in health care consuming almost 30% of the nation's entire output of goods and services (Fuchs, 1997).

The Health Maintenance Organizations (HMOs), which are the best known example of managed care outside the US, are often discussed as if they were simple, homogeneous organizations, easily replicated, and well understood. In reality, each HMO is a highly complex organization of economic incentives, bureaucratic structures, and personalities. HMOs are specifically defined for the purposes of federal and state regulatory agencies, but a generic definition includes the contractual responsibility to assure the delivery of a range of medical services (not just to reimburse the patients for their costs) to an enrolled population, which is periodically offered a choice of plan. Furthermore, HMO revenue comes mainly from premiums rather than from fee-for-service payments, and the HMO assumes at least part of the financial risk and/or gain in the provision of services.

The definition purposely allows for considerable variation in the organization of HMOs. For example, physicians could practice together in a clinical setting, either as employees of the HMO or as a legally distinct medical group contracting with the HMO. The first is often termed a *staff model* and the second, a *group model* plan. Both varieties are sometimes lumped together under the label 'prepaid group practice'. Alternatively, the HMO could contract with physicians who also maintain substantial fee-for-service practices; this model is often called an individual practice association (IPA). In some cases, IPAs contract primarily with groups of fee-for-service physicians, and this is often termed a network model (Luft, 1991)

Reinhardt (1996) has presented a simple ordering of the economic arrangement between health insurance plans and those who provide health care to the insured (see Table 1.5.4). Cell G represents the traditional economic arrangement in American health care. It is commonly referred to now as the 'old fashioned indemnity plan'. Under this arrangement, the providers of health care are paid on a fee-for-service basis, at prices largely dictated by the providers. There is virtually no direct or even indirect control over the volume of services going into the treatment of particular medical conditions. This arrangement, whose total lack of control had always astounded foreign observers, is now fast disappearing in the United States, although it is still more prevalent than is widely supposed, especially in the Southern states. Cell G represents the 'unmanaged' segment of American health care.

At the other extreme, in cell C, are arrangements under which an integrated network of health care providers—now commonly called a Provider Service

Table 1.5.4. Contractual arrangement between health plans and providers

Direct control over volume of services	Payment of provision		
	Fee for service	Fee for service and capitation	Capitation
Tight	A	B	C
Some	D	E	F
None	G	H	I

Source: Uwe E. Reinhardt, A social contract for 21st century health care: three-tier health care with bounty hunting, *Health Economics* (1996), **5**, 479–499. © John Wiley & Sons Ltd. Reproduced with permission.

Network (PSN)—is prepaid a flat annual capitation and then assumes the full financial risk for the insureds' morbidity. The traditional American health maintenance organization (HMO), such as the Kaiser Foundation Health Plan in California or the Health Insurance Plan of Greater New York, fits this model. Cell C represents fully 'managed' health care.

In between cells G and C are a host of alternative arrangements that now claim the label 'managed care', but are about as descriptive of the actual arrangement being so labeled as the term 'animal' would be in the description of a Schnauzer.

If it were not for low hospital occupancy rates, semi-idle lithotripters, magnetic resonance imagers (MRIs), and other expensive equipment, and a plethora of physicians in many specialities, managed care would not have grown so rapidly. The dominant motivation has been containment of expenditures. Spending has been slowed in three ways: reducing services to patients, providing services more efficiently, and squeezing the incomes of physicians and other health care professionals (Fuchs, 1997).

One of the reasons that managed care has been so debated outside the US has probably to do with the fact that from 1993 health care spending has stabilized around 14% of GDP. Real per capita health expenditure, which takes into account general inflation and population growth, went up only 1.4% in 1995, compared with a 4.8% annual rate through the 1980s. For the first time in more than three decades, however, stability in health spending as a percentage of GDP in the 1993–1995 period was precipitated by a slowdown in the rate of growth of health care spending, rather than an upswing in overall economic growth (Levit et al, 1996).

The positive trend for the last few years has lowered the Congressional Budget Office's estimates of national health expenditure in 2003 from 20% of GDP to 15% (ProPAC, June 1997b).

Managed care plans use a variety of methods to control their outlays: selective contracting with providers, negotiations for price discounts, payment methods that shift some risk to providers, and utilization control. Enrollment in managed care plans has skyrocketed. As can be seen in Table 1.5.5, by

Table 1.5.5. Share of employees in selected health plans 1992–1996 in firms with 200 or more employees, (%)

Year	Indemnity	Preferred provider organization	Point of service	HMO
1992	45	26	8	22
1996	26	26	16	33

Source: Medicare and the American health care system. Report to the Congress. Prospective Payment Assessment Commission (ProPAC, June 1997b).

1996, 75% of insured employees in firms with at least 200 workers enrolled in managed care plans, up from 56% in 1992.

The proportion of the nonelderly population with employer-based health insurance coverage dropped between 1988 and 1995, from 73% to 67%. This cost was offset partially by an increase in Medicaid recipients, from 9% to 13% of the population under 65. Between 1988 and 1993, the share of the nonelderly population without insurance at a given point in time grew from 15% to 17% (ProPAC, June 1997). Around 42 million Americans, about one in six, have no health insurance (anonymous, 1997).

In April 1997 more than 5 million Medicare beneficiaries were enrolled in managed care, a figure that has risen by more than 25% in each of the past years (ProPAC, June 1997b).

Medicare continues to employ cost-based reimbursement and fee-for-service payment methods, which create few financial incentives to furnish services efficiently and encourage overutilization. Moreover, since payment approaches vary by type of provider, Medicare may pay substantially different amounts for comparable services furnished to similar patients in alternative settings. Further, with each provider receiving separate payments, there are few incentives to manage patients' total needs and coordinate care across sites. Consequently, spending may be higher than necessary (ProPAC, June 1997b).

Controlling expenditures in individual settings, however, creates incentives to shift care to other sites. Without volume controls that encompass all services delivered across all sites, though, Medicare expenditures could continue to rise unchecked. A key factor in the private sector's success in curbing expenditure is the use of managed care techniques, which control the volume of service provided (ProPAC, June 1997b).

The implementation of either consistent prospective payment systems or payments for broader units of service depends on an adequate case-mix measurement system that can be used for multiple providers. Such adjusters are not yet available, however. Appropriate resource use is hard to determine because patterns of care vary widely across providers. Understanding these differences is critical to developing and implementing policies that will effectively control Medicare spending for post-acute care (ProPAC, June 1997b).

Similar to the diffusion of DRGs outside the United States during the 1980s there is probably an equivalent expansion of the managed care concept in many countries in the world. Several American managed care organizations are trying to expand their markets around the world: Russia, South Africa, Singapore, Australia, most western European countries, and Latin America (Hagland, 1996; Meyer, 1997; Kertesz, 1997a). 'Russians distrust managed care plans or anything that limits their control. They pay for their BMWs out of pocket, and they want to pay for health care up front, too' (Possehl, 1997). Underlying all this is a growing trend toward privatization. And even if the countries in question will not import the American health care system they are interested in the toolkit of managed care.

In recent years, the health care industry has experienced considerable growth in organizations that are national in focus—organizations that operate in multiple markets not clustered in one geographic region. The number of HMO enrollees increased from 35 million in 1990 to over 50 million in 1994. National HMOs increased by 85% during this period, of which 75% are for profit HMOs. In 1994 there were 79 million enrollees in the Preferred Provider Organizations (PPOs), a less restrictive form of managed care. Factors that influence growth of national managed companies may be categorized into three groups: access to capital, economies of scale, and legal and regulatory structures (Corrigan et al, 1997).

It seems that the increased competitive health care market in the US has lowered the costs. Areas with high managed care penetration have tended to have much lower rates of increase in their costs. One good example of that is California (Zwanziger and Melnick, 1996).

According to a study by Gaskin and Hadley (1997) hospitals in areas with high rates of HMO penetration and growth had a slower rate of growth in expenses (8.3%) than hospitals in low penetration areas (11.2%) during the period 1985–1993. The estimation implies that the cumulative effect of HMO growth on hospital costs has been a $56.2 billion reduction (in 1993 dollars).

Physicians who practice in managed care systems might be asked to make clinical decisions that benefit stockholders, while physicians in fee-for-service systems might make clinical choices that benefit their income. (Holleman et al, 1997)

The development of managed care is an unexpected product of competition between public and private purchasers of health care. Although the so-called managed care revolution has reduced the rate of increase in health care costs by creating a more competitive price environment, it is simply a start toward a more effective health care market. It is very much a work in progress that will affect and be affected by both political and market changes occurring over the remainder of this century (Drake, 1997). The author ends 'unless employees, who have borne the principal costs of change through reduced choice and/or higher costs, share in the benefits of reduced employer costs or, at least, receive good value in health care services, their support for these changes and for employer-sponsored health benefits could be threatened with significant political and market consequences.'

A study of 20 HMOs in California showed that overall, some 77% of the surveyed enrollees said they were satisfied with their HMOs. For individual plans, the satisfaction rate ranged from a low 67% to a high of 85% (Kaiser Permanente-Northern California).

To assess physicians' attitudes about the effects of gatekeeping compared with traditional care a cross-sectional survey of primary care physicians in outpatient facilities in the metropolitan area in Boston was performed. Overall, 32% of physicians rated gatekeeping as better than traditional care, 40% the same, 21% gatekeeping as worse, and 7% were of mixed opinion (Halm et al, 1997).

BACKLASH AGAINST HMOs

The success of managed care in containing health expenditure has had some, temporally or not, backlashes. In 1996 more than 1000 bills were introduced in state legislatures to control managed care practices and 56 laws were passed in 35 states (Mechanic, 1997). Cynics may contend that doctors mainly want to protect their incomes by preventing HMOs from lowering capitation payments. In California, where 75% of its insured citizens are in managed-care plans, the average earnings of a primary-care physician dropped from $172 100 in 1993 to $146 000 in 1995 (Church, 1997). One highly publicized issue is resistance to HMO 'gag rules.' These clauses in contracts between HMOs and physicians prevent physicians advocating treatment for which the HMO will not approve payment, disclosing bonuses physicians may receive as a result of denying services to their patients, or both (Bodenheimer, 1996). One very talked about issue is the coverage of postpartum hospital care to a period of 24 hours—'drive-through delivery,' as it is popularly known.

The ideals that guided the earliest health plans are slipping away: a tight medical staff, a clear social mission, affordable premiums for the entire community. Over the last 10 years, managed care has evolved from social movement to corporate colossus (Green, 1997).

The enthusiasm of employers for managed care arrangements is likely to be weakened by the passage of additional government rules and regulations restricting cost-reducing practices by managed care companies. This stems from the possibility that employer purchasing groups will join together to negotiate directly with large hospital and multispeciality physicians' groups, thereby completely bypassing the managed care companies (Ginzberg, 1997).

The current trend toward the invasion of commerce into medical care, an arena formerly under the exclusive purview of physicians, is seen as an epic clash of cultures between commercial and professional traditions in the United

States (McArthur and Moore, 1997). These authors propose a national agency in the private sector, the National Council on Medical Care, to set standards and provide an approval mechanism that would then be the basis for state enforcement through licensing.

Another important issue is what will happen to medical research as a result of the expansion of managed care. Two studies in the *Journal of the American Medical Association* showed that medical school faculties in a market with high managed care penetration published fewer scientific articles, and that 13 medical schools in high-penetration markets lost ground with National Institute of Health grants compared with their peers in other markets (Hudson, 1997).

Appendix 1.5.5 summarizes the pros and cons regarding the implications of managed care for health systems, clinicians and patients.

DIAGNOSIS RELATED GROUPS (DRGs)

Starting on 1 October 1983 there was a dramatic shift in paying the cost of hospital care for the Medicare population in the United States. From that day the hospitals were paid a prospective price per discharge. The prospective payment system (PPS) used for reimbursement was the Diagnosis Related Groups, or DRGs, which were developed during the 1970s by professors Robert B. Fetter and John Thompson at Yale University (Fetter, 1980, 1991). The DRG system classifies patients into groups based on the principal diagnosis, type of surgical procedure, presence or absence of significant comorbidities or complications, and other relevant criteria. DRGs are intended to categorize patients into groups that are clinically meaningful and homogeneous with respect to resource use. Medicare's PPS currently uses 490 mutually exclusive DRGs, each of which is assigned a relative weight that compares its costliness to the average for all DRGs. Providers are paid these rates regardless of the costs they actually incur.

It is also worth noting that the share of total spending accounted for by hospital services fell from 41.5% in 1980 to 35.5% in 1995. And in 1995 only 70% of spending on community hospital services was for inpatient care compared with 87% in 1980.

Even though the prospective payment system was phased in during several years there was an immediate drop after the first year in the number of admissions and the average length of stay.

According to a study by Russell and Manning (1989) the prospective payment system (PPS) was estimated to have contributed to a reduction on health care spending of about 17 billion dollars in the 1990 year's prices. But total health care spending continued to increase. It is, however, important to note that the PPS covered only about 17% of the total health care costs in the United States.

A study by Coularn and Gaumer (1991) showed that the unexpected and substantial decline in admission continued up to the end of the 1980s. The initial sharp decline in length of stay was mainly limited to the first two years. According to this study the reduction of the rate of increase of hospital expenditures was substantial, and only minor evidence of cost shifting could be demonstrated. There was no large or systematic reduction in technology diffusion, and no significant changes in access to care, mortality or readmission. The organization culture was more businesslike and management techniques more sophisticated.

This new way of financing hospitals was tested and evaluated in many countries in Europe and in Australia during the 1980s (Kimberly and Pouvourville, 1993; Håkansson et al, 1988, 1994).

Since the fiscal year 1983, payments for ambulatory services (excluding those for physician services) have risen an average of 14% annually, reaching $16.3 billion in 1995. HCFA estimates that about 70% of these payments were made to hospitals for services provided in outpatient departments (ProPAC, 1 March 1997a).

The prospective payment assessment commission have urged that case-mix based prospective payment systems for hospital outpatient services, skilled nursing facilities, home care agencies, rehabilitation hospitals and long-term care hospitals should be developed and implemented as soon as possible (ProPAC, 1 March 1997a).

Coffey (1997), in an overview of the impact of DRGs, says that they helped to decrease the growth rate in health spending, transferred patients to an outpatients' setting and included home care in post acute services. But the prospective payment system did not solve the overriding problem of ever increasing health care spending ('a payment system designed only for hospital services cannot solve runaway spending in the total health care system').

According to Coffey, patient classification system work is beginning to focus on comprehensive per capita payment that can apply to all settings and services: 'Unless we link classification systems for different settings together or design one system that comprehensively accounts for everything we do in health care, we will not be prepared to build a comprehensive system-wide payment plan with incentives for achieving the goal of reasonable spending on health care.'

EQUITY WITHIN DIFFERENT HEALTH CARE SYSTEMS

One important issue influencing how health systems are viewed by the citizens is the question of equity or fairness of distribution of health services between different segments of the population. From the project 'Equity in the Finance and Delivery of Health Care in Europe' (known as the ECuity Project) some very interesting results have recently been published.

A study of income-related inequalities in self-assessed health care in nine industrialized countries (Finland, West Germany, East Germany, The Netherlands, Spain, Sweden, Switzerland, United Kingdom and the United States) with data from the end of the 1980s to 1992 showed that inequalities in healthcare favored the higher income groups and were statistically significant in all countries. Inequalities were particularly high in the United States and the United Kingdom. Amongst the other European countries, Sweden, Finland and the former East Germany had the lowest inequality. Across countries, a strong association was found between inequalities in health and inequalities in income. According to the results 'the United Kingdom has a slightly higher level of inequality in health than one would expect on the basis of its income inequality, while the opposite is true for Sweden' (van Doorslaer et al, 1997).

Another part of the same project aimed to study the correlation between inequality in health and two indicators of socioeconomic status: education (morbidity and mortality; men, women), and occupational class (morbidity and mortality; men). Data of self-reported morbidity were obtained from 11 countries during the period 1985 to 1992. Data on mortality were obtained for 9 countries for about 1980 to 1992. The study found that Sweden and Norway had larger inequalities than most other countries in both morbidity and mortality, whereas Switzerland and Spain had smaller than average inequalities in both outcomes. France had the largest inequalities in mortality but average inequality in morbidity (Mackenbach et al, 1997a).

Taken together, these two studies show that, for example, Sweden's favorable position for income-related inequalities in health was more than balanced by unfavorable positions for inequalities related to education and occupation. The results challenge the widely held view on the relation between societal characteristics and the size of inequalities in health: 'Our data do not support the hypothesis that inequalities in health care are smaller in countries whose social, economic, and health-care policies are more influenced by egalitarian principles, such as Sweden and Norway.'

This study has been criticized (Vågerö and Erikson, 1997; Wilkenson, 1997). One potential cause of the large inequalities in Sweden and Norway could be the north-south gradient in mortality in cardiovascular diseases, particularly ischaemic heart disease in Europe: the north has large inequalities in ischaemic heart disease mortality, the south has not. But this has little to do with egalitarian policies (Mackenbach et al, 1997b).

EXPERIENCES OF HEALTH CARE REFORMS

There are many examples of health care reforms in the OECD countries during the last 15 years. Earlier we discussed the prospective payment system and the dramatic increase in 'managed care' in the United States and their impact on the health care system. But a lot of other examples are worth noting. The Clintons' proposal for health care reform in the early 1990s was a fiasco mainly because of a lack of necessary political leadership and managerial competence, and special-interest groups' manipulation, but ultimately because the American people did not support it (Blumenthal, 1995).

Ham (1997) has identified four approaches to the process of reform. The first is what has been described as *big-bang reform* (UK, Israel and New Zealand). The second is *incremental reform* (Holland and Germany). The third is the *bottom-up reform* (Sweden), and the fourth is '*reform without reform*' (USA, where managed care has revolutionized the health care system).

In the late 1980s and early 1990s there were many countries that experimented with the separation of purchaser and provider. One important inspiration for this came from professor Alain Enthoven at Stanford University in the United States. During the 1980s he did some case studies in the United Kingdom, The Netherlands and Sweden, which laid the framework for future reforms (Enthoven, 1989). But the first place in Europe to introduce a purchaser–provider split was Leningrad, the present St Petersburg, where the dramatic change took place in May 1988. In Leningrad the hospitals were reimbursed by their activities according to a fixed price list, a short version of DRGs (Håkansson et al, 1989, 1991).

In a study of the NHS reforms on English hospital productivity Söderlund et al (1997) found real productivity gains during the period 1991–1994 for NHS hospitals on average. Casemix adjustment drastically improved cross-sectional comparisons between hospitals. But it is important to note that no adjustment for potential changes in quality could be made. In a study of fundholders' prescribing costs from 1990 to 1996 Harris and Scrivener (1996) found a reduction in costs of about 6% relative to continuing fundholders, and this saving seemed to be retained during the study. But according to Keeley (1997) general practice fundholding overall has not succeeded in containing the rise in prescription costs, nor in reducing the use of expensive specialist hospital facilities. According to Dixon and Glennerster (1995) fundholding has curbed prescription costs but fundholding practices may have received more money than nonfundholding practices. The impact of fundholding on transaction costs, equity, and quality of care is unknown.

In Sweden there has been considerable experimentation regarding the purchaser–provider split and hospital service reimbursement. In 12 of the 26 counties in Sweden there has been a purchaser–provider split. Between 1992 and 1995 a new way of financing and organizing health care, the so-called Stockholm model, was gradually implemented in the Stockholm county council (population 1.7 million). Fundamental to the new system is that patient needs and their choice of health care provider determine the allocation of resources, that the roles of the purchasers (the health district) and providers (the hospitals) are separate, and that hospitals and primary care services (the family physician) compete in attracting the patients. The patients can freely choose their doctor, health center, or hospital, and may choose a private doctor. In the Stockholm model, hospital inpatient care is paid by a prospective fixed price list per DRG. The result for the first year (1992) was a success. Inpatient care increased by 8%, day surgery by 50% and outpatient visits by 15%. Taken all together, activities increased by 11%. Because there was a 10% decrease in DRG prices from 1 January 1992, the total costs decreased by 1% due to fewer personnel. Later on the county experienced problems with increased spending. There was a budget deficit of 4% for 1994. The reason for this was that the total health care supply was higher than could be bought from the total budget. The system has a built-in propensity to increase production. And from the end of that year when a new social democratic government took office the focus was on health care cutting. The focus went from competition to collaboration. In Bruce and Jonsson (1996) an evaluation of the productivity between so-called 'model counties' and a group of 14 counties that had not used the purchaser–provider split showed that the model counties increased their productivity more than the 'control counties'. The difference was due one quarter to cost reduction and three quarters to increased output (Håkansson, 1997; Bruce and Jonsson, 1996).

Broadly speaking, I think that the presumed positive expectations of the health care reforms in many countries during the last decade have been shadowed by what really happened. In several countries there has been a shift from competition to cooperation, see for example the United Kingdom, New Zealand and Sweden where Labour governments have come back to power (Malcolm, 1997; Warden, 1997; Hornblow, 1997).

In New Zealand the new government favours collaboration over competition, and its health policy is to abolish the market oriented Crown health enterprises and replace them with regional hospital and community service units, which will be required to improve the health of their communities. The bottom line is not profit; it is better health outcomes.

In the United Kingdom in December 1997 the new government presented its 10 year plan for the NHS. The competitive internal market, which was introduced by the Conservatives, will be replaced by a system of 'integrated care' based on partnership driven by performance. But the separation between purchasers and providers will be retained; cooperation, however, will replace competition. More attention will focus on the quality of care and less on finance. Trusts will have to publish the costs of treatments to expose inefficiency. National standards of care will be guaranteed. Computer technology, including telemedicine, will be diverted from administration to patient care. Health authorities will devolve responsibility for district commissioning of services to new 'primary care groups' comprising all GPs in an area together with community nurses. They will replace fundholding in 1999. In the meantime there will be no new admissions to the fundholding scheme.

DISCUSSION

As it has been shown above, any health care system is very dependent on the vitality of the economy. Since the 1980s the European countries have been lagging behind the United States in economic growth and employment (Eurosclerosis). High unemployment rates in Europe together with tough cost containment activities—because of the fact that many European countries cannot cope with a balanced budget requirement to the year 2000—have led to a rather stressed situation for people working in the health care sector. There is a strikingly close relationship between the economy's growth rate and the rate of change in the unemployment rate. In the United States, between 1980 and 1995, the rate of growth consistent with a steady unemployment rate was about 2.4%, which has been called 'Okun's law' (Krugman, 1997). This means that the growth rate in an economy has a tremendous impact on the situation of the health care sector.

Most of the health care reforms in the OECD countries took place in a time when there was a deep recession in the economies. And you must bear in mind that drawbacks in health care delivery have been associated with the backlash of the reforms and not with the fact that countries have been forced to cut down on public spending. In order to fulfill the requirements that the European Union has set up to be able to join the European Monetary Union, the countries must balance their expenditures and revenues.

New technologies, both at health care institutions and at home, an increasing aging of the population, new demands for patients' rights, will put severe pressure on health care systems in the future. Several health care reforms, however, have shown that there are never any 'quick fixes' in health care. There is a movement in many countries today towards integration and continuity of care with emphasis on collaboration between health and community services.

The trend is very clear worldwide: from hospital care to outpatient and home health care. Extensive technical innovations in home care technology and the use of telemedicine will probably dramatically change the health care environment in only a few years' time.

It is also probable that the use of managed care will have a potential in many countries with a health system quite different from that of the United States'. Several tools of managed care such as utilization review, disease management, clinical guidelines, publications of medical outcomes, costs and patient quality, together with evidence based medicine, can surely fit most of the health care systems of the industrialized world.

ACKNOWLEDGEMENT

I want to thank Erik Grönqvist, MSc(Econ), Spri, for valuable computations from the OECD health data file and Lena Wallgren, research assistant, Spri, for help with tables and secretarial assistance.

REFERENCES

Anonymous (1997). What price control? (Editorial), *Lancet*, **349**, 295.

Blendon, R. J., Leitman, R., Morrison, I., and Donelan, K. (1990). Satisfaction with health systems in ten nations, *Health Affairs*, **9**(2), 185–192.

Blendon, R. J., Benson, J., Donelan, K. et al (1995). Who has the best health system? A second look, *Health Affairs*, **14**(4), 220–230.

Blomqvist, Å. G., and Carter, R. A. L. (1997). Is health care really a luxury? *Journal of Health Economics*, **16**, 207–229.

Blumenthal, D. (1995). Health care reform: past and future, *New England Journal of Medicine*, **332**, 465–468.

Bodenheimer, T. (1996). The HMO backlash—righteous or reactionary? *New England Journal of Medicine*, **335**, 1601–1604.

Bruce, A., and Jonsson, E. (1996). *Competition in the Provision of Health Care: The experience of the US, Sweden and Britain*, Aldershot, UK, Arena, Ashgate Publishing.

Church, G. J. (1997). Backlash against HMOs: doctors, patients, unions, legislators are fed up and say they won't take it anymore, *Newsweek*, 21 April, 60–63.

Coffey, R. M. (1997). DRGs in the United States: fourteen years of management and clinical experience. Paper presented at the 13th International working conference on Patient Classification Systems/Europe (PCS/E). Florence, Italy, 1 October 1997. *Proceedings*, pp. 12–27.

Corrigan, J. M., Eden, J. S., Gold, M. R., and Pickreign, J. D. (1997). Trends toward a national health care marketplace, *Inquiry*, **34**, 11–28.

Coularn, R. F., and Gaurner, G. L. (1991). Medicare's prospective payment system: a critical appraisal, *Health Care Financing Review*, **13**, ann suppl, 45–77.

Dixon, J., and Glennerster, H. (1995). What do we know about fundholding in general practice? *British Medical Journal*, **311**, 727–730.

Doorslaer, E. van, Wagstaff, A., Bleichrodt, H. et al (1997). Income-related inequalities in health: some international comparisons, *Journal of Health Economics*, **16**, 93–112.

Drake, D. F. (1997). Managed care: a product of market dynamics, *Journal of the American Medical Association*, **277**, 560–563.

Ellwood, P. M., and Lundberg, G. D. (1996). Managed care: a work in progress, *Journal of the American Medical Association*, **276**, 1083–1086.

Enthoven, A. (1989). What can Europeans learn from Americans? *Health Care Financing Review*, **11**, ann suppl, 49–63.

Fairfield, G., Hunter, D. J., Mechanic, D., and Rosleff, F. (1997). Implications of managed care for health systems, clinicians, and patients, *British Medical Journal*, **314**, 1895–1898.

Fetter, R. B. et al (1980). Case-mix definition by diagnosis-related groups, *Medical Care*, **18** (suppl), 1–53.

Fetter, R. B. et al (Eds) (1991). *DRGs: Their Design and Development*, Ann Arbor, MI, Health Administration Press, Pennsylvania University Press.

Fuchs, V. R. (1997). Managed care and merger mania, *Journal of the American Medical Association*, **277**, 920–921.

Färe, R., Grosskopf, S., Lindgren, B., and Poullier, J-P. (1997). Productivity growth in health-care delivery, *Medical Care*, **35**, 354–366.

Gaskin, D. J., and Hadley, J. (1997). The impact of HMO penetration on the rate of hospital cost inflation 1985–1993, *Inquiry*, **34**, 205–216.

Gerdtham, U. G. (1992). Pooling international health care expenditure data, *Health Economics*, **1**, 217.

Ginzberg, E. (1997). Managed care and the competitive market in health care: what they can and cannot do, *Journal of American Medical Association*, **277**, 1812–1813.

Ginzberg, E., and Ostow, M. (1997). Managed care: a look back and a look ahead, *New England Journal of Medicine*, **336**, 1018–1020.

Green, J. (1997). Has managed care lost its soul? *Hospitals & Health Networks*, May, 36–42.

Hagland, M. (1996). Kaiser goes globe-trotting, *Hospitals & Health Networks*, Nov., 40–41.

Halm, E. A., Causino, N., and Blumenthal, D. (1997). Is gatekeeping better than traditional care? *Journal of the American Medical Association*, **278**, 1677–1681.

Ham C. (1997). *Healthcare Reform: Learning from International Experience*, Buckingham, UK, Open University Press.

Harris, C. M., and Scrivener, G. (1996). Fundholder prescribing costs: the first five years, *British Medical Journal*, **313**, 1531–1534.

Holleman, W. L., Holleman, M. C., and Moy, J. G. (1997). Are ethics and managed care strange bedfellows or a marriage made in heaven? *Lancet*, **349**, 350–351.

Hornblow, A. (1997). New Zealand's health reforms: a clash of cultures, *British Medical Journal*, **314**, 1892–1894.

Hudson, T. (1997). Is medical research doomed? *Hospitals & Health Networks*, 20 Oct., 41–44.

Håkansson, S. (1994). New ways of financing and organizing health care in Sweden, *International Journal of Health Planning and Management*, **9**, 103–124.

Håkansson, S., Paulson, E., and Kogeus, K. (1988). Prospects for using DRGs in Swedish hospitals, *Health Policy*, **9**, 177–192.

Håkansson, S., Majnono D'Intagnano de la Haye, B., Roberts, J. L., and Zöllner, H. (1989). *The Leningrad experiment in health care management*. Report of a WHO mission, Copenhagen, World Health Organization.

Håkansson, S., Majnono D'Intagnano de la Haye, B., Mooney, G. H., Roberts, J. L., Stoddard, G. L., Staehr-Johansen, K., and Zöllner, H. (1991). *Leningrad revisited*. Report of a second visit to the USSR, October 1989, Copenhagen, World Health Organization.

Håkansson, S., and Nordling, S. (1997). Sweden, in: M. W. Raffel (Ed.), *Health Care And Reform In Industrialized Countries*, Pennsylvania, PA, Pennsylvania University Press.

Keeley, D. (1997). General practice fundholding and health care costs, *British Medical Journal*, **315**, 139.

Kertesz, L. (1997a). Kaiser's success: Enrollees' good reports clash with unions' complaints, *Modern Healthcare*, Sept. 22, 28.

Kertesz, L. (1997b). The new world of managed care, *Modern Healthcare*, Nov., 114–142.

Kimberly, J., and Pouvourille, G. (Eds) (1993). *The Migration of Managerial Innovation: DRGs in Western Europe*, San Francisco, CA, Jossey-Bass.

Krugman, P. (1997). How fast can the US economy grow? *Harvard Business Review*, July–August, 123–129.

Leu, R. E. (1986). The public–private mix and international health care costs, in A. J. Culyer, and B. Jönsson (Eds), *Public and Private Health Services*, Oxford, Basil Blackwell.

Levit, K. R., Lazenby, H. C., and Braden, B. R. (1996). National health expenditures, 1995, *Health Care Financing Review*, **18**, 175–200.

Luft, H. S. (1991). Translating the US HMO experience to other health systems, *Health Affairs*, **10**(3), 172–186.

Mackenbach, J. P., Kunst, A. E., Cavelaars, E. J. M. et al (1997a). Socioeconomic inequalities in morbidity and mortality in western Europe, *Lancet*, **349**, 1655–1659.

Mackenbach, J. P., Cavelaars, E. J. M., and Kunst, A. E. (1997b). Author's reply, *Lancet*, **350**, 517.

Malcolm, L. (1997). GP budget holding in New Zealand: lessons for Britain and elsewhere? *British Medical Journal*, **314**, 1890–1894.

McArthur, J. H., and Moore, F. D. (1997). The two cultures and the health care revolution: commerce and professionalism in medical care, *Journal of the American Medical Association*, **277**, 985–989.

Mechanic, D. (1997). Managed care as a target of distrust, *Journal of the American Medical Association*, **277**, 1810–1811.

Meyer, H. (1997). Will US HMOs play in Pretoria? *Hospitals & Health Networks*, Jan., 66–67.

Mossialos, E. (1997). Citizens' views on health care systems in the 15 member states of the European Union, *Health Economics*, **6**, 109–116.

Newhouse, J. P. (1977). Medical-care expenditures: a cross-national survey, *Journal of Human Resources*, **12**, 115.

Nordic Social Statistical Committee (1997), *Social Protection in the Nordic Countries, 1997*, Copenhagen.

O'Connell, J. M. (1996). The relationship between health expenditures and the age structure of the population in OECD countries, *Health Economics*, **5**, 573–578.

OECD (1997). *OECD health data file*, OECD, Paris.

Parkin, D., McGuire, A., and Yule, B. (1987). Aggregate health care expenditures and national income: is health care a luxury good? *Journal of Health Economics*, **6**, 109.

Possehl, S. R. (1997). Russian rehab.: enterprising Westerners have imported managed care and one-stop clinics. That's pricey treatment for a tattered health system, *Hospitals & Health Networks*, Nov., 43–44.

Prospective Payment Assessment Commission, ProPAC (1997a). Report and Recommendations (1997, 1 March), Washington, DC.

Prospective Payment Assessment Commission, ProPAC (1997b). Medicare and the American health care system: Report to the Congress (1997, June), Washington, DC.

Raffel, M. W. (Ed.) (1997). *Health Care and Reform in Industrialized Countries*, Pennsylvania, PA, Pennsylvania University Press.

Reinhardt, U. (1996). A social contract for 21st century health care: three-tier health care without bounty hunting, *Health Economics*, **5**, 479–499.

Rublee, D. A., and Schneider, M. (1991). International health spending: comparisons with OECD, *Health Affairs*, **10**, 187–198.

Russell, L. B., and Manning, C. L. (1989). The effect of prospective payment on Medicare expenditures, *New England Journal of Medicine*, **320**(7), 439–444.

Saltman, R. B., and Figueras, J. (1997). European health care reform: analysis of current strategies, WHO Regional Publication, European Series, No 72, Copenhagen.

Schieber, G. J., and Poullier, J. P. (1991). Advancing the debate on international spending comparisons, *Health Affairs*, **10**, 199–201.

Schieber, G. J., Poullier, J. P., and Greenwald, L. M. (1994). Health system performance in OECD countries 1980–1992, *Health Affairs*, **13** (Fall), 100–112.

Söderlund, N., Csaba, I., Gray, A., Milne, R., and Raftery, J. (1997). Impact of the NHS reforms on English hospital productivity: an analysis of the first three years, *British Medical Journal*, **315**, 1126–1129.

Waldo, D. R., and Sonnefeld, S. T. (1991). US/Canadian health spending: methods and assumptions, *Health Affairs*, **10** (Summer), 159–164.

Warden, J. (1997). White paper puts GPs in the driving seat of the new NHS, *British Medical Journal*, **315**, 1561–1562.

Wilkenson, R. G. (1997). Socioeconomic inequalities in morbidity and mortality in western Europe (letter), *Lancet*, **350**, 516–517.
Zwanziger, J. K., and Melnick, G. A. (1996). Can managed care plans control health care costs? *Health Affairs*, **15**, 185–199.

GLOSSARY

Managed care Any system of health service payment or delivery arrangements in which the health plan or provider attempts to control or coordinate health service use to contain health expenditures, improve quality, or both. Arrangements often involve a defined delivery system of providers having some form of contractual relationship with the plan.

Capitation A method of paying health care providers or insurers in which a fixed amount is paid per enrollee to cover a defined set of services over a specified period, regardless of actual services provided.

Cost sharing A general term referring to payments made by health insurance enrollees for covering services. Examples of cost sharing include deductibles, coinsurance, and copayment.

Enrollee A person who is covered by health insurance.

Deductible A fixed dollar amount for covered services paid by a health insurance enrollee before additional services become payable by an insurer (e.g. the patient pays the first US$50 of the costs of a hospital stay, or pays the first US$200 of the year's outpatient care costs).

Evidence-based medicine (EBM) The conscientious, explicit and judicious use of current best evidence in making decisions about the care of individual patients. The practice of EBM means integrating individual clinical expertise with the best available external clinical evidence from systematic research.

Coinsurance A proportion of total payment for covered services paid by a health insurance enrollee after payment of a deductible (e.g. the patient pays 20% of the total charge for inpatient care).

Copayment A fixed dollar amount paid for a covered service by a health insurance enrollee (e.g. the patient pays US$5 per drug prescribed, or US$10 for each visit to the doctor).

Disease management An approach to patient care that coordinates medical resources for patients across the entire health care delivery system. There is a shift in focus from treating patients during discrete episodes of care to provision of high-quality care across the continuum.

Health Maintenance Organization (HMO) A managed care plan that integrates financing and delivery of a comprehensive set of health care services to an enrolled population. HMOs may contract with, directly employ, or own participating health care providers. Enrollees are usually required to choose from among these providers and in return have limited copayments. Providers may be paid through capitation, salary, per diem, or prenegotiated fee-for-service rates.

Point-of-Service Option (POS) A managed care option, usually offered by an HMO, that allows enrollees to choose among network and non-network providers at the time of service. Enrollees choosing non-network providers are subject to substantially higher coinsurance, copayments, or deductibles.

Preferred Provider Organization (PPO) A network of providers through which services are available to enrollees at lower cost than through non-network providers. PPO enrollees may self-refer to any network or non-network provider at any time.

Fee-for-Service A method of reimbursing health care providers in which payment is made for each unit of service rendered.

Physician–Hospital Organization (PHO) An organization, usually in the form of a joint venture, commonly owned by a hospital and a group of physicians, often the hospital's medical staff. The PHO can act as an agent for both parties in various activities, including contracting with managed care plan, owning a managed care plan, and providing administrative services.

Peer Review Organization (PRO) An organization that contracts with HCFA (Health Care Financing Administration) to investigate the quality of health care furnished to Medicare beneficiaries and to educate beneficiaries and providers. PROs also conduct targeted reviews of medical records and claims to evaluate the appropriateness of care provided.

Case Mix The mix of patients treated within a particular institutional setting, such as the hospital. Patient classification systems like DRGs can be used to measure hospital case mix.

Diagnosis Related Groups (DRGs) A system for determining case mix, used for payment under Medicare's PPS and by some other payers. The DRG system classifies patients into groups based on the principal diagnosis, type of surgical procedure, presence or absence of significant comorbidities or complications, and other relevant criteria. DRGs are intended to categorize patients into groups that are clinically meaningful and homogeneous with respect to resource use. Medicare's PPS currently uses 490 mutually exclusive DRGs, each of which is assigned a relative weight that compares its costliness to the average for all DRGs.

Prospective Payment A method of paying health care providers in which rates are established in advance. Providers are paid these rates regardless of the costs they actually incur.

Prospective Payment System (PPS)   Medicare's acute care hospital payment method for inpatient care. Prospective per case payment rates are set at a level intended to cover operating costs for treating a typical inpatient in a given diagnosis-related group. Payments for each hospital are adjusted for differences in area wages, teaching activity, care to the poor, and other factors. Hospitals may also receive additional payments to cover extra costs associated with atypical patients (outliers) in each DRG. Capital costs, originally excluded from PPS, are being phased into the system. By 2001, capital payments will be made on a fully prospective, per case basis.

Outliers   Cases with extremely long lengths of stay (day outliers) or extraordinarily high costs (cost outliers) compared with others classified in the same diagnosis-related group. Hospitals receive additional PPS payments for these cases.

Utilization Review (UR)   The review of services delivered by a health care provider to evaluate the appropriateness, necessity, and quality of the prescribed services. The review can be performed on a prospective, concurrent, or retrospective basis.

Gross Domestic Product (GDP)   A valuation of all goods and services produced within the boundaries of a country during a given period.

Productivity   The ratio of outputs (goods and services produced) to inputs (resources used in production). Increased productivity implies that the hospital or health care organization is either producing more output with the same resources or the same output with fewer resources.

Source: Medicare and the American Health Care System. Report to the Congress. June 1997. Prospective Payment Assesssment Commission (ProPAC). Washington, DC, 1997.

Appendices

Appendix 1.5.1. Total expenditure on health per capita (PPP in US$) as percentage of OECD average (ranks in parenthesis) 1970, 1980, 1990 and 1995

	1970		1980		1990		1995	
Australia	131	(7)	118	(9)	113	(12)	123	(9)
Austria	103	(11)	123	(7)	101	(15)	115	(12)
Belgium	81	(19)	104	(15)	107	(14)	118	(11)
Canada	158	(4)	129	(5)	145	(3)	146	(5)
Czech Republic	–	–	–	–	46	(23)	53	(23)
Denmark	133	(6)	105	(13)	92	(17)	97	(16)
Finland	102	(12)	92	(17)	111	(13)	97	(15)
France	129	(8)	126	(6)	132	(5)	139	(6)
Germany	143	(5)	152	(3)	141	(4)	151	(4)
Greece	37	(22)	34	(23)	33	(24)	50	(24)
Hungary	–	–	–	–	–	–	40	(25)
Iceland	86	(16)	112	(11)	118	(8)	125	(8)
Ireland	61	(20)	83	(18)	64	(21)	78	(20)
Italy	97	(13)	104	(14)	113	(11)	107	(14)
Japan	82	(18)	94	(16)	93	(16)	112	(13)
Korea	9	(25)	13	(25)	27	(25)	34	(26)
Luxembourg	93	(14)	109	(12)	128	(6)	156	(3)
Mexico	–	–	–	–	–	–	27	(27)
Netherlands	127	(9)	122	(8)	114	(10)	122	(10)
New Zealand	110	(10)	82	(19)	80	(19)	85	(19)
Norway	84	(17)	113	(10)	117	(9)	129	(7)
Poland	–	–	–	–	–	–	18[a]	(29)
Portugal	28	(23)	47	(22)	53	(22)	73	(22)
Spain	51	(21)	59	(21)	70	(20)	76	(21)
Sweden	170	(2)	153	(2)	128	(7)	96	(17)
Switzerland	167	(3)	150	(4)	153	(2)	168	(2)
Turkey	14	(24)	14	(24)	11	(26)	19[a]	(28)
United Kingdom	92	(15)	80	(20)	82	(18)	88	(18)
United States	211	(1)	185	(1)	230	(1)	258	(1)

[a] 1994 figures.

Source: OECD Health Data 97. Update 29 July 1997.

Appendix 1.5.2. Public expenditure on health as percentage of total expenditure on health 1970, 1980, 1990 and 1995

	1970	1980	1990	1995
Well-established tax-based system	*79.9*	*83.2*	*81.7*	*79.5*
Australia	56.7	62.9	68.1	66.7
Denmark	86.3	85.2	82.3	82.7
Finland	73.8	79.0	80.9	74.7
Iceland	81.7	88.2	86.6	84.2
Ireland	81.7	82.2	74.7	80.8
Norway	91.6	85.1	83.3	82.8
Sweden	86.0	92.5	89.9	81.6
United Kingdom	87.0	89.4	84.1	84.3
Well-established insurance-based system	*76.2*	*79.3*	*80.2*	*82.4*
Austria	63.0	68.8	75.0	75.6
Belgium	87.0	83.4	88.9	87.8
France	74.7	78.8	74.5	80.6
Germany	73.3	79.2	76.8	78.4
Luxembourg	–	92.8	93.1	92.8
Netherlands	84.3	74.7	72.7	77.1
In transition to tax-based system	*71.9*	*77.5*	*76.3*	*70.6*
Greece	53.4	82.2	82.3	75.8
Italy	86.9	80.5	78.1	69.6
Portugal	59.0	64.3	65.5	60.5
Spain	65.4	79.9	78.7	78.2
In transition to insurance-based system	*37.3*	*27.3*	*35.6*	*–*
Turkey	37.3	27.3	35.6	–
USA	37.8	42.4	40.8	46.2
OECD average	72.0	76.2	75.0	74.6

Source: OECD Health Data 97. Update 29 July 1997.

Appendix 1.5.3. Life expectancy, infant mortality and low weight at birth in the OECD
countries, 1995

	Life expectancy at birth Females (years)	Life expectancy at birth Males (years)	Infant mortality rate/1000 live births	Low weight at birth Hospital deliveries (%)
Australia	80.9	75.0	5.7	6.3[b]
Austria	80.1	73.5	5.4	5.7
Belgium	80.0	73.3	7.0	–
Canada	81.3	75.3	6.0	6.0[a]
Czech Republic	76.9	70.0	7.7	5.7
Denmark	77.8	72.5	5.5	5.2[a]
Finland	80.2	72.8	4.0	4.1
France	81.9	73.9	5.0	6.2
Germany	79.5	73.0	5.3	6.1
Greece	80.3	75.1	8.1	6.8[b]
Hungary	74.5	65.3	11.0	8.6[a]
Iceland	80.6	76.5	6.1	3.2[b]
Ireland	78.5	72.9	6.3	–
Italy	80.8	74.4	6.2	6.0[a]
Japan	82.8	76.4	4.3	7.1[a]
Korea	76.0	70.0	9.0	–
Luxembourg	79.5	72.5	5.0	–
Mexico	76.0	69.5	16.5	–
Netherlands	80.4	74.6	5.5	–
New Zealand	79.2	73.8	7.0	6.1
Norway	80.8	74.8	4.0	5.3
Poland	76.4	67.6	13.6	7.9[b]
Portugal	78.6	71.5	7.4	6.0
Spain	81.2	73.2	5.5	5.4[b]
Sweden	81.5	76.2	4.1	4.4
Switzerland	81.7	75.3	5.0	5.2[a]
Turkey	70.3	65.7	44.4	–
United Kingdom	79.7	74.3	6.0	7.0[a]
United States	79.2	72.5	8.0	7.2[b]

[a] 1994
[b] 1993

Source: OECD Health Data 97.

Appendix 1.5.4. Satisfaction from health systems in the 15 EU Member States in 1996

	A (%)	B (%)	C (%)	D (%)	E (%)
Denmark	54.5	36.0	3.8	4.5	1.2
Finland	15.2	71.7	7.0	5.3	0.7
Luxembourg	14.1	59.9	16.8	7.8	1.5
The Netherlands	14.3	59.2	8.9	13.8	3.8
Belgium	11.1	60.3	20.2	7.3	1.1
Sweden	13.3	55.2	17.0	11.6	2.8
Germany	13.0	54.1	21.8	10.0	1.2
France	10.2	56.0	19.0	13.0	1.9
Austria	17.8	48.4	28.9	4.2	0.7
Ireland	9.7	42.0	18.1	18.9	11.3
United Kingdom	7.7	40.9	10.1	26.0	15.4
Spain	3.8	32.5	34.6	20.8	8.4
Portugal	0.8	19.4	19.5	38.0	22.2
Greece	1.5	17.0	27.2	29.9	24.4
Italy	0.8	15.7	23.4	33.9	26.2
EU	8.9	42.1	20.2	19.1	9.7

A = Very Satisfied
B = Fairly Satisfied
C = Neither Satisfied/Nor Dissatisfied
D = Fairly Dissatisfied
E = Very Dissatisfied

Source: Mossialos, E. (1997). Citizens' views on health care systems in the 15 member states of the European Union, *Health Economics*, **6**, 109–116. © John Wiley & Sons Ltd. Reproduced with permission.

Appendix 1.5.5. Implications of managed care for health systems, clinicians, and patients

---

Implications of managed care for health systems

Positive: *Negative:*
Better outcomes   Increased costs and time
Lower cost   Need to overcome resistance to change
Better quality (evidence-based medicine)   Block to innovation
Improved allocation of resources   Research and education at risk
Seamless care   Vulnerable population at risk

Implications of managed care for doctors

Positive: *Negative:*
Increased professionalism   Reduced clinical freedom
Collaboration   Reduced status
Better information   Increased supervision
                                                      Conflicts of interest
                                                      Altered doctor–patient relationship

Implications of managed care for patients

Positive: *Negative:*
Better outcomes   Restriction of treatment or doctor
Better informed   Increased responsibility not wanted
Clearer expectations   Altered doctor–patient relationship
Patient-driven guidelines   Less satisfaction
Increased satisfaction

Source: Fairfield, G., Hunter, D., Mechanic, D., and Rosleff, F. (1997). Implications of managed care for health systems, clinicians, and patients, *British Medical Journal*, **314**, 1895–1898. Reproduced by permission of the BMJ Publishing Group.

Appendix 1.5.6. Percentage of population over 75 years

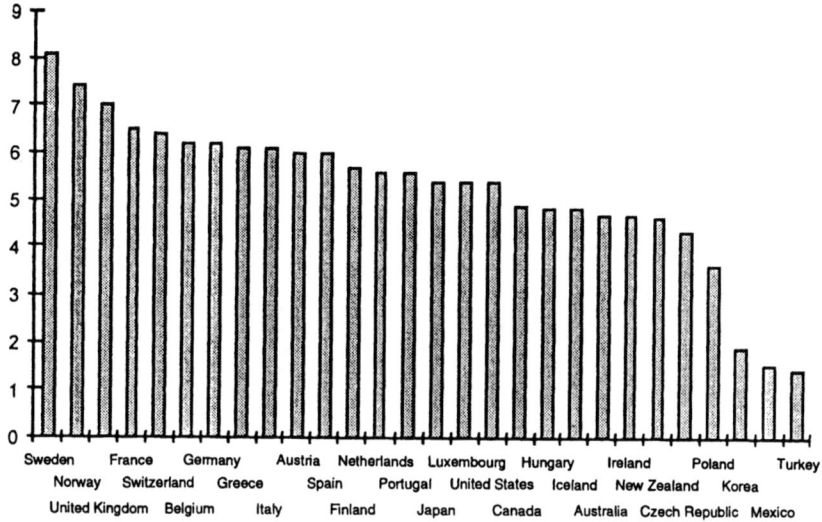

Source: OECD Health Data 97

Appendix 1.5.7. Total social and health expenditure as % of GDP in the Nordic countries and the European Union in 1994 (social) and 1995 (health)

Country	Social	Health	Total
Finland	34.7	7.7	42.4
Sweden	35.1	7.2	42.3
Austria	33.7	7.9	41.6
Germany	30.8	10.4	41.2
Netherlands	32.3	8.8	41.1
Denmark	34.2	6.4	40.6
France	30.5	9.9	40.4
Norway[a]	28.0	8.0	36.0
United Kingdom	28.1	6.9	35.0
Belgium	27.0	8.0	35.0
Italy	25.3	7.7	33.0
Luxembourg	24.9	7.0	31.9
Spain	23.6	7.6	31.2
Portugal	19.5	8.2	27.7
Ireland	21.1	6.4	27.5
Iceland[a]	18.6	8.2	26.8
Greece	16.0	5.8	21.8

[a] Not member of the European Union.

Source: Social Protection in the Nordic Countries 1995. Nordic Social Statistical Committee 1997 (NOSOSCO). Copenhagen, 1997, and OECD, Health Data 97.

1.6 Cultural Concepts of Care for the Demented

BERNARD INEICHEN

Imperial College School of Medicine, London, UK

DISTRIBUTION AND IDENTIFICATION OF DEMENTIA

The definition of dementia is not universally agreed, but may include some consideration of how mental function is influenced by the social and cultural setting of the patient (Wallin, 1996). Symptomatology is by and large universal: similarities revealed by epidemiology and detailed local research outweigh the differences. The growing body of epidemiological studies, now around a hundred in number, has been reviewed (Jorm, 1990; Henderson, 1994, Ineichen, in press). Further studies continue to appear, recently from Sweden (Aevarsson and Skoog, 1996) and Italy (Ferini-Strambi et al, 1997). Despite differences in sampling and criteria for 'caseness' most show a roughly similar pattern of age-related rates. Carefully detailed meta-surveys in a dozen European countries have revealed broadly similar international patterns of prevalence both for Alzheimer's disease (Rocca et al, 1991) and for all types of dementia (Hofman et al, 1991).

Divergence from the prevalence norm is most marked in poor countries with relatively low life-expectancy. In such settings, serious physical illness may produce dementia as part of the symptomatology, causing sufferers to die prematurely; and those who develop dementia while in good health may also die early, usually from pneumonia, hip fractures or diarrhoea (Chandra et al, 1994). The result of these trends will be to shorten the life-expectancy of sufferers still further, and produce lower prevalence rates for dementia when surveys are carried out.

Few studies have been done of different ethnic groups sharing a common territory. Those we have are fraught with methodological difficulties. Comparisons of whites, Hispanics and African-Americans in the USA, for example, have consistently shown lower rates in the white groups (Gurland et al, 1995), but must take account of the different demography and levels of health of the groups. Accurate identification of cases may be particularly difficult among old people who speak minority languages (McCracken et al, 1997). An ambitious

Health Economics of Dementia. Edited by Anders Wimo, Bengt Jönsson, Göran Karlsson and Bengt Winblad.
© 1998 John Wiley & Sons Ltd.

exercise was conducted by Silverman et al (1992) who compared the presence of dementia in the family history of elderly Chinese, Italian, Jewish and Puerto Rican New Yorkers. Italians and Jews showed an increased risk compared to Chinese and Puerto Ricans. However, methodological weaknesses make the study suggestive rather than definitive.

The subtypes of dementia have also been shown to be prevalent in roughly similar proportions in different countries, although some divergencies from the common pattern have been noted. In most surveys, Alzheimer's disease is diagnosed more often than multi-infarct dementia. The proportion has been reversed in a number of surveys of Oriental populations, chiefly from China and Japan; Silverman et al (1992) also suggest a lower rate of Alzheimer's among Chinese than among some other ethnic groups in New York. Suggested explanations have included diet, but defective case-identification and the shifting demography of the elderly are more likely; as elderly populations age, more cases of Alzheimer's appear until these become a majority (Ineichen, 1996a). A similar situation has been reported from Russia, and here the explanation of over-diagnosis of vascular (or multi-infarct) dementia has been offered (Shefer, 1987).

A number of studies from China (Ineichen, 1996b), Nigeria (Hendrie et al, 1994, 1995; Hall et al, 1994), and of Cree Indians in Canada (Hendrie et al, 1993) have reported low rates for dementia, especially Alzheimer's disease. The most likely explanation appears to be under-reporting of cases, but further work is needed to clarify this point.

Other differences have been shown in the composition of populations and subpopulations which result in a different pattern of dementia subtypes. The large European meta-study of all types of dementia mentioned earlier (Hofman et al, 1991) found the largest differences in the rates of MID for males. The authors suggest this may be the result of different patterns of heart and circulation illnesses among males in the different European countries involved. Richards and Brayne (1996) report an excess of strokes, hypertension and diabetes among African-Americans. Surveys from Korea (Park et al, 1994) and some from Scandinavia report higher rates than elsewhere for alcohol-related dementia, largely among males.

Case identification cross-culturally presents difficulties (Pollitt, 1996) which have been faced up to, for example by the translation of one of the best-used tests, the MMSE, into many languages (Chandra et al, 1994). Cultural differences in its performance remain, affected by education level and by culture: Chinese have better recall, but Finns and Americans did better when asked to copy a figure (Salmon et al, 1989). Gurland et al (1995) applied a range of scales to a sample of white, black and Hispanic Americans. They found marked variation in the estimates of dementia generated in the three groups by the various scales. The greatest agreement between the scales occurred when the measures for identifying the lowest rates of dementia were used.

Other experimental difficulties remain. The recording of precise age cannot be guaranteed: under-reporting of age is commonly reported, for example, in one sample from India (Srinivasan et al, 1993) and Chinese informants may add an extra year (Kua et al, 1996). Such doubts must remain from any country which has not had written registration of births from early in this century.

Other sources of error include: informants may offer responses they perceive to be acceptable to the interviewer, rather than accurate; they may expect questions to be addressed to the head of the household; wives may be reluctant to answer in front of their husbands; questions about matters deemed personal may be resisted (Pollitt, 1996).

Folk views of dementia have received almost no attention from researchers. Do different cultures differ in identifying what constitutes dementia? Universal distinctions are made between 'intact' old people, 'who are likely to be accorded high status and deference and who have been the subject of most of the work on the anthropology of old age', and 'decrepit' old people, who 'even in those societies in which old age is honoured . . . may be mistreated or even killed' (Pollitt, 1996). In some societies (Pollitt quotes the Eskimo, the Marind Amin of South New Guinea, and the Tiwi of Northern Australia) physically helpless old people were killed. She also quotes studies of South Sea Island societies where the mentally impaired elderly were considered 'socially dead' or received at best minimal care. Other Oceanic societies regard their demented elderly very differently, as neither mad nor diseased, but simply as subject to an inevitable process of life. Pollitt concludes that dementia is coterminous neither with abnormality nor decrepitude. Other descriptions of folk views are rare. Relatives in Benares, India, were more willing to identify personality changes, rather than memory loss, as signs of senile decline (Cohen, 1995).

ACCEPTING THE MEDICAL MODEL

Is dementia accepted universally as a medical problem, and if so, which professionals are more appropriate to provide care and assistance to the demented and their relatives in the first instance? None will be consulted if relatives do not perceive dementia in the sufferer, or are fatalistic about old-age decline (Chandra et al, 1994; Iliffe, 1997).

European studies reveal differences in the level of acceptance of the medical model of dementia. In Britain, recourse to medical help is not sought in every case: some relatives do not see dementia as a medical problem, but rather a normal aspect of ageing (Pollitt, 1994). Social class may be an influence on this decision: middle-class carers tend to regard the GP as an ally with a wider social role than do working-class people, who see him or her in narrower, more medical terms (Atkin, 1992). Only a small minority of elderly people who suffered from forgetfulness or confusion in one working-class area of London had reported their symptoms to their GP (Bowling, 1989). Iliffe (1997) reports that research from Italy and Belgium found a variety of reasons why the diagnosis of dementia was delayed, by patients or their primary physicians: respect for the elderly patient; the attribution of problems to normal ageing; and the negligible effect of the problem on daily living. Once made (often because of some crisis event), the diagnosis might be greeted by relatives with disbelief or fear. British GPs may prefer to keep patients under medical control by referring them to a psycho-geriatrician, and resist involving non-medical sources of help, which are outside their control. Patients and their carers may resist psychiatric referral because of its perceived stigma (Ineichen, 1994).

Not all groups consider that Western doctors are the best people to consult. Many Africans, Japanese and Koreans feel this way (Leighton et al, 1963; Chandra et al, 1994). The Yoruba in Nigeria, according to Leighton et al, see mental illness as 'African' illness and possess no word for senility.

The Chinese are particularly interesting in this respect. In China they seek medical help for strokes more readily than for Alzheimer's (Liu et al, 1994; Park et al, 1994) and do not seek medical help at all for failing memory (Ineichen, 1996b). Even Chinese-Americans retain many values from their homeland, holding beliefs about the cause of dementia lying in retribution for past sins, spirit possession, inbalance of yin and yang, and the consequences of astrological activity. They are more likely to seek help from a Chinese rather than a Western doctor (Elliott et al, 1996).

CONCEPTS OF CARE: AT HOME

The number of old people who live alone has been rising steadily in all European countries for which figures are available, Australia, New Zealand, Japan and the USA, throughout the second half of the twentieth century, although the rates for different countries remain well distanced. Scandinavian and German-speaking countries rose from about 20 to 35% during this period. Japan increased from 7% at the 1975 Census to 10% in 1985. Rates are particularly high among the very elderly, rising to 66% of over-80s in Denmark (Sundstrom, 1992).

As a corollary, the proportion of elderly people who live with their children has been decreasing in almost every developed country; in a number of cases this has been happening very dramatically, the figure for Finland, for example, falling from 55% in 1950 to 14% in 1987; even in Japan from 82% in 1960 to 65% in 1985 (Sundstrom, 1992, Table 2.2). Nevertheless, many surveys have shown that over half of the elderly people who do not live with their children have one living within half-an-hour's travelling (Sundstrom, 1992, p.32).

However, the majority of over-65s live with other people in every country for which figures are available. A number of European and North American studies have found that 'informal' carers look after two or three times as many elderly people as do 'formal' professional carers. In the Scandinavian countries, about 25% of women can expect to care for one or both parents at some time (Sundstrom, 1992). The most immediate source of help for dementia sufferers is their family member (spouse, daughter or whoever) who lives with them.

Many of those caring for a demented elderly relative find the experience stressful (Donaldson et al, 1997; Lightbody and Gilhooly, 1997), and many will have competing commitments: care of their own children and grand-children, and the need to work. The proportion of middle-aged women who work has risen markedly in every developed country for which figures are available, between 1971 and 1990 (Sundstrom, 1992, Table 2.5, p. 34) although rates for women aged 55–64, probably the peak age-group for caring for the elderly, are appreciably lower than those aged 45–54.

Many old people continue to live with their spouses, and the importance of such sources of help has been recognised by some governments (in Finland, Norway and Sweden) who pay spouses a cash allowance for looking after their dependent partner. These countries are, along with Denmark, those that provide the highest level of professional home help for elderly people (Sundstrom, 1992, Table 2.8, p. 41). Against charges that this makes people too dependent on the state, Sipila (1994) points out that many women are in paid employment in these countries, and thus carers who stay at home may make a considerable financial sacrifice; many women are politically active; and keeping old people out of institutional care saves money for the authorities. In Britain and some other countries carers may be eligible for an Attendance Allowance paid to someone who cares constantly for a dependent. Other countries vary in the extent to which relatives are liable for the upkeep of elderly family members, or have to pay for services provided by the State.

The number of elderly people living with their children has probably been decreasing steadily in poorer countries also. Allied with this is a decrease in respect for the elderly in developing countries once their health begins to fail (Levkoff et al, 1995).

Even in societies where the status of the elderly has traditionally been seen as high, there is evidence of change. This has been reported from China (Ineichen, in press) and Japan (Nakomo et al, 1996). Filial piety may inhibit children from taking a parent to a Western trained psychiatrist (Sung, 1990). Research in Seoul (Choi, 1993) and Tokyo (Koyano, 1996) finds that caring for elderly parents by the oldest son is increasingly compromised. Yet a preference of elderly people for caring by the extended family remains, according to evidence from Japan; but studies from a number of Western countries have found elderly people do not relish this situation, and support for 'formal' public services such as home helps may be growing (Sundstrom, 1992; Lock, 1993).

Three other reasons inhibit the help that relatives may provide: a fatalistic view that nothing can be done (Chandra et al, 1994); fear of the supernatural (Pollitt, 1996); and the fear that the family will be stigmatised, reported from Japan (Maeda et al, 1989) and India (Cohen, 1995), or its honour damaged in many Asian cultures by having a member with a 'weak mind' (Smith, 1996).

Differing concepts of care are likely within countries such as the US, which have large ethnic minorities. By 2020, an estimated 22% of Americans over 65 will be native Americans, African-Americans, Asian-Americans or Hispanics. Such groups may vary in their abilities with the English language, making the assessment of dementia difficult; cultural attitudes towards behaviour change in old age, attitudes within families, and towards professional workers all may differ (Yeo, 1996).

US ethnic minorities, according to Smith (1996), vary in their approach to caring for a demented elderly relative. African-American caregivers have more support from their extended families than whites, leading them to regard the experience generally more favourably. They are reluctant to use formal services, especially those involving residential care. Religion helps them to cope. Hispanics also enjoy good support from extended families, but those who adhere too strongly to the norm of filial respect find their burden difficult. Native Americans cope well with their frail elderly parents, according to one study (nothing has been written about dementia); among Asian-Americans much of the burden falls on young married women, who may find themselves caring for their husband's parents, and having to juggle this demand on their time with those from their husbands and children. Hispanics and Asians, the newly arrived groups, may find the younger generations assuming more mainstream US life-styles, and adopting the primacy of nuclear over extended family values.

Relatively little evidence has been gathered on ethnic variations in the way the burden of caring in other culturally diverse societies such as Israel, South Africa, or the United Kingdom has been reported. Cultural influences on the extent of help provided by informal carers, the type of assistance they are expected to provide, and the role of non-household kin, and neighbours, are also relatively neglected subjects. Donaldson et al (1997) review the impact of dementia on caregivers in 17 surveys, but do not mention cultural differences, nor even list the countries in which these surveys took place.

Help provided in sufferers' homes by paid workers depends on the culture, or more specifically on the kind of service organisation that exists, which will differ from country to country, and in some countries from area to area. In the United Kingdom, for instance, home helps were introduced in 1945 to provide assistance with matters such as shopping and cleaning the home, and have now spread to many other countries. By 1985 they were assisting 9% of the British elderly population; in Sweden they helped almost 40% of the over-80s in 1975, although now the figure is below 25% (Malmberg, 1997).

An increasing proportion of their clients suffer from a degree of dementia. The level of service provision, and the cost to users, varies from country to country, and in Britain from one local authority to another. Service refusal among demented old people and their carers is common. Reasons given include the carer's refusal to admit the need for help, a refusal to pay charges, the refusal of the demented person to admit a stranger into the house, the carer's feelings of shame at the state of the house, or that the kind of help offered was not appropriate (Ineichen, 1989; Levin et al, 1989).

Other workers who might feature in the help offered to a demented old person in Britain are various kinds of nurses, social workers and workers provided by a variety of voluntary (i.e. non-State) organisations. The mix of such workers varies greatly from one part of the country to another, and service refusal affects them all (Ineichen, 1989); some may work on experimental, short-term schemes. Some may work exclusively with demented clients, others with a wider range of old people or the mentally ill. A specialised service of community mental health nurses who work with the elderly has been found to be very successful. Social workers are valued for their emotional support, and their help in achieving access to other kinds of desired help, but have been criticised by other workers for their slowness of response (Ineichen, 1994).

Day care is provided for large numbers of demented old people: 12 000 in Sweden, for example. They relieve relatives and home helps of the caring task for part of the day, and attempt to preserve the intellectual and social functioning of their clients (Malmberg, 1997).

In a number of countries, either the State or charitable sources provide temporary 'Respite care' by providing holiday breaks for demented elderly people, either with or without the caring relative accompanying them.

CONCEPTS OF CARE: AWAY FROM HOME

The help available from family members is influenced by the extent to which institutional care is available. In developed countries, about 30% of old people spend their last days away from their home, in some kind of institutional care. Age, and level of frailty, at admission, is probably growing, and the period of residence probably shortening (Sundstrom, 1995). Of course, elderly people may be admitted to institutions earlier on a temporary basis.

The number of places in old peoples' homes and hospitals varies hugely from country to country. Even in Europe, the proportion of old people in long-stay care at any one time is 11–12% in the Netherlands, but less than half that figure in neighbouring France and Belgium. Very little of this variation can be explained by differences in age-structure (Cooper, 1994).

In poorer countries, the percentage is much lower, and subject to even greater variation. In some, institutional care is scarcely present. Relatives are expected to look after the oldest family members, including the demented. For example, all of Shaji et al's (1996) Indian sample of demented old people were cared for at home by relatives. Of a Taiwanese sample of carers 10% anticipated institutional care for their elderly relative (Wu and Chu, 1996).

There is a variety of types of care away from home, ranging from the scarcely separated 'granny annexe' in which the old person lives in a separate household within the same building as younger kin, to the long-stay hospital ward. Granny annexes and sheltered housing are found increasingly in Western countries. They may be suitable for an elderly relative suffering from mild to moderate dementia, but are in short supply, and unlikely to be used for a dementing elder unless he or she is in residence before the dementia develops. The growing popularity in Britain of 'very sheltered housing' which provides a higher level of support than a daily visit from a warden may prove to be a very valuable service for demented old people, enabling them to preserve an independent way of life.

Retirement communities are popular in the USA. The degree of support they offer demented residents is debatable: each community may develop an idiosyncratic response.

One important consequence of the growing numbers of demented old people in developed countries has been the establishment of forms of residential care specifically designed for their needs. Innovative schemes have come from France, Sweden, Australia, and the United Kingdom. All emphasise the desirability of a 'homelike' environment.

In France the 'cantou' (the word means 'fireside') has been described as typically consisting of 'individual rooms opening on to a large combined kitchen and living area. Residents are encouraged to bring their own furnishings. Meals are prepared by the house mothers in the common area and residents are encouraged to participate as far as possible in the preparation and cleaning up. It is generally assumed that the cantou resident will stay until his death, with additional medical and nursing care being provided if necessary in the terminal stages of the illness.' Times for dressing and washing are flexible (Ritchie et al, 1992).

Group homes in Sweden have very similar aims. Small units are preferred, each providing six to eight flats clustered round a shared living room and kitchen. Common areas are furnished with old-fashioned items, and residents are encouraged to bring their own possessions with them. A homely atmosphere is fostered, and results suggest that group homes are cheaper than the alternatives (Wimo et al, 1997) and are successful with residents who are neither severely disruptive nor very demented (Malmberg, 1997).

In Australia, 'lodges' providing for dementia sufferers to live as a family group were set up in the State of Victoria in the 1970s. Parallel developments have been the creation of special hostels for mobile dementia sufferers, and the establishment of CADE (confused and disturbed elderly) units providing a homelike residential atmosphere for small groups of dementia sufferers (Cooper, 1994). Cooking on CADE premises, and involving residents in food purchase and preparation, helps to prevent the 'de-skilling' that so often accompanies the entry into institutional life (Malone, 1997).

A deliberate attempt to cater for cultural diversity in Australia is the Old Timers' Hostel in Alice Springs, designed for the different needs of demented people of Aboriginal and non-Aboriginal background, all of whom had lived their lives in the bush, and for whom a residential home in a city would not have been desirable. 'Family' living is not considered appropriate. 'Good neighbouring' is the prime concept. Privacy may be less important than the ability to share life in public for such a clientele, especially the Aboriginals, and the design of the hostel reflects this. Bedrooms cluster around a central sitting area which opens directly to the outside. In this way, this area can be a meeting place, and the comings and goings of residents can be observed. People may interact with those who choose to sit outside around the campfire. Sitting outside may be preferred to sitting in a lounge (Bennett, 1997).

The British version of a residential home designed specifically for demented residents is known as a 'domus'. Residents are encouraged to do as much as possible for themselves, even if this entails risk. It has been shown to provide a higher quality of care than a hospital ward, although it can be more expensive (Ineichen, submitted).

Residents in residential homes for the elderly have been admitted at ever-older ages, with rising levels of disability, according to evidence in the United Kingdom. Numbers suffering from dementia or confusion have ranged from 14 to 87% (Ineichen, submitted). This experience is likely to be mirrored in many other countries: in the county of Jonkoping, in Sweden, for instance, only about one third of its 5200 residents are rated mentally alert (Malmberg, 1997).

One key debate has centred on the relative merits of segregating or integrating demented residents. Arguments for segregation include the easier recruitment of interested staff, the possibility of specially designed environments, more effective treatment and better research, and reduced risk to non-demented residents. Those against include lower cost; problems in deciding admission criteria and recruiting staff; unduly low staff expectations of residents; and the provision of care closer to residents' homes, with a lower likelihood of having to move once admitted (Ineichen, submitted).

Nursing homes provide for a huge market in the USA. Many incorporate special care units. By some estimates about half of all residents are demented; given its size and heterogeneity, assessing the quality of nursing home care for the demented is not easy (Ineichen, submitted).

The number of hospital beds for the mentally ill has declined sharply in most Western countries over the past three or four decades (Cooper, 1994). However, hospitals remain the traditional location of care for many of the most severely afflicted dementia patients, and those with major accompanying physical problems.

CONCLUSION

Treatment of the elderly appears to vary in many cases with the level of affluence a society enjoys. In very poor societies, elderly people may be left to die (Pollitt, 1996). In nomadic societies, they may be seen as a burden. In peasant societies, little may be expected of them, with consequences for the identification and care of the demented. Chandra et al (1994) state that in such settings 'many potentially treatable sources of disability, including memory loss, are tolerated as part of natural ageing' leading to non-reporting, non-intervention, and potentially worse outcomes. It seems likely that even in wealthy societies, some demented old people are still left to die, but this may be due increasingly to their difficult personalities, or to inefficiency within the services, rather than by deliberate policy.

Mild dementia may be accommodated, severe dementia not, in both Western and non-Western societies; though the distinction may not correspond to Western clinical practice (Pollitt, 1996). Cultural influences on responses to dementia in many non-Western societies remain relatively unexplored.

The rising number of elderly with dementia has been fuelled by higher life expectancy, and has been accompanied by rising levels of State welfare. Cultural variations influence this activity too.

It is probably generally agreed that State provision for dependent elderly, including the demented, is most advanced in Scandinavia. Sundstrom (1992, p. 48) has described the process of growth there of welfare:

> the product of culturally homogeneous societies with relatively minor social cleavages, and an above-average belief in the concept of 'the good State'. In these countries the labour movement, and the liberal political parties, wanted to free individuals from what they saw as the tight harness of informal relationships. This has slowly transformed patterns of solidarity, leading to a sharing between family and State of the responsibility for old and frail persons.

Yet simultaneously, the high costs of the welfare state in developed countries, due among other things to the increasing proportion of the population that is elderly, is causing a rethink of benefits such as universal old-age pensions. This is happening even in Scandinavia. At the same time, Sundstrom's 'tight harness of informal relationships' appears to be weakening everywhere. This is happening especially in developing societies, where young people may prefer the enticements of city living to a relatively unchanging life in a rural extended family.

For demented old people, for whom a need for assistance, once a certain level of cognitive decay has occurred, is absolute, the future looks ominous: their children and grandchildren disappearing down the road in the direction of the bright lights, and little prospect of growing State assistance. Organised mutual help, through voluntary groups such as the Alzheimer's Disease Society, may have an increasing role to play.

REFERENCES

Aevarsson, O. and Skoog, I. (1996). A population-based study of the Incidence of Dementia Disorders between 85 and 88 years of age, *J. Am. Ger. Soc.*, **44**, 1455–1460.

Atkin, K. (1992). Similarities and differences between informal carers, in J. Twigg (Ed.), *Carers: Research and Practice*, London, HMSO.

Bennett, K. (1997). Cultural issues in designing for people with dementia, in M. Marshall (Ed.), *State of the Art in Dementia Care*, pp. 164–169, London, Centre for Policy on Ageing.

Bowling, A. (1989). Contact with general practitioners and differences in health among people over 85 years, *Journal of Royal College of General Practitioners*, **39**, 52–55.

Chandra, V., Ganguli, M., Ratcliff, G. et al (1994). Studies of the epidemiology of dementia: comparison between developed and developing countries, *Ageing Clin. Exp. Res.*, **6**, 5, 307–321.

Choi, H. (1993). Cultural and noncultural factors as determinants of caregiver burden for the impaired elderly in South Korea, *Gerontologist*, **33**, 1, 8–15.

Cohen, L. (1995). Toward an anthropology of Senility: anger, weakness and Alzheimer's in Banaras, India, *Med. Anth. Quart.*, **9**, 3, 314–334.

Cooper, B. (1994). Health-care policy and planning for dementia: an international perspective, in F. A. Huppert et al (Eds), *Dementia and Normal Aging*, pp. 519–551, Cambridge, Cambridge University Press.

Donaldson, C., Tarrier, N. and Burns, A. (1997). The impact of the symptoms of dementia on caregivers, *Br. J. Psychiatry*, **170**, 62–68.

Elliott, K. S., Di Minno, M., Lam, D. and Tu, A. M. (1996). Working with Chinese families in the context of dementia, in G. Yeo and D. Gallagher-Thompson, *Ethnicity and the Dementias*, pp. 89–108, Washington, DC, Taylor & Francis.

Ferini-Strambi, L., Marcone, A., Garancini, P. et al (1997). Dementing disorders in North Italy: prevalence study in Vescovato, Cremona Province, *European J. Epidemiology*, **13**, 201–204.

Gurland, B., Wilder, D. E., Cross, P. et al (1995). Screening scales for dementia: toward reconciliation of conflicting cross-cultural findings, in E. Murphy and G. Alexopulos (Eds), *Geriatric Psychiatry: Key Research Topics for Clinicians*, pp. 57–70, Chichester, Wiley.

Hall, K., Ogunniyi, A., Hendrie, H. et al (1994). Community screening for dementia in Indianapolis and Ibadan, Nigeria, *Neurobiology of Aging*, **15**, Suppl 1, S42.

Henderson, A. S. (1994). *Dementia*, Geneva, WHO.

Hendrie, H. C., Hall, K., Pillay, N. et al (1993). Alzheimer's rare in Cree Indians? *Int. Psychogeriatrics*, **5**, 1, 5–14.

Hendrie, H. C., Osuntoken, B., Hall, K. et al (1994). A comparison of the prevalence of dementia and Alzheimer's disease in community dwelling residents of Ibadan, Nigeria and Indianapolis, USA, *Neurobiology of Aging*, **15**, Suppl 1.

Hendrie, H. C., Osuntoken, B., Hall, K. et al (1995). Prevalence of Alzheimer's disease and Dementia in two communities: Nigerian Africans and African Americans, *Am. J. Psychiatry*, **152**, 10, 1485–1492.

Hofman, A., Rocca, W. A., Brayne, C. et al (1991). The Prevalence of Dementia in Europe: a collaborative study of 1980–90 findings, *Int. J. Epidemiology*, **20**, 3, 736–748.

Iliffe, S. (1997). Problems in recognising dementia in general practice: how can they be overcome? In M. Marshall (Ed.), *State of the Art in Dementia Care*, pp. 67–72, London, Centre for Policy on Ageing.

Ineichen, B. (1989). *Senile Dementia: Policy and Services*, London, Chapman & Hall.

Ineichen, B. (1994). Managing demented old people in the community: a review, *Family Practice*, **11**, 2, 210–215.

Ineichen, B. (1996a). Senile dementia in Japan: prevalence and response, *Soc. Sci. Med.*, **42**, 2, 169–172.

Ineichen, B. (1996b). The prevalence of dementia and cognitive impairment in China, *Int. J. Geriatric Psychiatry*, **11**, 695–697.

Ineichen, B. (in press). The geography of dementia: an approach through epidemiology, *Health and Place*.

Ineichen, B. (submitted for publication). Mental Illness in Elderly Residential Care.

Jorm, A. F. (1990). *The Epidemiology of Alzheimer's disease and Related Disorders*, London, Chapman & Hall.

Koyano, W. (1996). Filial piety and intergenerational solidarity in Japan, *Aust. J. on Ageing*, **15**, 2, 51–56.

Kua, E. H., Ko, S. M., Fones, S. L. C. and Tan, S. L. (1996). Comorbidity of Depression in the Elderly: an epidemiological study in a Chinese Community, *Int. J. Geriatric Psychiatry*, **11**, 699–704.

Leighton, A. H., Lambo, T. A., Hughes, C. C. et al (1963). *Psychiatric Disorder among the Yoruba*. Ithaca, NY, Cornell University Press.

Levin E., Sinclair, T. and Gorbach, P. (1989). *Families, Services and Confusion in Old Age*. Aldershot, UK, Avebury.

Levkoff, S. E., Macarthur, I. W. and Bucknall, J. (1995). Elderly mental health in the developing world, *Soc. Sci. Med.*, **41**, 7, 983–1003.

Lightbody, P. and Gilhooly, M. (1997). The continuing quest for predictors of breakdown of family care of elderly people with dementia, in M. Marshall (Ed.), *State of the Art in Dementia Care*, pp. 211–216, London, Centre for Policy on Ageing.

Liu, H. C., Chou, P., Lin, K. N. et al (1994). Assessing cognitive abilities and dementia in a predominantly illiterate population of older individuals in Kinmen, *Psych. Med.*, **24**, 763–770.

Lock, M. (1993). Ideology, female midlife and the greying of Japan, *J. Japanese Studies*, **19**, 43.

Maeda, D., Teshima, K., Sugisawa, H. and Asakura, Y. S. (1989), Aging and mental health in Japan, *J. Cross-Cultural Gerontology*, **4**, 2, 143–162.

Malmberg, B. (1997). Group homes: an alternative for older people with dementia, in M. Marshall (Ed.), *State of the Art in Dementia Care*, pp. 78–82, London, Centre for Policy on Ageing.

Malone, L. (1997). Mealtime experiences, in M. Marshall (Ed.), *State of the Art in Dementia Care*, pp. 175–178, London, Centre for Policy on Ageing.

McCracken, C. F. M., Boneham, M. A., Copeland, J. R. M. et al (1997). Prevalence of dementia and depression among elderly people in Black and ethnic minorities, *Brit. J. Psychiatry*, **171**, 269–273.

Nakamo, I., Shimizu, Y., Hiraoka, K. et al (1996), Measuring the social-care service needs of impaired elderly people in Japan, *Ageing and Society*, **16**, 315–332.

Park, J., Ko, H. J., Park, Y. N. and Jung, C-H. (1994). Dementia among the elderly in a rural Korean community, *Brit. J. Psychiatry*, **164**, 796–801.

Pollitt, P. A. (1994). The meaning of dementia to those involved as carers, in F. A. Huppert et al (Eds), *Dementia and Normal Aging*, pp. 257–271, Cambridge, Cambridge University Press.

Pollitt, P. (1996). Dementia in old age: an anthropological perspective, *Psych. Med.*, **26**, 1061–1074.

Richards, M. and Brayne, C. (1996). Cross-cultural research into cognitive impairment and dementia: some practical consequences, *Int. J. Geriatric Psychiatry*, **11**, 383–387.

Ritchie, K., Colvez, A., Ankri, J. et al (1992). The evaluation of long-term care for the dementing elderly, *Int. J. Geriatric Psychiatry*, **7**, 549–557.

Rocca, W. A., Hofman, A., Brayne, C. et al (1991). Frequency and distribution of

Alzheimer's Disease in Europe: a collaborative study of 1980–1990 prevalence findings, *Ann. Neurol.*, **30**, 381–390.

Salmon, D. P., Riekkinen, P. J., Katzman, R. et al (1989). Cross-cultural studies of dementia: a comparison of MMSE performance in Finland and China, *Arch. Neurol.*, **46**, 769–772.

Shaji, S., Promodu, K., Abraham, T. et al (1996). An epidemiological study of dementia in a rural community in Kerala, India, *Brit. J. Psychiatry*, **168**, 745–749.

Shefer, V. F. (1987). Hypo- and hyperdiagnosis of senile dementia and Alzheimer's Disease in psychiatric practice, *J. Neuropathology and Psychiatry*, **87**, 897–898.

Silverman, J. M., Li, G., Schear, S. et al (1992). A cross-cultural family history study of primary progressive dementia in relatives of nondemented elderly Chinese, Italians, Jews and Puerto Ricans, *Acta Psychiatrica Scandinavica*, **85**, 211–217.

Sipila, J. (1994). Why do the Scandinavian governments compensate family members who care for elderly kin? *Care in Place*, **1**, 3.

Smith, A. (1996). Cross-cultural research on Alzheimer's Disease: a critical review, *Transcultural Psychiatric Research Review*, **33**, 3, 247–276.

Srinivasan, T. N., Suresh, T. R. and Rajkumar, S. (1993). Age estimation in the elderly: relevance to geriatric research in developing countries, *Indian Journal of Psychiatry*, **35**, 1, 58–59.

Sundstrom, G. (1992). Care by families; an overview of trends, in *Caring for Frail Elderly People*, Paris, OECD.

Sundstrom, G. (1995). Ageing is riskier than it looks, *Age and Ageing*, **24**, 373–374.

Sung, K. (1990). A new look at filial piety: ideals and practices of family-centered parent care in Korea, *Gerontologist*, **30**, 5, 610–617.

Wallin, A. (1996). Current definition and classification of dementia diseases, *Acta Neurol. Scand.*, Suppl. 168, 39–44.

Wimo, A., Lunggren, G. and Winblad, B. (1997). Costs of dementia and dementia care, *Int. J. Geriat. Psychiat.*, **12**, 841–856.

Wu, S. C. and Chu, C.-M. (1996). Public attitudes toward long-term care arrangements of the elderly in Taiwan, *Australian J. Ageing*, **15**, 2.

Yeo, G. (1996). Background, in *Ethnicity and the Dementias* (Eds G. Yeo and D. Gallagher-Thompson), pp. 3–7, Washington DC, Taylor & Francis.

1.7   Interaction with People Suffering Severe Dementia

ASTRID NORBERG

Department of Nursing, Umeå University, Sweden

People develop and maintain their sense of self in interaction with other people. In old age people are struggling to achieve an experience of integrity, that is wholeness and meaning (Erikson, 1982). This is no easy task even for healthy elderly people who often use reminiscence as a means of achieving this sense of integrity. This method, however, presupposes memory of past events as well as anticipations about the future. Interaction and communication with others can facilitate the process. Dementia symptoms, however, make every aspect of the task very difficult and mean a risk that the patient feels isolated. In this paper the term dementia will denote Alzheimer's disease and the paper will especially concern people suffering severe dementia.

Difficulties with interaction are connected with problems of memory, especially short-term episodic memory, with language, perception, attention, comprehension, and so on (APA, 1994). In the final stage of Alzheimer's disease the patient is often mute (Bayles et al, 1992). Non-verbal communication may be hindered, for example by the fact that facial expressions may be reduced (APA, 1994, p. 134; Asplund et al, 1993, 1995). All these symptoms make communication difficult. There is, however, evidence that some people suffering severe dementia express a range of affective signals (e.g. Magai et al, 1996) which makes it possible to reach them by means of emotional communication. One consequence of the fact that people suffering severe dementia are considered to be context-bound and find abstract thinking a problem (APA, 1994) and that they are very sensitive to environmental influences (e.g. Corcoran and Gitlin, 1991) is that their competence to interact varies in relation to the physical and psychological environment (cf. Svensson, 1984, p. 36 based on Lawton, 1982).

A MEANING BEHIND BEHAVIOUR

Several researchers have pointed to the lack of research about the lived experience of people suffering severe dementia, for example the experience

Health Economics of Dementia. Edited by Anders Wimo, Bengt Jönsson, Göran Karlsson and Bengt Winblad.
© 1998 John Wiley & Sons Ltd.

behind so-called behavioural disturbances (e.g. Ballard and Oyebode, 1995). Some attempts to interpret the experience have been made. Hallberg and Norberg (1990) for example made an assumption that patients with vocally disruptive behaviour and severe dementia expressed an experience of primitive types of anxiety, such as anxiety about abandonment and separation, by screaming. Hurley et al (1992) suggest that expressions of well-being and ill-being could be understood. Aggressive behaviour has been shown to be related to invasion of the private sphere, for example during bathing and feeding (e.g. Cohen-Mansfield et al, 1989; Rossby et al, 1992; Hallberg et al, 1995). Patients suffering severe dementia often search for their home and display a feeling of not being at home (Zingmark et al, 1993). A similar phenomenon has been described by Miesen (1992) as 'a strange situation' in which the patients feel unsafe. In such a situation the patients exhibit attachment behaviour, for example by trying to be close to carers, touching and calling after them. When the memory dysfunction increases the patient is in a situation that is reminiscent of bereavement, and may enter a phase similar to parent fixation, that is behaves as if the parents were present (Miesen, 1993). This can happen in the state in which the patient loses the awareness of a boundary between the inner and the outer world.

OUTLOOK ON THE DEMENTIA SUFFERER

The way carers perceive people suffering severe dementia seems essential for whether or not they try to interpret behaviour as carrying messages about the patients' lived experience. The presence or lack of such interpretations is of crucial importance for their interaction with the patients.

There are care providers who see the patient suffering severe dementia as an object and those who see the patient as a subject (Athlin et al, 1990). Too often the carers focus on the patients' losses and deficits. Liukkonen (1992) has found that the carers at ward in an institution regarded the patients from the perspective of their missing abilities and the problems they caused rather than from the perspective of remaining abilities, such as humour and the abilities to communicate through touch. The losses are often valued negatively. Asplund and Norberg (1993) report that professional carers responded differently to a picture of a person suffering severe dementia and to a picture of an infant. A person suffering severe dementia was described by means of negatively loaded words such as being apathetic, weak, cold, dark, rough, and ugly whereas the infant evoked positive responses.

The carers' outlook on the patients will influence whether or not they will try to understand their communicative cues and thereby influence the patients' well-being. It seems reasonable that the carers' view of the patients will affect the patients directly by the fact that it will be mirrored in their eyes (cf. Barnett, 1995). Angus et al (1991) describe mutual gaze as validating/invalidating the existence of another and as the most direct means of communication. Carers of patients suffering severe dementia sometimes feel that they can understand what the patient means by eye contact (e.g. Norberg et al, 1986).

INGRESSION

The negative view of the patient with dementia is mirrored in the term demented (no soul). The fact that patients suffering severe dementia have been said to regress to a second childhood is another indication of the devaluation of the patient. Berg-Brodén (1992) has suggested that the term 'ingression' would be a more proper term than 'regression' to describe adult use of early developed behaviour.

Thus people suffering severe dementia can be seen as ingressing to a state that in many respects resembles that of infancy (e.g. Hurley et al, 1992; Sandman et al, 1990; Sclan et al, 1990). For example they exhibit clinging and demanding behaviour that can be understood as attachment-seeking behaviour (Wright et al, 1995). This, however, does not mean that the patients are like infants, they just use primitive (early developed) ways of communicating when ways which demand abilities that are blocked by the disease are not available.

EPISODES OF PSYCHOLOGICAL LUCIDITY

Patients suffering severe dementia may suddenly and unexpectedly utter a few comprehensible phrases that show that they are aware of the situation, sometimes even aware of their own situation. These kinds of phenomena can be labelled episodes of lucidity (Norberg, 1996). Such experiences have been described by, for example, Norberg et al (1986) based on video-recordings of sensory stimulation of a mute patient suffering severe dementia, by Åkerlund and Norberg (1986) based on video-recordings of patients with moderate and severe dementia communicating with other patients; by Bleathman and Morton (1992) from validation therapy; by Bright (1992) in connection with listening to music; by Kitwood and Bredin (1992) when intersubjectivity was established with the care provider; by Sabat and Harré (1992, p. 452) in a 'heightened emotional state'; by Kitwood (1993) in settings where care was centred on the person; by Gibson (1994) in connection with reminiscence work; and by Ekman et al (1993) and Kihlgren et al (1994, 1996) based on video-recordings during integrity-promoting interaction with carers.

POSITIVE INTERACTIONS BETWEEN DEMENTIA SUFFERERS AND CARERS

There are many descriptions of negative interaction between dementia sufferers and carers, that is interactions that make the patients agitated, withdrawing and the like. In this paper however, I will describe a few reports about positive interactions, that is interactions that enhance the patients' sense of well-being and overt competence

Kihlgren et al (1994, 1996) trained the staff working in a ward at a nursing home in integrity-promoting care, that is care that promotes the patient's experience of trust, autonomy, initiative, industry, identity, intimacy, generativity and integrity (wholeness and meaning) during all care activities. The model was inspired by the Erikson (1982) theory of the 'eight stages of man'. Patients who communicated in a fragmented way changed and appeared to be much more integrated in the integrity-promoting climate, even disclosing competence and strengths that had previously been hidden. Kihlgren (1992) interpreted the findings as being related to motherly support and preservative love and confirmation of the person suffering severe dementia as a valuable human being. It is evident that the care providers in this study were focusing on the experiences of their patients.

Ekman et al (1993) compared video-recordings of interaction during morning care sessions between bilingual patients with moderate or severe dementia and carers who spoke the patients' mother tongue and those who did not, and found that the patients disclosed a competence that had hitherto been hidden in interaction with the bilingual carers. An interpretation of the interactions showed that the positive interactions could be understood as promoting integrity in the same manner as the interactions described by Kihlgren et al (1994).

PROMOTION OF INTERACTION

There are several suggestions in the literature of how interaction between patients suffering severe dementia and carers can be promoted.

People with dementia have problems keeping track of who said what in a conversation involving more than one participant (Alberoni et al, 1992). They have problems simultaneously comprehending spoken language and making a spatial and facial identification of the speakers. This is especially difficult when the dementia sufferer is not addressed directly. These problems make it difficult for them to take part in group activities. These people communicate better in face-to-face interaction.

Harlan (1993) describes how art work can be used to communicate with people with dementia in order to preserve a sense of identity, to facilitate the venting of emotions and to counteract social isolation. Her idea is that although the patient's art may be characterised by 'simplicity, regression, disorganisation, and confusion of perspective' it can be seen from the point of view of how it expresses any remaining strengths and attempts to cope, for example by painting images associated with safety. It can help the carer to gain access to the patient's inner world both through its content and through the carer listening to the patient's comments while the art work is being accomplished. There are several reports that patients suffering severe dementia can be reached through music (e.g. Norberg et al, 1986; Casby and Holm, 1994).

Reminiscence therapy seems to facilitate communication, for example by working individually and focusing on automatic processes rather than on conscious, effortful strategies (for review see Woods, 1996). Mills and Coleman (1994) report on conversations aimed at stimulating nostalgic memories in a patient with moderate to severe dementia. They started with the assumption that emotions can be well preserved and support the patient in recalling past memories. They emphasised that an emotionally loaded memory gives a meaning to life. The authors stress that given time and patience it was possible to help them remember. They also emphasise that some knowledge of the patient's social history is necessary in order to interpret fragmented messages and also provide adequate cues and prompts during the conversation. They believe that remembering emotionally loaded personal events leads to well-being and an experience of meaning and thus enhances personhood. Such activities also help carers to see the patient as a 'whole' human being.

Crisp (1995) describes a case and discusses the meaning of story telling in people with dementia. She emphasises that although the patient may confabulate and mix reality and fantasy the fact that they are able to narrate, that is let events occur in a time sequence linked by cause and effect and relate the end of the story to the opening situation, is an indication of a preserved ability. She has also made the observation that the telling of a story may give the teller amusement and pleasure. It may be possible to grasp the main point—the underlying message or thematic and metaphoric meaning of the story. It may foster interaction and help create an experience of order and sense (wholeness and meaning) and of identity and self-worth.

Research has claimed that people suffering severe dementia may simultaneously be and not be aware of their situation (Miesen, 1993). They may communicate about the present by using material from their past. Kitwood (1993) and Kitwood and Bredin (1992), Harrison (1993) as well as Gibson (1994) argue that care providers should listen with an open mind and try to grasp the emotional content of the message. By listening again and again to the patient the message may become more and more fully expressed and the carer can gradually build up an understanding of its content. The carer helps the patients to fill in missing parts in their message, to create a whole of fragments. The carers thus fulfil the patients' initiated actions.

COMMUNION

Sometimes it does not seem possible to get into cognitive contact with the patient, but still an emotional contact may be possible. This contact can be labelled communion.

There were for example sequences in video-recordings of the interaction of Finnish speaking carers with Finnish immigrants suffering severe dementia which indicated that the patients reacted to the melody of the speech rather than to the words, that is a kind of communion occurred (Ekman, 1993, p. 139). This observation is reminiscent of observations that infants react to the tone of their mothers' voices (cf. Fernald et al, 1989), which can also be seen as communion (cf. Stern 1985, p. 148). The term 'communion' denotes a deep contact with no demands being made on the other. The quality of this contact seems to be 'love'.

Carers at a group dwelling for people with moderate and severe dementia, who were also observed caring for residents, often referred to their personal experiences of being mothers of children or being daughters of mothers when they tried to explain how they could understand what the residents expressed (Häggström and Norberg, 1996).

Communion seems to occur even if the parties relate to a different time and space. The important prerequisite for communion seems to be a shared affective state, rather than a shared cognitive interpretation of that state.

In situations that occurred at a group dwelling characterised by communion, there was an understanding without words in a calm atmosphere where no demands were made on the patients, who seemed to experience a feeling of 'being at home' (Zingmark et al, 1993). In these situations the carers were observed to move flexibly in 'time' and 'space'.

Although it is not possible to get into a cognitive contact with some patients suffering severe dementia, the carers can interpret the patient's behaviour and her own feelings in a way reminiscent of a mother's imputation of meaning in her infant's cues (Pawlby, 1977). Carers can start with a preunderstanding that there is a meaning in the patient's communicative cues and create a narrative that discloses the meaning through the carers participating, actively filling in missing pieces in the puzzle of meaning based on knowledge of the situation and of the patient's life history and care history (cf. Jansson et al, 1993).

There seem to be several means available for carers to interact with patients suffering severe dementia, helping them to maintain their sense of self and achieve an experience of integrity, that is wholeness and meaning, even when they seemingly have lost cognitive abilities. More research is needed on this impalpable subject.

REFERENCES

Alberoni, M., Baddeley A., Della-Sala, S., Logie, R. et al (1992). Keeping track of a conversation: impairments in Alzheimer's disease, *International Journal of Geriatric Psychiatry*, 7, 639–646.

Angus, N. M., Osborne, J. W. and Koziey, P. W. (1991). Window to the soul: a phenomenological investigation of mutual gaze, *Journal of Phenomenological Psychology*, **22**, 142–162.

APA (American Psychiatric Association) (1994). *Diagnostic and Statistical Manual of Mental Disorders Prepared by the Task Force on DSM-IV*, 4th edn, Washington, DC, American Psychiatric Association.

Asplund, K., Jansson, L. and Norberg, A. (1995). Expressive facial behaviour in patients with severe dementia of the Alzheimer type (DAT). A comparison between unstructured naturalistic judgements and analytic assessment by means of the Facial Action Coding System (FACS), *International Psychogeriatrics*, **7**, 527–534.

Asplund, K. and Norberg, A. (1993). Caregivers' reactions to the physical appearance of a person in the final stage of dementia as measured by semantic differentials, *International Journal of Aging and Human Development*, **37**, 205–215.

Athlin, E., Norberg, A. and Asplund, K. (1990). Caregivers' perceptions and interpretations of severely demented patients during feeding in a task assignment care system, *Scandinavian Journal of Caring Sciences*, **4**, 147–156.

Ballard, C. and Oyebode, F. (1995). Psychotic symptoms in patients with dementia, *International Journal of Geriatric Psychiatry*, **10**, 743–752.

Barnett, E. (1995). Broadening our approach to spirituality, in T. Kitwood and S. Benson, *The New Culture of Dementia Care*, pp. 40–43, London, Hawker Publications in Association with the Bradford Dementia Group.

Bayles, K. A., Tomoeda, C. K. and Trosset, M. W. (1992). Relation of linguistic communication abilities of Alzheimer's patients to stage of disease, *Brain and Language*, **42**, 454–472.

Berg-Brodén, M. (1992). *Psykoterapeutiska interventioner under spädbarnsperioden.* (Swedish) (Psychotherapeutic interventions during the period of infancy), Trelleborg, Förlagshuset Swedala.

Bleathman, C. and Morton, I. (1992). Validation therapy: extracts from 20 groups with dementia sufferers, *Journal of Advanced Nursing*, **17**, 658–666.

Bright, R. (1992). Music therapy in the management of dementia, in G. Jones and B. M. L. Miesen (Eds), *Caregiving in Dementia. Research and Applications*, pp. 162–180, London, Routledge.

Casby, J. A. and Holm, M. B. (1994). The effect of music on repetitive disruptive vocalizations of persons with dementia, *American Journal of Occupational Therapy*, **48**, 883–889.

Cohen-Mansfield, J., Marx, M. S. and Rosenthal, A. (1989). A description of agitation in a nursing home, *Journal of Gerontology*, **44**, M77–84.

Corcoran, M. and Gitlin, L. N. (1991). Environmental influences on behaviour of the elderly with dementia: principles for intervention in the home, *Occupational Therapy in Geriatrics*, **9**, 5–20.

Crisp, J. (1995). Making sense of the stories that people with Alzheimer's tell: a journey with my mother, *Nursing Inquiry*, **2**, 133–140.

Ekman, S. L. (1993). *Monolingual and bilingual communication between patients with dementia diseases and their caregivers*, Umeå, Umeå University, Medical Dissertations, New Series No 370.

Ekman, S. L., Robins, Wallin T. B., Norberg, A. and Winblad B. (1993). Relationship between bilingual demented immigrants and bilingual/monolingual caregivers, *International Journal of Aging and Human Development*, **37**, 37–54.

Erikson, E. H. (1982). *The Life Cycle Completed. A Review*, New York, W. W. Norton.

Fernald, A., Taeschner, T., Dunn, J. and Papousek, M. (1989). A cross-language study of prosodic modifications in mothers' and fathers' speech to preverbal infants, *Journal of Child Language*, **16**, 477–501.

Gibson, F. (1994). What can reminiscence contribute to people with dementia? in J. Bornat (Ed.), *Reminiscence Reviewed, Perspectives, Evaluations, Achievements*, pp. 46–60, Buckingham, UK, Open University.

Hallberg, I. R., Holst, G., Nordmark, Å. and Edberg, A. K. (1995). Cooperation during morning care between nurses and severely demented institutionalized patients, *Clinical Nursing Research*, **4**, 78–104.

Hallberg, I. R. and Norberg, A. (1990). Staff's interpretation of the experience behind vocally disruptive behaviour in severely demented patients and their feelings about it, an explorative study, *International Journal of Aging and Human Development*, **31**, 295–305.

Harlan, J. E. (1993). The therapeutic value of art for persons with Alzheimer's disease and related disorders, *Loss, Grief and Care*, **6**, 99–106.

Harrison, C. (1993). Personhood, dementia and the integrity of a life, *Canadian Journal on Aging*, **12**, 428–440.

Hurley, A. C., Volicer, B. J., Hanrahan, P. A., Houde, S. and Volicer, L. (1992). Assessment of discomfort in advanced Alzheimer patients, *Research in Nursing and Health*, **15**, 369–377.

Håggström, T. and Norberg, A. (1996). Maternal thinking in dementia care, *Journal of Advanced Nursing*, **24**, 431–438.

Jansson, L., Norberg, A., Sandman, P. O., Athlin, E. and Asplund, K. (1993). Interpreting facial expressions in patients in the terminal stage of Alzheimer's Disease, *Omega*, **26**, 319–334.

Kihlgren, M. (1992). *Integrity promoting care of demented patients*, Umeå, Umeå University, Medical Dissertations, New Series No 351.

Kihlgren, M., Hallgren, A., Norberg, A. and Karlsson, I. (1994). Integrity promoting care of demented patients. Patterns of interaction during morning care, *International Journal of Aging and Human Development*, **39**, 303–319.

Kihlgren, M., Hallgren, A., Norberg, A. and Karlsson, I. (1996). Disclosure of basic strengths and basic weakness in demented patients during morning care, before and after staff training. Analysis of video-recordings by means of the Erikson theory of 'eight stages of man', *International Journal of Aging and Human Development*, **43**, 219–233.

Kitwood, T. (1993). Towards a theory of dementia care: the interpersonal process, *Ageing and Society*, **13**, 51–67.

Kitwood, T. and Bredin, K. (1992). Towards a theory of dementia care: personhood and well-being, *Aging and Society*, **12**, 269–287.

Lawton, M. P. (1982). Competence, environmental press and the adaptation of older people, in M. P. Lawton, P. G. Windley and T. O. Byerts (Eds), *Aging and the Environment. Theoretical Approaches*, New York, Springer.

Liukkonen, A. (1992). The models of nursing activity in the basic care of demented patients living in institutions, *Vård i Norden*, **12**, 4–8.

Magai, C., Cohen, C., Gomberg, D., Malatesta, C. and Culver C. (1996). Emotional expressions during mid- to late-stage dementia, *International Psychogeriatrics*, **8**, 383–395.

Miesen, B. M. L. (1992). Attachment theory and dementia, in G. Jones and B. M. L. Miesen (Eds), *Caregiving in Dementia. Research and Application*, pp. 38–56, London, Routledge.

Miesen, B. M. L. (1993). Alzheimer's disease, the phenomenon of parent fixation and Bowlby's attachment theory, *International Journal of Geriatric Psychiatry*, **8**, 147–153.

Mills, M. A. and Coleman, P. G. (1994). Nostalgic memories in dementia—a case study, *International Journal of Aging and Human Development*, **38**, 203–219.

Norberg, A. (1996). Caring for demented people, *Acta Neurologica Scandinavica*, **165**, 105–108.

Norberg, A., Melin, E. and Asplund, K. (1986). Reactions to music, touch and object presentation in the final stage of dementia. An exploratory study, *International Journal of Nursing Studies*, **23**, 315–323.

Pawlby, S. J. (1977). Imitative interaction, in H. R. Scaffer, *Studies in Mother-Infant Interaction*, pp. 203–224, London, Academic Press.

Rossby, L., Beck, C. and Heacock, P. (1992). Disruptive behaviors of a cognitively impaired nursing home resident, *Archives Psychiatric Nursing*, **6**, 98–107.

Sabat, S. R. and Harré, T. (1992). The construction and deconstruction of self in Alzheimer's disease, *Ageing and Society*, **12**, 443–461.

Sandman, P. O., Norberg, A., Adolfsson, R., Eriksson, S. and Nyström, L. (1990). Prevalence and characteristics of persons with dependency on feeding at institutions for elderly, *Scandinavian Journal of Caring Sciences*, **4**, 121–127.

Sclan, S. G., Foster, J. R., Reisberg, B., Franssen, E. and Welkowitz, J. (1990). Application of Piagetian measures of cognition in severe Alzheimer's disease, *Psychiatric Journal of the University of Ottawa*, **15**, 223–228.

Stern, D. N. (1985). *The Interpersonal World of the Infant*, New York, Basic Books.

Svensson, T. (1984). *Aging and Environment. Institutional Aspects*, Studies in Education, Dissertations No 21, Linköping, Linköping University, Department of Education and Psychology.

Woods, R. T. (1996). Psychological 'therapies' in dementia, in R. T. Woods (Ed.), *Handbook of the Clinical Psychology of Ageing*, pp. 575–600, Chichester, UK, John Wiley.

Wright, L. K., Hickey, J. V., Buckwalter, K. C. and Clipp, E. C. (1995). Human development in the context of aging and chronic illness: the role of attachment in Alzheimer's disease and stroke, *International Journal of Aging and Human Development*, **41**, 133–150.

Zingmark, K., Norberg, A. and Sandman, P. O. (1993). Experience of at-homeness and homesickness in patients with Alzheimer's disease, *American Journal of Alzheimer's Care and Related Disorders and Research*, **8**, 10–16.

Åkerlund, B. M. and Norberg, A. (1986). Group psychotherapy with demented patients, *Geriatric Nursing*, **7**, 83–84.

1.8 Distress and Burden for Family Caregivers

CAROL J. WHITLATCH

Benjamin Rose Institute, Cleveland, Ohio, USA

Providing care to an older adult with a dementing condition is often associated with a variety of physical and mental health conditions. Substantial empirical evidence indicates that caregivers are in poorer physical health and experience depressed immunologic functioning (Kiecolt-Glaser et al, 1987; Stone et al, 1987; Schulz et al, 1995; Tennstedt et al, 1992), use prescription drugs for depression, anxiety, and insomnia two to three times as often as the rest of the population, and report higher levels of depression, anger, and anxiety (Anthony-Bergstone et al, 1988; Gallagher et al, 1989; Haley et al, 1987). As a result of over 20 years of research, it is now widely accepted that providing care for a person with dementia is stressful and demanding.

Caregiver burden, the term often used to describe the stress experienced by caregivers who provide hands-on care to impaired relatives, has received a great deal of attention from the research, practice, and policy communities. What was once a unidimensional concept reflecting a family caregiver's general level of stress has evolved over the years into a multidimensional phenomenon that applies to both informal and formal caregivers. In describing this transformation, the present chapter will first provide a brief history of family caregiving research and burden. Next, more recent advancements in the study of burden will be presented with an emphasis on innovations in research and intervention. The chapter ends with discussion of future directions for research and intervention.

BRIEF HISTORY OF CAREGIVING AND THE CONCEPT OF CAREGIVER BURDEN

Caregiving is broadly defined as the provision of assistance or care to a family member, friend, or client which enables the care receiver to maintain an optimal level of independence. Caregivers provide assistance that is instrumental, affective, financial, or otherwise of value or necessity to the care receiver.

Health Economics of Dementia. Edited by Anders Wimo, Bengt Jönsson, Göran Karlsson and Bengt Winblad.
© 1998 John Wiley & Sons Ltd.

Caregiving varies in its intensity and duration; care can be provided for one hour per day, for one entire weekend per year, or for 24 hours a day for years at a time. The effects of providing assistance to persons with dementia can be long-term, lasting for many years after care responsibilities have ended.

The care received by millions of older adults comes from a wide variety of sources. Informal care, that is, the care provided or managed by a family member or friend, typically unpaid, is the most preferred and frequently used source of assistance for older adults worldwide (Bris, 1993; Johansson, 1991; Olson, 1994). Yet formal caregivers, that is, paid professionals associated with a service organization or independent contractor, are also responsible for a great deal of support, especially for the millions of older adults who live alone or who have no family or friends available to provide assistance.

The increasing prevalence of family caregiving stems from major social and demographic changes occurring throughout this century. Most notable is the growing percentage of adults aged 65 and older, and particularly those over the age of 85. In the United States, for example, 11% of the 1980 population was 65 years of age or older, whereas in 1993 this percentage had increased to nearly 13%. Moreover, it is projected that by the years 2000 and 2050, 13% and 20%, respectively, of the US population will be at least 65 years old (Subcommittee on Human Services, 1987).

These changes are not unique to the United States. Throughout the world the number of older adults, particularly the oldest old who are most in need of assistance, continues to grow (Freed, 1990; Olson, 1994). One reason for this growth is the development of medical technology that prolongs life without restoring functioning. In turn, families, who provide the majority of assistance with hands-on care and emotional and financial support, must care for their impaired relatives for a longer period. In the United States, for example, 71% of all long-term care is provided in the community, and 85% of all in-home care is provided by family members and friends. Between 5 and 8 million informal caregivers assist community dwelling disabled elderly (American Association of Retired Persons, 1988; Schulz et al, 1995; Stone et al, 1987; Stone and Kemper, 1989). Similarly, in Israel, Sweden, and elsewhere, at least two-thirds of the care needed by frail and disabled elders is provided by family and friends (Guttman, 1994; Johannson and Thorslund, 1991). In addition, because families are becoming smaller and more diversely structured, it is likely that family care will change in its construction and provision. It may be that there will be fewer family members available to provide care. It is also possible that step-children, in-laws, and extended kin will become more involved in caregiving. With changes in family size and structure, it is important that we broaden our view of how family caregiving occurs. In turn, there will be a greater need to develop strategies to care for the growing number of older adults, especially those with dementing conditions.

The outcome of these demographic trends has been viewed by planners and policy makers as a potential 'social problem': with the burgeoning number of elderly in need of long-term care, families would be less willing or able to assume this responsibility. In turn, it was expected that there would be increasing economic pressures on the public sector due to escalating expenditures for long-term care. Consequently, research on family caregiving became a priority for federal funders in the United States during the 1970s and 1980s. Many of the early investigations were primarily descriptive, designed to provide information about the prevalence, nature, and negative consequences of family caregiving (Zarit et al, 1980). Reports from a significant number of caregivers in the study samples lent support to the perspective that caregiving had adverse effects on health and personal well-being, employment, financial status, and family relationships. Later studies commonly applied conceptual models that reinforced a focus on caregiving as a problem or source of stress (Kahana et al, 1994; Lazarus and Folkman, 1984; McCubbin and Patterson, 1983).

As a result of these dramatic changes, research on caregivers, whether formal or informal, paid or unpaid, has grown enormously in both quality and quantity over the past decades. With increasing sophistication in both methodology and theory, caregiving research in the 1990s is characterized by its continued advances in theory, methodology, and application. One noteworthy advancement has been the delineation of the many dimensions of caregiver burden. The burden a caregiver experiences is now viewed as being comprised of feelings of being overwhelmed, trapped, angry, anxious, and torn between caregiving and other responsibilities (e.g., work, family). As well, research has shown that caregiving is a dynamic process with multiple domains and developmental transitions (Pearlin et al, 1990). After the initial onset of caregiving, the care receiver experiences a continued and long-term period of progressive decline to which the caregiver must constantly adapt. Once in-home care becomes unmanageable and placement becomes a reality, caregivers go through another transition as they adapt to their new role in the institutional setting. With the death of the care receiver comes another transition for the caregiver. And while bereavement may appear to be the final stage of adjustment and signal the end of their caregiving career, it is not uncommon for caregivers to take on the responsibility of providing care to another family member at some point later in their lives. Finally, although they may face many of the same transitions and stressors as they provide care over the long term, caregivers are a heterogeneous group with unique experiences. The following section describes the varied experiences of caregivers by highlighting specific research findings related to the experience of stress and burden of providing care to persons with dementing conditions.

RESEARCH ON CAREGIVER DISTRESS AND BURDEN

Research documents the wide variety of predictors of distress and burden depending on characteristics of both the caregiver and care receiver. These include the severity of the older adult's impairment, the caregiver's financial and work strain, gender differences, and racial, ethnic, and cultural factors.

LEVEL OF IMPAIRMENT

One of the most important factors in determining the magnitude of distress and burden a caregiver feels is linked to the type and severity of the elder's functional and cognitive impairment. The importance of illness severity is similar for caregivers of persons with stroke, dementia, cancer, and other debilitating illnesses. Cognitive impairment associated with dementia requires that caregivers provide substantial assistance with self-care activities such as bathing, eating, dressing, and walking. When the impaired person's behavior becomes unpredictable and ambiguous, caregiver distress is often further compromised. In addition, caregivers spend a great deal of time and energy dealing with their relative's problem behaviors (e.g., agitation, memory deficits, wandering, and inappropriate behaviors), behaviors which are associated with increased caregiver burden (Deimling and Bass, 1986).

Caregiver burden also varies depending upon the care recipient's level of impairment and stage of illness. Persons in the initial stages of dementia exhibit more deficits in memory and personality than in self-care tasks. As the disease progresses, cognitive functioning further deteriorates, leading to deficits in self-care activities. With most dementing illnesses, physical difficulties occur later in the disease progression and it is unlikely that the care receiver's mental or physical condition will improve. Cognitive impairment during the early stages of a disease appears to be more stressful to caregivers than the cognitive impairment of the later stages (Miller et al, 1986).

FINANCIAL AND WORK STRAIN

It is not uncommon for caregivers to experience financial strain as a result of providing care over the long term. Whether living at home or in an institution, the cost of providing care to a disabled or demented family member can be exorbitant. In some areas of the US the combined formal and informal costs of caring for an adult with Alzheimer's disease in 1990 have been estimated at US$47 000 or more per year (Rice et al, 1993). Compared to their same age peers in the general population, caregivers are more likely to report adjusted family incomes below the poverty line. Adding to this financial strain is the fact that the responsibilities of caregiving often lead to changes in work status. Caregivers often lose time from work, choose to retire early, or give up work entirely while they are helping their impaired relative (Enright and Friss, 1987; Scharlach, 1989).

GENDER DIFFERENCES

By and large, studies of caregiving families indicate that once a family member requires assistance, it is most likely the wife or daughter of the impaired relative who will become their caregiver (Stone et al, 1987). Among men, husbands are most likely to be caregivers; sons and sons-in-law are much less likely to take on the role. In fact, it is more common for an older woman to be cared for by her daughter-in-law than by her own son. Similarly, women caregivers, whether employed or not, spend more time providing care than do male caregivers (Stoller, 1983; Wilson, 1988). Research findings typically indicate that caregiving women report greater distress than men, regardless of the care receiver's diagnosis and level of impairment. This finding is consistent for employed and not employed caregivers and across different cultures (e.g., Sweden, Japan; Grafstrom et al, 1994; Harris and Long, 1993).

One explanation for these gender differences draws upon studies of health and well-being in the general population indicating that women commonly score higher than men on indicators of stress (Biegel et al, 1991). Alternatively, women may be more comfortable than men with expressing feelings of stress (Neal et al, 1993). It has also been suggested that the nurturant role developed by men in later life may be rewarding or act as a form of repayment for the care they received in the past, which in turn helps to counteract the otherwise negative effects of caregiving (Rustand, 1984; Williamson and Schulz, 1990).

DIFFERENCES ASSOCIATED WITH RACE, ETHNICITY, AND CULTURE

Until recently, little was known about the experience of caregivers with diverse cultural and ethnic identities. Advances in cross-cultural research have demonstrated the diversity among caregivers throughout the world including differences between developing and developed countries, urban and rural settings, and different class or caste structures.

Within the US, research focusing on ethnic diversity among caregivers indicates both similarities and differences among caregivers (Horowitz, 1985; Cantor, 1979; Stone and Short, 1990). Some work suggests that for family members caring for relatives with a variety of disabilities, there is no clear relationship between the caregivers' ethnicity and the amount of stress they experience (Neal et al, 1993). Yet, no matter what the ethnic background or identity of a caregiver, it is clear that across all ethnic groups family care is the most preferred and relied upon source of assistance. Extensive and supportive kin networks have been documented in Americans of all ethnic backgrounds, including Mexican Americans, African Americans, Asian Americans, and Euro-Americans (e.g., Jewish, Greek, Italian, Polish, Irish, etc.).

Currently, most research from the US focuses on the differences between Euro- and non-Euro-American caregivers paying little attention to the great heterogeneity within different ethnic groups. For example, Euro-American caregivers are frequently compared to Asian, Hispanic, or African American caregivers. Growing evidence indicates that differences between these groups are less pronounced than differences within the groups. In addition, it has been suggested that group differences may be more related to the length of time since immigration than to specific ethnic background (Guttman, 1979). As a result, there has been a call to shift efforts away from inter-group study and instead to focus attention on intra-group differences.

These and other research studies provide ample evidence that providing care for an elder with dementia has numerous negative physical and mental health consequences for family caregivers throughout the world (Kosberg, 1985). The long-term and unpredictable nature of dementia, coupled with the financial stress and potential for social isolation, makes caregiving especially problematic. Clearly, caregiving stress and burden and their antecedents are multidimensional and complex (MaloneBeach and Zarit, 1995; Zarit, 1989). Researchers and practitioners have responded to the needs of caregivers by developing programs and interventions to alleviate the burden associated with providing long-term care. The following sections highlight recent advances in program development, intervention, and evaluation.

STRATEGIES TO ALLEVIATE CAREGIVER BURDEN AND DISTRESS

Researchers and practitioners have made great efforts to design appropriate and effective interventions which combat the negative consequences of long-term caregiving. The following sections describe the services and interventions that have been developed to alleviate caregiving stress throughout the many transitions caregivers experience.

SERVICE USE

The stressful nature of caregiving has led many researchers to examine the impact of service use on caregiver well-being. Andersen and his colleagues (Andersen and Aday, 1978) have developed a theoretical model which includes both individual and social factors to predict the use of physician and other health care services. The Andersen Model views service use as a function of three categories of predictors. The first, predisposing factors, typically include socio-demographics (e.g., age, race, and health beliefs) which exist prior to the illness and can be related to the individual's propensity to use service. Second are enabling characteristics, the resources that facilitate service use including individual, family or community characteristics such as level of education, household income, and the availability of nursing home beds. The third category, need characteristics, often precipitate service use and represent illness conditions, symptoms and functional losses. Bass and Noelker (1987) have expanded the Andersen Model to include predisposing, enabling, and need characteristics of both the older individual and the primary caregiver. Chronically ill or disabled older persons receive most care from family members and other informal caregivers who, in turn, influence the older person's use of formal assistance. This can occur directly when the family caregiver seeks out a service on behalf of the impaired person, or indirectly when the caregiver's needs influence the decision to provide formal help. This approach also reflects the impact that an older person's illness and disability has on the family system and the methods by which the family manages the treatment of the ill member. Research findings lend support to the significance of caregiver characteristics, particularly care-related strains, as predictors of the elderly's use of home health care.

PLACEMENT

Many families rely on long-term institutional care once they are no longer able to care for their impaired relatives at home. Specifically, 25–35% of older Americans can expect to spend some time during their later life in a nursing home (Van Nostrand et al, 1979). The conservative use of nursing homes reflects generally unfavorable attitudes toward institutionalization and the high cost of nursing home care.

Assisted living, one alternative to skilled residential care, is becoming increasingly popular with moderately impaired older persons and their families. This service arrangement maximizes the older persons' life style choices in less restrictive housing environments that also provide supportive services. Typically, these services include housekeeping, transportation, and meals, although some facilities also provide supervision of medications and limited personal care.

The elderly's use of community-based and nursing home care is predicted by many of the same factors which predict in-home care. These factors include: advanced age, gender (female), cultural background (Euro-American), marital status (unmarried), living arrangement (alone), and level of functional disability. Additionally, the absence of a willing, able and proximate informal caregiver is a major factor in nursing home placement. This is particularly salient when the older individual has a neurological condition such as a stroke (Jette et al, 1992). Generally, family members control the timing of nursing home entry and physicians exert a major influence on the decision, particularly when it follows the older person's hospitalization.

Until recently, the tasks and responsibilities of caregivers were thought to end once an impaired elder was placed in an institutional setting. Current research indicates that caregivers continue to remain very active in the lives of their impaired family members once institutionalization becomes necessary. Family caregivers visit often and frequently travel great distances in order to spend time with their relatives. Caregivers of nursing home residents often perform many of the same tasks they did while caring at home, including assistance with eating, personal care, and walking. In fact, a large majority of caregivers remain very active in the lives of their placed relatives for many years after the initial placement has occurred (Zarit and Whitlatch, 1993).

With continued involvement in the care of their impaired relative comes the potential for additional distress and burden (Townsend, 1990). Once their family member is institutionalized, caregivers must restructure and redefine their lives and adjust to their new role. Recent research indicates that the stresses of caregiving are not alleviated by placement. Although these caregivers are relieved of the day-to-day demands of in-home care, many continue to feel distress. While some caregivers are less distressed, many exhibit symptoms well above their pre-placement levels of distress. It is now clear that placement alters rather than eliminates the stresses of caregiving (Aneshensel et al, 1995).

CAREGIVER INTERVENTIONS

Over the last 20 years, services targeted to informal caregivers have been developed and become more widely available based on the demonstrated stressful effects of long-term caregiving. These services include: respite care, support groups, education programs in care-related skills, training in problem-solving skills and behavioral techniques for patient management, and counseling and psychotherapy.

Respite services are presumed to help alleviate the stress of caregiving by providing 'time away' from caregiving duties to reduce the time and effort spent by family members in providing care. Families often identify respite care as one of their most pressing needs (Crossman et al, 1981; Friss, 1990; Lawton et al, 1989). Yet, studies examining the ability of respite care to decrease stress and burden have reported mixed results. Respite care may improve a caregiver's quality of life, but it has been found to have no influence on caregiver burden and mental health (Lawton et al, 1989). More recent research, however, suggests that use of adult day care can reduce care-related stress and improve a caregiver's psychological well-being (Zarit et al, 1996). One reason for these discrepant findings may be because families often delay the usage of respite care (Gwyther, 1994) which makes them particularly vulnerable to the chronic stress of long-term caregiving (Deimling, 1991; Whitlatch et al, 1997). Respite may have a limited role in giving caregivers time away from care responsibilities, but the mechanisms through which it helps families remain unknown (Berry et al, 1991).

Support groups, psycho-educational interventions, and counseling are also used to alleviate the stress of family caregiving. These interventions can be time-limited or ongoing, peer- or professionally led, structured or unstructured. Some programs are designed to help families caring for persons with specific diagnoses or for specific family caregivers only (e.g., wives caring for husbands). Unfortunately, intervention evaluation studies using control groups have reported modest or insignificant results (Haley et al, 1987; Toseland et al, 1989). Research has examined the effects of caregiving interventions on distress and well-being generally and depression specifically (Gage and Kinney, 1995;

Silven et al, 1986; Whitlatch et al, 1991; Zarit et al, 1987). Unfortunately the amount of change found among study participants has been relatively small.

One difficulty commonly encountered in evaluations of caregiver interventions is enrolling sufficient numbers of caregivers in study samples, even when the service is provided free of charge (Lawton et al, 1989). Various explanations offered for the apparent under-utilization of care-related services include unfamiliarity with the service, lack of perceived need, reliance on informal helpers for care-related assistance, absence of culturally relevant services, and barriers to the service system and the delivery of services.

A second problem common to intervention research is the lack of thorough economic evaluations of caregiver support programs. Few intervention studies include an economic evaluation component because of the methodological complexities involved. The handful of studies which do provide economic data show promising results. For example, research by Kyle et al (1987) indicates that caregiver support programs can be less costly than institutional care. More recently, Drummond et al (1991) report that a comprehensive six-month caregiver support program is associated with an 'implied incremental cost per quality adjusted life year' of Canadian $20 000. These studies demonstrate the feasibility of including rigorous economic evaluations of caregiver interventions as well as the implied cost of improving the quality of life of family caregivers.

A final problem is that many studies have focused on the effects of single, time-limited interventions designed specifically to lessen caregiver distress (Knight et al, 1993). An exception, however, is the work of Mittelman and colleagues (Mittelman et al, 1993; Mittelman et al, 1994) who have reported on the positive effects of multi-component interventions adapted to changing caregiver needs over time. Further research is needed to examine the impact of caregiver interventions, assess the impact of service use on caregiver well-being over an extended period of time, and determine the most efficient intervention for specific types of caregivers, the most effective timing of these interventions, the most appropriate duration of use, and the cost implications of the interventions.

FUTURE DIRECTIONS IN RESEARCH AND INTERVENTION

Recent advances in theory have been instrumental in delineating the mechanisms by which interventions are helpful to family caregivers. The first step in furthering our knowledge about caregiving and how to ameliorate its negative effects is to draw on theory which examines multiple components of the caregiving process. Pearlin and his colleagues (Pearlin et al, 1990) have presented the Stress Process Model of Family Caregiving which has its roots in sociological and psychological theories of stress and coping (Aneshensel et al,

1995). Within the Stress Process Model the experience of caregiving is conceptualized as a chronic stressor which, as with other chronic stressors, proliferates and reconfigures over time. The model provides a framework for the development and empirical testing of caregiver interventions designed to contain the proliferation of caregiving stressors.

Research shows that specific components within the Stress Process Model are related and that different types of social support work to alleviate many of the negative effects between stressors. To illustrate, instrumental social support, both formal and informal, as well as the emotional support provided to the caregiver by friends and family, acts to moderate or buffer the deleterious effects of stress at specific points within this model. Formal support lessens the negative effects of a care receiver's functional loss on a caregiver's feeling of role overload (i.e., the feeling of burnout or fatigue from caregiving). On the other hand, informal support lessens the negative effects of a care receiver's problematic behavior on a caregiver's feeling of role overload (Pearlin et al, 1995). Interventions designed to supplement or enhance specific elements of a caregiver's support network may help to alleviate specific components of caregiver distress and burden. The use of the Stress Process Model illustrates the potential utility of interventions based on related theory and empirical findings.

A second step that will increase our understanding of caregiving stress is the inclusion of caregivers in intervention studies who have the 'problem' that the intervention addresses. In this way it is possible to detect meaningful change so that the effect of the intervention is not underestimated. To illustrate, a sample of depressed caregivers is the most appropriate group to be enrolled in a study that tests the effectiveness of an intervention for depression. If caregivers are enrolled who are not depressed (e.g., low scores on measures of depression), then it is nearly impossible to show that they have improved. Because the caregivers are at the floor of the measure, their scores cannot decrease and the effectiveness of the intervention is underestimated (Whitlatch et al, 1991).

Third, drawing upon the methodology used in clinical outcomes research, it may prove fruitful for researchers to determine the amount or 'dosage' of an intervention a caregiver receives (Knight et al, 1993; Kosloski and Montgomery, 1995). Some caregivers do not attend all sessions of an intervention. Those who attend less often or sporadically might likely experience fewer positive gains. If, in an analysis, caregivers are regarded as if they all received equal amounts of an intervention, even though some caregivers attended more often than others, then the intervention's effectiveness is underestimated. Similarly, it may prove useful to include family caregivers in clinical trials of patient drug interventions. In other words, researchers would develop two sets of protocols (i.e., one protocol for the patient and one for the family caregiver) that might evaluate quality of life and resource utilization (i.e., service use, social costs, etc.). Including caregivers in clinical trials and insuring the careful monitoring of the entire sample's exposure to the intervention will aid in determining the effects of the larger intervention, its components, and both direct and indirect effects on patients and family caregivers.

A final step towards increasing our understanding of caregiving stress and burden is for researchers to specify and evaluate treatment outcomes that are directly relevant to the intervention (Bass et al, 1996; Bourgeois et al, 1995). To evaluate a treatment designed to help caregivers better manage problem behaviors, it is imperative to measure the caregiver's ability to manage these behaviors before and after the intervention. In addition, a secondary or indirect benefit to an intervention that helps caregivers manage disruptive behaviors may be that caregiver stress and depression are alleviated. By assessing both the direct and indirect effects of an intervention we gain a broader understanding of the mechanisms underlying caregiver burden and appropriate ways to intervene.

Providing care to a relative with a dementing condition is a dynamic and frequently long-term process. As the stressors of the caregiving process proliferate and intensify, so do their negative consequences. This chapter has described a variety of the consequences and stressors experienced by family caregivers who provide long-term care to a relative with a dementing condition. Scholarly work within the literature is rich with a greater understanding of the process of caregiving. Recent advances in theory, methodology, and intervention have propelled the literature forward and laid the foundation for further debate, critical thinking, and innovative intervention. Research and interventions which are clearly grounded in theory and informed by the successes and failures of applied work will contribute greatly to our understanding of the process of caregiving and how to ameliorate the burden experienced by families.

REFERENCES

American Association of Retired Persons (1988). *A National Survey of Caregivers: Final report*, Washington, DC, Author.

Andersen, R. and Aday, L. (1978). Access to medical care in the US: realized and potential, *Medical Care*, 4, 533–546.

Aneshensel, C. S., Pearlin, L. I., Mullan, J. L., Zarit, S. H. and Whitlatch, C. J. (1995). *Profiles in Caregiving: The Unexpected Career*, New York, Academic Press.

Anthony-Bergstone, C. R., Zarit, S. H. and Gatz, M. (1988). Symptoms of psychological distress among caregivers of dementia patients, *Psychology and Aging*, 3, 245–248.

Bass, D. M. and Noelker, L. S. (1987). The influence of family caregivers on elders' use of in-home services, *Journal of Health and Social Behavior*, **28**, 184–196.

Bass, D. M., Noelker, L. S. and Rechlin, L. R. (1996). The moderating influence of service use on negative caregiving consequences, *Journal of Gerontology*, **51B**, S121–S131.

Berry, G. L., Zarit, S. H. and Rabatin, V. X. (1991). Caregiver activity on respite and nonrespite days: a comparison of two service approaches, *Gerontologist*, **31**(60), 830–835.

Biegel, D. E., Sales, E. and Schulz, R. (1991). *Family Caregiving in Chronic Illness*, Newbury Park, CA, Sage.

Bourgeois, M. S., Schulz, R. and Burgio, L. (1995). Improving outcomes by monitoring the intervention process, *Gerontologist*, **35**, Special Issue 1, 189.

Bris, H. J. (1993). *Care for family carers: trends and innovations*, Netherlands Institute of Gerontology; European Center for Social Welfare Policy and Research, Bunnik, Netherlands, pp. 59–69.

Cantor, M. (1979). The informal support system of New York's inner city elderly: is ethnicity a factor? in D. E. Gelfand and A. J. Kutzik (Eds), *Ethnicity and Aging: Theory, Research and Policy*, pp. 153–174, New York, Springer.

Crossman, L., London, C. and Barry, C. (1981). Older women caring for disabled spouses: a model for supportive services, *Gerontologist*, **21**, 464–470.

Deimling, G. T. (1991). Respite use and caregiver well-being in families caring for stable and declining Alzheimer's patients, *Journal of Gerontological Social Work*, **18**(1/2), 177–134.

Deimling, G. T. and Bass, D. M. (1986). Symptoms of mental impairment among elderly adults and their effects on family caregivers, *Journal of Gerontology*, **41**(6), 778–784.

Drummond, M. F., Mohide, E. A., Tew, M., Streiner, D. L., Pringle, D. M. and Gilbert, J. R. (1991). Economic evaluation of a support program for caregivers of demented elderly, *International Journal of Technology Assessment in Health Care*, **7**, 209–219.

Enright, R. B. and Friss, L. R. (1987). *Employed caregivers of brain-impaired adults: An assessment of the dual role* (Final report to the Gerontological Society of America), San Francisco, Family Caregiver Alliance.

Freed, A. O. (1990). How Japanese families cope with fragile elderly, *Journal of Gerontological Social Work*, **15**(1–2), 39–56.

Friss, L. R. (1990). A model state-level approach to family survival for caregivers of brain-impaired adults, *Gerontologist*, **30**, 121–125.

Gage, M. J. and Kinney, J. M. (1995). They aren't for everyone: the impact of support group participation on caregiver's well-being, *Clinical Gerontologist*, **16**(2), 21–34.

Gallagher, D., Rose, J., Rivera, P., Lovett, S. and Thompson, L. W. (1989). Prevalence of depression in family caregivers, *Gerontologist*, **29**, 449–456.

Grafstrom, M., Fratiglioni, L. and Winblad, B. (1994). Caring for an elderly person: predictors of burden in dementia care, *International Journal of Geriatric Psychiatry*, **9**(5), 373–379.

Guttman, D. (1979). Use of informal and formal supports by White ethnic aged, in D. E. Gelfand and A. Kutzik (Eds), *Aging and Ethnicity*, pp. 246–262, New York, Springer.

Guttman, D. (1994). The 'graying' of Israel, in L. K. Olson (Ed.), *Graying of the World: Who Will Care for the Frail Elderly?* pp. 103–126, New York, Hawthorne Press.

Gwyther, L. P. (1994). Service delivery and utilization: research directions and clinical implications, in E. Light, G. Niederehe and B. D. Lebowitz (Eds), *Stress Effects on Family Caregivers of Alzheimer's Patients*, pp. 293–300, New York, Springer.

Haley, W. E., Levine, E. G., Brown, S. L., Berry, J. W. and Hughes, G. H. (1987). Psychological, social and health consequences of caring for a relative with senile dementia, *Journal of the American Geriatrics Society*, **35**, 405–411.

Harris, P. B. and Long, S. O. (1993). Daughter-in-law's burden: an exploratory study of caregiving in Japan, *Journal of Cross-Cultural Gerontology*, **8**(2), 97–118.

Horowitz, A. (1985). Family caregiving to the frail elderly, in M. P. Lawton and C. Maddox (Eds), *Annual Review of Gerontology and Geriatrics*, Vol. 5, pp. 194–246, New York, Springer.

Jette, A. M., Branch, L. G., Sleeper, L. A., Feldman, H. and Sullivan, L. M. (1992). High-risk profiles for nursing home admission, *Gerontologist*, **32**(5), 634–640.

Johansson, L. (1991, March). Informal care of dependent elderly at home: some Swedish experiences, *Aging and Society*, **11**(1), 41–58.

Johansson, L. and Thorslund, M. (1992). Care needs and sources of support in a nationwide sample of elderly in Sweden, *Zeitschrift für Gerontologie*, **25**, 57–62.

Kahana, E., Biegel, D. E. and Wykle, M. L. (Eds) (1994). *Family Caregiving Across the Lifespan*, Thousand Oaks, CA, Sage.

Kiecolt-Glaser, J. K., Glaser, R., Shuttleworth, E. C., Dyer, C. S., Ogrocki, P. and Speicher, C. E. (1987). Chronic stress and immunity in family caregivers of Alzheimer's disease victims, *Psychosomatic Medicine*, **49**, 523–535.

Knight, B. G., Lutsky, S. M. and Macofsky-Urban, F. (1993). A meta-analytic review of interventions for caregiver distress: recommendations for future research, *Gerontologist*, **33**, 240–248.

Kosberg, J. I. (1985). Family care of the aged in the United States: policy issues from an international perspective, University of South Florida, International Exchange Center on Gerontology, Tampa, FL.

Kosloski, K. and Montgomery, R. J. V. (1995). The impact of respite use on nursing home placement, *Gerontologist*, **35**, 67–74.

Kyle, D. R., Drummond, M. F. and White, D. M. D. (1987). The Hereford District Department of Mental Health of the Elderly: a preliminary evaluation, *Community Medicine*, **9**, 35–46.

Lawton, M. P., Brody, E. M. and Saperstein, A. R. (1989). A controlled study of respite service for caregivers of Alzheimer's patient, *Gerontologist*, **29**, 8–16.

Lazarus, R. L. and Folkman, S. (1984). *Stress, Appraisal and Coping*, New York, Springer.

MaloneBeach, E. E. and Zarit, S. H. (1995). Dimensions of social support and conflict as predictors of caregiver depression, *International Journal of Psychogeriatrics*, **7**(1), 25–38.

McCubbin, H. and Patterson, J. (1983). The family stress process: the doubled ABCX model of adjustment and adaptation, in H. McCubbin, M. Sussman and J. Patterson (Eds), *Social Stress and the Family: Advances and Developments in Family Stress Theory and Research*, New York, Haworth.

Miller, B. (1987). Gender and control among spouses of the cognitively impaired: a research note, *Gerontologist*, **27**, 447–453.

Mittelman, M. S., Ferris, S. H., Steinberg, G., Shulman, E., Mackell, J. A., Ambinder, A. and Cohen, J. (1993). An intervention that delays institutionalization of Alzheimer's disease patients: treatment of spouse-caregivers, *Gerontologist*, **33**, 730–740.

Mittelman, M. S., Ferris, S. H., Shulman, E., Steinberg, G., Mackell, J. A. and Ambinder, A. (1994). Efficacy of multicomponent individualized treatment to improve the well-being of Alzheimer's disease caregivers, in E. Light, G. Niederehe and B. Lebowitz (Eds), *Stress Effects on Family Caregivers of Alzheimer's Patients*, New York, Springer.

Montgomery, R. J. V. (1996). Next steps for social and behavioral research related to Alzheimer's disease, *International Psychogeriatrics*, **8**(1), 103–107.

Neal, M. B., Chapman, N. J., Ingersoll-Dayton, B. and Emlen, A. C. (1993). *Balancing Work and Caregiving for Children, Adults and Elders*, Newbury Park, CA, Sage.

Olson, L. K. (1994). *The Graying of the World: Who Will Care for the Frail Elderly?* New York, Hawthorne Press.

Pearlin, L. I., Aneshensel, C. S., Mullan, J. L. and Whitlatch, C. J. (1995). *Handbook of Aging and the Social Sciences*, 4th edition, New York, Van Nostrand Reinhold.

Pearlin, L. I., Mullan, J. L., Semple, S. J. and Skaff, M. M. (1990). Caregiving and the stress process: an overview of concepts and their measures, *Gerontologist*, **30**, 583–594.

Rice, D. P., Fox, P. J., Max, W., Webber, P. A., Lindeman, D. A., Hauck, W. W. and Segura, E. (1993). The economic burden of Alzheimer's Disease care, *Health Affairs*, **12**, 164–176.

Rustand, L. C. (1984). Family adjustment to chronic illness and disability in mid-life, in M. G. Eisenberg, L. C. Sutkin and M. A. Jansen (Eds), *Chronic Illness and Disability Through the Life Span*, pp. 222–242, New York, Springer.

Scharlach, A. E. (1989). A comparison of employed caregivers of cognitively impaired adults and physically impaired elderly persons, *Research on Aging*, **11**, 225–243.

Schulz, R., O'Brien, A. T., Bookwala, J. and Fleissner, K. (1995). Psychiatric and physical morbidity effects in Alzheimer's disease caregiving: prevalence, correlates and causes, *Gerontologist*, **35**, 771–791.

Silven, D., DelMaestro, S., Gallagher, D., Lovett, S., Benedict, A., Rose, J. and Kwong, K. (1986). Changes in depressed caregivers symptomatology through psychoeducational interventions. Paper presented at the annual scientific meeting of the Gerontological Society of America, Chicago, November.

Stoller, E. P. (1983). Parental caregiving by adult children, *Journal of Marriage and the Family*, **45**, 851–858.

Stone, R. I., Cafferata, G. and Sangl, J. (1987). Caregivers of the frail elderly: a national profile, *Gerontologist*, **27**, 616–626.

Stone, R. I. and Kemper, P. (1989). Spouses and children of disabled elders: how large a constituency for long-term care reform? *Millbank Quarterly*, **67**, 486–506.

Stone, R. I. and Short, P. F. (1990). The competing demands of employment and informal caregiving to disabled elders, *Medical Care*, **28**, 513–526.

Subcommittee on Human Services of the Select Committee on Aging, US House of Representatives (1987). *Exploding the Myths: Caregiving in America* (Committee Publication No. 99-611), Washington, DC, Government Printing Office.

Tennstedt, S., Cafferata, G. L. and Sullivan, L. (1992). Depression among caregivers of impaired elders, *Journal of Aging and Health*, **4**, 58–76.

Toseland, R. W., Rossiter, C. M. and Labrecque, M. S. (1989). The effectiveness of peer-led and professionally led groups to support family caregivers, *Gerontologist*, **29**, 465–471.

Townsend, A. L. (1990). Nursing home care and family caregivers' stress, in M. A. P. Stephens, J. H. Crowther, S. E. Hobfoll and D. L. Tennenbaum (Eds), *Stress and Coping in Later-Life Families*, New York, Hemisphere.

US Bureau of the Census (1991). Current population reports: Marital status and living arrangements: March 1990 (Series P-20 No. 450), Washington, DC, Government Printing Office.)

Van Nostrand, J., Zappolo, A., Hing, E., Bloom, B., Hirsch, B. and Foley, D. J. (1979). The national nursing home survey: 1977 summary for the United States. *Vital and Health Statistics*, Series 13-1, No. 43, US Department of Health, Education, and Welfare, DHEW Publications No. (PHS) 79-1794. Washington, DC: Government Printing Office.

Whitlatch, C. J., Feinberg, L. F. and Sebesta, D. (1997). Depression and health in family caregivers: adaptation over time, *Journal of Aging and Health*, **9**, 222–243.

Whitlatch, C. J., Zarit, S. H. and von Eye, A. (1991). Efficacy of interventions with caregivers: a reanalysis, *Gerontologist*, **31**, 9–14.

Williamson, G. M. and Schulz, R. (1990). Relationship orientations, quality of prior relationship and distress among caregivers of Alzheimer's patients, *Psychology and Aging*, **5**, 502–509.

Wilson, R. E. (1988). Intergenerational programs, in D. E. Friedman (Ed.), *Issues for an Aging America: Elder Care: Highlights of a Conference*, pp. 37–39, New York, Conference Board.

Zarit, S. H. (1989). Do we need another 'stress and caregiving' study? *Gerontologist*, **29**, 147–148.

Zarit, S. H., Anthony, C. R. and Boutselis, M. (1987). Interventions with caregivers of dementia patients: comparisons of two approaches, *Psychology and Aging*, **2**, 225–232.

Zarit, S. H., Reever, K. E. and Bach-Peterson, J. (1980). Relatives of the impaired elderly: correlates of feelings and burden, *Gerontologist*, **20**, 649–655.

Zarit, S. H., Stephens, M. A. P., Townsend, A. and Greene, R. (1996, August). *Stress reduction for family caregivers: Effects of adult day care use*, Paper presented at the Annual Conference of the American Psychological Association.

Zarit, S. H., Todd, P. A. and Zarit, J. M. (1986). Subjective burden of husbands and wives as caregivers: a longitudinal study, *Gerontologist*, **26**, 260–266.

Zarit, S. H. and Whitlatch, C. J. (1993). The effects of placement in nursing homes on family caregivers: short and long-term consequences, *Irish Journal of Psychology*, **14**(1), 25–37.

2 Health Economics Approaches to Dementia

2.1 Principles of Pharmacoeconomics

MICHAEL DRUMMOND
Centre for Health Economics, University of York, UK

INTRODUCTION

There is a growing interest in undertaking economic evaluations of pharmaceuticals (often known as 'pharmacoeconomic studies'). This reflects a recognition within the pharmaceutical industry and elsewhere, that health care decision makers are placing increasing emphasis on the value for money from health care interventions. The published literature has grown rapidly (Luce and Elixhauser, 1990) and many pharmaceutical companies have established an in-house capability in health economics.

Economic evaluation is a way of establishing the value for money of health care technologies, including pharmaceuticals. In economic evaluation studies the costs of health care interventions are compared with their consequences, in terms of improvement in the length or quality of life, and in savings in other health care resources. There are a number of forms of economic evaluation, including cost-effectiveness, cost-utility and cost-benefit analysis. These will be discussed briefly below and are described in fuller detail elsewhere (Warner and Luce, 1982; Drummond et al, 1987; Kamlet, 1992; Drummond, 1991).

There are a number of possible objectives when commissioning, or undertaking, an economic evaluation of a given product. First, economic evaluations may be performed early in the product development process in order to estimate the likely pay-off should the clinical promise of the medicine be fulfilled. Similarly, a burden of illness study may be conducted to estimate the full economic potential of an effective product in a given therapeutic area.

Secondly, an economic evaluation may be performed in order to delineate the range of prices for a given medicine that could be justified in terms of value for money. The economic data will then be *one* input to the final pricing decision, which obviously depends on a number of factors.

Thirdly, an economic evaluation may be undertaken to provide essential data for negotiations on price or reimbursement status in those jurisdictions where this is necessary. Finally, it may be undertaken in order to help in the marketing of the medicine, by demonstrating value for money to individual prescribers or formulary committees.

Health Economics of Dementia. Edited by Anders Wimo, Bengt Jönsson, Göran Karlsson and Bengt Winblad.
© 1998 John Wiley & Sons Ltd.

Those undertaking or commissioning economic evaluations have an interest in following well-established methodological principles. This is true both for internally conducted studies, where accurate estimates of economic value are required for business planning and for studies intended for outside use, where data are likely to be subjected to close scrutiny. There are a number of published sources of methodological standards for economic evaluation. Often these are summarized in the form of a checklist of questions to ask about a published study (Drummond et al, 1987; Udvarhelyi et al, 1992; Adams et al, 1992).

The overall conclusion in the published literature is that, while a number of general methodological principles have emerged, many details require more discussion and debate. Therefore, the objective of this paper is to outline the basic methods underlying pharmacoeconomic studies, given the current state of our knowledge. The next section discusses the basic forms of economic evaluation, and subsequent sections discuss methodological issues in study design, data collection and analysis and reporting of results.

BASIC FORMS OF ECONOMIC EVALUATION

There are a number of forms of economic evaluation, but they have the common feature that some combination of the inputs to a health care programme are compared with some combination of the outputs (Figure 2.1.1). The inputs include the direct costs of providing care (C_1 in Figure 2.1.1), which fall mainly (though not exclusively) on the health care sector, and the indirect costs (in production losses) arising when individuals are withdrawn from the workforce to be given therapy (C_2). Although not strictly an 'input', there may also be intangible costs, in pain or suffering, associated with therapy (C_3).

The simplest form of analysis considers only costs. This approach is justified where it can reasonably be assumed, or has been previously shown, that the alternative programmes or therapies being compared produce equivalent medical results. This was the approach used by Davies and Drummond (1990) in their study of prostaglandin PGE_2 in the induction of labour. Such a study is called a *cost-minimization analysis*. Some analyses confine themselves to consideration of direct costs only, others consider also the indirect costs.

One particular form of cost analysis deserves further mention since it has had wide application. The *cost of illness* study calculates all the direct and indirect costs of a particular disease or illness, such as dementia (Gray and Fenn, 1993; Ernst and Hay, 1994). These studies can serve two purposes, depending on how they are carried out. First, by providing an estimate of the economic impact of a given disease, they can alert policy makers to the importance of the problem and suggest that investments should be made in interventions to ameliorate its effect. Secondly, they can provide a baseline

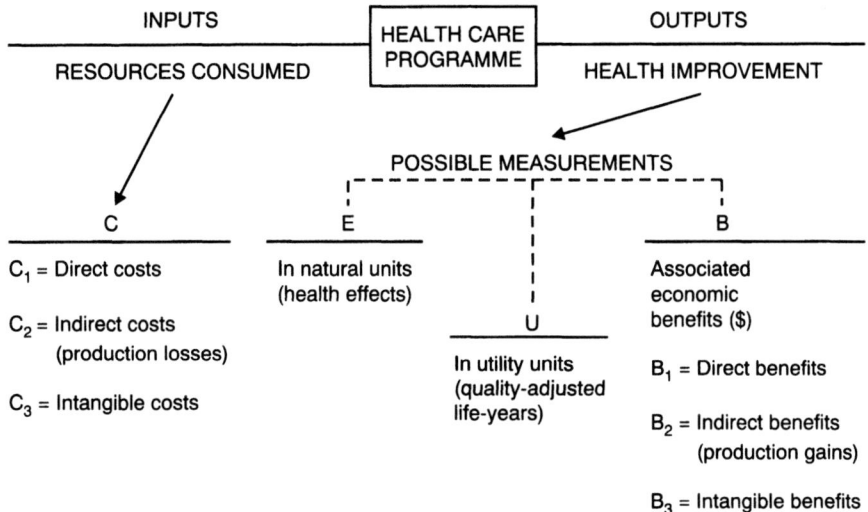

Figure 2.1.1. Components of economic evaluation

estimate of costs against which the potential economic impact of a new medicine can be judged.

However, most forms of economic evaluation require explicit measurement of the outputs of the programmes or therapies being compared. They differ mainly in the method of measuring the outputs. The earliest forms of analysis concentrated on the benefits of interventions in terms of the resulting savings in other direct medical care costs (direct benefits, B_1), and the production gains from an earlier return to work (indirect benefits, B_2). Typically, in a *cost-benefit analysis*, these benefits were expressed in money terms in order to make them commensurate with the costs of the intervention. However, other more intangible benefits, such as the value to patients of feeling healthier (B_3), are obviously more difficult to express in money terms. Therefore cost-benefit analyses have often been criticized for ignoring important benefits from health care programmes and for concentrating on items that are easy to measure. Many of the early studies were therefore very narrow assessments, considering only direct and indirect costs and benefits. However, more recently there have been some good examples of studies valuing health improvements in money terms (Johannesson and Jönsson, 1991).

Instead of attempting to measure outputs in money terms, other analysts have preferred to assess them in the most convenient natural units (health effects), such as 'cases successfully treated' or 'years of life gained'. For example, Oster and Epstein (1987) estimated the cost per life-year gained of different strategies to lower elevated cholesterol by drugs. Such analyses are known as *cost-effectiveness analyses*.

Of course, many health technologies are concerned with improving the *quality*, not quantity, of life. In addition, some therapies, such as cancer chemotherapy or hypertension treatment, may bring about slight reductions in the quality of life in order to extend life. Therefore, there has been a growth in interest in *cost-utility analysis*, where the life-years gained from treatment are adjusted by a series of utility weights reflecting the relative values individuals place on different states of health (Drummond et al, 1987). The output measure most frequently used in cost-utility analysis is known as the *quality-adjusted life-year* (QALY).

DESIGN OF ECONOMIC EVALUATION STUDIES

As in all fields of scientific enquiry, the design of economic evaluation studies is critical to the production of reliable data. Two features in particular will be highlighted, the selection of alternatives for evaluation and the perspective (or viewpoint) adopted.

SELECTION OF ALTERNATIVES

Other than in the case of burden of illness studies, economic evaluations of health care interventions compare alternative treatments for programmes. In evaluating a given medicine, the choice of comparator is a key strategic decision. In the case of 'breakthrough' products such as tacrine (Knapp et al, 1994) there may be no satisfactory treatment for the condition concerned. Here the comparator is implicitly 'current care' or 'doing nothing'. However, for most new pharmaceuticals there are normally a number of relevant comparator products on the market. Some of these may be out-moded and relatively inexpensive; others may be recently developed products more comparable to the new medicine of interest.

In selecting the comparator therapy one should resist the temptation to choose a particularly expensive or relatively ineffective medicine. Rather, the comparator should be the most widely used medicine for the condition concerned in the setting where the evaluation is being undertaken. The logic is that this would be the therapy which most prescribers would replace in practice (Commonwealth of Australia, 1992). This approach does raise practical problems, however. First, the most widely used medicine may vary over time and from place to place. Secondly, there may not be a 'head-to-head' comparison with the drug concerned among the available Phase III clinical trials. Therefore, the economic evaluation may need to rely on a synthesis of clinical data from a number of trials.

If a comparison is made with the most widely used medicine for the condition concerned, the economic evaluation is unlikely to be heavily criticized.

Other potential sources of criticism relate to having too narrow a focus for the evaluation. For example, the evaluations of misoprostol, a drug that has been shown to reduce the incidence of NSAID-associated ulcers in people on long-term therapy experiencing symptoms, were criticized for not including, as one option, stopping the NSAID. Similarly, some evaluations of cholesterol-lowering drugs have been criticized for not including non-pharmacologic interventions such as dietary advice, or for not considering the broader impacts on casefinding and/or screening. It is understandable that some evaluations have adopted a narrow focus, since this merely mirrors the tradition in controlled trials. However, in designing economic studies companies should consider whether key decision makers are likely to require that a wider range of options be considered.

PERSPECTIVE OF STUDY

It was mentioned earlier that there are a number of potential objectives in economic evaluations. Sometimes a given study may be designed to meet a range of objectives. In doing so it has to be recognized that different decision makers have different perspectives on costs and consequences, depending on whether they be individual prescribers, hospital managers or government policy makers.

Typically, economists argue that evaluations should be performed from a broad, societal viewpoint, but it is not clear who takes decisions on this basis. Certainly part of the purpose of economic evaluation is to encourage decision makers to take a broad view of costs and consequences, beyond the impacts on their own budget. However, it is also prudent to design the study so that the various budgetary impacts can be assessed, thereby satisfying a number of viewpoints.

DECISION ANALYTIC FRAMEWORKS

In designing a study it is often useful to set out the options in a decision analytic framework. A *decision tree* sets out the key decisions, and their consequences, under each alternative. The decision tree used in the evaluation of misoprostol is given in Figure 2.1.2 as an example. This approach helps clarify the analyst's thoughts about the alternatives being compared and forms the basis of a model that can be used for extrapolation of the results to different settings. For example, in the case of the example given, different estimates were used for compliance rates, rates of hospitalization, surgery rates and costs in order to estimate the costs and consequences in four different countries (Drummond et al, 1992). The logical nature of decision trees means that they are amenable to computerization. This greatly facilitates generalization of results and the exploration of the impact of different assumptions. (This will be discussed further later.)

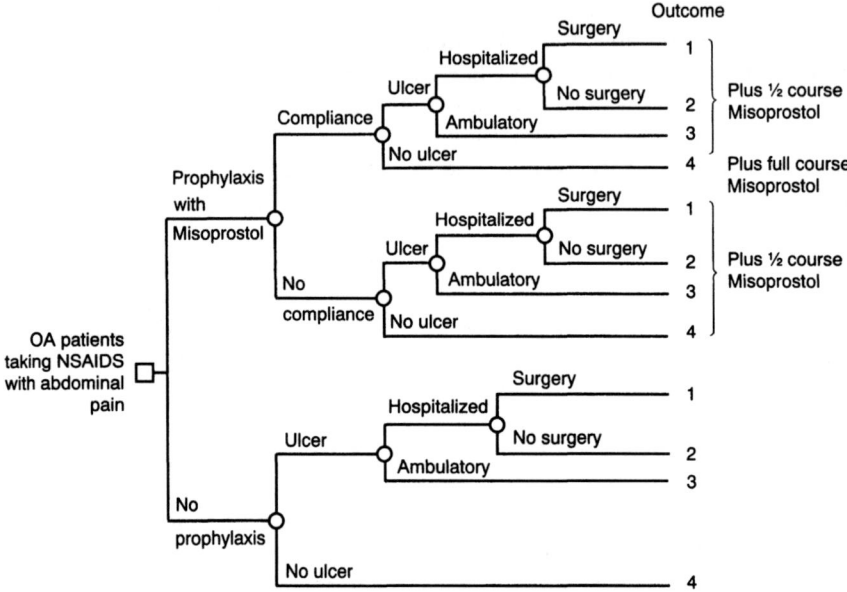

Figure 2.1.2. Presentation in decision-tree format to facilitate extrapolation. *Source*: adapted from Drummond et al (1992)

BOX 2.1.1: ISSUES TO CONSIDER IN STUDY DESIGN

- Have non-pharmacologic alternatives been considered, including the option of 'doing nothing'?
- Does the evaluation include, as the main comparator, the most widely used medicine(s) for the condition concerned in the relevant setting(s)?
- Has adequate consideration been given to the target audience(s) for the study and the items of costs and consequences that would be most important to them?
- Has consideration been given to setting out the options in a decision-tree format in order to facilitate the generalization of results?

DATA COLLECTION

Economic evaluations typically require three data elements: (1) efficacy of the therapies concerned; (2) resource use and cost; (3) impact on quality of life. These are discussed in turn.

EVIDENCE OF EFFICACY

The main source of efficacy evidence is, of course, the controlled clinical trials of the medicine(s) concerned, although trial data may be supplemented by data from actual clinical use where these are available. Economic evaluations tend to use trial data in one of three ways. First, the evaluation may be undertaken *retrospectively*, after a clinical trial, but will use the published trial results. For example, the evaluations of tacrine (Lubeck et al, 1995; Wimo et al, 1997) were all based on the results of a clinical trial undertaken in the USA by Knapp et al (1994). Data on the use of resources and their costs were then extracted from routine data sources. Thus in this approach clinical trial data are synthesized, along with cost data, to produce an economic evaluation result. It is not normal for the cost data to relate to the patients included in the original clinical trial although on occasions retrospective data are collected through chart review.

The second approach also involves synthesis of data. However, instead of the economic evaluation being based on efficacy data from a single trial, it is based on a meta-analysis or overview of a number of trials. For example, Goldman et al (1988) used data from a meta-analysis in their cost-effectiveness analysis of post-infarction prophylaxis with beta-blockers. This approach has more external validity than the former one, but is crucially dependent on the quality of the underlying meta-analysis (Sacks et al, 1987). It is also rare to find a meta-analysis for a new product at the time the economic evaluation is performed, since often only a few trials will have been undertaken. A meta-analysis may be available for the comparator therapy, however.

The third approach is to combine data on efficacy with those on resource use and cost by undertaking economic data collection *prospectively*, alongside a given clinical trial. This has the advantage that data on cost are collected on the same patients for whom the efficacy data are available. Thus the same quality standards, in data collection and analysis, can be applied. This approach is increasingly being followed for new medicines, partly because of the quality of the data thus obtained and partly because economic evidence is increasingly being required early in product development, prior to launch.

Despite the obvious advantages, prospective data collection alongside clinical trials is not a panacea for the generation of efficacy data for inclusion in economic evaluations (Drummond and Davies, 1991). Problems arise because of the atypical nature of the setting for many Phase III trials (e.g. specialist centres), the clinical alternatives evaluated (e.g. placebo or baseline therapy, not current best practice), the short period of follow-up and the small sample size, which may be adequate for the assessment of the primary clinical endpoint but not for some of the key economic variables. Also, if data on use of resources are being collected, some of the resource use (e.g. tests) may be protocol-driven. In principle, these would be easy to exclude from the economic evaluation, although other protocol effects, arising from the more careful monitoring of patients, may be more difficult to detect or adjust for.

Therefore all three approaches to the generation of efficacy data for economic evaluations have disadvantages. It is likely that most evaluations in the future will use a combination of approaches, undertaking prospective evaluations alongside clinical trials where the opportunity exists, but in addition using other efficacy data reflecting normal clinical use in order to extrapolate trial findings. However, it is clear from the draft government guidelines for cost-effectiveness studies that good quality efficacy data, however obtained, are essential for a credible economic evaluation. This view is further reinforced when one considers that the majority of economic evaluations are published in clinical journals, thereby having to pass the review process. Economic studies cannot make good any gaps in the efficacy data; rather they demonstrate the value in broader economic and social terms, of improved efficacy or a superior side-effect profile.

DATA ON RESOURCE USE AND COSTS

The first methodological issue to resolve when undertaking an economic evaluation is to determine the range of costs that is considered to be relevant. To a major extent this depends on viewpoint, as was discussed above. However, most economic evaluations consider *direct costs*. These are the changes in resource use, borne mainly though not exclusively by the health care system, in providing the therapy. A major item of direct cost in drug studies is usually the medicine itself, but there are also the resources required to administer the therapy (e.g. medical time) and, for some treatments, hospitalization. In their economic evaluation of an oral gold preparation for arthritis, Thompson et al (1988) collected data on medical procedures, laboratory tests, concomitant medications, hospitalization and nursing home care. Not all the resource changes arising from the use of a new medicine will be in the same direction. For example, a more effective antibiotic may lead to a reduction in hospitalization for the patient.

In the case of some therapies, significant resource inputs are made by the patient or family, in terms of travel time, expenditure on medications, home adaptations and informal nursing care. Some time commitments may mean forgone work opportunities (see below). The existence of these costs is usually recognized by economic analysts, but they are rarely quantified and valued. Therefore, they usually receive less emphasis than those direct costs borne by the health care system. Given the inevitable emphasis on health care budgets it is usually difficult to make a case for a more expensive medicine on the grounds that it reduces costs to the patient or the family, although from a societal perspective these impacts are relevant.

There are two components to data collection for direct costs: the physical quantities (e.g. hours of nursing time, or number of procedures) and their unit costs or prices in money terms. Frequently economic evaluations merely report that the cost of hospitalization was (say) $3000, although clearly this calculation would have involved both prices and quantities.

There are a number of advantages in reporting prices and quantities separately. First, it greatly facilitates the extrapolation of results to other settings. Whereas generalization of economic data is not without its pitfalls (Drummond et al, 1992), the fact that the average length of hospitalization was five days means more to a decision maker in another setting than reporting that it cost $3000.

Secondly, separate reporting of price and quantity data enables the quality of data sources to be more easily evaluated. For example, it is relevant to know whether the quantities of resources consumed were gathered alongside a clinical trial, obtained from routine hospital records or patients' charts, or were merely based on assumptions. Similarly, for unit cost data it is relevant to know whether these were obtained from detailed costing studies in the institution where the patients were treated, were based on charges or payments, or calculated from national routine data sources.

Each of the sources of unit cost data has its advantages and disadvantages. However, one needs to be particularly careful in interpreting data based on charges, which may bear no relation to real costs (Finkler, 1982). Nevertheless, if the main perspective adopted is that of the third party payer, the actual payments (which often differ from charges) may be relevant.

In general there is a tendency to pay too little attention to detail in the estimation of resource use and cost in economic evaluations, although this is changing now that more studies are being conducted alongside clinical trials. The days when a 'cost-effectiveness study' consisted of a clinical trial with some 'back-of-the-envelope' costing attached are rapidly becoming a thing of the past. Therefore, it is important to estimate resource quantities as carefully as possible and to be explicit about the sources of the unit cost data.

The other major category of resource changes in economic evaluation relates to the impacts on productive activity. These are known as *indirect costs.* Although the patient is often taken out of work to be given therapy, changes in productive activity usually occur on the benefit side of the equation in economic evaluations of pharmaceuticals. That is, more efficacious medicines, or those with fewer wide effects, may enable the patient, or the person caring for him or her, to return to work quicker.

There is considerable discussion and debate about the relevance of indirect costs and benefits in economic evaluations. This uncertainty is reflected in the government guidelines for cost-effectiveness studies (Drummond, 1992). The Australian guidelines state that they should be excluded unless a good case can be made. The Ontario guidelines tacitly allow their inclusion as part of a societal analysis. The arguments for and against indirect costs and benefits are conducted on two levels. On one level it is argued that productivity may not actually be lost when a person is away from work; for short-term absences the work may be covered by others, for long-term absences the worker can be replaced by someone who was previously unemployed. On another level it is argued that inclusion of indirect costs and benefits would place a relatively higher value on therapies for employed persons in highly paid occupations, at the expense of those for the elderly or for homemakers. Although this problem could be countered by valuing a day's lost productivity at the same amount, no matter what the person's income. (Gross salary is the most common approach to valuing productivity losses.)

Whether or not indirect costs and benefits are included is far from being a trivial matter. For example, Osterhaus et al (1992) estimated the indirect costs of migraine in the USA to be between $5.6 and $17.2 billion annually, through individuals being off work or operating at reduced productivity. Conversely, there would be few savings in direct health care costs from more effective therapies for conditions such as migraine. Therefore, the economic case for many more expensive medications often rests on arguments of increased productivity and improved quality of life (see below).

Given the current degree of confusion over inclusion or exclusion of indirect costs, it is advisable to estimate the indirect costs and benefits separately from the direct changes in health care resources. It would also make sense to estimate the number of work days lost as well as attempting to *value* the changes in production by applying daily wage rates or estimating social security payments. This approach allows the decision maker to give the appropriate weight to productivity changes, depending on the perspective he or she chooses to adopt.

EVIDENCE OF IMPACT ON QUALITY OF LIFE

A minority of medicines may be able to make their economic case in terms of overall cost savings, or in terms of their impact on survival. (For example, comparisons are often made between life-saving therapies in terms of their relative cost per life-year saved [Schulman et al, 1991].) However, most modern medicines are more expensive than their predecessors and have an impact on quality of life rather than survival. Therefore, assessments of the impact on quality of life are an important feature of many current economic evaluations of medicines.

In some areas of medicine the clinical trials of the medicines may include quality of life measures, either because improved quality of life is the most appropriate measure of efficacy, or because therapies are known to have detrimental effects on quality of life owing to side-effects. Therefore, on some occasions it may be possible for economic evaluations to draw on evidence gathered in the clinical programme. On other occasions additional data gathering may be required, either outside the clinical trial or by modifying the trial protocol if data are being gathered prospectively.

There are three broad types of quality of life measures: disease-specific scales, general scales or profiles (e.g. SF-36 or Nottingham Health Profile) and health state preference valuations (e.g. health 'utilities'). Each type of measure has its own prime purpose and it is often common to include more than one in a given prospective study (see Figure 2.1.3). Economists tend to favour health state preference valuations since these enable an overall assessment of the benefit of therapy to be obtained. For example, in one approach survival and quality of life data are combined to calculate the quality-adjusted life-years (QALYs) gained by treatment (Drummond et al, 1987). Comparisons of the relative value for money of therapies of, for instance, dementia are then made in terms of cost per QALY or equivalents (Drummond et al, 1992).

Deciding on the most appropriate way of assessing the quality of life impact of therapy is one of the most difficult choices to make, especially in view of the costs of gathering the data. All the issues cannot be discussed here, but they revolve around: (1) which categories of quality of life measure to employ; (2) which particular instruments to use (e.g. SF-36 or NHP for a general measure; visual analogue scale or standard gamble for health state preference valuation); and (3) whether to collect data in the clinical trial itself, from other sources. Figure 2.1.3 illustrates that there are interrelationships between the various measures and that, in particular, there are a number of ways of generating data on health 'utilities'.

The overall trend is towards more inclusion of disease-specific and general quality of life measures in the clinical trials themselves. Most analysts argue for inclusion of both types of measure. They counsel strongly against developing one's own measure, at least before carefully examining all existing measures in order to be sure that they are inappropriate. (A common failing is to reject all existing measures, on the grounds that they are 'too insensitive to change' for the condition concerned, without sufficient empirical evidence.) The main problem with developing a new measure is the time and expense, particularly if it is required in a number of languages. Another difficulty is that even when the data are reported, possibly showing a beneficial change as measured by the new instrument, the decision maker has nothing to relate it to. The development of new quality of life measures, or their translation and validation in different languages, are not tasks to be undertaken lightly.

Whereas the descriptive quality of life measures, whether general or disease-specific, is more often being included in clinical trials, the position with health state preference valuation is less clear (Feeny and Torrance, 1989). First, it is not clear *whose* preferences should count. Measurement of preference values within trials enables these to be obtained from patients. However, it might also be argued that, for health care resource allocation decisions, it should be the preferences of the general public (who pay the taxes) that should count. Secondly, the most widely used approach, to estimate the QALYs gained by

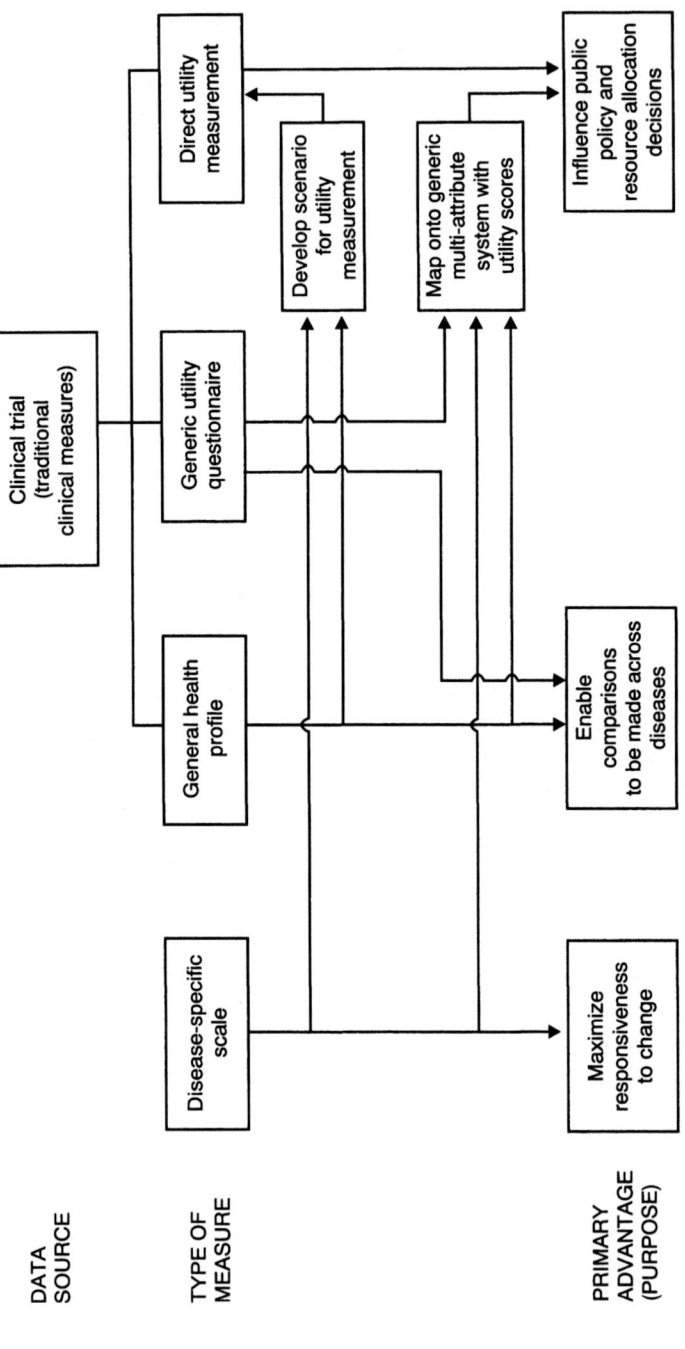

Figure 2.1.3. Interrelationships between health-related quality of life measures. *Source:* adapted from Drummond and Davies (1991)

valuing health state preferences and multiplying them by the time spent in a given state, has been criticized (Loomes and McKenzie, 1989; Mehrez and Gafni, 1989).

Therefore, it is important to consider the options carefully before investing large amounts of resources in health state preference valuation alongside clinical trials. Issues that need to be considered are: (1) can health state preference valuations be reliably derived by a secondary analysis; (2) whose preferences should count; and (3) how much criticism will there be of the instruments used? Currently the risk/benefit trade-off from undertaking health state preference valuations alongside clinical trials is unclear.

Another approach, which is less resource-intensive, is to include a generic health state preference instrument in the clinical trial. These instruments, of which the EuroQoL (EQ-5D) (1995) and McMaster Health Utilities Index (1995) are examples, have the advantage that only a simple questionnaire is administered in the trial itself. The responses from patients can then be expressed as a health state preference value by reference to pre-scaled responses from a relevant reference group.

Finally, it should be mentioned that there has been a renewed interest in estimating the benefits of health care interventions in terms of what individuals would be *willing to pay* to have improved health (Johannesson and Jönsson, 1991). Given the fact that many of the benefits from more efficacious medicines, or those with fewer side-effects, are intangible, this approach is more likely to be applied in economic evaluations of medicines in the future. Most economists would agree that to estimate willingness-to-pay is the theoretically correct approach, since it is grounded in the principles of Paretian welfare economics (Birch and Gafni, 1991). The policy-making relevance of such estimations is less clear, however. First, most health insurance systems do not call upon individuals to pay for their health care at the time of consumption. Therefore, individuals not having much experience of actually being called upon to pay may have difficulty in answering such questions. Secondly, presenting government policy makers with evidence that individuals would be willing to pay more for their medications is fairly compelling evidence for increasing copayments for pharmaceuticals at a time when the government has a budgetary crisis! On the other hand, in settings like the USA, where most health care is provided through private health insurance, the amount that individuals would be willing to pay for increased benefits is probably one of the main pieces of information required by health insurers (Pauly, 1992).

ANALYSIS AND REPORTING OF RESULTS

No matter how well a study is conducted, the overall benefit will be lost if the results are not communicated effectively. A major aspect of analysing and reporting economic evaluations is to pay attention to the viewpoints of the relevant decision makers. Indeed it is likely that the same study should be communicated in different ways in order to meet the needs of governmental decision makers, hospital formulary committees and individual prescribers. There are, in addition, a number of technical points that need to be taken into account and these are discussed in turn below.

BOX 2.1.2: ISSUES TO CONSIDER IN DATA COLLECTION

- Which are the best clinical trial data upon which to base an economic evaluation?
- If a number of trials have been undertaken is a meta-analysis available?
- Are any of the existing clinical trials suitable vehicles for conducting an economic evaluation?
- Has a relevant range of costs been considered, bearing in mind the viewpoint(s) for the analysis?
- Have the physical quantities of the relevant resources been estimated and reported separately from the unit costs (prices)?
- Which measures of quality of life have been considered, bearing in mind the objectives of the economic evaluation?
- Which method has been chosen to estimate health state preference valuations and on whom?
- Which quality of life data would it be most appropriate to collect alongside the clinical trials themselves?

INCREMENTAL ANALYSIS

No matter what form of economic analysis is adopted, data will normally be available, for two or more alternative therapies, on comparative costs and comparative consequences (measured in life-years gained, improved quality of life, etc.). It is normally argued that the relevant data for decision making are derived from the *incremental* analysis of one therapy compared with the other. That is, the decision maker needs to know what *extra* is being gained, in desirable consequences, for the extra costs.

This being said, it is important to be aware that such incremental analyses can be greatly affected by the choice of baseline comparator. For example, is the relevant baseline 'no intervention', or 'current care'? If it is 'current care', has this option itself been evaluated for cost-effectiveness? These issues are most problematic where there are a number of stages of intervention, each more intensive than the last.

For example, consider the evaluation of the statins, a new class of lipid-lowering agents. One incremental analysis would compare the relative costs and consequences of treatment of known high-risk patients (e.g. individuals with familial hypercholesterolaemia, or a pre-treatment cholesterol level greater than 7.8 mmol/L) with statins instead of current medications (e.g. resins or fibrates). From a pharmaceutical company's point of view this is probably the most obvious comparison, since the new product may have been developed to replace existing drugs for the condition concerned. It would also probably have been compared with exiting medications in controlled clinical trials.

However, from the decision maker's point of view there are other relevant incremental analyses. One would relate to whether *any* drug therapy be given when dietary measures fail to reduce total cholesterol to the recommended target level (e.g. 6.5 mmol/L). Another incremental analysis would relate to the cost-effectiveness of expanding therapy to a wider range of individuals, based on age, pre-treatment cholesterol level or other risk factors. In this case, since more individuals would be brought into therapy, the costs of additional case finding may also be relevant to the economic analysis. Without necessarily stating which is the most relevant incremental analysis, it can be readily seen that different analyses among those outlined above are likely to generate quite different incremental cost-effectiveness ratios. Therefore, when it is claimed that a given medicine is 'cost-effective', this begs the questions 'compared to what?' and 'under what circumstances?' Good analyses make these issues explicit.

DISCOUNTING COSTS AND CONSEQUENCES OCCURRING IN THE FUTURE

It is a convention in economic analyses to discount costs and consequences occurring in the future to present values. A discount factor is applied, which reduces the quantitative significance, in the analysis, of events occurring in the future, compared with those occurring in the present. Discounting has its origins in the belief that as individuals, and as a community, we have a positive rate of time preference. That is, we prefer benefits sooner rather than later and prefer also to postpone costs. There is some empirical justification for a positive rate of time preference, at least at the individual level. In borrowing money we normally have to pay an interest rate above the rate of inflation in order to encourage others to postpone their own consumption.

The convention in economic evaluations in the heath care field is to discount both costs and consequences by an annual rate of 5% in real terms. There is little empirical basis for this, other than that the convention was widely applied in economic evaluations published in the *New England Journal of Medicine* in the late 1970s and early 1980s. Rates close to 5% per annum have also been operating in countries, like the UK, where the government announces a rate for the appraisal of public sector projects.

More recently the debate over discounting has been reopened in the literature, particularly in respect of whether consequences (which are typically not expressed in money terms) should be discounted at all, or discounted at a different rate from costs. This interest partly follows the UK government's decision not to discount the health benefits from health care interventions (e.g. the life-years saved). Savings in health care costs occurring in the future will still be discounted, however (Parsonage and Neuberger, 1992; Cairns, 1992). The most recent advice has come from the Public Health Service Panel on the Cost-Effectiveness of Health and Medicine in the USA, which recommended a rate of 3% (Gold et al, 1996).

The choice of discount rate is not a trivial matter, particularly in the case of preventive programmes, such as screening and treatment for hypertension. Applying a lower discount rate, or a zero rate for health benefits, makes investments in preventive programmes look much more attractive and can also change the cost-effectiveness rankings among different classes of anti-hypertensive medicines (Drummond and Coyle, 1992) and those for hyper-cholesterolaemia (Drummond et al, 1993). Given the current uncertainty, those undertaking studies should: (1) apply the conventional rate of 5% per annum to both costs and consequences; (2) also apply any rate advised by government or expert committees in a given jurisdiction; (3) explore the impact on the results of the evaluation of choosing different rates.

ALLOWING FOR UNCERTAINTIES IN THE ANALYSIS

The choice of discount rate is one of a number of uncertainties in current economic evaluation methodology in the health care field. Other uncertainties arise from a lack of precision in various estimates of costs and consequences. The approach usually employed to deal with uncertainty in economic evaluations is known as *sensitivity analysis*. Here key parameters or assumptions are varied, either singly or together, in order to explore the impact on study results. Although the *principle* of undertaking sensitivity analysis is well accepted by economic analysts, precisely *how* it is done varies greatly. Indeed the analyst has considerable freedom over how conservative or optimistic to be in making various assumptions about the likely values of key parameters, particularly in the case of those for which few measurements are available.

Despite the temptation to produce a positive result, analysts should consider carefully the balance of optimism and conservatism they wish to encourage in the studies they commission or undertake. As has been remarked elsewhere, 'a small solid piece of English cheddar cheese is sometimes worth much more than a large piece of Swiss emmental with lots of holes in it!' (Drummond, 1992). When undertaking studies it is always wise to consider the likely extent of scrutiny and criticism of the results once the study is published.

Although sensitivity analysis remains the dominant approach, now that more economic analyses are being undertaken alongside clinical trials it has been suggested that the economic data be subjected to the same statistical tests as the efficacy data. There is an inherent logic in this although a number of methodological issues remain unresolved (O'Brien et al, 1994). These include whether to undertake statistical tests on the physical quantities of resources or overall costs, how to undertake statistical tests on cost-effectiveness ratios and how to determine the 'economically important difference' in cost or cost-effectiveness.

Some of these issues will take some time to resolve. In the meantime analysts need to be aware of this growing requirement for statistical analysis of economic data and to keep abreast of methodological developments. Finally, it should be noted that, even though more economic studies will be conducted alongside clinical trials in the future, there will still be a role for sensitivity analysis. This is because some of the data in economic evaluations are not stochastic and thereby the application of statistic tests has no meaning. Variables in this category include the choice of discount rate and many of the prices (unit costs) of resources.

GENERALIZING ECONOMIC EVALUATION RESULTS TO DIFFERENT SETTINGS

The unit costs (or prices) of resources represent one item that can vary from place to place and could therefore conceivably affect the relative cost-effectiveness of therapies. Other relevant factors include geographical variations in demography or epidemiology of disease, clinical practice patterns and the availability of health care resources.

As more economic evaluations of medicines are being conducted, and as the level of international interest in study results increases, the issue of international transferability of economic data has been discussed. Clinical trial results are generally considered to be transportable from one setting to another, although this is probably more true of the evaluations of medicines than those of (say) surgical procedures. It would be particularly beneficial to both pharmaceutical companies and health care decision makers if economic study results could similarly be generalized from one setting to another. This would avoid having to repeat every study of each new medicine in every setting.

It is clear that the generalization of economic data is not straightforward. However, it is made easier if the alternatives being evaluated are set out in a decision-tree format, as discussed earlier. The limited experience to date suggests that it may be possible to transfer economic evaluation results from one setting to another, with manageable amounts of additional data collection (Drummond et al, 1992). As more economic studies are undertaken on an international level, perhaps alongside multinational clinical trials, our experience of this issue will greatly increase. In the meantime those planning studies in more than one country should explore the potential benefits of standardized protocols for the economic evaluation and the use of decision trees to facilitate generalization.

CONCLUDING REMARKS

It can be seen from the above that, despite a general methodology having emerged, there are currently many uncertainties surrounding the economic evaluation of medicines. The needs of health care decision makers for economic data remain despite the known imperfections in methods. Two jurisdictions, Australia and Ontario, have already proposed draft guidelines for cost-effectiveness studies to be submitted by companies in support of claims for government reimbursement of their products.

This paper has reviewed the current status of economic evaluation methods with the aim of providing general guidance to those undertaking, or commissioning, economic evaluations of their products. The approaches suggested do not constitute a blueprint for the perfect economic study, but it is hoped that by following the advice given analysts may be able to avoid the major pitfalls in undertaking research in this emerging field.

BOX 2.1.3: ISSUES TO CONSIDER WHEN ANALYSING AND
REPORTING RESULTS

- Has an appropriate form of economic evaluation been selected, given the advantages of the medicine over its competitors?
- Has careful consideration been given to the range of possible baseline comparison alternatives against which the incremental costs and consequences of the medicine can be assessed?
- Have costs and consequences occurring in the future been discounted at a rate considered relevant in the settings where the study will be reported?
- Has a sensitivity analysis been performed, exploring the impact on results of differing assumptions about key parameters (e.g. the discount rate)?
- Has enough consideration been given to the overall balance of conservatism and optimism in the analysis and reporting of study results?
- Where stochastic data are reported, has consideration been given to the appropriateness of tests of statistical significance?
- Has consideration been given to the most appropriate ways of extrapolating the study results to different settings?

ACKNOWLEDGEMENTS

An earlier version of this chapter was published in the *British Journal of Medical Economics* (1993), 6B, 1–18. I am grateful to the editors for allowing me to use the original text.

REFERENCES

Adams, M. E., McCall, N. T. and Gray, D. T. (1992). Economic analysis in randomized control trials, *Medical Care*, 30(3): 231–243.

Birch, S. and Gafni, A. (1991). Cost-effectiveness/utility analyses: do current decision rules lead us to where we want to be? *CHEPA Working Paper 91–6*, Hamilton (Ont.), McMaster University.

Cairns, J. (1992). Discounting and health benefits: another perspective, *Health Economics*, 1(1), 76–80.

Commonwealth of Australia (1992). *Guidelines for submissions to the Pharmaceutical Benefits Advisory Committee including economic analyses*, Woden (ACT), Commonwealth of Australia.

Davies, L. M. and Drummond, M. F. (1990). Management of labour: consumer choice and cost implications, *Journal of Obstetrics and Gynaecology*, 11 (Suppl. 1), 528–533.

Dolan, P., Gudex, C., Kind, P. and Williams, A. (1995). A social tariff for EuroQoL: results from a UK general population survey, Centre for Health Economics Discussion Paper 138, University of York, September.

Drummond, M. F. (1991). Common mistakes in the design of economic evaluations of medicines, *British Journal of Medical Economics*, 1, 5–14.

Drummond, M. F. (1992). Cost-effectiveness guidelines for reimbursement of pharmaceuticals: is economic evaluation ready for its enhanced status? *Health Economics*, 1, 85–92.

Drummond, M. F., Bloom, B. S., Carrin, G. et al (1992). Issues in the cross-national assessment of health technology, *International Journal of Technology Assessment in Health Care*, 8(4), 671–682.

Drummond, M. F. and Coyle, D. (1992). Assessing the economic value of antihypertensive medicines, *Journal of Human Hypertension*, 6, 495–501.

Drummond, M. F. and Davies, L. M. (1991). Economic analysis alongside clinical trials: revisiting the methodological issues, *International Journal of Technology Assessment in Health Care*, 7(4), 561–573.

Drummond, M. F., Heyse, J., Cook, J. and McGuire, A. (1993). Selection of endpoints in economic evaluations of coronary heart disease interventions, *Medical Decision Making*, 13(3), 184–190.

Drummond, M. F., Mohide, E. A., Tew, M., Streiner, D. L., Pringle, D. M. and Gilbert, J. R. (1992). Economic evaluation of a support program for caregivers of demented elderly, *International Journal of Technology Assessment in Health Care*, 7, 209–219.

Drummond, M. F., Stoddart, G. L. and Torrance, G. W. (1987). *Methods for the Economic Evaluation of Health Care Programmes*, Oxford, Oxford University Press.

Ernst, R. L. and Hay, J. W. (1994). The US economic and social costs of Alzheimer's disease revisited, *American Journal of Public Health*, 84, 1–4.

Feeny, D. and Torrance, G. W. (1989). Utilities and quality-adjusted life-years, *International Journal of Technology Assessment in Health Care*, 5, 559–575.

Finkler, S. (1982). On the distinction between costs and charges, *Annals of Internal Medicine*, 96, 102–109.

Gold, M. R., Siegel, J. E., Russell, L. B. and Weinstein, M. C. (Eds) (1996). *Cost-effectiveness in Health and Medicine*, New York, Oxford University Press.

Goldman, L., Sia, S. T. B., Cook, E. F. et al (1988). Costs and effectiveness of routine therapy with long-term beta-adrenergic antagonists after acute myocardial infarction, *New England Journal of Medicine*, 319(3), 152–157.

Gray, A. and Fenn, P. (1993). Alzheimer's disease: the burden of illness in England, *Health Trends*, 25, 31–7.

Johannesson, M. and Jönsson, B. (1991). Economic evaluation in health care: is there a role for cost-benefit analysis? *Health Policy*, 17, 1–23.

Kamlet, M. S. (1992). *A framework for Cost-utility Analysis of Government Health Care Programs*, Washington, DC, Department of Health and Human Services.

Knapp, M. J., Knopman, D. S., Solomon, P. R., Pendlebury, W. W., Davis, C. S. and Gracon, S. I. (1994). A 30-week randomized controlled trial of high-dose tacrine in patients with Alzheimer's disease, *Journal of the American Medical Association*, 271, 985–991.

Loomes, G. and McKenzie, L. (1989). The use of QALYs in health care decision making, *Social Science and Medicine*, 28, 299–308.

Lubeck, D. P., Mazonson, P. D. and Bowe, T. (1995). The potential impact of tacrine on expenditures for Alzheimer's disease, *Medical Interface*, 7, 130–138.

Luce, B. R. and Elixhauser, A. (1990). *Standards for Socio-economic Evaluations of Health Care Products and Services*, Berlin, Springer-Verlag.

Mehrez, A. and Gafni, A. (1989). Quality adjusted life years, utility theory and healthy years equivalents, *Medical Decision Making*, 9, 142–149.

O'Brien, B., Drummond, M. F. and Labelle, R. J. (1994). In search of power and significance: statistical issues in economic evaluations, *Medical Care*, 32, 150–163.

Oster, G. and Epstein, A. M. (1987). Cost-effectiveness of antihyperlipidemic therapy in the prevention of coronary heart disease: the case of cholestyramine, *Journal of the American Medical Association*, 258(17), 2381–2387.

Osterhaus, J. T., Gutterman, D. L. and Plachetka, J. R. (1992). Health care resource and lost labour costs of migraine headache in the US, *PharmacoEconomics*, 2(1), 67–76.

Parsonage, M. and Neuberger, H. (1992). Discounting and health benefits, *Health Economics*, 1(1), 71–75.

Pauly, M. (1992). Presentation at the DIA Meeting, Nice.

Sacks, H., Berrier, J., Reitman, D., Ancona-Berk, V. A. and Chalmers, T. C. (1987). Meta-analyses of randomized controlled trials, *New England Journal of Medicine*, 316, 450–455.

Schulman, K. A., Lynn, L. A., Glick, H. A. and Eisenberg, J. M. (1991). Cost-effectiveness of low-dose zidovudine therapy for symptomatic patients with human immunodeficiency virus (HIV) infection, *Annals of Internal Medicine*, 114, 798–802.

Thompson, M. S., Read, J. L., Hutchings, H. C. et al (1988). The cost-effectiveness of auranofin: results of a randomized clinical trial, *Journal of Rheumatology*, 15, 35–42.

Torrance, G. W., Furlong, W., Feeny, D. and Boyle, M. (1995). Multi-attribute preference functions: health utilities index, *PharmacoEconomics*, 7(6), 503–520.

Udvarhelyi, D., Colditz, G. A., Rai, A. and Epstein, A. M. (1992). Cost-effectiveness and cost-benefit analysis in the medical literature, *Annals of Internal Medicine*, 116, 238–244.

Warner, K. E. and Luce, B. R. (1982). *Cost-benefit and Cost-Effectiveness Analysis in Health Care*, Ann Arbor MI, Health Administration Press.

Wimo, A., Karlsson, G., Nordberg, A. and Winblad, B. (1997). Treatment of Alzheimer's disease with tacrine—a cost analysis model, *Alzheimer Disease and Associated Disorders*, 11, 191–200.

2.2 Methodological Issues in Health Economic Studies of Dementia

GÖRAN KARLSSON, BENGT JÖNSSON
Stockholm School of Economics, Stockholm, Sweden

ANDERS WIMO
Umeå University, Umeå and Karolinska Institute, Stockholm, Sweden

BENGT WINBLAD
Karolinska Institute, Stockholm, Sweden

INTRODUCTION

Dementia is a costly disease in terms of resources used and forgone due to the disease but also in terms of suffering for the patients and their relatives. In other parts of this book, cost-of-illness studies of dementia show that the economic burden of dementia is substantial. Analysts have pointed out that the economic burden may increase in the future because of an ageing population and an associated increase in prevalence of the disease (Jorm et al, 1987; Ritchie et al, 1992; Schneider and Guralnik, 1990).

However, recently new 'antidementia' drugs have been introduced on the market and further drugs are in the pipeline for introduction. The potential benefits of these drugs in terms of reduction in costs in the treatment and caring of dementia, and improvements in quality of life, are substantial. But now when we are facing the beginning of a drug treatment era of dementia, difficult balances are also imposed. The benefits of a drug have to be weighed against its costs in terms of resources and side-effects. And which one of several drugs should be used if benefits and costs differ?

As the economic and quality of life impacts of new treatment programmes are considerable, the need for economic evaluation is obvious. There is a well-developed methodology of economic evaluation of health care interventions. The basic principles of pharmacoeconomics have been described in more detail by Michael Drummond in the previous chapter. But are there specific methodological challenges in the economic evaluation of dementia? We believe there are. Many of these methodological challenges are also found in other disease areas but they are emphasised in the economic evaluation of dementia.

Health Economics of Dementia. Edited by Anders Wimo, Bengt Jönsson, Göran Karlsson and Bengt Winblad.
© 1998 John Wiley & Sons Ltd.

Intricate choices regarding the perspective of the economic study, type of study, study design, outcome measurement, data needed for modelling, how to handle costs of informal care and to what extent international comparisons can be made, are issues that characterise the economic evaluation of dementia. These issues are briefly outlined in this chapter and many aspects of them will be discussed further in later chapters of this book.

PERSPECTIVE

From which perspective should an economic evaluation of an intervention be performed? Is it from a societal perspective which includes all relevant costs, or is it from the perspective of a specific payer, such as a County Council, a municipality, the public sector in general, the patient's perspective or that of an insurance company? One characteristic of dementia is that there are many participants involved in covering the costs for the disease. The cost drivers of dementia care are costs for living and caring, while the costs for therapies are low. This means that the participant(s) who covers the cost for caring carries the main part of the economic burden. Who this participant actually is varies between countries, but in most countries it is the community/municipality or an informal, often unpaid, caregiver.

The cost implication of a new drug treatment is that the cost for the drug therapy is a part of the health care cost, while possible cost savings occur in the municipalities and through the informal caregiver. Limiting the economic analysis just to the health care sector or to the public sector means that important costs are excluded from the analysis. Therefore, a societal perspective where all costs are included regardless of where they occur and regardless of who pays is to be preferred.

However, incentives are important in analysing new therapies against dementia. If one participant is paying for the therapy—mainly the health care sector—and the benefits go to other participants, there is a risk that a new therapy will never be implemented even if it is profitable. Therefore, detecting inoptimal incentives is an essential part of economic analysis. But it is important to make a distinction between the financing of dementia care and the economic evaluation of dementia interventions. This chapter, and this book, mainly deal with the economic evaluation of dementia.

TYPE OF STUDY

An important purpose of economic evaluation is that it should serve as a tool for decision making regarding scarce resources. Cost-of-illness studies are descriptive and cannot be used for setting priorities. Such studies only describe the economic burden of a particular disorder in monetary terms. In order to assist decision making at least two treatment strategies have to be included. Therefore, at least a cost-minimisation study should be used. In such a study the cost implications of two or more alternatives are included. But an effective drug treatment has impact not only on costs but also on the quality of life of the patient. The problem is how improvements in quality of life can be incorporated in an economic evaluation.

One option is a cost-consequence analysis. Here costs and outcome are presented separately. Instruments for measuring quality of life can be used at different points in time. Generic quality of life instruments such as SF-36 or specific instruments for dementia can be used. A cost-consequence analysis gives information on costs as well as quality of life, but they are not integrated into one evaluation measure, which reflects efficiency. In order to do that the outcome has to be expressed in a single measure.

This is the case with cost-effectiveness and cost-utility analyses. An advantage with cost-effectiveness analysis is that it produces a measure of efficiency, that is the incremental cost-effectiveness ratio. However, the challenge in economic evaluation of dementia is to find an appropriate effectiveness measure. Quality-adjusted life-years—QALYs—are used as an effectiveness measure in cost-utility analysis. QALYs as an effectiveness measure facilitate efficiency comparisons with treatments in other disease areas. The US Panel for cost-effectiveness analysis recommends QALYs as an effectiveness measure in the case referred to by Gold et al (1996). But the construction of QALYs is not straightforward in dementia. Although there are advantages in using cost-effectiveness and cost-utility analysis there are also problems with finding and calculating an appropriate outcome measure. This leads us to a discussion regarding the outcome measure.

OUTCOME MEASURE

Mini Mental Stage Examination (MMSE), a measure of cognitive ability, and measures of ADL-capacity are often used in clinical trials. MMSE is an example of so-called surrogate endpoints, which is impossible to use in cost-effectiveness analysis (Johannesson et al, 1996). Measures of ADL-capacity are also difficult to use in economic evaluation.

Days spent outside institutional care units have been suggested as an effectiveness measure. This measure is also difficult to use in economic evaluation. The place of living is to a large extent determined by the organisation of care and the supply of different forms of care units, and not only by the patient's health state. This measure is therefore a combination of the organisation of dementia care and the patient's health status, which makes it difficult to interpret.

A health state can be defined as a dichotomous variable, for example whether or not the patient's cognitive ability is below a certain level. This level can be based on MMSE, for instance if the patient has an MMSE-score below 10. If an MMSE-score lower than 10 is defined as severe dementia, then the corresponding evaluation measure is incremental cost per day of severe dementia avoided. But this measure is not free from weaknesses either. It implicitly means that all MMSE-scores above 10 have the same value for the patient and all MMSE-scores below 10 have the same value. This is obviously a simplification.

QALYs are a good candidate for an outcome measure. The main problem with QALYs is how the preference score for a specific health state should be measured. When the patient's cognitive ability has deteriorated she cannot evaluate her health state herself. Therefore, somebody else has to evaluate the health state; some kind of indirect (proxy) measurement has to be used, for example with the help of instruments such as EuroQol or the Health Utility Index—Mark 2. Indirect measurement is not necessarily a problem—the US Panel for cost-effectiveness actually recommends that the general public should evaluate their health states and then an indirect measurement procedure is necessary (Gold et al, 1996). A problem, however, is that the patient cannot fill in the questionnaire herself. Furthermore, severe dementia may be regarded as worse than death and this creates ethical as well as methodological problems, especially when these states are located in the latest phase of life.

There is no obvious choice of outcome measure in the economic evaluation of dementia. As different outcome measures give different pieces of information, several outcome measures and evaluation measures can be used. The fact that there are weaknesses with all outcome measures also has implications for the choice of type of economic study. A cost-consequence analysis should not be excluded as a candidate for the economic evaluation of dementia.

INFORMAL CARE

Informal care by persons, mostly spouses or daughters of the patient but also volunteers, is one of the most important resources in dementia care. There is enormous support in the literature for the view that dementia has a very heavy impact on the caregiver's situation in terms of burden, quality of life, coping, stress, and so on. There are studies that indicate that the share of informal care may be as high as 70–90% of total home care costs (Wimo et al, 1997a).

Informal care should be valued and incorporated in an economic evaluation of dementia treatment. Otherwise an important part of the total burden of dementia is excluded from the analysis. Whether or not the caregiver is paid for the care does not matter in the economic evaluation; it has impact on the distribution of the burden but not on the total societal cost. The relevant cost is the opportunity cost, that is the benefits that are forgone because a resource—in this case the caregiver's time—is not used in the best possible way.

A key issue, therefore, is to determine what the alternative use of the caregiver's time actually is. If the alternative for the caregiver is working on the labour market, the cost for informal care should be valued as the production lost when he or she is absent from work. This should be valued by methods that are traditionally used in the estimation of labour cost.

It is more difficult to value the caregiver's time if the alternative is leisure. In the health economics literature there is no consensus how this should be performed. Koopmanshap and Brouwer suggest in this book (Chapter 2.8) that the loss of leisure time should be measured as a reduction of the caregiver's quality of life. They mean that quality of life instruments such as EuroQol and SF-36 can be used. However, it is unclear how a reduction in quality of life for the caregiver should be integrated into an economic evaluation. SF-36 cannot be used for measuring preference scores in the calculation of QALYs (Gold et al, 1996) so this approach may reduce the economic evaluation to a cost-consequence analysis. This means that costs and consequences, including reduction in quality of life for the caregiver and maybe also quality of life for the patient, are reported separately. As pointed out above, it is not then possible to present the economic evaluation as one efficiency measure. EuroQol, on the other hand, can be used for calculating QALYs. However, it is not clear if the proposers of this approach mean that the caregiver's quality of life should be incorporated in QALYs in a cost-utility analysis. If so, the issue as to how to aggregate the patient's and the caregiver's quality of life into one measure remains. To measure the caregiver's time as a reduction in quality of life, therefore, leaves many problems unresolved.

The alternative is to include the caregiver's leisure time in the cost side. The problem is how this time should be valued. One option is to value it against the cost of professional formal care, for example the cost of professional home help. The idea is that the alternative to informal care is professional home help; the informal caregiver's time and the professional caregiver's time are assumed to be perfect substitutes. The valuation of the informal caregiver's leisure time is then based on the cost-savings due to a reduced need for professional time.

However, such an approach is not based on the opportunity cost of the informal caregiver's time. In an opportunity-cost approach the cost of the caregiver's time is the value of the time used as leisure time. The main problem is that there is no such market price available. There are survey methods—for example the contingent valuation method—that may be fruitful in the valuation of the caregiver's leisure time. As far as we know no such empirical estimates have yet been performed.

Should the caregiver's leisure time be incorporated in the cost side, or as a consequence in terms of quality of life reductions, in an economic evaluation of dementia? To include it in both means double-counting and is not allowed.

We have to choose between the methods. A major problem with valuing lost leisure time as a quality of life reduction for the caregiver is that it seems to exclude the use of traditional cost-effectiveness and cost-utility analysis, where the effectiveness measure is linked to the patient. Therefore, in our opinion it seems to be more fruitful to include the caregiver's time in the cost side of the economic study. However, unresolved methodological and empirical issues remain in this field.

STUDY DESIGN

Demented patients may live 10 years or more after diagnosis. Furthermore, dementia is a chronically progressive disease. A drug intervention means that the scenario of the disease changes; the deterioration rate in cognitive ability and maybe also survival are affected by the drug. For example, the tacrine studies show improvements in MMSE-score but there was also a tendency for improved survival although it was non-significant (Knopman, 1996). Therefore an economic evaluation has to take into account impacts on costs and outcomes during the whole life-span.

The problem is that there are no clinical studies where patients are followed for such a long time period. Most existing clinical studies last for 6–12 months. A major purpose of economic evaluation is that it should serve as an input for decision making regarding allocation of resources. When new drugs for dementia are available and decisions regarding resources have to be made we need information on their cost-effectiveness. It is, obviously, not possible to start a prospective health economic study lasting for more than 10 years and wait for the results before we decide on which treatment strategy should be used.

Some kind of modelling—using clinical, economic, and epidemiological data—is therefore unavoidable. So-called Markov models (see the next chapter, 2.3) are frequently used for this purpose. In such a model (health) states, or Markov states, are defined. A Markov state can for instance be defined in terms of cognitive ability, for example intervals of MMSE-scores. To each state a cost and, in case, a preference score is associated. A cohort of patients are run through the model, where there are ongoing risks that the patients will move to worse Markov states with a higher cost and a lower utility. A Markov model is a tool for describing how the disease develops over time and can be used for simulating interventions.

The major body of costs in dementia care is linked to the patient's position in the care organisation and not to pure medical treatment. The cost that is associated to a specific Markov state is therefore determined by the organisa-tion of care. There have been great changes in the care organisation and conditions for care in many countries over time. Such changes include both a change of resources (such as deinstitutionalisation) and organisational changes

Table 2.2.1. Number of beds in different care alternatives in Sweden

	No.	1992 per 1000 80+	No.	1996 per 1000 80+	1992–96[a] (%)
Geriatric care	7 983	21	4 699	11	−41
Hospital care	29 473	77	21 750	52	−26
Psychiatric care	11 846	31	7 276	17	−38
Others[b]	8 476	22	1 679	4	−80
Total	57 778	172	35 404	84	−39

[a] Absolute figures.
[b] Public health care.

Sources: Annual statistics for county councils, *Statistical Yearbook of Health Care 1996*, Statistics Sweden (data on file), The National Board of Health and Welfare, Annual Report of the Care for the Elderly, 1997.

as outlined in the White Paper in England (Secretaries of State for Health, Social Security, Wales and Scotland, 1989) and the Ädelreform in Sweden (Äldredelegationen, 1989). For example, in Sweden the number of resources changed considerably during the 1980s. Between 1980 and 1991, the number of institutional beds (long-term care, hospital care, psychiatric care and homes for the aged) decreased from 170 000 to 126 000 (−26%). If this change is expressed as number of beds per 1000 80+, there was a decrease from 645 to 332 beds per 1000 80+. This deinstitutionalisation trend has continued during the 1990s (Table 2.2.1).

There is also a shift in care concepts, such as the implementation of Special Care Units in the USA (Volicer et al, 1994) and Group Living Units in Sweden (Wimo et al, 1995). It is also very important in the discussion of efficacy vs effectiveness to include a judgement of how the distribution of patients in a clinical trial reflects the dementia care organisation in a country (Wimo et al, 1997b). The conclusion is that a Markov model is linked, implicitly or explicitly, to a specific organisation of care. If the organisation of care, and as a result also the cost and the utility associated to a Markov state, changes over time the modelling has to be modified.

INTERNATIONAL COMPARISONS

A related issue is whether or not an economic evaluation of dementia care can be transferred between countries; there are differences in care organisation and care concepts between countries. Existing care concepts that are used in dementia care, such as nursing homes, can include a wide range of resources in terms of staff density, competence, physical environment, technical equipment, leading to different costs. Day care can be associated with specific units outside institutions, designed for demented patients only, and with a special care philosophy, but it may also be associated with care focused on somatic problems and with a mixture of patients. There are also care concepts that are used in just one or a few countries, such as SCU (Volicer et al, 1994) or DOMUS care (Beecham et al, 1993) or Group Living (Wimo et al, 1995). 'Home care' may be associated with social services with poorly educated staff, but also with specific teams focused on demented patients only. Even if care can roughly be divided into levels (such as nursing home care—intermediate care alternatives—home care), such an approach includes simplifications that threaten the validity of the analysis of a multinational intervention study.

Not only the resources associated with a specific form of care differ between countries but the relative supply of different forms of care also varies. Therefore, the cost associated with a specific Markov state probably differs substantially between countries. Not only costs but the outcome associated to a certain Markov state may vary between countries due to differences in care concepts. It is probably more difficult to transfer economic studies regarding dementia between countries than studies for many other disease areas. The characteristics of organising dementia care in a specific country have to be taken into account in an economic evaluation.

CONCLUDING REMARKS

The basic principles of economic evaluation of health care programmes also apply for dementia. An overview of these principles is given in Chapter 2.1 by Michael Drummond in this book. On most issues regarding methods for economic evaluation there is agreement among economists; see for example the US Panel regarding cost-effectiveness analysis (Gold et al, 1996) and a recently issued textbook (Drummond et al, 1997). However, there are choices that have to be made in all evaluations. In some disease areas they are more intricate than in others. Dementia care has some characteristics that challenge the skill and carefulness of the investigators.

Choice of type of study and choice of outcome measure are two issues that are closely related. There are good reasons for choosing a cost-effectiveness or a cost-utility analysis but the choice and calculation of an effectiveness measure are not obvious. The importance of informal care is emphasised in dementia care. The valuation of informal care is still a methodological issue that has to be solved. Modelling, where economic, clinical and epidemiological data are brought together, is an important part of economic evaluation of dementia. The modelling cannot be performed without taking into account the availability of data and the characteristics of organising dementia care. The assessors of dementia care have to have good knowledge of economic evaluation, modelling and the organisation of dementia care. Finally, to transfer an economic study from one country to another is probably more complicated than to do so for many other disease areas. Economic evaluation of dementia care is country-specific.

REFERENCES

Beecham, J., Cambridge, P., Hallam, A. and Knapp, M. (1993). The costs of domus care, *Int. J. Geriatr. Psychiat.*, **8**, 827–831.

Drummond, M. F., O'Brien, B., Stoddart, G. L. and Torrance, G. W. (1997). *Methods for the Economic Evaluation of Health Care Programmes*, Oxford, Oxford University Press.

Gold, M. R., Siegel, J. E., Russel, L. B. and Weinstein, M. C. (Eds) (1996). *Cost-effectiveness in Health and Medicine*, New York, Oxford University Press.

Johannesson, M., Jönsson, B. and Karlsson, G. (1996). Outcome measurement in economic evaluation, *Health Economics*, **5**, 279–296.

Jorm, A. F., Korten, A. E. and Henderson, A. S. (1987). The prevalence of dementia: a quantitative integration of the literature, *Acta. Psychiatr. Scand.*, **76**, 465–479.

Knopman, D. (1996). Long-term tacrine (Cognex) treatment: effects on nursing home placement and mortality, *Neurology*, **47**, 166–177.

Mace, N. L. and Rabins, P. V. (1991). *The 36-Hour Day: A Family Guide to Caring for Persons with Alzheimer's Disease, Related Dementing Illnesses, and Memory Loss in Later Life*, revised edn. Baltimore, Johns Hopkins University Press.

Ritchie, K., Kildea, D. and Robine, J. M. (1992). The relationship between age and the prevalence of senile dementia: a meta-analysis of recent data, *Int. J. Epidemiol.*, **21**, 763–769.

Schneider, E. L. and Guralnik, J. M. (1990). The aging of America. Impact on health care costs, *JAMA*, **263**, 2335–2340.

Secretaries of State for Health, Social Security, Wales and Scotland (1989). *Caring for people: community care in the next decade and beyond*, London, HMSO.

Statistics Sweden. *Hälso och sjukvårdsstatistisk årsbok 1996 (Statistical Yearbook of Healthcare in Sweden)*, Statistics Sweden, Stockholm, Sweden (in Swedish).

Volicer, L., Collard, A., Hurley, A., Bishop, C., Kern, D. and Karon, S. (1994). Impact of special care unit for patients with advanced Alzheimer's disease on patient's discomfort and costs, *J. Am. Geriatr. Soc.*, **42**, 597–603.

Wimo, A., Eriksson, T., Mattsson, B., Krakau, I., Nelvig, A. and Karlsson, G. (1995). Cost-utility analysis of Group Living in dementia care, *Int. J. Technol. Assess. Health Care*, **11**, 49–65.

Wimo, A., Ljunggren, G. and Winblad, B. (1997a). Costs due to dementia and dementia care—a review, *Int. J. Geriatr. Psychiatr.*, **12**, 841–856.

Wimo, A., Karlsson, G., Nordberg, A. and Winblad, B. (1997b). Treatment of Alzheimer's Disease with tacrine: a cost analysis model, *Alzheimer. Dis. Assoc. Disord.*, **11**, 39–45.

Äldredelegationen. *Ansvaret för äldreomsorgen* (The responsibility for the care of the elderly), Stockholm, Socialdepartementet 1989 (Ds S 1989:27) (in Swedish).

2.3 Modeling Disease Progression with Markov Models

FRANK A. SONNENBERG AND ELAINE A. LEVENTHAL

UMDNJ Robert Wood Johnson Medical School, New Brunswick, NJ, USA

INTRODUCTION

Decision models compare competing strategies by modeling the prognosis of a patient subsequent to each strategy. Prognosis can be measured both in terms of health effects and costs. For example, a strategy involving surgery may model the events of surgical death, surgical complications, and various outcomes of the surgical treatment itself. For practical reasons, the analysis must be restricted to a finite time frame, often referred to as the *time horizon* of the analysis. This means that, aside from death, the outcomes chosen to be represented by terminal nodes of the tree may not be final outcomes, but may simply represent convenient stopping points for the scope of the analysis. Thus, every tree contains terminal nodes that represent 'subsequent prognosis' for a particular combination of patient characteristics and events.

There are various ways in which a decision analyst can assign values to these terminal nodes of the decision tree. In some cases the outcome measure is a crude life expectancy. One method for estimating life expectancy is the declining exponential approximation DEALE (Beck et al, 1982) which calculates a patient-specific mortality rate for a given combination of patient characteristics and comorbid diseases. Life expectancies may also be obtained from Gompertz models of survival (Gompertz, 1825) or from standard life tables (National Center for Health Statistics, 1991). This paper explores another method for estimating life expectancy, the Markov model. In considering the prognosis of dementia, quality of life is at least as important as quantity and therefore prognosis is measured in terms of *quality-adjusted* life-expectancy (Mehrez and Gafni, 1989) which weights each period of life according to its associated quality of life.

In 1983, Beck and Pauker described the use of Markov models for determining prognosis in medical applications (Beck and Pauker, 1983). Since that introduction, Markov models have been applied with increasing frequency in published decision analyses (Eckman et al, 1990; Wong et al, 1990; Hillner et

Health Economics of Dementia. Edited by Anders Wimo, Bengt Jönsson, Göran Karlsson and Bengt Winblad.
© 1998 John Wiley & Sons Ltd.

al, 1992; Birkmeyer et al, 1992). Microcomputer software has been developed to permit constructing and evaluating Markov models more easily.

Markov models are particularly useful when a decision problem involves clinical changes that are ongoing over time. The progression of dementia with time is a good clinical example. Other examples are the risk of hemorrhage while on anticoagulant therapy, the risk of rupture of an abdominal aortic aneurysm and the risk of mortality in any person whether sick or healthy. There are two important modeling consequences of ongoing clinical changes. First, the time at which events occur is uncertain. This has important implications because the health value (utility) of an outcome often depends on when it occurs. For example, a stroke which occurs immediately may have a different impact on the patient than one which occurs 10 years later. For economic analyses, both costs and utilities are discounted (Weinstein and Stason, 1977; Detsky and Haglie, 1990) such that events that are more distant in time have less impact on a decision than events occurring sooner. The second consequence is that a given event (e.g. clinical worsening) may occur more than once. As the following example shows, representing events that are repetitive or that occur with uncertain timing is difficult using a simple tree model.

A SPECIFIC EXAMPLE

Consider a patient with the earliest stages of dementia. Over the course of the patient's life, dementia will advance, resulting in progressive disability. At any stage of the illness, the patient may become sufficiently disabled to require entering a nursing home. In the case of some dementing illnesses (e.g. Parkinson's disease) later stages of the disease are also associated with increases in mortality. Treatment may modify the progression of dementia by slowing the rate of development of disability. The decision tree fragment in Figure 2.3.1 shows one way of representing the prognosis for such a patient. The first chance node labelled DEMENTIA has three branches, labelled DIE, WORSEN and NO CHANGE. Thus, both WORSEN and NO CHANGE may lead to entering a nursing home, although with different probabilities. We assume that patients who worsen become disabled. Thus, there are five ultimate outcomes; DEAD, disabled in a nursing home (DISABLED NH), disabled at home (DISABLED), non-disabled in a nursing home (NURSING HOME) and non-disabled still at home (DEMENTIA).

There are several shortcomings with this model. First, the model does not specify when events occur. Second, the structure implies that if one outcome occurs (e.g. entering a nursing home without worsening) that no other outcome will subsequently occur. In fact, regardless of which clinical event occurs first, another event may occur later. Finally, at the terminal nodes labeled DISABLED, DISABLED NH, NURSING HOME and DEMENTIA, the

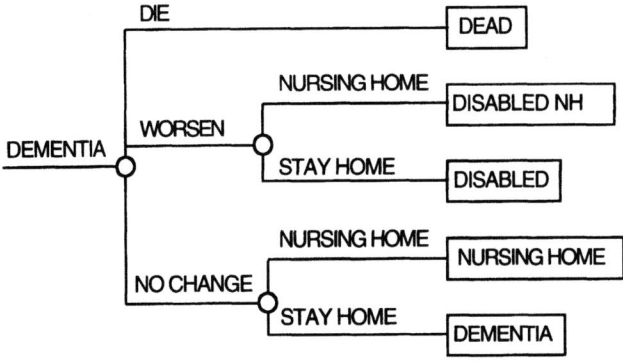

Figure 2.3.1.

analyst still is faced with the problem of assigning utilities, a task equivalent to specifying the prognosis for each of these non-fatal outcomes.

The first problem, specifying when events occur, may be addressed by using the tree structure in Figure 2.3.1 and making the assumption that either worsening or entering a nursing home occurs at the average time consistent with the known rate of each complication. For example, if the rate of becoming disabled is a constant 0.10 per person per year, then the average time before the occurrence of a hemorrhage is 1/0.1 or 10 years. However, if the patient is very old, their normal life expectancy may be less than 10 years. Thus, clinical worsening would have the paradoxical effect of improving the patient's life-expectancy. Other approaches, such as assuming that the worsening occurs half-way through the patient's normal life-expectancy, are arbitrary and may lessen the fidelity of the analysis.

Both the timing of events and representation of events that may occur more than once can be addressed by using a recursive decision tree (Lau et al, 1983). In a recursive tree, some nodes have branches which have appeared previously in the tree. Each repetition of the tree structure represents a convenient length of time and any event may be considered repeatedly. A recursive tree that models the dementia problem is depicted in Figure 2.3.2.

Here, the nodes representing the previous terminal nodes DISABLED NH, DISABLED, NURSING HOME and DEMENTIA are replaced instead with the branch DEMENTIA which appeared previously at the root of the tree. Each generation of this tree represents a distinct time period so the recursive model can represent the timing of events. However, despite this relatively simple model and carrying out the recursion for only two time periods, the tree in Figure 2.3.2 is 'bushy' with 14 terminal branches. If each level of recursion represents one year, then carrying out this analysis for even five years would result in a tree with hundreds of terminal branches. Thus, a recursive model is tractable only for a very short time horizon.

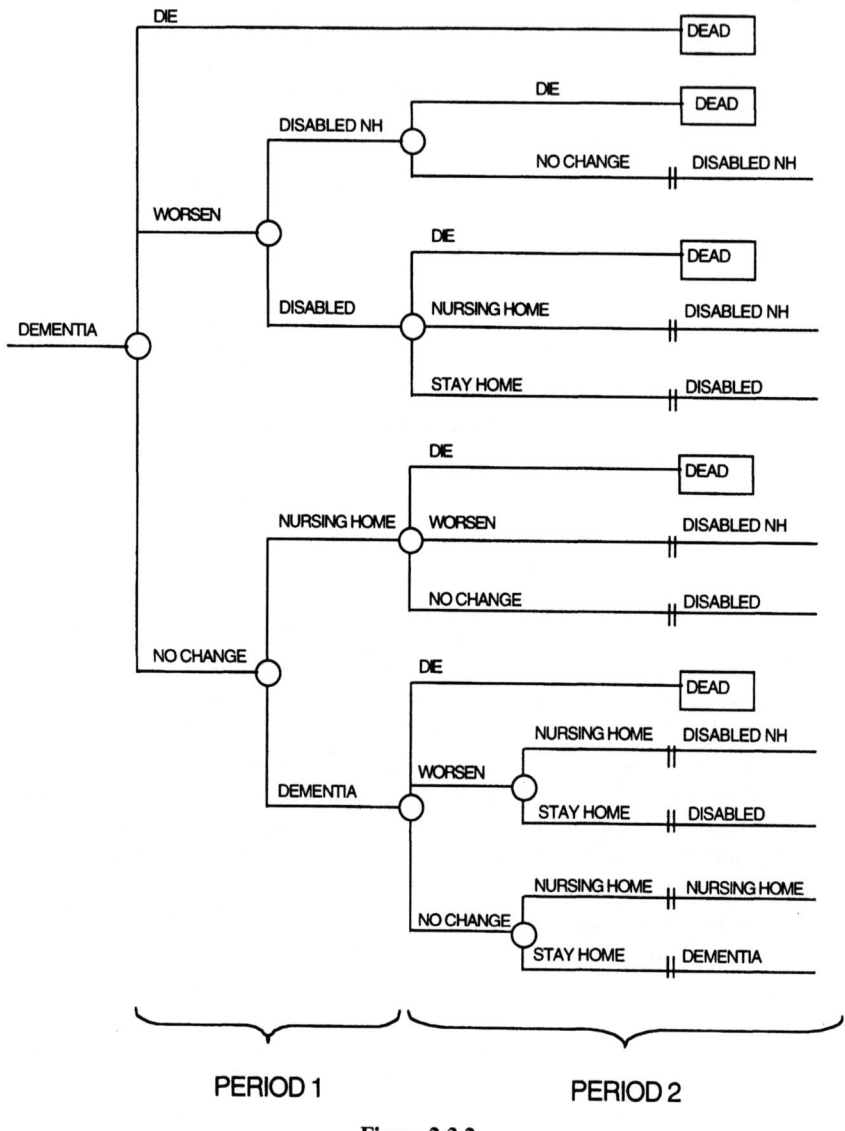

Figure 2.3.2.

THE MARKOV MODEL

The Markov model provides a far more convenient way of modeling prognosis for clinical problems with ongoing risk. The model assumes that the patient is always in one of a finite number of states of health referred to as *Markov states*. All events of interest are modeled as transitions from one state to

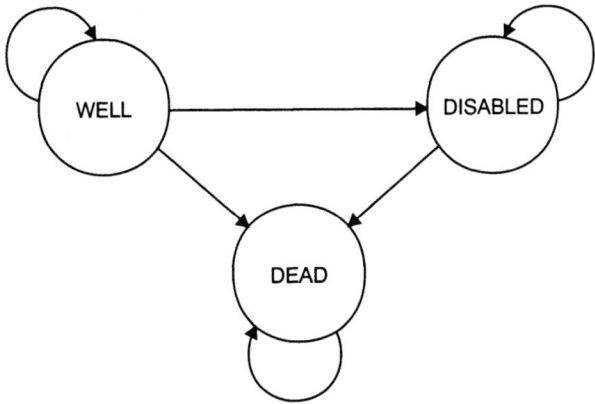

Figure 2.3.3.

another. Each state is assigned a utility and the contribution of this utility to the overall prognosis depends on the length of time spent in the state. In our example of a patient with dementia these states are WELL, DISABLED (at home), DISABLED (in a nursing home), NURSING HOME (not disabled) and DEAD. For the sake of simplicity in this example, we will consider only the development of disability and assume that disability from dementia is permanent.

The time horizon of the analysis is divided into equal increments of time, referred to as *Markov cycles*. During each cycle, the patient may make a transition from one state to another. Figure 2.3.3 shows a commonly used representation of Markov processes called a *state transition diagram* in which each state is represented by a circle. Arrows connecting two different states indicate allowed transitions. Arrows leading from a state to itself indicate that the patient may remain in that state in consecutive cycles. Only certain transitions are allowed. For example, a person in the WELL state may make a transition to the DISABLED state, but a transition from DISABLED to WELL is not allowed. A person in either the WELL state or the DISABLED state may die and thus make a transition to the DEAD state. However, a person who is in the DEAD state, obviously, cannot make a transition to any other state. Therefore, a single arrow emanates from the DEAD state leading back to itself. It is assumed that a patient in a given state can make only a single state transition during a cycle.

The length of the cycle is chosen to represent a clinically meaningful time interval. For a model that spans the entire life history of a patient and relatively rare events the cycle length can be one year. On the other hand, if the time frame is shorter and models events which may occur much more frequently, the cycle time must be shorter, for example monthly, or even weekly. The cycle time also must be shorter if a rate changes rapidly over time.

An example is the risk of perioperative myocardial infarction (MI) following a previous MI that declines to a stable value over six months (Goldman, 1983). The rapidity of this change in risk dictates a monthly cycle time. Often the choice of a cycle time will be determined by the available probability data. For example, if only yearly probabilities are available, there is little advantage to using a monthly cycle length.

INCREMENTAL UTILITY

Evaluation of a Markov process yields the average number of cycles (or analogously, the average amount of time) spent in each state. Seen another way, the patient is 'given credit' for the time spent in each state. If the only attribute of interest is duration of survival, then one need only add together the average time spent in each state to arrive at an expected survival for the process.

Where t_s is the time spent in state s

$$\text{Expected utility} = \sum_{s=1}^{n} t_s$$

Usually, however, the quality of survival is considered important. Each state is associated with a quality factor representing the quality of life in that state relative to perfect health. The utility which is associated with spending one cycle in a particular state is referred to as the *incremental utility*. Consider the Markov process depicted in Figure 2.3.3. If the incremental utility of the DISABLED state is 0.7, then spending one cycle in the DISABLED state contributes 0.7 quality-adjusted cycles to the expected utility. Utility accrued for the entire Markov process is the total number of cycles spent in each state, each multiplied by the incremental utility for that state.

Let us assume that the DEAD state has an incremental utility of zero, and that the WELL state has an incremental utility of 1.0. (For medical examples, the incremental utility of the absorbing DEAD state must be zero, because the patient will spend an infinite amount of time in the DEAD state and if the incremental utility were non-zero, the net utility for the Markov would be infinite.) This means that for every cycle spent in the WELL state the patient is credited with a quantity of utility equal to the duration of a single Markov cycle. If the patient spends, on average, 2.5 cycles in the WELL state and 1.25 cycles in the DISABLED state before entering the DEAD state, the utility assigned would be $(2.5 \times 1) + (1.25 \times 0.7)$ or 3.9 quality adjusted cycles. This number is the quality-adjusted life-expectancy of the patient.

When performing cost-effectiveness analyses, a separate incremental utility may be specified for each state, representing the financial cost of being in that state for one cycle. The model is evaluated separately for cost and survival.

The calculation of cost-effectiveness ratios is performed as for a standard decision tree.

TYPES OF MARKOV PROCESSES

Markov processes are categorized according to whether the state transition probabilities are constant over time or not. In the most general type of Markov process, the transition probabilities may change over time. For example, the transition probability for the transition from WELL to DEAD consists of two components. The first component is the probability of dying from unrelated causes. In general, this probability changes over time because, as the patient gets older, the probability of dying from unrelated causes will increase continuously. The second component is the probability of dying from causes directly related to the dementia. In some cases, dementia is caused by illnesses (e.g. Parkinson's disease) that are themselves associated with a higher risk of mortality.

A special type of Markov process in which the transition probabilities are constant over time is called a *Markov chain*. If it has an absorbing state, its behavior over time can be determined as an exact solution by simple matrix algebra as we will see below. The declining exponential approximation of life expectancy (DEALE) can be used to derive the constant mortality rates needed to implement a Markov chain. However, the availability of specialized software to evaluate Markov processes and the greater accuracy afforded by age-specific mortality rates has resulted in greater reliance on Markov processes with time-variant probabilities.

The net probability of making a transition from one state to another during a single cycle is called a *transition probability*. The Markov process is completely defined by the probability distribution among the starting states and the probabilities for each allowed transition. For a Markov model of n states, there will be n^2 transition probabilities. When these probabilities are constant with respect to time they can be represented by an $n \times n$ matrix as shown in Table 2.3.1. Probabilities representing disallowed transitions will, of course, be zero. This matrix, called the *P matrix*, forms the basis for the fundamental matrix solution of Markov chains described in detail by Beck and Pauker (1983).

THE MARKOV PROPERTY

The model illustrated in Figure 2.3.3 is compatible with a number of different models collectively referred to as *finite stochastic processes*. In order for this model to represent a Markov process, one additional restriction applies. This restriction, sometimes referred to as the *Markovian assumption* (Beck and Pauker, 1983) or the *Markov property* (Kemeny and Snell, 1976), specifies that the behavior of the process subsequent to any cycle depends only on its

Table 2.3.1. P matrix

		TO:		
		WELL	DISABLED	DEAD
	WELL	0.6	0.2	0.2
FROM:	DISABLED	0	0.6	0.4
	DEAD	0	0	1

description in that cycle. That is, the process has no memory for earlier cycles. Thus, in our example, if someone is in the DISABLED state after cycle n, we know the probability that they will end up in the DEAD state after cycle $n + 1$. It does not matter how much time they spent in the WELL state before becoming DISABLED. Put another way, all patients in the DISABLED state have the same prognosis regardless of their previous history. For this reason, a separate state must be created for each subset of the cohort that has a distinct utility or prognosis. If we want to assign different utilities for different levels of disability, then we must create a separate state for each level of disability. The Markovian assumption is not followed strictly in medical problems. However, the assumption is necessary in order to model prognosis with a finite number of states.

MARKOV STATES

In order for a Markov process to terminate, it must have at least one state which the patient cannot leave. Such states are called *absorbing states* because, after a sufficient number of cycles have passed, the entire cohort will have been absorbed by those states. In medical examples the absorbing states must represent death because it is the only state which a patient cannot leave. There is usually no need for more than one DEAD state, because the incremental utility for the DEAD state is zero. However, if one wishes to keep track of the causes of death, then more than one DEAD state may be used.

Temporary states are required whenever there is an event which has only short-term effects. Such states are defined by having transitions only to other states and not to themselves. This guarantees that the patient can spend, at most, one cycle in that state. Figure 2.3.4 illustrates a Markov process the same as that shown in Figure 2.3.3 except that a temporary state has been added, labelled STROKE. An arrow leads to STROKE only from the WELL state and there is no arrow from STROKE back to itself. This ensures that a patient may spend no more than a single cycle in the STROKE state. Temporary states have two uses. The first use is to apply a utility or cost adjustment specific to the temporary state for a single cycle. The second use is to assign temporarily different transition probabilities. For example, the

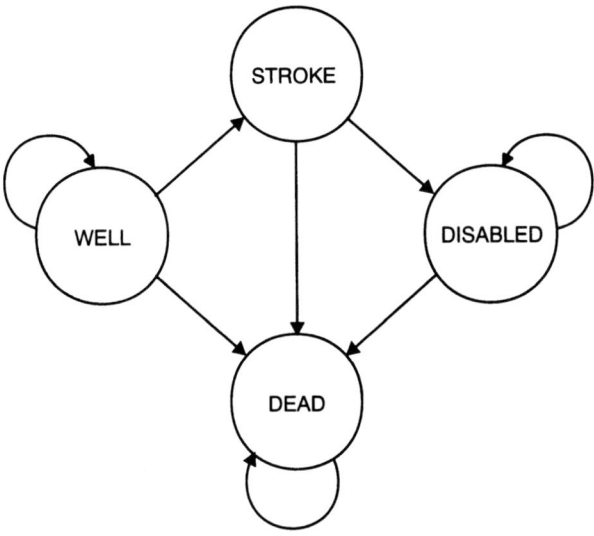

Figure 2.3.4.

probability of death may be higher in the STROKE state than in either the WELL or DISABLED states.

A special arrangement of temporary states consists of an array of temporary states arranged so that each has a transition only to the next. These states are called *tunnel states* because they can be visited only in a fixed sequence, analogous to passing through a tunnel. The purpose of an array of tunnel states is to apply an adjustment to incremental utility or to transition probabilities that is temporary, but lasts more than one cycle.

An example of tunnel states is depicted in Figure 2.3.5. The three tunnel states, shaded in Figure 2.3.5 and labelled POST MI1 through POST MI3, represent the first three months following an MI. The POST MI1 state is associated with the highest risk of perioperative death. POST MI2 and POST MI3 are associated with successively lower risks of perioperative death. If a patient passes through all three tunnel states without having surgery, he or she enters the POST MI state in which the risk of perioperative death is constant.

Because of the Markovian assumption, it is not possible for the prognosis of a patient in a given state to depend on events prior to arriving in that state. Often, however, patients in a given state, for example WELL, may actually have a different prognosis depending on previous events. For example, consider a patient who is WELL but has a history of gallstones. Each cycle, the patient has a certain probability of developing complications from the gallstones. Following a cholecystectomy, the patient will again be WELL but no longer has the same probability of developing biliary complications. Thus, the state WELL actually contains two distinct populations of people, those with gallstones and

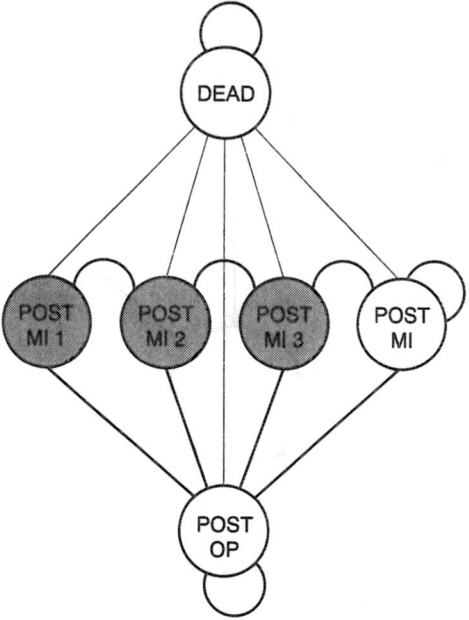

Figure 2.3.5.

those who have had a cholecystectomy. In order for the model to reflect the different prognosis for these two classes of well patients, it must contain two distinct well states, one representing WELL WITH GALLSTONES and the other representing WELL, STATUS-POST CHOLECYSTECTOMY. In general, if prognosis depends in any way on past history, it requires that there be a distinct state for each different history.

USE OF THE MARKOV PROCESS IN A DECISION ANALYSIS

The Markov process models prognosis for a given patient and therefore is analogous to a utility in an ordinary decision tree. For example, if we are trying to choose between surgery and medical therapy, we may construct a decision tree like that shown in Figure 2.3.6A. In this case, events of interest, such as operative death and cure, are modelled by tree structure 'outside' of the Markov process. The Markov process is being used simply to calculate survival for a terminal node of the tree. This structure is inefficient, because it requires that an entire Markov process be run for each terminal node of which there may be dozens or even hundreds. A far more efficient structure is shown in Figure 2.3.6B. In this case, the Markov process incorporates all events of interest and the decision analysis is reduced simply to comparing the values

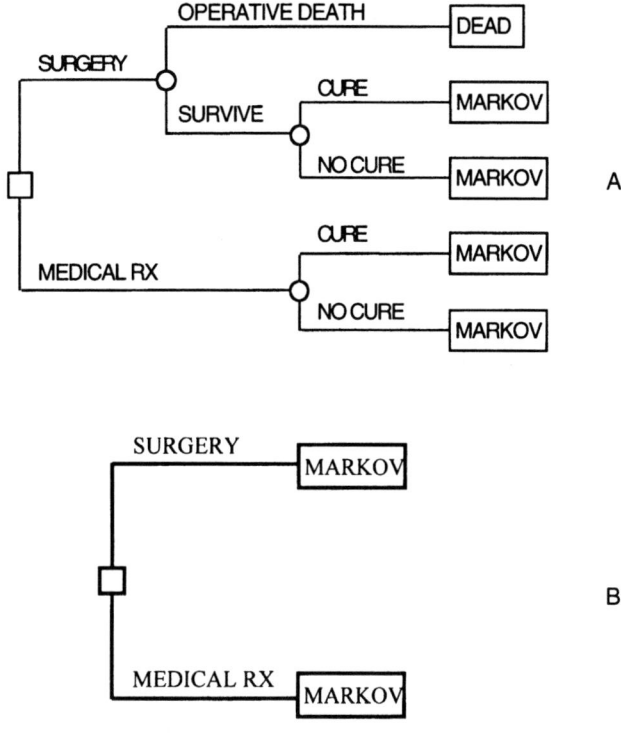

Figure 2.3.6.

of two Markov processes. The use of the cycle tree representation (discussed in detail below) permits representing all relevant events within the Markov process.

REPRESENTATIONS OF MARKOV MODELS

THE FUNDAMENTAL MATRIX SOLUTION

When the Markov process has constant transition probabilities (and constant incremental utilities) for each state, the expected utility may be calculated by matrix algebra to yield the *fundamental matrix* which shows, for each starting state, the expected length of time spent in each state. The matrix solution is fast and provides an 'exact' solution that is not affected by the cycle length. There are three main disadvantages of the matrix formulation. The first is the difficulty in performing matrix inversion. However, this is less of a problem than when Beck and Pauker (1983) described the technique because many commonly available microcomputer spreadsheet programs now perform matrix algebra. The second disadvantage is the restriction to constant transition probabilities. The third disadvantage is the need to represent all the possible ways of making a transition from one state to another as a single transition probability. At least for medical applications, the matrix algebra solution has been largely relegated to the history books. For more details of the matrix algebra solution the reader is referred to Beck and Pauker (1983).

MARKOV COHORT SIMULATION

The *Markov cohort simulation* is the most intuitive representation of a Markov process. The difference between a cohort simulation and the matrix formulation may be thought of as analogous to the difference between determining the area under a curve by dividing it into blocks and summing their areas, versus calculating the area by solving the integral of the function describing the curve. The simulation considers a hypothetical cohort of patients beginning the process with some distribution among the starting states. Consider again the prognosis of a patient who has mild dementia, represented by the Markov state diagram in Figure 2.3.3. Figure 2.3.7A illustrates the cohort at the beginning of the simulation. In this example, all patients are in the WELL state. However, it is not necessary to have all patients in the same state at the beginning of the simulation. For example, if the strategy represents surgery, a fraction of the cohort may begin the simulation in the DEAD state as a result of operative mortality.

The simulation is 'run' as follows. For each cycle, the fraction of the cohort initially in each state is partitioned among all states according to the transition probabilities specified by the P matrix. This results in a new distribution of the cohort among the various states for the subsequent cycle. The utility accrued for the cycle is referred to as the *cycle sum* and is calculated by the formula

$$\text{Cycle sum} = \sum_{s=1}^{n} f_s \times U_s$$

where n is the number of states, f_s is the fraction of the cohort in state s and U_s is the incremental utility of state s. The cycle sum is added to a running total that is referred to as the *cumulative utility*. Figure 2.3.7B shows the distribution of the cohort after a few cycles: 50% of the cohort remains in the WELL state: 30% of the cohort is in the DISABLED state; and 20% in the DEAD state. The simulation is run for enough cycles so that the entire cohort is in the DEAD state (Figure 2.3.7C).

The cohort simulation can be represented in tabular form as shown in Table 2.3.2. This method may be implemented easily using a microcomputer spreadsheet program. The first row of the table represents the starting distribution.

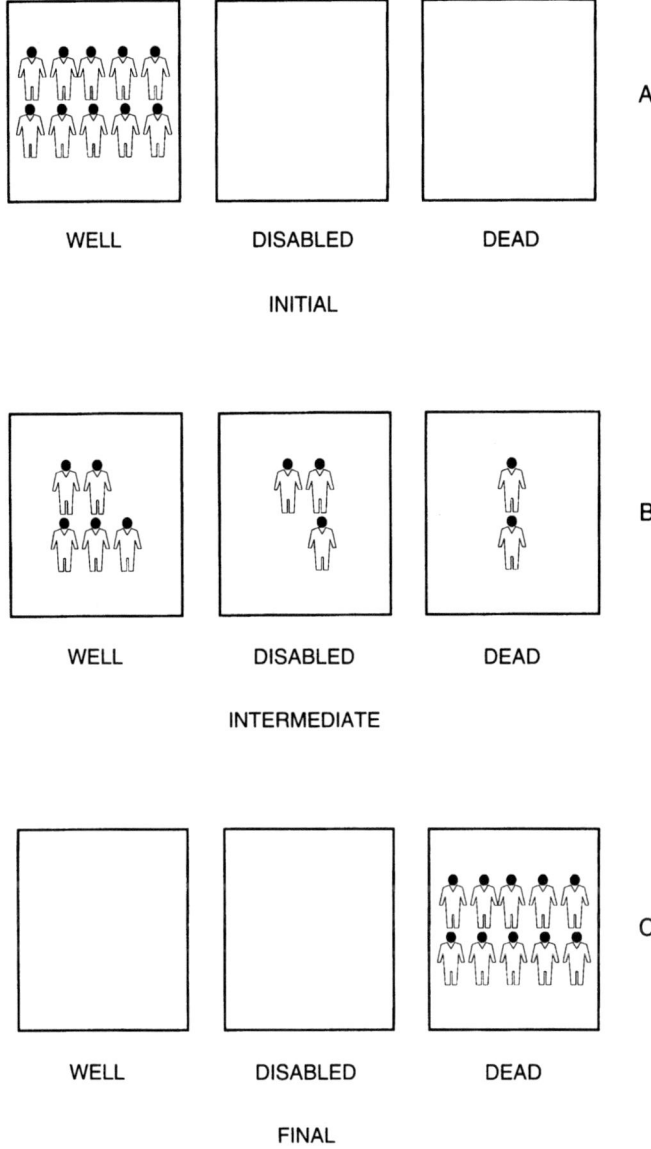

Figure 2.3.7.

Table 2.3.2. Markov cohort simulation

Cycle	WELL	DISABLED	DEAD	Cycle sum	Cumulative utility
Start	10 000	0	0	–	–
1	6 000	2 000	2 000	7 400	7 400
2	3 600	2 400	2 000	5 280	12 680
.	.	.	.	.	.
.	.	.	.	.	.
23	0	1	9 999	7	23 752
24	0	0	10 000	<1	23 752
Totals	15 000	12 500		23 752	23 752

A hypothetical cohort of 10 000 patients begins in the WELL state. The second row shows the distribution at the end of the first cycle. In accordance with the transition probabilities specified in the P matrix (Table 2.3.1), 2000 patients (20% of the original cohort) have moved to the DISABLED state and another 2000 patients to the DEAD state. This leaves 6000 (60%) remaining in the WELL state. This process is repeated in subsequent cycles. The fifth column in Table 2.3.2 shows the calculation of the cycle sum which is the sum of the number of cohort members in each state each multiplied by the incremental utility for that state. For example, because the incremental utility of the DISABLED state is 0.7, the cycle sum during Cycle 1 is equal to (6000 × 1) + (2000 × 0.7) = 7400. The DEAD state does not contribute to the cycle sum because its incremental utility is zero. The sixth column shows the cumulative utility following each cycle.

Because the probability of leaving the WELL and DISABLED states is finite and the probability of leaving the DEAD state is zero, more and more of the cohort ends up in the DEAD state. The fraction of the cohort in the DEAD state actually is always less than 100% because, during each cycle, there is a finite probability of a patient remaining alive. For this reason, the simulation is stopped when the cycle sum falls below some arbitrarily small threshold (e.g. 1 person-cycle), or when the fraction of the cohort remaining alive falls below a certain amount. In this case, the cycle sum falls below 1 after 24 cycles. The expected utility for this Markov cohort simulation is equal to the cumulative utility when the cohort has been completely absorbed divided by the original size of the cohort. In this case, the expected utility is 23 752/10 000 or 2.3752 quality-adjusted cycles. The unadjusted life-expectancy may be found by summing the entries in the columns for the WELL and DISABLED states and dividing by the cohort size. Note that the cohort memberships at the start do not contribute to these sums. Thus, the cohort members will spend, on average, 1.5 cycles in the WELL state and 1.25 cycles in the DISABLED state, for a net *unadjusted* life-expectancy of 2.75 cycles.

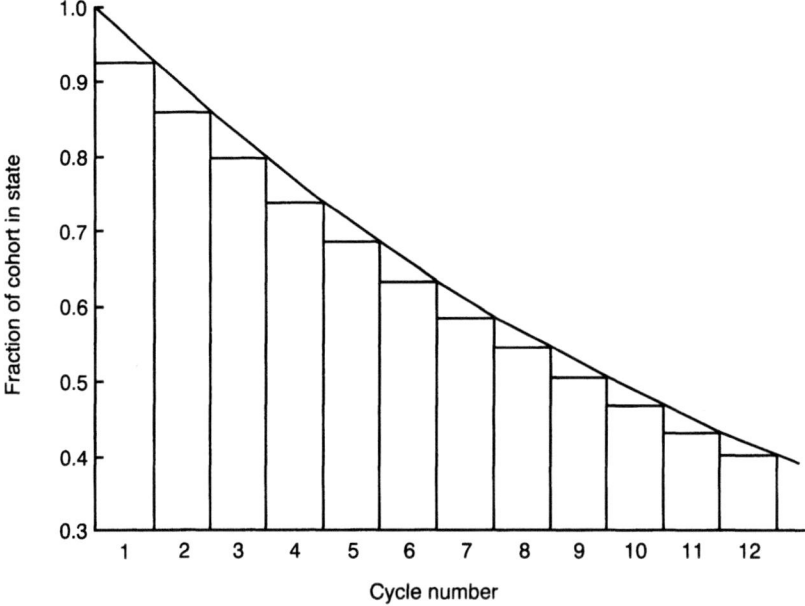

Figure 2.3.8.

THE HALF-CYCLE CORRECTION

The Markov model assumes that during a single cycle, each patient undergoes no more than one state transition. One way to visualize the Markov process is to imagine that a clock makes one 'tick' for each cycle length. At each tick, the distribution of states is adjusted to reflect the transitions made during the preceding cycle. The Markov cohort simulation requires explicit bookkeeping (as illustrated in Table 2.3.2) during each cycle to give credit according to the fraction of the cohort in each state. In the example illustrated in Table 2.3.2, the bookkeeping was performed at the *end* of each cycle.

In reality, transitions occur not only at the clock ticks, but continuously throughout each cycle. Therefore, counting the membership only at the beginning or at the end of the cycle will lead to errors. The process of carrying out a Markov simulation is analogous to calculating expected survival which is equal to the area under a survival curve. Figure 2.3.8 shows a survival curve for members of a state. The smoothness of the curve reflects the continuous nature of state transitions. Each rectangle under the curve represents the accounting of the cohort membership during one cycle when the count is performed at the end of each cycle. The area of the rectangles consistently underestimates the area under the curve. Counting at the beginning of each

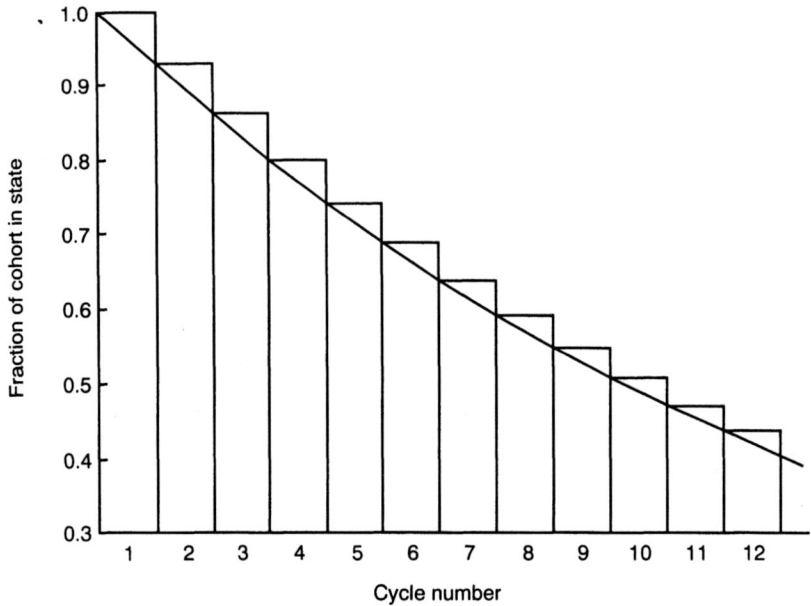

Figure 2.3.9.

cycle, as in Figure 2.3.9, consistently overestimates the survival. To more accurately reflect the continuous nature of the state transitions, we make the assumption that state transitions occur, on average, *half-way through* each cycle. There is no way to determine the state membership in the middle of the cycle. However, if we consider the count at the end of each cycle to be in the middle of a cycle that begins half-way through the previous cycle and ends half-way through the subsequent cycle, as in Figure 2.3.10, then the under- and overestimation will be balanced. This is equivalent to shifting all cycles one half-cycle to the right. We must then add a half-cycle for the starting membership at the beginning to compensate for this shift to the right. Adding a half-cycle for the example in Table 2.3.2 results in an expected utility of 2.875 quality-adjusted cycles and a life-expectancy of 3.25 cycles.

The shift to the right makes no difference at the end of the simulation if the cohort is completely absorbed because the state membership at that time is infinitesimally small. However, if the simulation is terminated prior to the absorption of the cohort, the shift to the right will result in overestimation of the expected survival. Therefore, for simulations that terminate prior to absorption, an additional correction must be made by subtracting a half-cycle for members of the state who are still alive at the end of the simulation. The importance of the half-cycle corrections depends on cycle length. If the cycle length is very short relative to average survival, the difference between actual

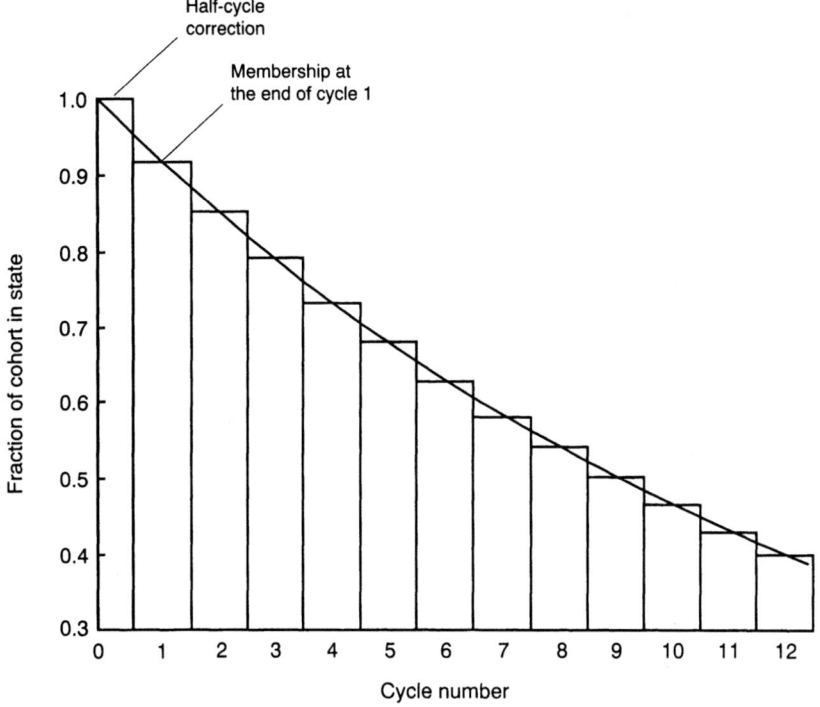

Figure 2.3.10.

survival and simulated survival will be small. If the cycle time is larger relative to survival, the difference will be more significant. The interested reader should note that the fundamental matrix representation is equivalent to counting state membership at the *beginning* of each cycle. Therefore, the correction that should be applied to the result of a matrix solution is *subtraction* of one half-cycle from the membership of each starting state.

THE MARKOV CYCLE TREE

In the preceding discussion, transition probabilities were provided as if they were elemental data supplied with a problem. However, for actual clinical settings, transition probabilities may be quite complicated to calculate because transitions from one state to another may happen in a variety of ways. For example, a patient in the WELL state may make a transition to the DEAD state by having a fatal stroke, by having an accident or by dying of complications of a coexisting disease. Each transition probability must take into account all of these transition paths. Hollenberg (1984) devised an elegant representation of Markov processes in which the possible events taking place during each cycle are represented by a probability tree.

The probability tree corresponding to the dementia problem from Figures 2.3.1 and 2.3.2 is illustrated in Figure 2.3.11. The node with 2 circles connected by an arrow within a rectangle is the Markov node. Its branches represent the Markov states. Each branch connects to a subtree. Each subtree contains a chance node modeling the occurrence of death from age, sex and race (ASR), specific mortality, the branch labeled DIE ASR. If the patient does not die from natural causes, the branch labeled WORSEN leads to a chance node modeling whether the patient goes to a nursing home or not. If neither worsening nor nursing home admission occurs (the branch NO CHANGE) the patient remains in the DEMENTIA state. Note that because of the assumption that disability and nursing home admission are irreversible, the subtrees representing more advanced clinical states have fewer branches. Each terminal node in the probability tree is labeled with the name of the state in which a patient reaching that terminal node will begin the next cycle. Thus a patient reaching any terminal node labeled DEAD will begin the next cycle in the DEAD state. A patient who worsens but stays out of a nursing home will begin the next cycle in the DISABLED state. The probability tree for patients beginning in the DEAD state consists only of the terminal node labeled with the name of the DEAD state since no event is possible, and a patient in the DEAD state will always remain in that state.

The subtrees are attached to a special type of node designated a *Markov node* as depicted in Figure 2.3.11. There is one branch of the Markov node for each Markov state. Each probability from the Markov node to one of its branches is equal to the probability that the patient will *start* in the corresponding state. The Markov node together with its attached subtrees is referred to as a *Markov cycle tree* (Hollenberg, 1984) and, along with the incremental utilities and the probabilities of the branches of chance nodes, is a complete representation of a Markov process. Starting at any state branch, the sum of the probabilities of all paths leading to terminal nodes labeled with the name of a particular ending state is equal to the transition probability from the beginning state to the ending state.

EVALUATING CYCLE TREES

A cycle tree may be evaluated as a Markov cohort simulation. First, the starting composition of the cohort is determined by partitioning the cohort among the states according to the probabilities leading from the Markov node to each of its branches. Each subtree is then traced from its root to its termini ('folding forward') partitioning the subcohort for the corresponding state

DIE

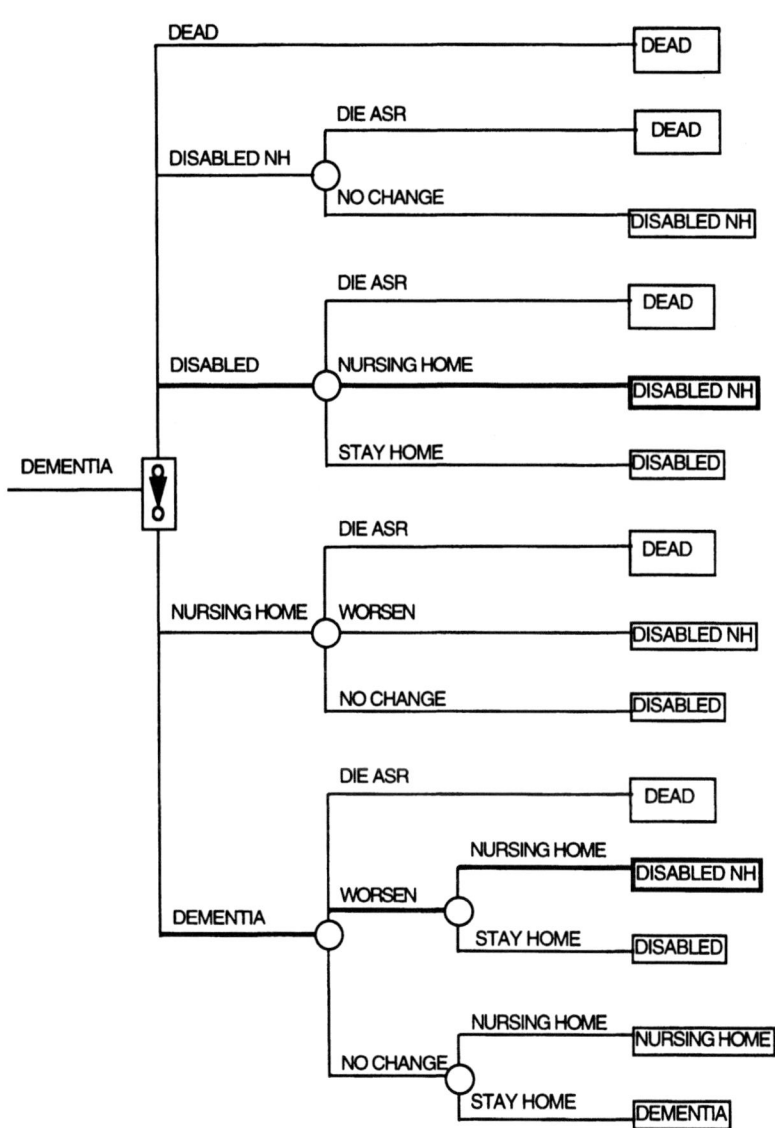

Figure 2.3.11.

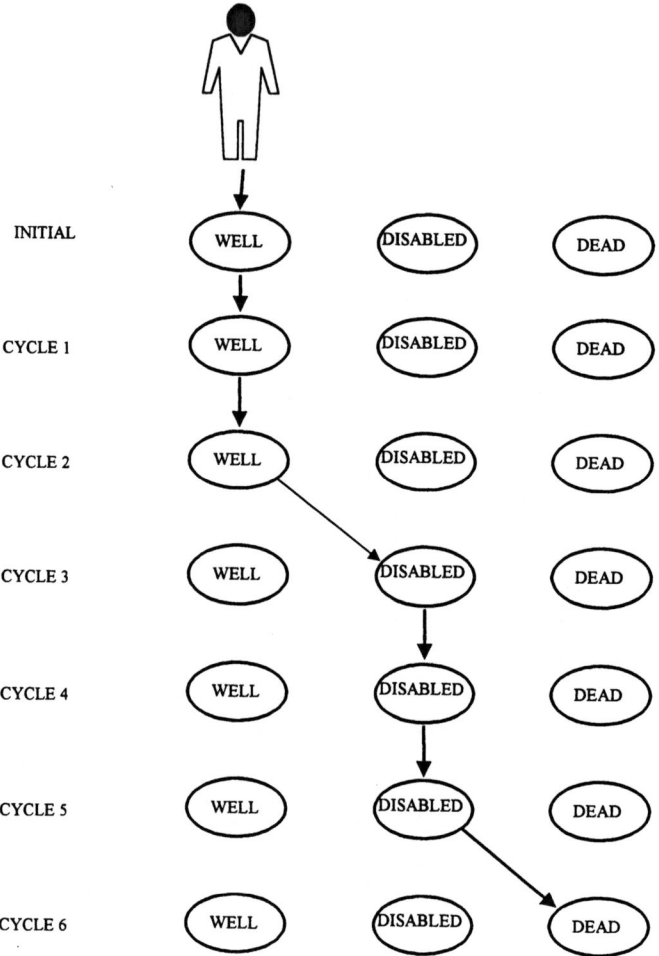

Figure 2.3.12.

according to the probability tree. The result is a new distribution of the cohort among the states, which reflects how the cohort appears after a single cycle. The fraction of the cohort currently in each state is then credited with the appropriate incremental utility to form the cycle sum which is added to the cumulative utility. The new distribution of the cohort is then used as the starting distribution for the next cycle. The process is repeated until some predetermined criterion is reached, usually when the quantity of utility accumulating for each state drops below some specified small quantity. This occurs when the fraction of the cohort in the DEAD state approaches one.

Advantages of the cycle tree representation

Cycle trees have many of the same advantages that decision trees have for modeling complex clinical situations. They allow the analyst to break up a large problem into smaller, more manageable ones. This clarifies issues for the analyst and for others trying to understand the results. The use of subtrees promotes appropriate symmetry among the various states, thus enhancing the fidelity of the model. The model provides a great deal of flexibility when changing or refining a Markov model. If a single component probability or a detail of a subtree needs to be changed this can be done without recalculating the aggregate transition probabilities. Finally, the disaggregation of transition probabilities permits sensitivity analysis to be performed on any component probability. Because of its advantages, the cycle tree representation has been used most often in recently published Markov decision analyses (Eckman et al, 1990; Wong et al, 1990; Hillner et al, 1992; Birkmeyer et al, 1992).

MONTE CARLO SIMULATION

As an alternative to simulating the prognosis of a hypothetical cohort of patients, the Monte Carlo simulation determines the prognoses of a large number of individual patients This is illustrated in Figure 2.3.12. Each patient begins in the starting state (e.g. the WELL state) and at the end of each cycle, a random number generator is used together with the transition probabilities to determine in which state the patient will begin the next cycle. Just as for the cohort simulation, the patient is given credit for each cycle spent in a non-DEAD state and each state may be adjusted for quality of life. When the patient enters the DEAD state, the simulation is stopped. For the example shown in Figure 2.3.12, the patient spends 2 cycles in the WELL state and 3 cycles in the DISABLED state before being 'absorbed', resulting in a utility of $(2 \times 1) + (3 \times 0.7)$ or 4.1 quality-adjusted cycles. The process is repeated a very large number of (on the order of 10^4) times. Each trial generates a quality-adjusted survival time. After a large number of trials these constitute a *distribution* of survival values. The mean value of this distribution will be similar to the expected-utility obtained by a cohort simulation. However, in addition to the mean survival, statistical measures such as variance and standard deviation of the expected utility may be determined from this distribution. It should be noted that a Markov cycle tree may be evaluated as a Monte Carlo simulation.

COMPARING THE DIFFERENT REPRESENTATIONS

Each representation has specific advantages and disadvantages for particular purposes. The simulations (Markov cohort, Monte Carlo and cycle tree) permit the analyst to specify transition probabilities and incremental utilities that vary

Table 2.3.3. Characteristics of Markov approaches

Feature	Model Type		
	Markov cohort simulation (including cycle tree)	Monte Carlo (including cycle tree)	Fundamental matrix
Transition probabilities	Time dependent	Time dependent	Constant
Incremental utilities	Time dependent	Time dependent	Constant
Accuracy	Dependent on cycle length	Dependent on number of trials	Cycle independent
Computation	Intermediate	Most	Least
Variability measures	No	Yes	Yes

Source: Adapted from Beck, J. R. and Pauker, S. G. (1983).

with time. Such variation is necessary to model certain clinical realities, such as the increase in baseline mortality rate with age. A disadvantage common to all simulations (cohort, cycle tree and Monte Carlo) is the necessity for repetitive and time-consuming calculations. However, the availability of specialized microcomputer software to perform these simulations has made this much less of an issue. The fundamental matrix solution is very fast because it involves only matrix algebra and provides an 'exact' solution which is not sensitive to cycle time (as in the cohort simulation) or number of trials (as in the Monte Carlo simulation). The major disadvantages of the matrix formulation are the restriction to problems with constant transition probabilities, the need to express each composite transition probability as a single number and the difficulty of performing matrix algebra. The matrix manipulations required for a Markov process with a large number of states may require special computational resources. The Monte Carlo method and the matrix solutions provide measures of variability, if these are desired. Such measures are not possible with a cohort simulation. The features of each representation are summarized in Table 2.3.3.

Time-dependence of probabilities

In the most general case, the transition probabilities in a Markov model vary with time. An obvious example is the probability of death which increases as the cohort ages. If the time horizon for the analysis is a long one, the mortality rate will increase significantly during later cycles. There are two ways of handling such changing probabilities. One is with a continuous function, such as the Gompertz function (1825). For each clock cycle, the appropriate mortality rate is calculated from a formula and converted to a transition probability.

Some rates are not easily described as a simple function. One example is the actual mortality rate over a lifetime which initially is high during early childhood, falls to a minimum during late childhood and then gradually increases during adulthood. Another example is the risk of acquiring a disease (such as Hodgkin's disease) which has a bimodal age distribution. In such cases, the necessary rates (or corresponding probabilities) may be stored in a table, indexed by cycle number and retrieved as the Markov model is evaluated. Some computer software used for evaluating Markov processes provides facilities for constructing and using such tables.

Discounting: time-dependence of utilities

Incremental utilities, like transition probabilities, may vary with time. One important application of this time-dependence is the discounting used in cost-effectiveness analyses (Weinstein and Stason, 1977). This is based on the fact that costs or benefits occurring immediately are valued more highly than those occurring in the future. The discounting formula is:

$$U_t = \frac{U_0}{(1 + d)^t}$$

where U_t is the incremental utility at time t, U_0 is the initial incremental utility, and d is the discount rate (Weinstein and Stason, 1977). Because of the time variance, discounting cannot be used when the fundamental matrix solution is used.

SUMMARY

Markov models consider a patient to be in one of a finite number of discrete states of health. All clinically important events are modeled as transitions from one state to another. Markov processes may be represented by a cohort simulation (one trial, multiple subjects), by a Monte Carlo simulation (many trials, single subject for each) or by a matrix algebra solution. The matrix algebra solution requires the least computation, but can be used only when transition probabilities are constant, a special case of the Markov process called a Markov chain. The Markov cycle tree is a formalism which combines the modeling power of the Markov process with the clarity and convenience of a decision tree representation. Specialized computer software (Sonnenberg and Pauker, 1987; Hollenberg, 1985) has been developed to implement Markov cycle trees.

The assignment of quality adjustments to incremental utility permits Markov analyses to yield quality-adjusted life-expectancy. Discounting may be applied to incremental utilities in cost-effectiveness analyses. The Markov model provides a means of modeling clinical problems in which risk is continuous over time, in which events may occur more than once and when the utility of an outcome depends on when it occurs. Most analytic problems involve at least one of these considerations. Modeling such problems with conventional decision trees may require unrealistic or unjustified simplifying assumptions and may be computationally intractable. Thus, the use of Markov models has the potential to permit the development of decision models that more faithfully represent a clinical problem.

REFERENCES

Beck, J. R., Kassirer, J. P. and Pauker, S. G. (1992). A convenient approximation of life expectancy (the 'DEALE'). I. Validation of the Method, *Am. J. Med.*, **73**, 883–888.

Beck, J. R. and Pauker, S. G. (1983). The Markov process in medical prognosis, *Med. Decis. Making*, **3**, 419–458.

Birkmeyer, J. D., Marrin, C. A. and O'Connor, G. T. (1992). Should patients with Bjork–Shiley valves undergo prophylactic replacement? *Lancet*, **340**(8818), 520–523.

Detsky, A. S. and Haglie, I. G. (1990). A clinician's guide to cost-effectiveness analysis, *Ann. Intern. Med.*, **113**, 147.

Eckman, M. H., Beshansky, J. R., Durand-Zaleski, I., Levine, H. J. and Pauker, S. G. (1990). Anticoagulation for noncardiac procedures in patients with prosthetic heart valves. Does low risk mean high cost? *JAMA*, **263**(11), 1513–1521.

Goldman, L. (1983). Cardiac risks and complications of noncardiac surgery, *Ann. Intern. Med.*, **98**, 504–513.

Gompertz, B. (1825). On the nature of the function expressive of the law of human mortality, *Philos. Trans. R. Soc. Lond.*, **115**, 513–585.

Hillner, B. E., Smith, T. J. and Desch, C. E. (1992). Efficacy and cost-effectiveness of autologous bone marrow transplantation in metastatic breast cancer. Estimates using decision analysis while awaiting clinical trial results, *JAMA*, **267**(15), 2055–2061.

Hollenberg, J. P. (1984). Markov cycle trees: a new representation for complex Markov processes, *Med. Decis. Making*, **4**, 529.

Hollenberg, J. (1985). *SMLTREE: The All Purpose Decision Tree Builder*, Boston, Pratt Medical Group.

Kemeny, J. B. and Snell, J. L. (1976). *Finite Markov Chains*, New York, Springer-Verlag.

Lau, J., Kassirer, J. P. and Pauker, S. G. (1983). DECISION MAKER 3.0: improved decision analysis by personal computer, *Med. Decis. Making*, **3**, 39–43.

Mehrez, A. and Gafni, A. (1989). Quality-adjusted life years, utility theory, and healthy-years equivalents, *Med. Decis. Making*, **9**, 142–149.

National Center for Health Statistics (1991). *Vital Statistics of the United States, 1988*, vol II, *Mortality*, Part A, Section 6, Washington, DC, Public Health Service.

Sonnenberg, F. A. and Pauker, S. G. (1987). Decision maker: an advanced personal computer tool for clinical decision analyis, *Proceedings of the Eleventh Annual Symposium on Computer Applications in Medical Care*, Washington, DC, IEEE Computer Society.

Weinstein, M. C. and Stason, W. B. (1977). Foundations of cost-effectiveness analysis for health and medical practices, *New Engl. J. Med.*, **296**, 716.

Wong, J. B., Sonnenberg, F. A., Salem, D. and Pauker, S. G. (1990). Myocardial revascularization for chronic stable angina: an analysis of the role of percutaneous transluminal coronary angioplasty based on data available in 1989, *Ann. Intern. Med.*, **113**, 852–871.

2.4   Cost of Illness of Dementia

WENDY MAX

Institute for Health & Aging, University of California, USA

INTRODUCTION

Dementia exacts a large economic toll on patients, their families, health care providers, and society in all nations of the world. Alzheimer's disease is the most common type of dementia, accounting for about two-thirds of all cases, followed by vascular dementia, which accounts for another 15% cases (Small et al, 1997). It is estimated that in the United States alone 4.0 million persons are currently afflicted with Alzheimer's disease and that this number will increase to 10.0 million by the year 2050 (Evans, 1990). According to one recent study, as many as 10% of all elderly, and 48% of those over age 85 may have Alzheimer's disease (Evans, 1990). The number of dementia patients is large and growing as the population ages and as life expectancy increases. As the number of patients with dementia increases, the number of those severely afflicted is also increasing. It has been reported that nearly half of all nursing home residents in the United States have severe dementia (Rovner et al, 1986).

This chapter describes the methodology used to estimate the economic cost of illness and reviews the research that has estimated the cost of dementia. The studies that assess the impact of disease severity on cost are included. The potential impact of drug therapies on cost is also discussed.

COST OF ILLNESS STUDIES

COST OF ILLNESS METHODOLOGY

The cost of dementia to society is the value of all goods and services that are given up in order to prevent, diagnose, treat, and otherwise cope with dementia. Costs are typically classified into direct and indirect costs. Direct costs consist of those goods and services that result in dollar expenditures. They are estimated by adding up the cost of individual components. Alternatively, if cost or expenditure data are not available, one can obtain data on units of each type of service used and assign a per unit cost. For example,

Health Economics of Dementia. Edited by Anders Wimo, Bengt Jönsson, Göran Karlsson and Bengt Winblad.
© 1998 John Wiley & Sons Ltd.

physician costs could be estimated by applying an average cost per visit to the total number of visits for the diagnosis under study. Direct costs for dementia patients include physician services, hospital care, nursing home care, medications, adult day care, homemaker services, respite care, transportation services, and many additional social and other services.

Indirect costs measure the value of resources used that do not involve dollar expenditures, such as the value of time lost from activities or the value of lives lost. Therefore, values must be imputed. Two methods that have been used to value indirect costs are the human capital approach and the willingness-to-pay approach. The human capital approach values lost productivity using forgone market earnings and an imputed value for lost household production. The willingness-to-pay approach values life using the amount that individuals would be willing to pay for a change that reduces the probability of illness or death (Schelling, 1968). The unpaid informal caregiver services provided by family members and friends are an important indirect cost of dementia. The value of caregiving services has been estimated using a replacement cost approach, in which time is valued according to what one would have to pay someone to provide the services (Max et al, 1995). Alternatively, informal care has been valued using an opportunity cost approach that values a caregiver's time according to their next best opportunity. Another indirect cost is the physical and emotional suffering experienced by patients and their families. Clearly, this cost is difficult to quantify.

Cost-of-illness studies represent a certain perspective, which could be that of the patient, the family, the health care provider, the payer, or the society at large. This perspective determines what costs should be included. For example, from the perspective of the family, only costs borne out of pocket are relevant. The perspective of the nursing home provider would only include costs incurred by the facility. From the social perspective all costs, including the value of lost time, should be included.

Two approaches are commonly used to estimate the costs of illness. Incidence-based costs are the lifetime costs associated with all cases of an illness diagnosed in a particular period of time. For example, one could follow a group of dementia patients over time and estimate all the costs incurred related to their dementing condition. Incidence-based costs are useful for ascertaining the cost-effectiveness of new therapies or treatment modalities. Prevalence-based costs represent the costs of all persons who have the illness in a given period of time regardless of when they were diagnosed. For example, one could estimate the total costs borne by a social insurance program in a given year that result from Alzheimer's disease. Prevalence-based costs are useful for predicting the impact of illness on public and private expenditures.

Estimates of the cost of illness can be generated from the 'top down' or from the 'bottom up'. A top-down approach would start with total expenditures and disaggregate them by disease. For example, Rice and colleagues estimated the economic burden of all illness in the US to be $455 billion in 1980 (Rice et al,

1985). They then estimated the proportion of the total attributable to specific diseases. The bottom-up approach is one in which estimates of the cost per case of different services for a specific illness are used to estimate the total cost of that illness. This approach is used in the studies of dementia described here.

It is difficult to accurately estimate the cost of dementia for several reasons. The definition of dementia used varies across studies, with some researchers including all types of dementia and others focusing on Alzheimer's disease alone. Care is provided to patients in many settings, including at home, nursing homes, mental hospitals, community mental health centers, and adult day care centers. However, the number of dementia patients cared for in each of these settings is not known, adding to the difficulty of assessing the true economic impact.

USE OF COST OF ILLNESS STUDIES

Cost of illness studies are used to understand the relative magnitude of different illnesses and how these have changed over time. They also show the potential benefit of preventing or eliminating a disease. Combined with measures of interventions and outcomes, cost of illness measures are used in cost effectiveness analyses that permit decision makers to direct resources to the areas where they will have the greatest impact per dollar spent.

ESTIMATES OF THE COST OF DEMENTIA

Studies of the total cost of dementia are few. Most of the work to date has been done in the United States; these studies are summarized in Table 2.4.1. In a pilot study of 44 institutionalized and community-residing patients, Hu et al (1986) estimated the cost of formal and informal care for persons with dementia. The researchers concluded that the 1983 annual costs of dementia per person were $22 458 for a nursing home resident and $11 735 for a demented person at home. This study included only nursing home costs, informal caregiving, and social services. Severely demented patients were found to require over twice as many hours of informal care as mildly demented ones. In a later paper, the authors estimated the national cost of dementia for 1985 to be $44.8 billion, including $13.3 billion for direct medical and social service costs and $31.5 billion for informal care costs (Huang et al, 1988). The costs of unpaid informal care were found to be twice as high as the direct care costs.

Hay and Ernst (1987) examined the costs of caring for persons with Alzheimer's disease using secondary data sources, including costs associated with medical care and informal care. They estimated the costs to society for all persons first diagnosed with Alzheimer's disease in 1983 to be between $27.9 and $31.2 billion. This approach differs from that of Hu and colleagues because it is incidence-based; that is they considered the lifetime costs of newly

Table 2.4.1. Estimates of the cost of care for dementia patients in the United States

Reference	Year of estimate	Methodology	Annual per person cost ($)	Annual total cost ($)
Hu et al	1983	Prevalence-based, AD and related dementias, primary data on 44 patients in eastern US	22 458 in nursing home 11 735 at home (informal care)	NA
Huang et al	1985	Prevalence-based, AD and related dementias, national, based on secondary data	NA	Direct care: 13.3 billion Informal care: 31.5 billion Total: 44.8 billion
Hay and Ernst	1983	Incidence-based, AD alone, includes direct costs and informal care, national, based on review of published research	18 517 first year, 17 643 per year in subsequent years	27.9–31.2 billion
Rice et al	1990	Prevalence-based, AD alone, northern California, primary data on 187 patients and their caregivers	At home Direct care: 12 565 Informal care: 34 518 Total: 47 083 In nursing home Direct care: 42 049 Informal care: 5 542 Total: 47 591	NA
Ernst and Hay	1991	Incidence-based, AD alone, includes direct cost, informal care, premature death	Lifetime direct cost: 47 581 Lifetime total cost: 173 932	Direct: 20.6 billion Total: 67.3 billion
Weinberger et al	1989	Cost of caring for dementia patients at home, includes imputed value for informal care provided by someone other than the caregiver, based on 141 caregiver diaries	Formal care: 10 700 Informal care (noncaregiver): 3 300 Informal care (by caregiver): 36 000 Total: 50 000	NA
Stommel et al	1989	Cost to families of caring for dementia patients at home (excluding reimbursed costs), including informal care, based on caregiver diaries for 264 patients	Cost to family: Paid: 5 800 Unpaid: 12 400 Total: 18 200	NA

diagnosed patients. It also differs in that the researchers limited their estimates to a specific diagnosis of Alzheimer's disease. Ernst and Hay (1994) updated their estimates and also included premature mortality. They estimated the lifetime cost per Alzheimer's patient in 1991 to be $47 581 for direct costs and $173 932 for total costs. Annual national direct and total costs were estimated to be $20.6 billion and $67.3 billion respectively.

Rice and colleagues (Rice et al, 1993) compared the costs of caring for northern California Alzheimer's disease patients in two settings. Data were collected from 94 patients in nursing homes and 93 patients in the community. The total social costs of care per person for 1990 were found to be almost the same in the two settings—approximately $47 000 per year. However, the cost breakdowns differed substantially in the two settings. The expenditures for formal care provided to Alzheimer's patients in the community consisted primarily of social services (76%) and hospital care (13%), while the expenditures for patients in nursing homes were largely accounted for by the institution itself (93%). The imputed value of informal care comprised almost three-quarters of the costs for noninstitutionalized patients, and only 12% of costs for patients in nursing homes. Caregivers of patients in the community spent more time managing behaviors than in any other activity (Max et al, 1995). Severely demented patients were found to receive more formal and informal care than mildly to moderately demented patients in both settings. In fact, most mild to moderately demented patients were cared for at home.

Welch et al (1992) analyzed nursing home and hospitalization costs in a prospective study of Alzheimer's patients. While they did not consider the total cost of Alzheimer's care, they conclude that high rates of nursing home admission and lengthy stays make institutional care the most costly component of Alzheimer's disease.

Weinberger and colleagues (1993) estimated the cost of caring for a dementia patient at home to be $50 000 (in 1990 dollars), including $10 700 for paid services and $39 300 for the unpaid informal care provided by family and friends. Most of these expenses were borne by patients and their families

A study by Stommel et al (1994) found that the burden of dementia care borne by families, including out-of-pocket expenses and unpaid informal care, averaged over $18 000 per year in 1989. The informal care costs were more than twice the paid formal costs. Note that the costs of hospitalization and nursing home care are excluded to the extent that these costs are reimbursed.

In recent years, a number of international studies of the cost of Alzheimer's disease or dementia have appeared in the literature. These are summarized in Table 2.4.2.

Souêtre and colleagues assessed the cost of Alzheimer's disease in France, and analyzed the impact of severity on cost (Souêtre et al, 1995). They found the 1991 annual cost (in US dollars) including an imputed value for caregiver's time to range from $5156 for mildly/moderately demented patients to $8400 for severely demented patients. For the severe patients, the informal care costs

Table 2.4.2. International estimates of the cost of care for dementia patients

Reference	Country and year of estimate	Methodology	Annual per person cost	Annual total cost
Soêtre et al	France—1991	Prevalence-based study of 51 AD patients seen in 2 university outpatient centers, includes direct and informal care costs	Severe AD: $8400 Mild/moderate AD: $5156	NA
Wimo et al	Sweden—1991	Prevalence-based study based on review of published studies, including direct costs and cost of lost income	SEK166 200	SEK30.7 billion
Østbye and Crosse	Canada—1991	Net economic cost of caring for dementia patients in the community and institutions, based on Canadian Study of Health & Aging, includes informal care in the community	NA	$3.9 billion
Gray and Fenn	England—1990/91	AD only, review of published studies, including home and institutional care and informal care paid by the Dept. of Social Security		£1039 million

represent about one-third of the total; for the mildly/moderately demented patients informal care costs are 41% of the total.

Swedish researchers estimated the cost of dementia in 1991 to be SEK30.7 (Wimo et al, 1977). Most of this cost, 94%, is for those who are moderately and severely demented. Over half of the total is for institutional care, including nursing home care, geriatric care, and psychiatric care.

The cost of dementia in Canada in 1991 was estimated using the Canadian Study of Health and Aging, a survey of over 10 000 Canadians (Østbye and Crosse, 1994). The study included formal and informal care provided in the community as well as nursing home care. Total costs were estimated at $3.9 billion (US dollars), including $1.25 billion to care for those in the community. Half of the community care was unpaid informal care.

A British study (Gray and Fenn, 1993) estimated the annual burden of caring for Alzheimer's patients in England to be £1039 million in 1990/91 prices. Converted to dollars, this equals $1845 million for formal and informal care costs. Most of this cost was incurred in institutions: 66% in residential facilities or nursing homes and an additional 25% for hospital based care.

There is a wide range of estimates of the cost of dementia across countries and over time. Nonetheless, several common results emerge. First and foremost, dementia is a costly illness regardless of how it is measured and what costs are included. Costs of formal care are dominated by institutional care, particularly nursing home care. However, for patients cared for at home the unpaid cost of informal care is typically several times as large as the paid cost of formal care. Furthermore, most of the care provided to patients at home is borne by their families either in the form of out-of-pocket payments for services or in the form of hours of time spent caring for the patients without reimbursement.

POTENTIAL IMPACT OF DRUG THERAPIES ON COST OF DEMENTIA

There is no cure or known means of preventing dementia at present. Currently, two cholinesterase inhibitors—tacrine and donepezil—are approved for the treatment of cognitive impairment of Alzheimer's patients. These two drugs have been shown to result in some improvement in cognition in mildly to moderately demented patients, but their impact on severely demented patients has not been established (Small et al, 1997). One study characterized the improvement seen in patients taking tacrine as equivalent to reversing 6–12 months of deterioration (Knapp et al, 1994). However, in the short term it appears that cognitive function returns to placebo levels when treatment ceases (Small et al, 1997). There are also side-effects, including hepatotoxicity, gastrointestinal disturbances, headache, myalgia, and ataxia (Watkins et al, 1994). Donepezil, a second-generation cholinesterase inhibitor, shows promise in that it appears to have similar cognitive effects to tacrine but without hepatoxicity

(Small et al, 1997). Other drug therapies are very much in the development stage at present. Dementia patients are also treated with many other medications for various symptoms, including depression, anxiety, paranoia, agitation, and psychosis (Wolf-Klein, 1993).

Drug therapies for dementia are likely to have three impacts of relevance to economic cost: they may permit a delay in the institutionalization of the patient, may reduce the number of hours of informal caregiving required in the short run, and may therefore improve the quality of life for patients and caregivers (Max, 1996). Outcomes associated with drug therapies for dementia should be measured using psychometric instruments that assess patient abilities, either directly or by relying on observations of health care providers or caregivers. For purposes of economic analysis, it is difficult to translate an improvement on such an instrument into economic benefit because the improvement is qualitative in nature. While it has been shown that less demented patients are more likely to be cared for at home and require fewer hours of informal care (Hu et al, 1986), there is no evidence that any of these therapies will lead to longer life or improved health status. Furthermore, the highest costs of dementia occur late in the disease course where there is little evidence of drug effectiveness.

Several US studies have analyzed the potential cost savings from delayed institutionalization associated with the use of tacrine. The costs considered include community-based medical care and social services, nursing home care, the drug therapy, and monitoring. Expert opinions and published research were used to estimate time to nursing home placement under different drug doses. The authors concluded that tacrine could reduce direct expenditures by 7–30% over the patient's lifetime by delaying institutionalization for 9–15 months (Henke and Burchmore, 1997; Mundell, 1993; Lubeck et al, 1994). Similar studies are underway in the United Kingdom (Mundell, 1993).

A recent study estimated the dollar savings in cost from a hypothetical treatment that would stop or reverse the loss of cognitive functioning in Alzheimer's disease (Ernst et al, 1997). The authors found that the savings are greatest for moderately demented patients and would range from $3700 to $7100 per year depending on the impact of the treatment on an index of patient cognitive functioning.

Delaying nursing home placement by caring for patients at home longer reduces the formal cost of institutionalization. However, when patients live at home longer, the burden borne by the family may increase, both in terms of out-of-pocket expenditures and time spent caregiving. Therefore, a drug therapy that delays institutionalization will reduce the direct cost, cause the patient and family to incur other direct costs that are more likely to be borne out-of-pocket, and increase the indirect cost of informal care. While improved patient functioning may reduce the time spent caregiving at home on a daily basis, especially in the area of behavior management, the total caregiving hours may increase because the patient remains at home longer. Maintaining a patient at home is often considered a desirable goal by families, and therefore this trade-off may be one that families will be willing to make. Furthermore, the quality of life of both the patient and caregiver are important objectives, and may well be enhanced by delaying institutionalization. The indirect costs of caregiving need to be measured in a way that incorporates both the quantitative and qualitative dimensions.

CONCLUSION

The economic impact of dementia is large and likely to become larger. Studies of the cost of illness of dementia need to consider direct costs as well as the cost of unpaid caregiving by family and friends. Drug therapies that delay institutionalization are likely to reduce direct cost. However, informal care costs may increase thereby shifting the burden of care to the family.

REFERENCES

Ernst, R. L. and Hay, J. W. (1994). The US economic and social costs of Alzheimer's disease revisited, *Am. J. Public Health*, **84**, 1261–1264.

Ernst, R. L., Hay, J. W., Fenn, C., Tinklenberg, J. and Yesavage, J. A. (1997). Cognitive function and the costs of Alzheimer disease. An exploratory study, *Arch. Neurol.*, **54**, 687–693.

Evans, D. (1990). Estimated prevalence of Alzheimer's disease in the United States, *Millbank Q.*, **68**, 267–289.

Gray, A. and Fenn, P. (1993). Alzheimer's disease: the burden of the illness in England, *Health Trends*, **25**(1), 31–37.

Hay, J. W. and Ernst, R. L. (1987). The economic costs of Alzheimer's disease, *Am. J. Public Health*, **77**, 1169–1175.

Henke, C. J. and Burchmore, M. J. (1997). The economic impact of tacrine in the treatment of Alzheimer's disease, *Clinical Therapeutics*, **19**(2), 330–345.

Hu, T., Huang, L. and Cartwright, W. (1986). Evaluation of the costs of caring for the senile demented elderly: a pilot study, *Gerontologist*, **26**, 158–163.

Huang, L., Cartwright, W. and Hu, T. (1988). The economic cost of senile dementia in the United States, 1985, *Public Health Rep.*, **103**, 3–7.

Knapp, M. J, Knopman, D. S., Solomon, P. R. et al (1994). A 30-week randomized controlled trial of high-dose tacrine in patients with Alzheimer's disease, *JAMA*, **271**, 985–991.

Lubeck, D. P., Mazonson, P. D. and Bowe, T. (1994). Potential effect of tacrine on expenditures for Alzheimer's disease, *Medical Interface*, **7**(10), 130–138.

Max, W. (1996). The cost of Alzheimer's disease. Will drug treatment ease the burden? *PharmacoEconomics*, **9**(1), 5–10.

Max, W., Webber, P. A. and Fox, P. J. (1995). Alzheimer's disease. The unpaid burden of caring, *Journal of Aging and Health*, **7**(2), 179–199.

Medical Letter for Drugs and Therapy (1993). Tacrine for Alzheimer's disease, *Med. Lett. Drugs Ther.*, **35**, 87–88.

Mundell, I. (1993). Is tacrine worth the price? *Inpharma*, **910**, 3–4.

Østbye T. and Crosse, E. (1994). Net economic costs of dementia in Canada, *Can. Med. Assoc. J.*, **151**(10), 1457–1464.

Rice, D. P., Hodgson, T. A. and Kopstein, A. N. (1985). The economic costs of illness: a replication and update, *Health Care Financing Review*, **7**(1), 61–80.

Rice, D. R., Fox, P. J., Max, W. et al (1993). The economic burden of Alzheimer's disease care, *Health Affairs*, **12**, 165–176.

Rovner, B, Kafonek, S., Filipp, L. et al (1986). Prevalence of mental illness in a community nursing home, *American Journal of Psychiatry*, **143**(11), 1446–1449.

Schelling, T. C. (1968). The life you save may be your own. In S. B. Chase (Ed.), *Problems in Public Expenditure Analysis*, Washington, DC, Brookings Institution.

Small, G. W., Rabins, P. V., Barry, P. P. et al (1997). Diagnosis and treatment of Alzheimer disease and related disorders. Consensus statement of the American Association for Geriatric Psychiatry, the Alzheimer's Association, and the American Geriatrics Society, *JAMA*, **278**(16), 1363–1370.

Soûetre, E. J., Qing, W., Vigoureux, I., Dartigues, J. F., Lozet, H., Lacomblez, L. and Derouesne, C. (1995). Economic analysis of Alzheimer's disease in outpatients: impact of symptom severity, *International Psychogeriatrics*, **7**(1), 115–122.

Stommel, M., Collins, C. E. and Given, B. A. (1994). The costs of family contributions to the care of persons with dementia, *Gerontologist*, **34**(2), 199–205.

Watkins, P. G., Zimmerman, H. J., Knapp, M. J. et al (1994). Hepatotoxic effects of tacrine administration in patients with Alzheimer's disease, *JAMA*, **271**, 992–998.

Weinberger, M., Gold, D. T., Divine, G. W. et al (1993). Expenditures in caring for patients with dementia who live at home, *Am. J. Public Health*, **83**, 338–341.

Welch, H. G., Walsh, J. S. and Larson, E. B. (1992). The cost of institutional care in Alzheimer's disease: nursing home and hospital use in a prospective cohort, *JAGS*, **40**, 221–224.

Wimo, A., Karlsson, G., Sandman, P. O., Corder, L. and Winblad, B. (1997). Cost of illness due to dementia in Sweden, *International Journal of Geriatric Psychiatry*, **12**, 857–861.

Wolf-Klein, G. P. (1993). New Alzheimer's drug expands your options in symptom management, *Geriatrics*, **48**(8), 26–36.

2.5 Costs of Dementia in The Netherlands

MARC A. KOOPMANSCHAP
Institute for Medical Technology Assessment, Erasmus University, Rotterdam, The Netherlands

JOHAN J. POLDER, WILLEM J. MEERDING, LUC BONNEUX, PAUL J. VAN DER MAAS
Department of Public Health, Erasmus University, Rotterdam, The Netherlands

INTRODUCTION

For the Netherlands we performed a general, comprehensive cost of illness study, allocating Dutch health care costs for 1994 to diseases, age, sex and health care sector (Polder et al, 1997). In this chapter we present the health care costs for dementia, compared with costs of other diseases and total health care cost. Absence from work and disability are included as indicators of indirect cost of disease. The outcomes for 1994 are compared to similar cost estimates for 1988 (Koopmanschap et al, 1994).

Future costs of dementia are projected, based on the expected changes of the age distribution of the Dutch population. The cost estimates for the Netherlands are briefly compared with results for other countries.

METHODS AND DATA

The total costs of Dutch health care in 1994 amounted to 59.5 billion guilders, about 9.5% of the Gross National Product (VWS, 1996). These costs comprise all health care sectors, including nursing homes and homes for the elderly. A complete overview of Dutch health care sectors and costs is given in Appendix 2.5.1. We did not include indirect costs of dementia, that is costs of production lost or time sacrificed by patients and/or informal caregivers.

For each of the 22 health care sectors, we allocated total costs to 62 disease categories (covering the entire International Classification of Diseases (ICD)

Health Economics of Dementia. Edited by Anders Wimo, Bengt Jönsson, Göran Karlsson and Bengt Winblad.
© 1998 John Wiley & Sons Ltd.

version 9), age (five-year groups) and sex, using a *top-down procedure*. For each health care sector we defined the best available production parameter(s) of that sector: outpatient visits for outpatient hospital care, inpatient days for nursing home care, and so on. Total costs of each health care sector were allocated to disease, age and sex, using the volumina of the production parameter(s) for each subgroup. We only used the primary diagnosis to facilitate comparability of results among diseases and to prevent double counting costs of diseases. The drawback is a possible underestimation of costs of diseases which occur relatively often as comorbidity.

Using aggregated data and following this top-down procedure provides broad estimates of disease costs, but it guarantees comparability among disease categories. Exact cost estimates for particular types of dementia patients require 'bottom-up' cost calculation: prospective data collection of all types of medical consumption of individual patients and estimated resource costs per unit for the medical services delivered.

In this study, dementia was defined as ICD-code 290, and International Classification of Primary Care (ICPC) code P70 in cases of primary care and pharmaceutical care, including Alzheimer's disease and other types of dementia.

For most health care sectors, the Netherlands has (nearly) complete registries or large national samples of medical consumption, by disease, age and sex. An overview of registrations and samples used for dementia, together with the production parameters, is presented in Table 2.5.1. For most care sectors the cost allocation is quite straightforward. The estimation of costs of pharmaceuticals and homes for the elderly needs further explanation.

The costs of pharmaceuticals prescribed for non-hospital consumption were assigned in two steps. A national sample covering 20% of Dutch inhabitants contained the total costs by age, sex and type of medicine (ATC-clusters, third level) for 1994. For each of these cells the link with diagnosis was established by using a large sample of general practitioners' care for 1988, that combined prescriptions with diagnosis.

Homes for the elderly have two functions, a residential function and a nursing function. In the Netherlands, people are admitted to homes for the elderly, partly for medical reasons. About 80% of the residents are 80 years and more old. Groenenboom and Huisman (1995) estimated for the Netherlands that 41% of total costs of homes for the elderly can be assigned to the nursing function. These nursing costs amount to 41% of 5388 = 2209 million guilders. The latter costs were assigned to disease, age and sex. No exact information was available on the diagnosis of the patients living in homes for the elderly. The exact fraction of patients having dementia is unknown, but it is presumably substantial. Therefore, for each combination of age and sex, we assumed the proportion of inpatient days for dementia to be equal as for nursing homes. Costs were estimated at current prices for 1994 and, where applicable, compared to costs for 1988 in current prices.

Table 2.5.1. Data and production parameters per health care sector for dementia

Care sector	Type of data source	Year	Cost allocation key
General and teaching hospital	nationwide registration	1994	inpatient days day cases outpatient visits medical procedures
General practitioner	regional sample	1994	contact reasons
Home (nursing) care	regional samples	1988	contacts
Pharmaceuticals	nationwide samples	1994, 1988	costs by ATC & GP prescriptions by ATC
Inpatient psychiatric care	nationwide registration	1994	inpatient days day cases
Outpatient psychiatric care	nationwide sample	1994	patients & contacts
Homes for the elderly	nationwide registration	1994	residents (inpatient days nursing homes)
Nursing homes	nationwide registration	1994	inpatient days
Patient transport	regional registration	1994	ambulance rides

RESULTS

EPIDEMIOLOGY

The prevalence of dementia in the Netherlands is 6.3%, varying from 0.4% at the age of 55–59 to 40.7% at the age of 90 years and older, see Table 2.5.2. Between 60 and 85 years of age the prevalence doubled every 5 years approximately. The most frequently found sub-diagnosis is AD (72%), followed by vascular dementia (14%) and dementia from Parkinson's Disease (6%). The prevalence of dementia rises exponentially over the age of 55 (Ott et al, 1995).

HEALTH CARE COSTS

Of total health care costs, 81% could be assigned to specific diseases and 11% is not related to specific diagnoses, such as administrative costs and residential costs of homes for the elderly. For 8% of costs information on diagnosis was lacking: for home help (presumably important for dementia), preventive care and several small care sectors.

The total costs of dementia were estimated to be 3309 million guilders: 5.6% of total health care costs. Dementia is the second most expensive disease in the Netherlands, after mental handicap, causing 8.1% of total costs. For women it is the most expensive disease, responsible for 7.4% of their total costs, for men it ranks sixth, causing 2.9% of their total costs.

Table 2.5.2. Prevalence of dementia in the Netherlands
(Ommoord Rotterdam) by age and sex in %

Age	Women	Men	Total
55–59	0.6	0.2	0.4
60–64	0.4	0.5	0.4
65–69	1.0	0.8	0.9
70–74	2.1	2.0	2.1
75–79	6.2	6.0	6.1
80–84	19.3	13.7	17.6
85–90	32.7	28.4	31.7
90+	40.6	41.2	40.7
Total	7.9	3.8	6.3

Source: Ott et al, 1995.

COSTS BY AGE AND SEX

The majority of costs of dementia is concentrated in women (79%) and in the
oldest ages, as can be seen in Table 2.5.3. This partly reflects the age- and sex-
distribution of the Dutch population: 66% of people aged 75 and older are
women. Adjusted for the prevalence (Ott et al, 1995), the costs per woman
with dementia as primary diagnosis are consistently higher (25–70% higher
depending on the age-group) than per demented man of the same age. This
may be explained by the fact that older women are more often single, since on
average they live 6 years longer than men and they are often married to older
men: if their partner still lives, he is often not capable of caregiving. These
circumstances increase the risk for institutionalisation for women as compared
to men (Huisman, 1990).

From age 75 onwards, costs of dementia become quite substantial. The fact
that dementia is typically a disease of the oldest old is illustrated by the
dementia costs as a fraction of age-specific total costs: for age 0–64: 0.2%; age
65–74: 3.7%; age 75–84: 14.2% and for age 85 and older 22.2% of total costs is
due to dementia.

COSTS BY CARE SECTOR

The care for demented patients is concentrated in nursing homes and homes
for the elderly (see Table 2.5.4). These sectors together are responsible for 96%
of total dementia costs and within these sectors a substantial fraction of costs
is caused by dementia. The costs of general practitioners' care and district
nursing are remarkably modest. The costs for home help could not be assigned
to disease, however it is plausible that a substantial share of this sector's
production is actually related to (mild and moderate) dementia.

Table 2.5.3. Health care costs for dementia by age and sex, in millions of guilders, Netherlands 1994

Age-group	Men	Women	Total	
0–59	16	13	28	(1%)
60–64	17	21	39	(1%)
65–69	32	52	84	(3%)
70–74	69	147	216	(7%)
75–79	130	377	507	(15%)
80–84	197	711	909	(27%)
85–89	164	778	942	(28%)
90–94	68	400	468	(14%)
95+	16	97	113	(3%)
Total	710	2599	3309	(100%)

Table 2.5.4. Costs of dementia by health care sector in millions of guilders, Netherlands 1994

Care sector	Sectoral dementia costs (% of sector total)	% of total dementia costs
Hospitals	36 (0.2%)	1.1%
General practitioner	3 (0.2%)	0.1%
Home (nursing) care	35 (3.2%)	1.1%
Pharmaceuticals	3 (0.1%)	0.1%
Inpatient psychiatric care	42 (1.3%)	1.3%
Outpatient psychiatric care	29 (3.1%)	0.9%
Homes for the elderly	985 (18.3%)	29.8%
Nursing homes	2176 (41.0%)	65.8%
Patient transport	1 (0.1%)	0.0%
Total health care	3309 (5.6%)	100%

Table 2.5.4 obscures the fact that a substantial proportion of demented patients are staying at home, being cared for by informal care and possibly professional care. The burden and costs of informal care are undoubtedly substantial, but these could not be estimated in this study.

COSTS FOR 1994 VERSUS 1988

Since we performed a comparable study of Dutch health care costs in 1988, the costs for dementia in 1994 can be related to costs for 1988. We amended the costs for 1994 by deleting the costs of dementia in homes for the elderly, as these costs were not included in 1988. Together with some minor corrections the 'comparable costs' for dementia amount to 2336 million guilders in 1994 and 1361 million in 1988. This implies an average annual cost increase of 9.4%

for dementia, which is significantly more than the average cost increase of 5.2%. The costs of dementia have risen particularly in nursing homes. The average annual cost increase for nursing homes was 5.2%, whereas the costs of dementia in nursing homes increased at 10.6% per year, twice the average rate. Together with AIDS/HIV and coronary heart disease, the cost increase of dementia during 1988–1994 was the highest of all diseases.

We broke down the total cost increase during 1988–1994 into a price component, a demographic component and a residual component, the latter containing a mixture of epidemiology, technology and other factors. Demographic development increased total health care costs during 1988–1994 by 1.3%. For dementia this was 2.1%. The residual component for total health care is estimated to be 1.0%, for dementia 4.2%. The remainder is due to price- and wage-increase.

It can be concluded that dementia costs are already substantially being affected by the ageing population. The explanation for the high residual component is not straightforward: there is no evidence that the prevalence rates of dementia have risen substantially during these 6 years. Possible explanations may be: the capacity of psychogeriatric nursing homes was increased; dementia symptoms may be more often being labelled (and hence registered) as dementia than before.

FUTURE COSTS OF DEMENTIA

We performed a demographic projection of future costs, using the age-, sex- and disease-specific health care costs per inhabitant for 1994 and the mid-variant of the 1996 population forecast (CBS, 1997). We assumed the age- and sex-specific prevalence and the age and the treatment structure and unit costs to be constant.

Health care costs were projected for 2015 and 2035 respectively. The latter year was chosen, because by then the Dutch post-World War Two baby boom will have reached the oldest age. On average the real total health care costs (constant 1994 prices) rise by 0.9–1.0% per year until 2015, during 2015–2035 the rate is 1.0–1.1%. Dementia costs are projected to increase at 1.6% during 1994–2015 and 2.4% during 2015–2035; ranking third among diseases with the largest cost increase. It can be concluded that future dementia costs will be strongly affected by ageing, especially in the second period.

INDIRECT COSTS

Since dementia is primarily a disease for people older than age 65, the indirect costs related to paid work are limited. In the Netherlands, the fraction of total absence from work due to dementia is 0.0%. Only 0.1% of the total prevalence of disability is due to dementia (Polder et al, 1997). These indirect costs of paid work are negligible, as compared to the health care costs. To what degree dementia affects productivity of unpaid work at home is unknown, but it could be substantial.

INTERNATIONAL COMPARISON

As stated above, we estimated the direct health care costs of dementia in the Netherlands to be 3309 billion guilders: 5.6% of total health care costs. For Canada the results are similar, as Østbye and Crosse (1994) estimated direct dementia costs in 1991 as 3.3 billion CAN$: 4.9% of total health care costs. Ernst and Hay (1994) estimated for the United States $20.6 billion: 3% of total health care costs. This cost fraction is substantially lower, but these authors only studied Alzheimer's disease.

For Sweden direct health care costs for dementia, including nursing homes and excluding housing, amounted to SEK23.4 billion, being 19% of total health care costs (Wimo et al, 1997). This fraction is much higher than for other countries. A part of the difference is due to the relatively aged Swedish population. In addition, the Swedish estimate contains costs of home help for dementia, whereas for the Netherlands home help costs could not be allocated to disease. However, these differences may not entirely explain the substantial gap between Sweden and other countries.

For the United States Schneider and Guralnik (1990) analysed the future costs of dementia, using demographic projections. According to the middle demographic scenario, dementia costs would increase at 1.9% during 1985–2020 and 2.6% during 2020–2040. This pattern of substantial cost increase, accelerating after 2020 as a result of the post-World War Two baby boom becoming very old, is strikingly similar to our results for the Netherlands. It appears that in developed countries, dementia takes a substantial share of health care costs, which is expected to grow substantially in the following decades, due to ageing.

ACKNOWLEDGEMENT

We thank Elles Goes for her valuable comments and suggestions.

REFERENCES

CBS (Central Office for Statistics) (1997). Population prognosis 1996 (mid-variant). Monthly Population Statistics 97/1, Voorburg/Heerlen.
Ernst, R. L. and Hay, J. W. (1994). The US economic and social costs of Alzheimer's disease revisited, *AJPH*, **84**(8), 1261–1264.

Groenenboom, G. K. C. and Huisman, R. (1995). *Care for the Elderly in Economic Perspective: Costs Scenarios* (in Dutch), Utrecht, STG.

Huisman, R. (1990). A simulation model for the care for the elderly (dissertation in Dutch), Maastricht, University of Limburg.

Koopmanschap, M. A., Roijen, L. van, Bonneux, L., Bonsel, G. J., Rutten, F. F. H. and Maas, P. J. van der (1994). Cost of diseases in international perspective, *European Journal of Public Health*, **4**, 258–264.

Østbye, T. and Crosse, E. (1994). Net economic costs of dementia in Canada, *Can. Med. Assoc. J.*, **151**(10), 1457–1464.

Ott, A., Breteler, M. M. B., Birkenhager-Gillesse, E. B., Harskamp, F. van, Koning, I. de and Hofman, A. (1995). Prevalence of Alzheimer's disease and vascular dementia: association with education. The Rotterdam Study, *Br. Med. J.*, **310**, 970–973.

Polder, J. J., Meerding, W. J., Koopmanschap, M. A., Bonneux, L. and Maas, P. J. van der (1997). Costs of diseases in the Netherlands 1994 (in Dutch), Institute for Public Health/Institute for Medical Technology Assessment, Rotterdam, Erasmus University.

Schneider, E. L. and Guralnik, J. M. (1990). The aging of America: impact on health care costs, *JAMA*, **263**(17), 2335–2340.

VWS (Government Department of Health, Welfare and Sport) (1996). Annual overview of care 1997 (in Dutch), The Hague.

Wimo, A., Karlsson, G., Sandman, P. O., Corder, L. and Winblad, B. (1997). Cost of illness due to dementia in Sweden, *International J. of Geriatric Psychiatry*, **12**, 857–861.

Appendix

Appendix 2.5.1. Overview of Dutch health care sectors and costs in 1994

Care sector	Cost in mln Dfl	% of total
Hospital care	19 080	32.1
General and teaching hospitals	18 067	30.4
Special hospitals	1 013	1.7
Non-hospital somatic care	9 683	16.3
General practitioners' care	1 959	3.3
Dental care	2 407	4.0
Physical therapy	1 398	2.4
Maternity services	497	0.8
Psycho-social assistance	219	0.4
Home (nursing) care	3 204	5.4
Pharmaceutical care	5 259	8.8
Appliances	833	1.4
Psychiatric care	4 208	7.1
Inpatient psychiatric care	3 264	5.5
Outpatient psychiatric care	945	1.6
Care for the disabled	5 121	8.6
Nursing home care	5 309	8.9
Homes for the elderly	5 388	9.1
Governmental public health care	818	1.4
Patient transport	585	1.0
Administration	3 180	5.3
Total health care	59 463	100.0

2.6 Cost of Treatment and Care of Alzheimer's Disease in Germany

J.-M. GRAF V.D. SCHULENBURG, INES SCHULENBURG
Hanover University, North German Center for Health Services Research HSR

ROLF HORN
Bad Honnef, Germany

HANS-JÜRGEN MÖLLER
Munich University, Germany

THOMAS BERNHARDT, ANDREAS GRASS, OLIVER MAST
Bayer Vital GmbH and Co. KG, Leverkusen, Germany

INTRODUCTION

Resources in medical care are scarce (Drummond et al, 1993), yet health insurers have to make decisions on how financial funds should be distributed across different patient groups or different health service suppliers. These decisions can only be made if there is knowledge about the cost of the treatment and care of certain diseases, but such data are rarely available. This study aims to close the information gap on the cost of dementia of the Alzheimer's type in Germany.

In (West) Germany there are 932 500 to 1.26 million patients suffering from dementia, based on a projection by the Federal Ministry of Health (Beske, 1993). This number will increase further because of an ageing population. Whilst only 2.4% to 5.1% of Germans suffer from dementia in the age group 65 to 69 years, the prevalence of dementia rises to 10–12% for the group 75 to 79 years and 20–24% for the group of 80 to 90 years of age (Beske, 1993).

The most common form of dementia is Alzheimer's disease, followed by vascular dementia (15%) and mixed type dementia (20%). About 10% of patients suffer from secondary dementia caused by hydrocephalus, inflammatory diseases, infections, intoxication, metabolic diseases, tumours, and so on. In the present study only patients with dementia of Alzheimer's type (DAT) are included since this is the most common form, accounting for 60% to 70% of all cases.

Health Economics of Dementia. Edited by Anders Wimo, Bengt Jönsson, Göran Karlsson and Bengt Winblad.
© 1998 John Wiley & Sons Ltd.

ECONOMIC CONSEQUENCES OF DEMENTIA

The economic consequences of treatment and care for patients with dementia are dramatic. Beske (1993) produced a rough estimate for Germany of DM4.1 billion annual direct cost for treatment and care of demented patients in 1987, equalling US$2.9 billion (an exchange rate of 1.40 DM/US$ in 1995 is assumed throughout this paper). Adding indirect cost, the total is US$19 billion. A large share (85%) of these costs are not reimbursed and therefore are the burden of caregivers. If all patients were to be institutionalised, and if the large burden for home care was not carried by the patients' families, total direct costs for treatment and care would be substantially higher. In this case financing nursing care by the relevant insurance for all patients with dementia would be virtually impossible.

Three retrospective American studies reported an economic burden from DAT of US$13.6 billion as direct health expenditures and US$43.2 billion as indirect cost. Indirect cost resulted mainly from care provided by family caregivers, for example patients' spouses or children, caring for their relatives (Hay and Ernst, 1987). A cross-sectional analysis of a small group of patients showed that the annual costs per patient are either US$11 735 or US$22 458, depending on whether the patient is looked after by relatives or in a nursing home (Hu et al, 1986). Another American study confirms these high costs: dementia and hip fractures account for the bulk of health care costs among the elderly (Schneider and Guralnik, 1990). A Swedish study reports an average annual direct cost of US$20 000 versus US$23 125 per patient, depending on whether care is provided in day care centres or at home by professional nurses (Wimo et al, 1994).

A French study (Souêtre et al, 1993) was based on a retrospective cost assessment of 51 patients and showed that the average total costs for three months were US$2100 for more severe demented patients with an MMSE score of 15 or below and US$1289 for less severe demented patients scoring above 15. Indirect cost accounted for an average of 36%, non-medical costs for 30% and medical costs for 34% of total costs.

Within an initial German study involving 65 patients, Schulenburg et al (1995) calculated a three-month total cost of US$2421 for an MMSE score of 15 or below and US$915 for an MMSE above 15. These 65 patients are also included in the present study. These American, French, Swedish and German findings demonstrate that dementia is not merely a medical issue but also a major challenge for society, with enormous economic implications.

STUDY OBJECTIVES

The aim of this study is to assess the average cost for treatment and the possible range of average cost for care of patients with dementia of the Alzheimer's type by the severity of the disease in Germany. The study focuses only on costs that were covered by the German statutory health insurance (SHI) and the social nursing insurance (SNI) in 1995. Therefore results represent a public payer perspective. Cost are assessed in a bottom-up design.

About 90% of the German population is covered by both SHI and SNI. The remainder is either covered by a private health insurance or by other insurance plans (e.g. civil servants). The social nursing insurance was recently introduced in Germany. It provides financial support for persons requiring care given by either family members or nurses. Its financial contribution depends on the amount or degree of care needed (three different categories) and the place where care is given—at home (e.g. by family members) or in a nursing home.

STUDY DESIGN AND METHODS

SUBJECTS

From 158 patients with dementia of Alzheimer's type (DAT) medical resource utilisation data were collected retrospectively over a three-month period in a cross-sectional analysis. Patients were recruited via 10 office-based physicians, all working in collaboration with three university psychiatric departments. Patient inclusion criteria were: diagnosis of DAT based on ICD 10 and the availability of retrospective data for the last three months at least. Patients with primary dementia of vascular origin and patients with secondary dementia caused by inflammatory diseases, infections, intoxication, metabolic diseases or tumours were excluded. Within practices patients were selected randomly. No patients were hospitalised at the time of inclusion, but those in nursing homes were included. Interviews with general practitioners and clinicians revealed that the vast majority of DAT patients are managed by family doctors.

SEVERITY OF DEMENTIA

The severity of dementia is classified according to the Mini-Mental State Examination (MMSE; Folstein et al, 1975). The MMSE is commonly used in general practice as well as in international studies. The basis of this test is a structured, easy to manage interview of patients, including questions about orientation, memory and other neuropsychological areas which demented people find difficult or impossible to cope with. A maximum of 30 points can be awarded by this method and, according to the literature, a score of less than 26 is often considered as a threshold for dementia. In the present study a cut-off point of MMSE = 15 was defined prior to the study to differentiate between more severe dementia (MMSE $\leq$ 15) and less severe dementia (MMSE > 15). This cut-off point, the middle of the 30-point scale, is defined arbitrarily, but has already been used in a French study by Souêtre (1993). MMSE was assessed after patients were included in the study. According to the above predefined cut-off criterion, 88 patients had less severe dementia and 70 patients were classified into the category 'more severe dementia'. In 9 patients with diagnosed DAT in the less severe group dementia is very mild due to an MMSE above 25.

TREATMENT COSTS

All medical services provided to the patient specifically for the treatment of their DAT have been recorded retrospectively for three months, aligned to a physician's accounting quarter. Physicians' services as consultants, laboratory tests and diagnostic procedures were assessed using the EBM, the German classification scheme for physicians' professional fees within the statutory health insurance. The EBM lists a number of value-points for each service. The monetary value of a point is variable due to a fixed SHI budget. It is adjusted quarterly; for this study a point value of US$0.064 is assumed. Drug prescriptions were recorded in detail and costed according to the 'Rote Liste 1995', a price list for drugs sold in Germany. Referrals to specialists, hospital stays and rehabilitation services were also recorded and are analysed on a patient-by-patient basis. The cost for a day in hospital is based on the average German hospital bed-day-rate in 1994 of US$288.

All cost figures are presented as annual figures and were extrapolated from three-month resource utilisation data by multiplying the three-month cost by 4. This reflects the underlying assumption that the same pattern of resource consumption would also be found over a twelve-month period of observation.

COST OF CARE

Both doctors and relatives were asked about the time required in hours per day for the care of a given patient. Patients were then categorised into three different groups, depending on the amount of care needed. This was done in accordance with the patient classification scheme within the new German social nursing insurance (for definitions see Table 2.6.1). In contrast to the more common approach of estimating cost for care based on a single threshold of dependency (e.g. need for hospitalisation), three gradual levels of dependency are applied, this allowing for a more precise and adequate calculation of cost from a payer perspective.

Costs for care are calculated from two different perspectives:

1. Minimum social nursing insurance expenses (MIN)
   MIN cost estimates are based on the SNI refunds given to family care-givers, which is based on level of dependency and not on the actual time a family caregiver spends.

Table 2.6.1. Definition of dependency stages and assumed cost for care

Dependency	Definition	MIN Cost/Month (US$)	MAX Cost/Month (US$)
Independent	No need for care	none	none
Stage I	Minor effort for care needed; patient requires help at least once a day	286	286
Stage II	Moderate effort for care needed; patient requires help at least three times a day at various times of the day	571	1786
Stage III	Major effort for care needed; patient requires care for 24 hours	928	2000

2. Maximum social nursing insurance expenses (MAX)
    MAX cost estimates are based on SNI refunds for professional residential care. They are based on the three different levels of dependency as above.

The *MIN cost* estimate is based on the benefit scheme for home care as provided by relatives in the new social nursing insurance (SNI), founded and effective since 1 April 1994. Within this scheme three categories of care requirement are distinguished: I (minor), II (moderate) and III (major). The monthly benefits for family caregivers are US$286, US$571 and US$928 respectively.

MIN cost for care underestimates the actual direct costs for care as refunded by the SNI since there is assumed to be no professional care.

The *MAX cost* is based on the same benefit scheme, but for professional residential care. In dependency stage I it is the same amount as in the MIN cost scheme, since this amount of care is assumed to be manageable by almost any family caregiver. However for patients in dependency stage II and III the need for professional support is given and therefore SNI refunds are higher: US$1786 per month in stage II and US$2000 per month in stage III.

MAX cost for care overestimates the actual direct costs for care as refunded by the SNI since there is assumed to be professional care only.

TOTAL COST

Direct costs and either MIN or MAX cost for care are added to calculate the annual total cost.

COMPARISON OF GROUPS

Comparisons of frequencies between the two severity groups are performed using the Chi-Square-test, comparisons of means are performed using the t-test.

Table 2.6.2. Characteristics of patients with different severity of DAT

Patient characteristics	Total	Severity of dementia (MMSE)	
		above 15 (less severe)	15 or below (more severe)
Number of patients	158	88	70
Covered by private health insurance	28	17	11
Demographics			
Age of patients in years	78.5^a	75.5	82.2
Percentage of women	70.3^a	62.2	80.0
Provider of care			
Family care in %	29.3^a	31.8	26.1
Nursing home care in %	34.4^a	14.8	59.4
Outpatient care services in %	8.9^a	6.8	11.6
Without care in %	27.4^a	46.6	2.9
Degree of Dependency			
Non-dependent	27.2^a	46.6	2.9
Dependency stage I in %	20.9^a	35.2	2.9
Dependency stage II in %	19.6^a	13.6	27.1
Dependency stage III in %	32.3^a	4.5	67.1

N = 158

^{a} Significant difference: $p < 0.01$.

RESULTS

CHARACTERISTICS OF PATIENTS WITH DIFFERENT SEVERITY OF DAT

Table 2.6.2 lists characteristics of the 158 patients included in this study. Patients with more severe dementia (MMSE $\leq$ 15) are significantly older than those with MMSE-scores above 15 ($p < 0.01$). The percentage of women is also significantly higher in this group ($p < 0.01$). As expected, disease severity has significant impact on the degree of care needed: the majority of patients with higher MMSE are living without care, whereas the majority of patients with lower MMSE do require nursing home care. In the group of patients with more severe dementia there is a significantly lower proportion of patients without any care or with family care ($p < 0.01$), but a significantly higher share of patients with nursing home care or outpatient care ($p < 0.01$).

Care dependency stages are also significantly different between groups. Patients with less severe DAT are more often classified as non-dependent or dependency stage I ($p < 0.01$), whereas patients with more severe DAT are more often assigned to dependency stage II or III ($p < 0.01$). The share of patients in stage III shows most difference between the two groups: 67.1% in the MMSE $\leq$ 15 group and only 4.5% in the MMSE > 15 group.

Table 2.6.3. Number of patients by degree of dependency and provider of care

Degree of dependency	Nature of care			
	Relatives	Outpatient care service	Nursing home/ hospital	Total
I	20 (60.6%)	5 (15.2%)	8 (24.2%)	33 (100%)
II	14 (45.2%)	4 (12.9%)	13 (41.9%)	31 (100%)
III	12 (23.5%)	5 (9.8%)	34 (66.7%)	51 (100%)
Total	46 (40.0%)	14 (12.2%)	55 (47.8%)	115 (100%)

PROVIDERS OF CARE BY DEGREE OF DEPENDENCY

The effect of the degree of dependency on the type of care provider, which ultimately determines the amount of *cost for care*, is presented in Table 2.6.3 where 43 patients without care and therefore without an attributable degree of dependency have been excluded. As is to be expected there is a similar association between the degree of dependency and the type of care provided: with higher degrees of dependency, the share of family caregivers and out-patient care services declines, whereas an increase in care provided by nursing homes and hospitals is observed. In particular, as 61% of patients classified into dependency stage I are looked after by relatives, 67% of patients in stage III receive residential care.

In the present patient sample, there is a particularly high number of cases classified to dependency stage III (32.3%). Regarding care providers, the pro-portion of patients on outpatient services (12.2%) is low in relation to family care and residential care options (40% and 47.8%) in the subgroup of dependent patients.

THREE-MONTH TREATMENT RESOURCE UTILISATION

The impact of the severity of DAT on the use of treatment resources, which ultimately determines the amount of *costs for treatment*, is underlined by Table 2.6.4. As expected, the amount of outpatient medical services, expressed in number of EBM points per patient, is higher for those patients suffering from a more severe dementia ($p < 0.01$). In the group of patients with less severe dementia, there are more hospitalisations ($p < 0.01$), most of them for diagnostic purposes. The higher average number of days per case in the high-severity group ($p < 0.01$) was caused by one patient who was hospitalised for 42 days while waiting for a place in a nursing home. Diagnostic procedures are significantly more often performed in patients with less severe dementia ($p < 0.01$) and therefore closer to the onset of the disease. Interestingly, there is no significant difference in the number of patients receiving drugs.

Table 2.6.4. Resource utilisation (3-month) by severity of DAT

Resources	All	Severity of dementia (MMSE)	
		above 15 (less severe)	15 or below (more severe)
N	158	88	70
Outpatient care			
EBM points per patient	2861[a]	2584	3208
Hospitalisations			
number (%) of patients	13 (8%)[a]	11 (13%)	2 (3%)
days per case	9.1[a]	6.5	23.5
days per patient	0.75[a]	0.82	0.67
Diagnostic procedures			
number (%) of patients	47 (30%)[a]	35 (40%)	12 (17%)
Drug prescriptions			
number (%) of patients	118 (75%)	67 (76%)	51 (73%)

[a] Significant difference: $p < 0.01$.

COST PER DAT PATIENT PER YEAR FOR TWO LEVELS OF SEVERITY OF DAT

Annual cost calculations were done according to the calculation model as described above: the estimation of treatment cost is based on data on treatment resource utilisation (Table 2.6.4). The estimation of cost for care is based on dependency stage information (Table 2.6.2). Costs are listed as average cost per patient and year by severity of the disease in Table 2.6.5.

Concerning the *treatment costs*, costs for diagnostics, costs for hospitalisations and costs for medication are significantly higher in less severe cases ($p < 0.05$). Costs for outpatient consultations are significantly higher in the group of more severe DAT patients ($p < 0.05$). Total treatment cost are slightly higher in less demented patients.

Both care and total costs are calculated in two different ways as described above. *MIN costs for care* in less demented patients are less than a third of costs for severe cases ($p < 0.01$). A similar relationship applies for *MIN total cost*. Costs for care (both MIN and MAX) exceeded costs for treatment, but the ratio depends on the degree of severity: for less severe cases, there is a *MIN care-to-treatment-cost ratio* of about 1:1, compared to approximately 4:1 in the more severe group. *MAX cost for care* and *MAX total cost* are three to four times higher in severely demented patients. Both differences reached statistical significance ($p < 0.01$).

The *MAX care-to-treatment-cost ratio* is 2:1 in less severe cases as compared to 10:1 in the group with MMSE below 16.

In summary, the cost of care is at least twice as high as treatment costs. Both increasing severity of disease and an increasing share of patients in residential care enlarge the gap up to 10-fold treatment cost.

Table 2.6.5. Effects of the severity of dementia on the average cost of dementia per patient and year in US$

Annual costs in US$	All	Severity of dementia (MMSE)	
		above 15 (less severe)	15 or below (more severe)
N	158	88	70
Treatment costs			
outpatient doctors' costs	750[a]	665	825
hospital costs	883[a]	941	772
medication costs	506[a]	532	451
diagnostic costs	182[a]	245	96
Total treatment cost	*2 321*	*2 383*	*2 144*
Cost for care			
MIN	5 767[b]	2 649	9 441
MAX	12 912[b]	5 221	22 029
Total cost			
MIN	8 088[b]	5 032	11 585
MAX	15 233[b]	7 604	24 173

[a] Significant difference: $p < 0.05$.
[b] Significant difference: $p < 0.01$.

SENSITIVITY ANALYSIS: COST PER PATIENT PER YEAR BY SEVERITY OF DAT

For a more detailed analysis of the correlation between cost and severity, patients were subdivided into five subgroups (very mild, mild, moderate, severe and advanced dementia) according to their MMSE scores (Table 2.6.6).

No significant differences in *treatment costs* were observed between groups. However with increasing severity there is a declining trend in medication cost. Expenses for diagnosis peak in mild to moderate cases. Even though hospitalisation costs were somewhat higher in less severe cases in Table 2.6.5, the detailed analysis shows that hospitalisations do continuously increase until MMSE has declined to 11. The drop in the last group is probably attributable to increasing nursing home care with increasing dependence, this providing continuous care and control of advanced patients.

In contrast, the cost for care and total cost are positively correlated to DAT severity, both increasing in line with severity. This applies for the conservative MIN estimate as well as for the MAX estimate.

The MIN cost for care ranged from US$380/US$1551 for questionable/mild dementia to US$10 428 for advanced cases, meaning a continuous and up to 27-/7-fold increase with progressing disease. The *MAX cost for care* ranged from US$381/US$2592 for questionable/mild dementia to US$23 571 for advanced cases, this meaning a continuous and up to 62-/9-fold increase with progressing disease.

Table 2.6.6. Effects of the degree of severity on average cost of dementia per patient and year in US$

Severity MMSE	Very mild 30–26	Mild 25–21	Moderate 20–16	Severe 15–11	Advanced 10–0
N (%)	9 (6%)	42 (27%)	37 (23%)	22 (14%)	48 (30%)
Treatment costs					
outpatient doctors' costs	623	634	709	637	911
hospital costs	0	574	1 686	2 197	120
medication costs	620	526	517	434	460
diagnostic costs	94	240	286	137	77
Total treatment costs	*1 337*	*1 974*	*3 198*	*3 405*	*1 568*
Cost for care					
MIN		380	1 551	4 449	7 286	10 428[b]
MAX		381	2 592	9 382	18 662	23 571[b]
Total cost					
MIN	1 717	3 525	7 647	10 691	11 996
MAX	1 718	4 566	12 580	22 067	25 139

[a] significant difference: $p<0.05$
[b] significant difference: $p<0.01$

With respect to total cost, the pattern of results is similar due to the dominance of cost for care. The *MIN total cost* ranges from US$1623 to US$11 800, and the *MAX total cost* ranges from US$1624 to US$24 948 for advanced dementia—about 15 times the total costs for questionable cases.

Differences in cost of care are significant ($p < 0.01$) between different severity categories. The same applies for total corrected cost.

DISCUSSION

Dementia of the Alzheimer's type is a progressive disease, associated with a loss of competence for activities of daily living and an increase in disability. Therefore it is to be expected that an increase in disease severity is accompanied with an increasing need for care, resulting in rising cost. If so, early measures for slowing down the progression of DAT should delay the progression of need for care and hence reduce the resulting financial burden.

In the process of empirically supporting the above hypothesis, the first step is to investigate the relationship between cost and the severity of the disease. Therefore the aim of this study was to estimate the average treatment cost and cost for care for patients with DAT of different severity in Germany. Severity is defined by different MMSE ranges. One special feature of the present study is that the calculation of cost for care is not, as usually done, based on a single threshold of care requirement (e.g. hospitalisation), but on three gradual levels of dependency on care. This results in an increase in precision of estimates and a better alignment to the German refund system.

Because of the immediate need for information, the assessment of dependency and costs alongside the progressive course of the disease in a longitudinal study with several years of duration was not feasible, although this approach would allow for the highest precision and reliability.

Therefore, costs in DAT patients were empirically investigated using a cross-sectional study design. It is assumed that the empirical data on the treatment and care for DAT patients with MMSE above 15 are representative for an early stage of dementia with a lower severity, whereas data from DAT patients with MMSE equal or below 15 are representative for conclusions on later stages of the disease with higher severity. On this basis, a comparison between patients of different degrees of severity was performed to evaluate both differences in the method of treatment and the provision of care, in line with different structures of cost. The difference of mean MMSE between the two groups was more than 10 points in the present sample.

The study sample was not planned to be representative for Germany. The focus is rather on the relationship between cost for care and cost for treatment than on representativity of the estimates of cost in absolute terms. There might be regional differences in the provision of care which cannot be covered in a study focusing on just one region in Germany. Study population demographics match patient characteristics from other German studies (Federal Ministry of Health, 1986; Cooper and Sosner, 1983).

The utilisation of *treatment resources*, which determines *treatment costs*, does not, as might be expected, increase with the severity of dementia. Even though outpatient consultations increase, costs for both hospitalisation and medication are higher in less severe patients. Longer hospitalisations are mainly found in patients with higher severity of DAT who are living alone or without care. Physicians reported that these patients are often referred to hospital where they then have to stay for weeks until a free place is found in a nursing home. Short hospitalisations, as mainly found in less severe cases, go along with diagnostic procedures. Interestingly, prescriptions do not increase with severity, even though a seven-year difference in age between the two groups does make an increase very likely. This could result from some kind of therapeutic nihilism by physicians in general practice.

On the other hand, analysis of the relationship between degree of severity and different *care options* as determinants of *cost for care* revealed a significant increase according to a priori expectations. In the group of more severe demented patients, quite a low proportion of patients are able to manage living without care as compared to the other group. They are particularly often supported by professional care as provided in nursing homes and by professional outpatient services. This is also reflected by consistently higher degrees of dependency in the group of more severe demented patients. Therefore the study descriptively confirms that an increase in dependency is associated with a shift in care providers from family care via outpatient services to expensive nursing homes. Therefore increasing dependency results in an increase in cost.

The increase in cost for care and total cost with an increase in severity of the disease, as demonstrated by this study, reconfirms findings from an intermittent analysis of 65 patients (Schulenburg et al, 1995). The results of the present investigation also replicate findings from Souêtre et al (1993). In that study the same MMSE threshold value of 15 was applied to separate groups by severity. However Souêtre found a lower increase in total costs of only 60% when progressing to the more severe group. This is probably due to the fact that the share of patients receiving costly nursing care was significantly lower in French patients with severe DAT.

When comparing studies it has to be considered that the definition of treatment costs and cost for care as used in the present study differs from the general concept of indirect and direct costs in literature. There indirect costs also cover non-monetary effects on society. Funding of care is also regulated differently in many countries, which has important implications on cost estimates. This study is aligned to the German social nursing insurance refund scheme. The difference between MAX and MIN costs indicates the savings to the health system due to family caregivers providing care at home and not asking for professional support. It also demonstrates the economic burden to families that are not able to provide care at home to a patient, but for whom the need for professional nursing care is not officially approved. In this case excessive costs have to be covered by the patients and their relatives. By this it does roughly approximate the socio-economic value of care provided by family caregivers. There are socio-economic costs due to a loss of productivity of caring relatives, who might for example give up work as a consequence of a demented relative needing care. From a human capital point of view this is, however, likely to be small because of the high average age of spouses and resulting high chance of retirement.

Treatment costs are distinctly below cost for care (<50%), even compared to the MIN estimates. Comparable results were found by Beske (1993) (care-to-treatment-cost ratio of 6:1) and Hay and Ernst (1987) (care-to-treatment-cost of 3:1). Only Souêtre et al (1993) reported higher medical treatment costs. Furthermore, the present study revealed that the care-to-treatment-cost ratio increases with increasing disease severity.

Subgroup analysis assuming five distinct categories of severity confirmed the results based on only two distinct groups: there is no linear relationship between treatment costs and severity, but cost for care is highly correlated with the severity of the disease. The care-to-treatment-cost ratio increased accordingly.

Because of the low numbers of cases per group treatment resource utilisation can only be interpreted qualitatively as an indicator for trends. Diagnostic costs mainly occur in mild to moderate cases. Hospitalisations peak in moderate to severe DAT patients (MMSE 11–20). Medication costs decline with severity, outpatient consultation fees increase in advanced cases.

However, the cost for care is the major determinant of cost in the treatment of DAT patients under current treatment practices.

If a lower degree of severity is representative for early stages of DAT and a higher severity for late stages of the illness, the reported results demonstrate that cost for care significantly increases as the disease progresses. However, treatment costs remain almost unchanged. The cost for care is the main component of total cost. This is attributable to the increasing need for care and a move towards professional care provision as a result of the disease progression.

The results of the present study support the hypothesis that even a gradual delay in the progression of severity results in a meaningful reduction of cost through lower proportions of patients requiring costly residential care. Early treatment aiming to slow down the progression of DAT will in the short term result in increased treatment costs from diagnosis and medication. However, it is to be expected that over a longer period of time a shift in care provision from cost-intensive residential care to family home-based care will compensate for the increase in direct costs for treatment, and it will reduce indirect costs. This should lead to a favourable impact on total cost as well. Mental exercise, physical therapy, dietary treatment and drugs such as cognition enhancers (nootropics) have been shown to be beneficial in slowing down the progression of the disease in the early stages of dementia. The cost-effectiveness of different treatment approaches needs to be analysed in the future by modelling studies or, if feasible, by longitudinal trials, aiming to reconfirm the above hypothesis.

REFERENCES

Beske, E., and Kunczik, T. (1993). Frühzeitige Therapie kann Milliarden sparen, *Der Kassenarzt*, pp. 3–6.

Bundesministerium für Jugend, Frauen, Familie und Gesundheit (1986). *Vierter Familienbericht*, Bonn.

Cooper, B., and Sosna, U. (1983). Psychische Erkrankungen in der Altenbevölkerung. Eine epidemiologische Feldstudie in Mannheim, *Der Nervenarzt*, **54**, 239–249.

Drummond, M. F., Rutten, F., Brenna, A., Pinto, C. G., Horisberger, B., Jönsson, B., Le Pen, C., Rovira, J., Schulenburg, M.v.d., Sintonen, H., and Torfs, K. (1993). Economic evaluation of pharmaceuticals: a European perspective, *Pharmaco-Economics*, **4**(3), 173–186.

Folstein, M. F., Folstein, S. E., and McHugh, P. R. (1975). 'Mini-Mental-State'. A practical method for grading the cognitive state of patients for the clinician, *J. Psychiat. Res.*, **12**, 189–198.

Hay, J. W., and Ernst, R. L. (1987). The economic cost of Alzheimer's disease, *Amer. J. Publ. Hlth*, **77**, 1169–1175.

Hu, T. W., Huang, L. F., and Cartwright, W. S. (1986). Evaluation of the costs of caring for the senile demented elderly: a pilot study, *Gerontologist*, **26**, 158–163.

Schneider, E. L., and Guralnik, J. M. (1990). The aging of America, impact on health care costs, *J. Amer. Med. Ass.*, **263**, 2335–2340.

Schulenburg, J.-M., Horn, R., Grobe-Einsler, R., Bernhardt, T., Möller, H.-J., and Schulenburg, I. (1995). Kostenanalyse der Behandlung hirnleistungsgestörter Patienten, *Geriatrie Forschung*, **5**(1), 31–40.

Souêtre, E. J., Qing, W., Vigoureux, I., Dartigues, J. F., Lozet, H., Lacomblez, L., and Derouesne, C. (1995). Economic analysis of Alzheimer's disease in outpatients: impact of symptom severity, *Int. Psychogeriatr.*, **7**(1), 115–122.

Wimo, A. et al (1994). Cost-effectiveness analysis of day care for patients with dementia disorders, *Health Economics*, **3**, 395–404.

2.7 Costing Community Care of People with Dementia

MARTIN KNAPP and RACHEL WIGGLESWORTH
London School of Economics and Political Science, UK

INTRODUCTION

Community-based care for elderly people with somatic or mental health problems is an explicit policy preference in a great many countries today. As earlier chapters have described, there are numerous reasons for this preference, including current economic pressures on available resources, and especially concerns about the future resource pressures. Consequently, the costs and cost-effectiveness of community care have attracted growing attention from national and local policy makers, service providers and funding bodies.

Dementia, particularly in the later stages of the illness, is associated with high levels of service utilisation and there is a common need for admission to some form of institutional or congregate care (residential or nursing homes, hospitals and similar). The ageing of the world population, and the associated increases in the numbers of people with dementia, have thus concentrated the minds of national governments and the managers of health and social care systems on affordable community alternatives to institutional care.

In this chapter we examine the service and cost characteristics of community care for people with dementia. We draw on evidence from a number of countries, although we will tend to privilege British experiences because of our own research perspectives. We first describe observed patterns of service provision in the community as revealed in recent research, noting the great variety of professions and agencies that tend to be involved. We then turn to the costs of these support arrangements, first setting out the principles of community care costing and of economic evaluations more generally, and second showing how these principles have been applied in recent research. We make the usual distinction between direct and indirect costs, and examine the cost consequences for different agencies in the community care system. We also examine the extent of cost variation in the community care context and its interpretation. In the concluding section we discuss how research and practice in this field should move forward.

Health Economics of Dementia. Edited by Anders Wimo, Bengt Jönsson, Göran Karlsson and Bengt Winblad.
© 1998 John Wiley & Sons Ltd.

PATTERNS OF CARE

Care and support for elderly people with dementia is delivered in a variety of different settings. The balance between settings will vary from country to country. However, there is generally a substantial proportion of people with dementia, especially with mild to moderate dementia, who live in their own homes (in private households, with or without a caregiver), where they are supported by community-based services. In Canada half the people suffering from dementia in 1991 were found to be living in the community (Østbye and Crosse, 1994). In the UK the proportion of elderly people with 'mild to severe confusion' living in private households was found to be as high as 63% (Kavanagh et al, 1993). Those elderly people with a higher level of intellectual impairment were less likely to live alone although many still lived with others. Four out of ten people with dementia in England lived with another elderly person (Melzer et al, 1996). In Spain and Italy the tendency of people to remain in the community is notably higher (Trabucci et al, 1995: Cabellero Garcia et al, 1993). In contrast, in countries such as Ireland, Japan, Canada, France and New Zealand, hospitals still provide substantial amounts of long-term care for elderly people generally (OECD, 1996).

The high number of elderly people with dementia receiving home-based care can be understood partly as the result of policy initiatives to encourage care in the community rather than in the more costly institutional settings, which are also often argued to be inappropriate. As a result of the search for alternatives to institutional care, a number of intermediate care arrangements have been developed. In this chapter we use the term *community care* to refer to care services in an ordinary domestic setting, performed either by formal services and/or informally by relatives and friends.

Home care services play a vital role in maintaining people in their own homes by providing practical help such as with housework, shopping, collection of social security benefits and personal care (Banerjee and Macdonald, 1996). In Britain, these tasks are usually performed by domiciliary care workers (formerly known as home helps) or by family or other informal caregivers. Elderly people with dementia also require significant medical services. In a survey of community care of people with mean age of 83, 96% of whom suffered from dementia, Black et al (1995) found that frail elderly people supported at home have significant mortality and morbidity rates and have high rates of inpatient admission.

In the early stages of dementia, and in the absence of debilitating comorbid conditions, the sufferer is likely to be able to lead a quite normal life, requiring minimal care. As the disease progresses, however, the amount of care that is needed increases. This care is predominantly palliative, in the absence of any cure for dementia, although the new cholinesterase inhibitor drugs such as tacrine and donepezil appear to be able to slow down the rate of cognitive decline associated with Alzheimer's disease (Knapp et al, 1994; Rogers et al,

1996). The high levels of morbidity mainly occur in the late stages of the disease when the mobility of the patient is also restricted. Physical illnesses associated with dementia include incontinence, pneumonia and infections. Confused elderly people living at home are also prone to self-neglect, falls, accidents and injuries as a result of wandering and defects in balance and coordination (Gauthier et al, 1996; Keady, 1994), which again generates needs for health and social care support.

Health and social care providers—in Britain, these are the National Health Service and local authority social services departments—find people with dementia among the most difficult to maintain at home, especially those people presenting challenging behaviours. A high level of supervision is often required when caring for people whose judgement is poor and whose behaviour can be dangerous (particularly to themselves). Although Alzheimer's disease and other dementias are non-curable, a number of treatments exist although they vary in availability. Apart from basic physical care, physiotherapy and occupational therapy there are several other treatment strategies, including reality orientation, reminiscence therapy and validation therapy and hermeneutics approaches (Wimo et al, 1997).

Care packages for people with dementia today often comprise a complex support network of formal and informal services. In England, Schneider et al (1993) found that 91% of elderly with dementia living in the community had seen their GP in the previous year, 36% a community nurse, 24% a home care worker, 16% a chiropodist, 14% a social worker and 13% a psychiatrist. With the exception of GP consultation the reported services received by people with dementia in the community could be seen as somewhat small. In order to coordinate these diverse services a number of countries have introduced forms of care or case management (Davies, 1992). Good care management has been found to enable elderly people with dementia who are on the margins of long-term hospital care to be discharged or to remain in their own homes (Challis, 1993). There is variation in services depending on whether the person with dementia is living alone or with someone else. People living with others use more respite care and sitting services, but also more day and nursing care and more health care in general. There are several explanations for this finding. One is that people living with others generally have higher levels of confusion (as found by Schneider et al, 1993), and another is that caregivers act as advocates or are better informed about which services are available. Levin et al (1988) also found that more home care was available to those elderly people living alone.

The extent of unmet need amongst dementia sufferers cared for at home is a cause for concern and represents a failure to relieve the burden of care of many elderly spouse carers. Service use and unmet need were estimated in a US study by Philp et al (1995) by asking supporters of Alzheimer's disease sufferers which of the locally available services they received and whether they would like to receive more of any of them. Philp found that the presence of dementia was associated with a high level of unmet need for mainstream medical services and domiciliary support. A high proportion of caregivers had not heard of the statutory service available. Over a third had not heard about the community psychiatric nurse service, 30% about private domestic help, 30% about relatives' support groups, 29% about health visitors, 27% about geriatricians, and 25% about respite care in hospitals. Of grave concern was the discovery in another study of a number of people with moderate to severe dementia who were living alone at serious risk (O'Connor et al, 1989).

As a result of gaps in community services, many people with dementia are admitted earlier than would otherwise be needed into institutional or hospital care. The resultant costs can be very high. In a longitudinal study of care-givers, Collins et al (1994) found that a third of the sample reported that at least one service issue (such as affordability, access or service quality) had an influence on the placement in a nursing home of the elderly person they had been supporting. Four out of ten caregivers said that the availability of at least one additional service in the community would have delayed the institutional admission of their relative.

However, despite the frequency and intensity of use of the various health and social care services available in most developed countries today, these formal services are—in aggregate—only a fraction of the informal care provided by family and other caregivers. The majority of informal care is provided by relatives, usually female relatives aged 45–64. A considerable commitment is required from these unpaid caregivers, in terms of time, labour and financial support, and the associated costs can be high. Often caregivers suffer high degrees of morbidity as a result of the demands of this role, especially as cognitive impairment advances in the early stages (Donaldson et al, 1997). For community care plans to operate successfully, the reliance of the care system on these unpaid caregivers needs to be recognised and the caregivers will need to be supported.

There are other providers of care which sit outside the public health and social services system. It is noticeable, for example, that a growing proportion of community and social care services are being carried out by both formal (through an organisation) and informal volunteering, other than by or for relatives. UK volunteering patterns were examined by Knapp et al (1996) and their findings show the importance of this source of human resources to the support for the elderly living at home. Formal volunteering through a health or social welfare organisation supporting elderly people was reported by 17% of those who had volunteered during the previous 12 months. Informal volunteering in the form of visiting an elderly or sick person—not through an organisation and not for a relative—was reported by a third of respondents who had volunteered in the previous 12 months, and a quarter had provided transportation or escorting services (often for frail elderly people). These statistics indicate the extent of the rarely quantified volunteer inputs to community care services. A number of factors were associated with a higher or lower probability of volunteering, including net wage (the higher the net wage, the lower the probability of volunteering), age, gender, ethnic group, family or household responsibilities, social networks and local public spending on certain kinds of social care service.

Voluntary organisations undoubtedly contribute invaluable services to people with dementia living in the community. Organisations such as Help the Aged, MIND and the Alzheimer's Disease Society both locally and nationally provide schemes of caregiver support, meals on wheels, sitter services and the loan of specialist equipment. Nationally, UK voluntary organisations for elderly people spent £424 million in 1990 (Kendall and Knapp, 1996), which may look small as a proportion of total public spending on this group of people, but the activities funded by these bodies can improve the quality of life of a great many dementia sufferers and their caregivers.

The private sector has grown to assume substantial care responsibilities for elderly people in the UK, including elderly people with dementia. It is the largest provider of residential care and nursing home places in the UK, having grown rapidly over a 20-year period. More recently, the private sector has become an important provider of domiciliary care, but it remains a very modest provider of health care treatments in the UK. Some of these private sector services are funded under contract by the health service and by local authority social services departments, and some are privately purchased. Both need to be included in examinations of community care costs.

COSTING COMMUNITY CARE

It is clear that elderly people with dementia need and generally use a large number of care services in the community. What do these services cost? In this section we first briefly set out the principles of calculating costs for community care services (which are described at greater length by Beecham, 1995, and reported on a regular basis in the annual *Unit Costs of Health and Social Care* volume published by the Personal Social Services Research Unit; see Netten and Dennett, 1997). We then set out a related set of principles to adopt in the analysis and interpretation of costs data which again characterises the research programmes of PSSRU and other groups.

COSTING METHODS

Economists distinguish various broad categories of cost. The most common distinction is between *direct costs*, which are the health and social services provided to people with dementia, and usually associated directly with the illness or need under study, and *indirect costs*, which include expenditures by families and other caregivers, volunteers working in health or social welfare agencies, together with any broader social impacts. As we shall see below, estimating values for these indirect costs is less straightforward than the costing of direct service inputs. The largest direct cost items are likely to be associated with inpatient admission or residence in a residential or nursing home, with others including community nursing and medications. Where possible, each of the relevant direct and indirect costs should be included in an evaluation. There might also be some *immeasurable costs*, although these might be better described as negative benefits or outcomes. Examples of these 'costs' which an economic evaluation might fail to measure are the consequences of premature mortality, family anxiety or the psychological impact of informal care on caregivers.

Cost estimates might be obtained directly from agency accounts or purchaser records, particularly in fee-for-service systems, but the most common need is to gather data on service use patterns and then to attach estimated unit cost measures. In PSSRU research in the fields of mental health, learning disability, elder care and child care we have found it helpful to use variants of the Client Service Receipt Inventory (CSRI; Beecham and Knapp, 1992). The CSRI collects data on employment, individual or household income, formal service use and informal care support.

The most appropriate monetary value to attach to each of the services identified by the CSRI or in other ways is its long-run marginal opportunity cost. This particular cost measure of the resource consequences is widely employed in economic evaluations. It helps to ensure that a long-term perspective on resource implications is employed, that only those effects on resources attributable to the programme or service user are counted, and that costs are reckoned as 'opportunities forgone', not just money expended. Beecham (1995) and Drummond et al (1997) offer useful and accessible explanations of the principles and practicalities of long-term marginal opportunity costing.

An example of an opportunity cost which might otherwise get missed—because of the absence of any formal monetary exchange—would be the time spent by a volunteer helper or family caregiver: no payment is made from one person to another, or one agency to another, but there are costs in terms of the lost opportunities to do other things (including working for a salary). We saw earlier how an individual's net wage is one of the determinants of the propensity to volunteer (in both formal and informal ways) in the support of elderly people (Knapp et al, 1996). Attaching costs to the informal inputs which are so important in the support of many elderly people with dementia is complicated by the fact that the motivations underpinning caregiver and volunteer activities are so varied (Knapp, 1990).

COST RESEARCH PRINCIPLES

When utilising cost measures of the kind outlined above it is advisable to attend to certain basic principles. These guide all of our own economic evaluations, even if there are studies in which it proves impossible for us to apply every principle fully. These principles are set out in more detail elsewhere (Knapp and Beecham, 1990), but are captured by four simple 'rules':

1. Costs should be comprehensively measured.
2. The cost variations that are almost always observed between individual people (patients), facilities, areas of the country and so on should not be overlooked, but should be explored and, if possible, analysed.
3. Variations encourage comparisons: this service is cheaper than that one, this group of patients is more costly to support than that group. The fourth principle argues that only like-with-like comparisons have full validity.
4. Finally, cost information should usually be integrated with information on outcomes.

These principles are honoured more in the breach than in the observance. For example, few studies approach the fully comprehensive costings which are generally needed if we are to understand the broad social consequences of a particular policy or mode of treatment. It remains comparatively rare to find studies which explore the sources or causes of variations in costs or outcomes between individuals, even though this can be very revealing (Knapp, 1997). Like-with-like comparisons are ensured in a well-conducted randomised control trial, but the literature includes plenty of examples of misplaced conclusions built on inappropriate comparisons between groups of people with somewhat different needs or characteristics. As regards the fourth principle—the need to integrate cost data with outcomes data—the accumulating research evidence on dementia is again disappointing, for relatively few economic studies to date have included outcome indicators, and few clinical studies have built an economics dimension into their design.

Notwithstanding these reservations about the dementia literature, in the next section we look at some of the recent evidence on the costs of community care.

THE COSTS OF COMMUNITY CARE

Caring for an elderly person with dementia in the community generally requires a huge commitment from informal caregivers. This commitment, sometimes referred to as the 'burden' of care, is considered in more detail in another chapter. Here we focus on formal care services and their costs. We will draw on the four 'rules' noted above to help to interpret the evidence.

As we saw earlier, in the section on patterns of care, the needs of elderly people for formal support services are often quite high, and certainly are usually higher than the needs of elderly people without dementia living in the community (Torian et al, 1992; Hu et al, 1986; Trabucci et al, 1994). We will show in this section that the comprehensively measured costs of dementia care fall to a range of stakeholders, which raises a number of issues about service coordination. It will also be seen that costs are positively linked to the increasing level of need found with disease progression.

Resource use and costs of care for elderly people with dementia in England have been calculated by Schneider et al (1993), based on secondary analyses of data collected in the large and nationally representative sample surveys of private households and institutional settings (residential homes, nursing homes, hospitals) conducted in the mid and late 1980s by the OPCS. Schneider costed all services reported as being used by survey respondents, using best available unit costs figures. Each such unit cost was a comprehensive measure (including where necessary, capital charges, travel costs and overheads). The costed packages of care were fairly comprehensive, but would have missed some (comparatively minor) services because the survey instruments did not cover them. Estimates were included for informal care costs. The packages of care and their costs were rather different for those people living alone and those living with others. For those living alone, mean cost per week of both direct and indirect costs was £237 at 1996/97 price levels, compared to £272 for elderly people with dementia living with others in private households. Costs were substantially higher in residential and nursing homes, and in hospital (where a number of elderly people with dementia reside long-term), but care should be taken to make like-with-like comparisons between settings, for the institutional groups usually have greater needs.

Projecting from the OPCS sample to the full national stage, Kavanagh et al (1995) estimated that the total annual costs of the balance of care for elderly people with dementia that prevailed in 1992 amounted to £5662 million (at 1996/97 price levels). One quarter of this total cost fell to the health service, 24% to local authority social services departments, and the bulk of the remainder to the social security budget, users and their families. Kavanagh projected the expenditure implication of altering the balance of care in various ways, such as extending the availability of respite care services or providing enhanced home care for those living alone.

A recent costing study by Livingston et al (1997) placed the cost for caring for people with dementia in the community in the context of the costs for other client groups. For example, the 5.6% of people who were found to have dementia within the sample of 700 people over the age of 65 interviewed in a household survey in the Islington area of North London used 15.6% of the community care resources. This study, and consequently the latter proportion, did not include caregiver costs or long-term care. Livingston and colleagues estimated the total costs of these formal community services received by the dementia group, and extrapolated to the whole of the UK to suggest that the annual expenditure amounted to over £1000 million at current price levels. This estimate—which excludes long-term care costs—compares to the figure presented by Gray and Fenn (1993) for the *total* costs of care for people with dementia in 1990/91—£1303m at 1996/97 prices—which now looks to have been a considerable underestimate.

In Canada the net annual costs of paid services for elderly people both with and without dementia living in the community were estimated by Østbye and Crosse (1994). The costs increased as expected with the severity of the illness. For the group without dementia the annual cost was $1790, for those with mild dementia $4506, with moderate dementia $8625 and with severe dementia $8109 (all costs in Canadian dollars at 1991 prices). The respective costs for the informal element of care for the same groups were estimated to be: mild $3543; moderate $5773; and severe $9476. The total annual net cost of community care for the estimated 123 900 elderly people with dementia in Canada was therefore $1.25 billion. A study in the USA by Weinberger et al (1993) estimated expenditure for patients that live at home on the basis of diaries recording services received by the primary caregivers of elderly people with dementia. They found the cost to be $13 972 for formal services and $1572 for informal care per annum. Private expenditure for day care, sitter services, visiting nurses and other such services was found to be significantly higher for high income families and those caring for people with more severe dementia (Stommel et al, 1994).

Although these formal service costs are high, as noted earlier the principal indirect costs of dementia care in the community are associated with family and other caregiver support (including out-of-pocket expenses on adaptations and medications, forgone income from employment given up, and the value of lost leisure time). The balance between the direct and indirect costs will vary with the stage of the illness, and will obviously also depend on a country's health and social care systems, the culture surrounding ageing, the degree to which families have remained nuclear, and so on. In the US it has been estimated that it costs families around $47 000 per annum (1990 prices) to care for a dementia sufferer at home including valuing informal care itself ($34 500 of total) (Rice et al, 1991). A survey in Lombardy found that someone with Alzheimer's disease needed 18 hours a week of paid non-medical services and 45 hours a week of personal care provided by a primary caregiver (Cavallo and Fattore, 1997). The annual cost per patient of this care using the replacement cost method was calculated to be 72.9m lire (US$ 44 700).

Due to the varied nature of the needs of elderly people with dementia living in the community the costs of community care fall upon a number of sectors and agencies. For people living in private households, whether alone or with others, the individual or their family meet the largest proportion of the costs—almost 75% of the total in England (Kavanagh et al, 1993). Figures show that those living alone require more use of social services support whilst those living with others tend to use more health authority resources. It has also been found, through service usage data from the Gospel Oak study in London, that elderly people living alone with dementia are generally supported by the social services whilst people suffering from depression tend to be treated by the health services (Cullen et al, 1993).

One trend across much of the developed world is the growing tendency for governments to encourage multiple sources of funding for health and social care, mixing the public with the private. This can create a number of incentive problems, for there generally are a number of interchangeable services for this group of clients which cut across agencies which can create incentives to shift costs onto other agencies (Melzer et al, 1996). There is also the need for the coordination of services by a case or care manager which will itself have its own costs, some of them potentially substantial (Petch et al, 1996; Davies and Challis, 1986).

We noted earlier that services and care professionals try to respond to the different needs of patients which will result in potentially wide variations in cost within the group of people with dementia. The severity of the illness is usually found to be directly correlated with service utilisation and cost. For example, the cost of care in different settings in relation to the degree of dementia progression was examined by Wimo et al (1994). The annual costs generated by care in a private household were found to be 241 179 SEK. The cost of this care in the community was found to increase as cognitive capacity, ADL capacity and behavioural disturbances deteriorated. In group living arrangements, however, costs were found to remain constant. Ernst et al (1997) reported links between costs and Mini-Mental State Examination (MMSE) scores, used as an index of cognitive function, albeit for a small sample of community-dwelling elderly people. Ongoing PSSRU research, reanalysing the national OPCS data previously used by Schneider et al (1993), has detected similar links between cost and cognitive function in both community and institutional settings. These associations have relevance when looking to project the resource consequences of the new cholinesterase inhibitors.

CONCLUSIONS

As the numbers of frail elderly people with dementia increase across the world, economic pressures in most countries will make it almost imperative that the proportion living in the community also increases if care for them is to be afforded. One consequence will inevitably be even greater demands for informal and formal care, demands which even now are not being adequately met. The cost of community care will rise considerably. If people living in the community also require high levels of day hospital or occasional inpatient stays in acute hospitals the costs can rise quite rapidly (O'Shea and Blackwell, 1993). For multiple service users it may then become more appropriate—for both health and quality of life, and also on cost-effectiveness grounds—to provide support in institutional care settings. It is evident therefore that although it may be desirable to help elderly people with dementia to remain at home if they and their families wish, it is not necessarily the most efficient option.

A number of issues about costing and its uses have been raised in this chapter. One set of issues relates to the need for multiple service inputs to support elderly people with dementia who live in the community. This will have an impact on a range of statutory and non-statutory agencies, and also on the families and other 'informal' caregivers of those with the illness. Recognition of this comprehensiveness is important, and action is likely to be needed to overcome the development of inequitable burdens (for example on informal caregivers) and the dangers of cost shifting. Case-level and strategic coordination of responsibilities and finances are prerequisites for successful community-based care.

Some other issues concern the timing of care or treatment interventions. Community-based care relies heavily on informal caregivers. If these people are to continue to provide the personal and individualised support which many of them want to offer to their relatives and friends, they will need support in the *early* stages of dementia to help them establish manageable and effective care routines. If the cholinesterase inhibitor drugs can slow down the rate of decline in cognitive function, these too will considerably assist caregivers to cope with what can quickly become an oppressive and lonely care task.

Finally, there is the question of the links between the resources of community care described here (and their costs) and the outcomes for dementia sufferers and their caregivers. Focusing simply on the *costs* of community-based care is not enough, for the outcomes achieved from those costs must also be taken into account. Despite the cost-cutting intentions of many decision makers, there could be a strong case for *increasing* expenditure on a particular dementia patient or group of patients if the benefits in terms of health status and quality of life are substantial. This is the theme of other chapters in this volume, and here we would simply emphasise the fundamental importance of weighing up both costs and outcomes in reaching decisions about treatments, care arrangements and policies.

REFERENCES

Alzheimer's Disease Society (1996). *Home Alone*, Alzheimer's Disease Society, London.

Banerjee, S. and MacDonald, A. (1996). Mental Disorder in an elderly home care population: associations with health and social services use, *British Journal of Psychiatry*, **168**, 750–756.

Beecham, J. K. (1995). Collecting and estimating costs, in M. R. J. Knapp (Ed.), *The Economic Evaluation of Mental Health Care*, Aldershot, Arena.

Beecham, J. K. and Knapp, M. R. J. (1992). Costing mental health services, in G. Thornicroft, C. Brewin and J. Wing (Eds), *Measuring Mental Health Needs*, London, Gaskell.

Black, D. A., Foster, C. J. and Maitland, N. (1995). Community care outcomes, *British Journal of Clinical Practice*, **49**, 19–21.

Cabellero Garcia, J. C., Garay Lillo, J., Guijarro Garcia, J. L. and Lozano Fernandez, R. (1993). Consideraciones sobre la enfermedad de Alzheimer: epidemiologia, diagnostico, asistencia y tratamiento, *Geriatrica*, **9**, 37–47.

Cavallo, M. C. and Fattore, G. (1997). The economic and social burden of Alzheimer's disease on families in the Lombardy region, Italy, *Alzheimer's Disease and Associated Disorders*, in press.

Challis, D. (1993). Lewisham care management project—preliminary report, in D. Robbins (Ed.), *Community Care: Findings from Department of Health Funded Research 1988–1992*, London, HMSO.

Collins, C., King, C. and Kokinakis, C. (1994). Community service issues before nursing home placement of persons with dementia, *Western Journal of Nursing Research*, **16**, 40–52.

Cullen, W., Blizard, R., Livingston, G. et al (1993). The Gospel Oak Project 1987–1990: provision and use of community services, *Health Trends*, **25**, 142–146.

Davies, B. P. (1992). *Care Management, Equity and Efficiency: The International Experience*, University of Kent at Canterbury, PSSRU.

Davies, B. P. and Challis, D. J. (1986). *Matching Resources to Needs in Community Care*, Aldershot, Gower.

Donaldson, C., Tarrier, N. and Burns, A. (1997). The impact of the symptoms of dementia on caregivers, *British Journal of Psychiatry*, **170**, 62–68.

Drummond, M. F., O'Brien, B., Stoddart, G. L. and Torrance, G. W. (1997). *Methods for the Economic Evaluation of Health Care Programmes*, Oxford, Oxford University Press.

Ernst, R. L. and Hay, J. W. (1994). The US economic and social costs of Alzheimer's disease revisited, *American Journal of Public Health*, **84**, 1261–1264.

Ernst, R. L., Hay, J. W., Fenn, C., Tinklenberg, J. and Yesavage, J. A. (1997). Cognitive function and the costs of Alzheimer's disease, *Archives of Neurology*, **54**, 687–693.

Gauthier, S., Baumgarten, M. and Becker, R. (1996). Dementia behaviour disturbance scale, *International Psychogeriatrics*, **8**, Suppl. 3, 325–327.

Gray, A. M. and Fenn, P. (1993). Alzheimer's disease: the burden of illness in England, *Health Trends*, **25**, 31–37.

Henke, C. J. and Burchmore, M. J. (1997). The economic impact of the tacrine in the treatment of Alzheimer's disease, *Clinical Therapeutics*, **19**, 330–345.

Hu, T. W., Huang, L. F. and Cartwright, W. S. (1986). Evaluation of the costs of caring for the senile demented elderly: a pilot study, *Gerontologist*, **26**, 158–163.

Kavanagh, S., Schneider, J., Knapp, M. R. J., Beecham, J. and Netten, A. (1993). Elderly people with cognitive impairment: costing possible changes in the balance of care, *Health and Social Care in the Community*, **1**, 2, 69–80.

Kavanagh, S., Schneider, J., Knapp, M. R. J., Beecham, J. and Netten, A. (1995). Elderly people with dementia: costs, effectiveness and balance of care, in M. R. J. Knapp (Ed.), *The Economic Evaluation of Mental Health Care*, Aldershot, Arena.

Keady, J. (1994) Living alone with dementia, *British Journal of Nursing*, **3**, 648–650.

Kendall, J. and Knapp, M. R. J. (1996). *The Voluntary Sector in the UK*, Manchester, Manchester University Press.

Knapp, M. J., Knopman, D. S., Solomon, P. R., Pendlebury, W. S., Davis, C. S. and Gracon, S. I. (1994). A 30-week randomized controlled trial of high-dose tacrine in patients with Alzheimer's disease, *Journal of the American Medical Association*, **271**, 985–991.

Knapp, M. R. J. (1990). *Time is Money: The Costs of Volunteering in Britain Today*, Berkhamsted, The Volunteer Centre.

Knapp, M. R. J. (1997). Making music out of noise? The cost function approach to evaluation, *British Journal of Psychiatry*, supplement, forthcoming.

Knapp, M. R. J. and Beecham, J. K. (1990). Costing mental health services, *Psychological Medicine*, **20**, 893–908.

Knapp, M. R. J., Koutsogeorgopoulou, V. and Davis Smith, J. (1996). Volunteer participation in community care, *Policy and Politics*, **24**, 2, 171–192.

Levin, E., Sinclair, I. and Gorbach, P. (1988). The effectiveness of the home help service with confused old people and their families, *Research Policy and Planning*, **3**, 1–7.

Livingston, G., Manela, M. and Katona, C. (1997). Cost of community care for older people, *British Journal of Psychiatry*, **171**, 56–69.

Max, W. (1993). The economic impact of Alzheimer's disease, *Neurology*, **43**, S6–S10.

Melzer, D., Hopkins, S., Pencheon, D., Brayne, C. and Williams, R. (1996). Dementia, in A. Stevens and J. Raftery (Eds), *Health Care Needs Assessment*, Oxford, Radcliffe.

Netten, A. and Dennett, J. (1997). *Unit Costs of Health and Social Care 1997*, University of Kent at Canterbury, PSSRU.

O'Connor, J. et al (1989). Distribution of services to elderly demented people living in the community, *International Journal of Geriatric Psychiatry*, **4**, 339–344.

OECD (1996). *Caring for Frail Elderly People*, Social Policy Studies, 19, Paris, OECD.

O'Shea, E. and Blackwell, J. (1993). The relationship between the cost of community care and the dependency of old people, *Social Science and Medicine*, **37**, 583–590.

Østbye, T. and Crosse, E. (1994). Net economic costs of dementia, *Canadian Medical Association Journal*, **151**, 10.

Petch, A., Cheetham, J., Fuller, R., MacDonald, C., Myers, F. with Hallam, A. and Knapp, M. R. J. (1996). *Delivering Community Care: Initial Implementation of Care Management in Scotland*, Edinburgh, The Stationery Office.

Philp, I., McKee, K. J., Meldrum, P., Ballinger, B. R., Golhooly, M. L. M., Gordon, D. S., Mutch, W. J. and Whittick, J. E. (1995). Community care for demented and non-demented elderly people: a comparison study of financial burden, service use, and unmet needs in family supporters, *British Medical Journal*, **310**, 1503–1506.

Rice, D. P., Fox, P., Hauck, W. et al (1993). The burden of caring for Alzheimer's disease patients. National Center for Health Statistics. *Proceedings of the 1991 Public Health Conference on Records and Statistics*. Washington, DC, US Department of Health and Human Servces, pp. 119–124.

Rogers, S. L., Friedhoff, L. T. and the Donepezil Study Group (1996). The efficacy and safety of donepezil in patients with Alzheimer's disease: results of a US multicentre, randomized, double-blind, placebo-controlled trial, *Dementia*, **7**, 293–303.

Schneider, J., Kavanagh, S. M., Knapp, M. R. J., Beecham, J. and Netten, A. (1993). Elderly people with advanced cognitive impairment in England: resource use and costs, *Ageing and Society*, **13**, 27–50.

Stommel, M., Collins, C. E. and Given, B. A. (1994). The costs of family contributions to the care of persons with dementia, *Gerontologist*, **34**, 199–205.

Torian, L., Davidson, E., Fulop, G., Sell, L. and Fillit, H. (1992). The effect of dementia on acute care in a geriatric medical unit, *International Psychogeriatrics*, **4**, 231–239.

Trabucchi, M., Govoni, S. and Bianchetti, A. (1995). Socio-economic aspects of Alzheimer's treatment, in E. Giacobini and R. Becker (Eds), *Alzheimer's Disease: Therapeutic Strategies*, Bolsoy, Bickhauser, pp. 459–463.

Weinberger, M., Gold, D. T., Divine, G. W. et al (1993). Expenditures in caring for patients with dementia who live at home, *American Journal of Public Health*, **83**, 338–341.

Wimo, A., Krakau, I., Mattsson, B. and Nelvig, A. (1994). The impact of cognitive decline and workload on the costs of dementia care, *International Journal of Geriatric Psychiatry*, **6**, 21–29.

Wimo, A., Grafstrom, M. and Winblad, B. (1997). The social consequences of Alzheimer's disease, forthcoming.

2.8 Indirect Costs and Costing Informal Care

MARC A. KOOPMANSCHAP and WERNER B. F. BROUWER
Institute for Medical Technology Assessment, Erasmus University, Rotterdam, The Netherlands

INTRODUCTION

Indirect costs of disease is an often discussed concept, in health economics generally and particularly in economic evaluation of health care programmes. As indirect costs relate to production loss as a result of illness, these costs may be substantial for many diseases. In addition, the impact of health care programmes on indirect costs is often an important outcome in economic evaluations. The discussion on indirect costs focuses on three questions:

- How to define indirect costs
- Whether to include indirect costs in economic evaluation of health care
- How to measure and value these costs in order to derive reliable estimates

This chapter first discusses the matter of definition and inclusion of indirect costs. Two alternative methods to value indirect costs will be described (second section). In the third section we will outline the specific problems of estimating indirect costs of dementia in various circumstances, also paying some attention to informal care. The fourth section presents the available limited empirical evidence on indirect costs of dementia. The final section provides some suggestions on how to estimate the indirect costs of dementia in economic evaluations of health care programmes.

THE CONCEPT OF INDIRECT COSTS

DEFINITION OF INDIRECT COSTS

Indirect costs of disease have been defined in many ways, creating confusion about their meaning and their importance in economic evaluation of health

Health Economics of Dementia. Edited by Anders Wimo, Bengt Jönsson, Göran Karlsson and Bengt Winblad.
© 1998 John Wiley & Sons Ltd.

care. We propose the following definition of indirect costs of disease, using a societal perspective:

Costs due to production lost and/or replacement as a result of disease, absence from work, disability or mortality of productive persons, engaged in paid or unpaid work.

According to this definition, the impact of being ill on the sick individual's income is not of primary importance, what matters is the change in production and/or the costs of replacing sick workers in order to maintain production at the initial level. Income and production losses should never be added in estimating indirect costs, as this would induce double-counting. Furthermore, social security benefits may not be used as a proxy for indirect costs since these benefits represent only a redistribution of wealth, not a change in wealth.

Unpaid work is included in our definition, since unpaid work is an indispensable input for the reproduction of society's wealth and therefore should not be overlooked. The productivity loss that may occur when sick persons are still at work, being less productive than usual, is also included.

With respect to mortality, this definition only refers to the economic implications of workers dying, it does *not include the value of life as such.* The latter value may be an element in cost-benefit analysis. The definition of indirect costs as stated here is to be used in cost-effectiveness and cost-utility analyses, in which life as such is valued as an element of health: in natural units (lives and life-years gained) or in QALYs or DALYs, correcting for quality of life. 'Intangible costs' of pain, suffering, discomfort, and so on, aspects of illness that are sometimes labelled as indirect costs, are excluded here. These consequences of disease should preferably be measured as health effects, using quality of life instruments. The influence of illness on leisure time is not included in our definition of indirect costs, but this topic will be discussed in the third section.

In the following sections it will be discussed whether or not to include indirect costs in economic evaluations of health care and alternative ways to estimate indirect costs will be presented.

INCLUSION OF INDIRECT COSTS

Equity

Inclusion of production losses in economic evaluation may favour health care programmes directed to working people as compared to people without a paid job: an equal reduction of illness may save more indirect costs for (better salaried) working people. This result may conflict with equity considerations.

This situation could be avoided by excluding indirect costs from economic evaluations. However, this would deny that production losses influence the scarcity of resources and hence decrease the wealth of society. To give a full picture of indirect costs one should also value lost production related to unpaid work, diminishing adverse equity consequences. Furthermore, it would be advisable to report on possible equity implications of including indirect costs. It is the responsibility of decision makers to decide on the relative weight that they want to attach to the equity considerations, apart from the relative efficiency of interventions.

Opportunity costs versus QALYs

Recently, Gerard and Mooney argued that including non-health care costs in cost-utility analysis is wrong (Gerard and Mooney, 1993). According to them, the opportunity costs of health care resources are defined in terms only of the QALYs forgone. Hence, cost-utility analysis would be about generating QALYs and QALYs forgone by opportunities sacrificed. This would preclude considering indirect costs, which could only be considered in cost-benefit analysis. These authors interpret opportunity costs in a rather narrow sense. Clearly, when program A requires a similar health care budget to program B, but uses less resources than program B from a societal perspective, the additional resources becoming available when applying program A as compared to B could be added to the health care budget (or added to budgets for education, housing and working conditions, which may contribute to health status), and could produce QALYs. Therefore, the opportunity costs in terms of QALYs forgone of program B would be larger than those of program A. So, using a societal perspective, there is no specific requirement to use cost-benefit analysis, with its valuation problems, when considering indirect costs in an economic evaluation.

Guidelines

Canadian guidelines for economic appraisal in support of reimbursement decisions regarding pharmaceuticals do not object to including indirect costs in economic evaluation studies (CCOHTA, 1994). The most recent version of the Australian guidelines suggests that economic appraisals of pharmaceuticals should present results both with and without indirect benefits and costs included, but stresses that valuation of work time gained or lost should be made explicit (Henry, 1992).

Because French, German and British guidelines and the 'Washington Panel' (Gold et al, 1996) are in favour of including indirect costs in economic evaluation of health care, overall consensus seems to be growing.

MEASUREMENT OF INDIRECT COSTS

Most studies estimating indirect costs use the human capital approach. This method estimates the value of potentially lost production (measured as the potentially lost income) as a consequence of disease. In the event of absence from paid work, labour income during the period of absence is used as an estimate for indirect costs. With respect to disability, labour income during the entire period of disability is used for estimating indirect costs. If for example a 35-year-old person becomes permanently disabled, the total income forgone from age 35 onwards until the age of retirement is estimated as indirect costs. For mortality before the age of retirement, the estimation procedure is analogous.

Many authors have criticised the human capital approach. They state that the human capital method estimates the value of potential production lost, whereas the actual loss for society may be much smaller. Drummond (1992) commented in this respect: 'for short-term absences, a given person's work may be covered by others or made up by the sick person on his return to work. For long-term absences, an individual's work can be covered by someone drawn from the ranks of the unemployed. Therefore, while absence from work may cost the individual, or that person's employer, it may not cost society very much.' Thus the human capital method may overestimate the economic consequences of disease in various circumstances.

An alternative measurement method (the 'friction cost method') has been proposed to quantify indirect costs (Koopmanschap et al, 1995). The basic idea is that the amount of production lost due to disease depends on the time-span organisations need to restore the initial production level. If unemployment is beyond the level of frictional unemployment sick employees can be replaced, after a period necessary for adaptation. Production losses are assumed to be confined to the period needed to replace a sick worker: the friction period. Application of the friction cost method requires information on the *frequency and length of friction periods* and the *value of productivity lost*. In order to estimate the total number of friction periods one needs data on the frequency and length of absence spells and the incidence of disability and mortality. The length of the friction period can be based on the average vacancy duration. The friction cost method assumes that the production level is restored after (a part of) the friction period. The actual indirect costs of disease consist of the value of production lost and/or the extra costs to maintain production and, if an employee is to be replaced permanently, the costs of filling a vacancy and training new personnel. The friction cost method also takes into account several medium-term macro-economic effects of absence from work and disability. For more detailed information see Koopmanschap and Rutten (1996).

The friction cost method is still a broad instrument for estimating indirect costs (as is the human capital approach) and it needs more refinement in measuring the exact consequences of short-term absence from work for production and costs. The debate on the friction cost method is ongoing, see Johanneson and Karlsson (1997) and Koopmanschap et al (1997).

Recently, the US Panel on Cost-Effectiveness in Health and Medicine (Gold et al, 1996) proposed a rather unusual way to incorporate indirect costs related to paid work in cost-effectiveness analysis. They proposed to incorporate this in terms of quality of life. According to the Panel, respondents who value health states incorporate income changes due to the changed health state if this is not explicitly excluded in the quality of life instrument or the valuation process. This way, productivity changes should be incorporated in quality of life outcomes through income and any additional monetary valuation of productivity losses would then obviously lead to a double-count. Recently, the approach of the Panel has been criticised (Brouwer et al, 1997a, 1997b) and defended (Weinstein et al, 1997). The critique was two-fold; first, income should not be part of health-related quality of life and the most common quality of life instruments, such as EuroQol and SF-36, should avoid questions alluding to income. Second, if one still wanted to capture productivity losses through quality of life, the method proposed by the Panel would not lead to sound estimations of the true societal costs involved for several reasons. One is that social and private insurance will often influence (i.e. increase) income in the event of reduced productivity due to illness. Therefore the relation between productivity, income and quality of life will be affected, making income an unsuitable proxy for productivity. Another reason is that if income losses are considered to cause a decrease in quality of life, an income increase (of the person replacing the impaired patient) will lead to a quality of life increase. Taking a societal perspective, this 'balancing effect' should also be taken into account. Finally, production losses without absence often do not cause income decreases and therefore will go unnoticed in the approach of the Panel.

Estimates of indirect costs

Estimates of indirect costs for the Netherlands using both methods show that the results differ substantially, see Table 2.8.1. The short-term friction costs amount to 2.0–2.5% of net national income in 1988 and 1990 (Koopmanschap et al, 1995) and the medium-term economic consequences of absence and disability amount to 0.8% of NNI. The costs of absence from work predominate, since it is assumed that production losses are confined to the friction period; consequently disability and mortality hardly contribute to the costs. Indirect costs for 1988 according to the human capital approach amount to 18% of net national income. The huge difference compared to the friction costs is related to the cost of disability and mortality, which are assumed to cause production losses over a longer period. Costs of disability are very large, because the average duration of disability in the Netherlands is 15 years. The

Table 2.8.1. Indirect costs of disease in the Netherlands for 1988 and 1990 in billions of Dutch guilders (in parentheses as % of net national income)

Cost category	Friction costs 1988	Human capital costs 1988	Friction costs 1990
Absence from work	9.2	23.8	11.6
Disability	0.15	49.1	0.2
Mortality	0.15	8.0	0.2
Total indirect costs	9.5 (2.1%)[a]	80.9 (18%)	12.0 (2.6%)[a]

[a] In addition medium-term economic consequences of absence from work and disability amount to 0.8% of net national income.

costs of absence from work differ less dramatically. As the friction cost method assumes production loss to be limited to the short run, the friction costs for diseases that cause mainly disability and mortality are much lower than according to the human capital approach. For diseases entailing short-term absence, the difference is much smaller.

STANDARDISATION

Although some debate will remain, most authors accept that indirect costs are relevant to an economic evaluation framework and should in principle be included. They also tend to agree in their rejection of the human capital approach for quantifying these indirect costs as it has been applied in most studies to date. They also point out that preferably a method should be used which takes into account that after an adaptation period sick workers may be replaced by someone else if unemployment (both registered and hidden) is above the friction level. The Australian guidelines also allude to this phenomenon where it is stated that 'the Australian economy is constrained by macroeconomic factors rather than by the lack of healthy workers' (Commonwealth of Australia, 1990). Thus a method of estimating indirect costs should preferably be used which takes this transitory character of the associated opportunity costs to society into account.

INDIRECT COSTS APPLIED TO DEMENTIA

Whatever method is used to estimate indirect costs of disease, it should first be made clear under what circumstances indirect costs are relevant for dementia. In this section we will discuss indirect costs related to paid and unpaid work of patients and informal caregivers.

PATIENTS' INDIRECT COSTS

Paid work

In most Western countries, the normal age of retirement is between age 60 and 64. Consequently, the participation in paid labour of this age-group is limited. Furthermore, the prevalence of dementia for the age-group 55–64 is very low (in the Netherlands: 0.4%). In addition, dementia is rarely a primary cause of death below age 75. Consequently, the indirect costs of dementia, related to paid work, appear to be very limited, irrespective of the method used. For an estimate of indirect costs of dementia for the Netherlands, see the next section, on empirical evidence.

Unpaid work

Regarding unpaid work, dementia patients living at home may be less able to perform a substantial part of normal unpaid work in their household. As far as unpaid activities are not taken over by other people, production may be lost and indirect costs occur. The amount of unpaid work lost may be estimated using the Health and Labour questionnaire, analysing four categories of unpaid work: household activities, shopping, child care and odd jobs (van Roijen et al, 1996). The economic impact of home-production can best be valued by using the wage-rate of a professional housekeeper (Brouwer et al, 1998). If partners, other informal caregivers and/or professional caregivers (partly) take over these activities, (part of) the production loss in the household is compensated for, at the opportunity costs of the time invested by those persons. In the case of professional home care, these costs are clearly direct health care costs and should be measured accordingly. In the case of informal care matters become more complicated, as explained below.

Leisure time

In our opinion the patient's loss of leisure time due to illness can best be measured in terms of quality of life, instead of being valued monetarily; see the following section for a more extensive discussion.

INFORMAL CAREGIVERS' COSTS

In this section we will focus on the time input of informal caregivers in the intervention. Apart from this time input 'intangible effects' such as fatigue and disutility from having to perform unpleasant tasks may also be important. The valuation of these effects on informal caregivers is not discussed further here. Also, the illness may of course in itself affect the well-being of a spouse or close relative. These 'family effects' are naturally present in all diseases, whether there is informal care or not, and should therefore not be taken into account as being costs of informal care, although eventually they may be measured and taken into account. Gold et al (1996) encourage analysts to 'think broadly about the people affected by the intervention and begin to include health related quality of life effects of significant others in sensitivity analyses when they are important' (p. 67).

Paid work

If informal caregivers have to give up (a part of) paid work, temporarily or permanently, in order to care for the demented patient the distinction between direct and indirect costs becomes vague. Taking the viewpoint of the care-process, these activities are an indispensable element in caring for the demented and hence should be classified as *direct non-health care costs*. Taking an opportunity cost viewpoint, a reduction of paid work clearly incurs *indirect costs* as a result of absence from work. The exact classification of these costs becomes somewhat arbitrary and it should be noted that discussing these costs under the heading indirect costs is not unambiguous. A possible solution could be to value these costs according to the principles of estimating indirect costs and to report these costs separately under the heading 'costs of informal care'. For the primary caregiver, often the partner of the patient, the indirect costs of paid work may be limited as he/she is also often retired. For other informal caregivers, such as children of the demented, the indirect costs of paid work may not be negligible.

Unpaid work

If informal caregivers give up unpaid activities, in order to care for demented patients, again it is crucial whether unpaid work lost is taken over by other people. The amount and value of unpaid work lost may be estimated analogously to that for the demented patient.

Leisure time

Informal care often reduces leisure time substantially. For caregivers living in the same household, it may be very difficult to indicate how much leisure time is given up, since many tasks may be combined with normal household tasks (preparing meals) or with leisure activities (surveillance) (Busschbach et al, 1998). However, if the amount of leisure time sacrificed is known, the question remains how to value it. In our opinion leisure time may best be treated as time in which one can do the things that make life valuable: sporting, hobbies, socialising and so on (Brouwer et al, 1998). We feel that the loss of leisure time can only be captured meaningfully by measuring the reduction of quality of life from lost leisure time, instead of a monetary valuation. Quality of life questionnaires such as EuroQol and SF-36 explicitly ask about problems in performing leisure activities or social activities.

Following this option invokes one problem: the patient's quality of life is clearly *health-related*, whereas the caregiver's quality of life change is *care-related*. Because these 'QALYs' are not of the same type, they cannot be simply summed up in an economic evaluation. An alternative solution is to mention the influence of dementia on the quality of life of caregivers as a separate item, not entering the cost-utility ratio.

Explicit attention for caregiver quality of life makes it possible to give an appropriate weight to changes in caregiver quality of life. This is especially relevant for dementia, since the informal care activities appear to be very demanding and lengthy. Note that quality of life also seems to be an appropriate tool to capture 'intangible effects' such as fatigue and having to perform unpleasant tasks. In that sense the remark by Gold et al (1996) about the incorporation of quality of life effects of significant others seems especially relevant for informal caregivers, on whom the impact may be significant.

EMPIRICAL EVIDENCE

Empirical evidence on indirect costs of dementia is very scarce. Results labelled as indirect costs often appear to be a mixture of indirect costs *strictu sensu*, costs of informal care and costs of other family contributions.

THE NETHERLANDS

For the Netherlands, it is feasible to make a rough estimate of indirect costs of dementia due to absence from work, disability and mortality of patients having paid work. In 1993 only 11 cases (3000 absence days) of absence from work due to dementia were registered: 0.0% of total absence (Polder et al, 1997). In 1994, 446 persons were disabled due to dementia: 0.1% of total disability (Polder et al, 1997). Before age 65 only 25 persons died primarily through dementia: 0.0% of total age <65-mortality. Using these figures, according to the friction cost method indirect costs amounted to 0.8 million guilders in 1994, whereas applying the human capital approach gives 25 million guilders. In the latter estimate disability and mortality make up almost all costs. However, both indirect costs estimates are negligible as compared to the estimate of direct health care costs: 3309 million (Polder et al, 1997, and Chapter 2.5, this volume, on the cost of dementia in the Netherlands). It may be concluded that indirect costs incurred through paid work for patients are insignificant. With respect to indirect costs of unpaid work for patients and indirect costs related to informal caregivers no Dutch evidence is available.

OTHER COUNTRIES

Only a few studies have analysed non-health care costs of dementia, predominantly in the United States, Canada and Sweden. Indirect costs of paid and unpaid work for patients were only reported by Ernst and Hay (1994). Using an incidence-based cost model, they estimated lifetime earnings lost due to disability and mortality as US$50 000 per patient (discount rate 4% per year), using the age-income profiles of Rice and associates. The authors do not provide much detail on their calculation. For example it is not known if unpaid labour was included and what retirement age was used for paid labour. Given the relatively low prevalence of dementia below age 65, the estimate of $50 000 per patient seems rather high. According to Ernst and Hay, total lifetime costs per patient amounted to US$174 000, of which $48 000 were direct health care costs and $76 000 were for unpaid informal care, valued at the market wage of home health care workers.

Other studies only estimated costs of informal care, using the market wage for home health workers as a valuation. No information is available to what extent the time sacrificed for informal care was devoted to paid work, unpaid work and leisure time, precluding a valuation based on opportunity cost principles. Informal care costs as reported are substantial: Can$636 million for Canada in 1991, that is about 16% of total costs of dementia (Østbye and Crosse, 1994). Stommel et al (1994) estimated the annual costs of informal care for demented living at home to be US$12 456 per person per year (cost level 1989), whereas Rice et al (1991) calculated much higher costs: $34 518 per demented at home.

For Sweden indirect costs of patients only represented 0.1% of total direct and indirect costs of dementia in 1991 (Wimo et al, 1997). The costs of *paid informal care* were SEK2.07 billion, only 1.7% of total health care costs. The costs for unpaid informal care are unknown, but these were probably much higher.

HOW TO ESTIMATE INDIRECT COSTS OF DEMENTIA

In this section we offer some suggestions on how to estimate indirect costs of patients and informal care costs in prospective economic evaluation studies. First of all, it does not seem advisable to put much effort into estimating the indirect costs of paid work of dementia patients, since these costs appear to be very limited. For the unpaid labour of patients the impact has yet to be established. Instruments such as the 'Health and Labour' questionnaire may be administered repeatedly in order to collect data, and if necessary the patient's partner may fill out the questionnaire.

Since informal care has an important role for dementia, measurement and valuation of informal care needs more attention. The costs may be substantial and need to be documented extensively as well as the quality of life of the caregiver. It is advisable to collect data on the amount of informal care as often as possible. Preferably, diaries should be kept to register the daily amount of professional care and informal care, focusing on time spent on caregiving in addition to normal time use. The valuation of time sacrificed in providing informal care should preferably be based on the opportunity costs for each type of time-use. Hence, it is advisable to collect data on the nature of the time sacrificed by informal caregivers: to what extent paid work/unpaid work/leisure time is given up. For paid work, information on the type of job, income and the length of the period of (part-time) absence from work should be available. To get a complete picture on the burden of care, it seems worthwhile to collect data on the quality of life of informal caregivers, especially the primary caregiver.

REFERENCES

Brouwer, W. B. F., Koopmanschap, M. A. and Rutten, F. F. H. (1997a). Productivity costs measurement through quality of life? A response to the recommendations of the Washington Panel, *Health Economics*, **6**, 253–259.

Brouwer, W. B. F., Koopmanschap, M. A. and Rutten, F. F. H. (1997b). Productivity costs in cost-effectiveness analysis: numerator or denominator: a further discussion, *Health Economics*, **6**, 511–514.

Brouwer, W. B. F., Koopmanschap, M. A. and Rutten, F. F. H. (1998). Patient and informal caregiver time in cost-effectiveness analysis, *Int. J. Technology Assessment in Health Care* (in press).

Busschbach, J. J. V., Brouwer, W. B. F., Donk, A. van der, Passchier, J. and Rutten, F. F. H. (1998). An outline for a cost-effectiveness analysis of a drug for patients with Alzheimer's disease, *PharmacoEconomics*, **13**, 21–34.

CCOHTA (1994). *Guidelines for Economic Evaluation of Pharmaceuticals: Canada*, Ottawa, Ontario.

Commonwealth of Australia (1990). *Guidelines for the pharmaceutical industry on preparation of submissions to the Pharmaceutical Benefits Advisory Committee: including submissions involving economic analyses.* Department of Health, Housing and Community Services, Woden (ACT).

Drummond, M. F. (1992). Cost-of-illness studies: a major headache? *Pharmaco-Economics*, **2**, 1.

Ernst, R. L. and Hay, J. W. (1994). The US economic and social costs of Alzheimer's disease revisited, *AJPH*, **84**(8), 1261–1264.

Gerard, K. and Mooney, G. (1993). QALY league tables: handle with care, *Health Economics*, **2**, 59.

Gold, M. R., Siegel, J. E., Russell, L. B. and Weinstein, M. C. (Eds) (1996). *Cost-effectiveness in Health and Medicine*, Oxford, Oxford University Press.

Henry, D. A. (1992). The Australian guidelines for subsidisation of pharmaceuticals, *PharmacoEconomics*, **2**, 422.

Johanneson, M. and Karlsson, G. (1997). The friction cost method: a comment, *J. Health Economics*, **16**(2), 249–255.

Koopmanschap, M. A., Rutten, F. F. H., Ineveld, B. M. van and Roijen, L. van

(1995). The friction cost method for measuring indirect costs of disease, *J. Health Economics*, **14**, 171–189.

Koopmanschap, M. A. and Rutten, F. F. H. (1996). A practical guide for calculating indirect costs of disease, *PharmacoEconomics*, **10**(5), 460–466.

Koopmanschap, M. A., Rutten, F. F. H., Ineveld, B. M. van and Roijen, L. van (1997). Reply to Johanneson's and Karlsson's comment, *J. Health Economics*, **16**(2), 257–259.

Østbye, T. and Crosse, E. (1994). Net economic costs of dementia in Canada, *Can. Med. Assoc. J.*, **151**(10), 1457–1464.

Polder, J. J., Meerding, W. J., Koopmanschap, M. A., Bonneux, L. and Maas, P. J. van der (1997). *Costs of Diseases in the Netherlands 1994* (in Dutch). Erasmus University, Rotterdam, Institute for Public Health/Institute for Medical Technology Assessment.

Rice, D. P., Fox, P., Hauck, W. et al (1991). *The Burden of Caring for Alzheimer's Patients. National Center for Health Statistics*, pp. 119–124, Proceedings of the 1991 public health conference on records and statistics, Washington, DC, US Department of Health and Human Services.

Roijen, L. van, Essink-Bot, M. L., Koopmanschap, M. A., Bonsel, G. J. and Rutten, F. F. H. (1996). Labor and health status in economic evaluation of health care: the health and labor questionnaire, *Int. J. Technology Assessment in Health Care*, **12**(3), 405–415.

Stommel, M., Collins, C. E., Faan, R. N. and Given, B. A. (1994). The costs of family contributions to the care of persons with dementia, *Gerontologist*, **34**(2), 199–205.

Weinstein, M. C., Siegel, J. E., Garber, A. M., Lipscomb, J., Luce, B. R., Manning, Jr W. G. and Torrance, G. W. (1997). Productivity costs, time costs, and health-related quality of life: a response to the Erasmus Group, *Health Economics*, **6**, 505–510.

Wimo, A., Karlsson, G., Sandman, P. O., Corder, L. and Winblad, B. (1997). Cost of illness due to dementia in Sweden, *International J. of Geriatric Psychiatry*, **12**, 857–861.

2.9 The Resident Assessment Instrument (RAI) and Resource Use in Dementia Care

GUNNAR LJUNGGREN
Karolinska Institute and Stockholm County Council, Stockholm, Sweden

JOHN N. MORRIS
Hebrew Rehabilitation Center for the Aged, Boston, USA

INTRODUCTION

Dementia care is heavily influenced by our understanding of the individual. Expectations for decline predominate, rehabilitation can be difficult to justify, and narrow thinking abounds. Biased, superficial assessments are common, and if we are to move into a new realm of quality care, we must first scrutinize how we go about assessing the demented person. High-quality care cannot occur in an environment in which we fail to fully grasp issues of dependency, motivation, and social meaning. In short, we must redouble our efforts to ensure that we know the patient. This has implications not only on quality but also on resource use.

How this is to be achieved and the areas to be covered in any new, standardized assessment are crucial considerations. Our perspective should be global and not disease-limited. We would acquire information from the patient, the family, and the direct providers of care. Our perspective would begin with function, describing how the person is involved in ADLs, communication, planning, continence, and so on. We would look at physical as well as mental problems: delirium, depression, falls, pressure ulcers, weight loss. And we would not stop here. We would also require that there be global knowledge about the informal and formal resource utilization.

In taking this position, we recognize that there will be issues of time, interest, and values. We presume that the demented elder is still a valued member of the human community, albeit one who may require more instrumental supports within his/her environment.

We know much about the changing needs of the dementia patient. There are known correlations between patient characteristics and resource inputs, and if

Health Economics of Dementia. Edited by Anders Wimo, Bengt Jönsson, Göran Karlsson and Bengt Winblad.
© 1998 John Wiley & Sons Ltd.

care provision patterns are problematic, it cannot simply be said that we knew not what to do. To the extent that we seem to be in the dark, the most reasonable explanation is our failure to grasp the need for comprehensive patient assessment.

If we permit ourselves to know the patient, if we put the necessary resources into patient assessment, we will be in a powerful position to link resources to patient needs. This is as true for demented residents in nursing homes as it is for demented patients in the community.

Soon after the admission of a resident into a nursing home, the provider of a professional care must target the needs of the resident. The staff must get to know the resident in a cost-effective way, so that time is not wasted and the quality and quantity of care is proportional to the needs of the resident. This is particularly true for a person with cognitive dysfunction, who is also at risk through not being able to communicate or not being understood, or when there is an acute health status problem.

For this, as well as for other reasons, we need to do a comprehensive assessment of a demented person, soon after he or she has entered a nursing home or other type of institution for the elderly. One such an attempt is the Resident Assessment Instrument for Nursing Homes, now mandated for global use in the US, as well as in Iceland and in broad areas in Canada and Japan. With this assessment, we get a full picture of the resident, as well as many other spin-off effects regarding resource use, cognitive status, and the need for further education of the staff. For vertically integrated care systems, we also have a companion Minimum Data Set (MDS) for home care.

THE RAI FAMILY, COMPREHENSIVE ASSESSMENT INSTRUMENTS IN ELDERLY CARE

MDS Version 1.0/2.0

To develop the interaction between resident and carer in nursing homes in the US, and thus to improve the quality of care delivered, OBRA '87, a US law, requested a comprehensive assessment system to be developed and implemented for all Medicare nursing homes from 1992. Under a contract from HCFA (Health Care Financing Administration), researchers from four academic settings were charged with developing the Minimum Data Set for Nursing Home Resident Assessment and Care Screening (MDS/RAI) (Morris et al, 1990). MDS is the core functional assessment instrument in the RAI and covers such domains as physical functioning in the activities of daily living (ADLs), cognition, continence, mood, behaviors, nutritional status, vision and communication, activities, and psychosocial well-being. The purpose of the MDS assessment is to identify a resident's strengths, preferences, and needs in key areas, and provide a holistic and comprehensive picture of the resident's functional status.

A few years after the implementation of the MDS/RAI, the experiences of its use nationwide necessitated a second version, launched in 1995 (Morris et al, 1997). By then, the international community also had become aware of this new process of improving the quality of care in nursing homes and an international network, the interRAI, had been established with participants from many countries. Today, the MDS has been translated to 15 different languages and many of these versions have been tested for interrater reliability (Sgadari et al, 1997).

MDS-HC

Within this international ongoing research, the needs for new instruments that cover other areas of elderly care have been highlighted. One of these instruments is the MDS-HC, Minimum Data Set for Home Care.

The MDS-HC is a problem and care plan guideline-driven assessment instrument for use in community care settings. It is an extension of the MDS Version 2.0 for nursing homes and it is designed to assist clinicians in arriving at a comprehensive view of the needs and strengths of the population served, a view that is essential to the development of appropriate plans of care, allowing elders to achieve their functional potential. The MDS-HC can work in tandem with the MDS Version 2.0 to track elders within vertically integrated health care systems. This system thus forms the basis for a common core of key assessment items for following elderly persons from institutional to community settings.

The Resident Assessment Instrument for Acute Care (RAI-AC) and Others

The Resident Assessment Instrument for Acute Care (RAI-AC) has been under development for the past two years. This system was designed to supplement the traditional medically oriented approach to assessment of hospitalized persons with standardized measures in key domains of function, health behaviors, social support, and service use pertinent to quality of care and quality of life. The RAI-AC contains a large subset of core assessment items from the nursing home and home care instruments, some of which have been adapted for use in a more transitional setting with shorter lengths of stay.

Other instruments under construction by interRAI and collaborating centers are assessments in mental health patients, palliative care, and postacute care. They are all meant to be built around a common core of clinical knowledge that should follow the individual throughout an episode of care or in a particular setting.

COMMON CONSTRUCTION OF THE RAI INSTRUMENTS

Despite its name, the RAI is not just an assessment tool. Instead it could be called a second-generation tool, which includes three parts: the Minimum Data Set (MDS); triggers that could tell the existence of a problem; and the Resident Assessment Protocols (RAPs) that are in-depth clinical protocols to help the staff in the care planning process when a problem is triggered.

The MDS is a minimal requirement (let alone it now comprises approx. 450 items) for a comprehensive assessment of an elderly institutionalized person. Every item has been thoroughly scrutinized by clinicians and professionals (physicians, nurses, physical therapists, occupational therapists, social workers), trying to decide whether that particular item is reliable and valid and thus adds to, or is necessary for, the care planning process.

Among the items for the MDS, many help directly in the care planning process. When put together in logical patterns, many variables trigger the threat or existence of a clinical problem, such as pressure ulcers, or behavior problems. In the RAI system, 18 of the most frequent and important problems are identified through their triggers. The clinical protocols, RAPs, help the assessor to get deeper into a problem area, to see what further knowledge is required to be able to plan the care in a more professional way.

USES OF THE RAI INSTRUMENTS

The basis for the development of the RAI in nursing homes in the US was to improve the quality of care for the elderly in nursing homes and other institutional settings. This is done in several ways: the RAI assessment improves the quality of nursing documentation and the staff's knowledge of the resident, recently shown in a Swedish study (Hansebo et al, forthcoming). Since many of the items in the MDS have not earlier been systematically collected in the average nursing home, these new data give an opportunity to discuss quality in a new way, through comparisons either between institutions within the same organization/area or between assessments in the same facility over time. Since the cross-national reliability has been proven, comparisons between nursing homes in different countries are also possible to make, and since they often represent national traditions that are not possible to run as randomized trials in a clinical environment for ethical or other reasons, this could be a start to discussing and learning about better care in such areas as restraint use (Ljunggren et al, 1997), psychotropic drug use, prevention of falls, undernutrition in nursing homes, and so on.

KNOWN EFFECTS OF THE INSTRUMENTS

In the most recent field trials of the MDS in the US, most nurse assessors made positive, reaffirming statements regarding the MDS, although it was also believed to be a paper burden. Items were described as helpful, definitions were seen to be clear, while, for care planning purposes, most clinical assessors have been very positive in assessing the care planning utility of the full set of MDS items (Morris et al, 1997). Similar experiences have been reported from other countries.

In a study, process indicators of quality revealed improvement when using the RAI. As a consequence, it appears that:

- Functional decline was slowed after the implementation of the RAI, particularly for the most impaired
- Clinical outcomes ranging from nutritional status to corrected visual impairment were better post-RAI
- Finally, hospitalization rates dropped by 20%, largely associated with the most cognitively impaired, and there was no change in 6 month mortality (Hawes et al, 1997).

The RAI is problem-focused, emphasizes reducing unnecessary decline, and identifies those residents with multiple problems. At the same time, facilities have implemented the RAI in an environment with relatively stable levels of resources and increasing scrutiny of outcomes by regulators. In the areas of physical functioning, the RAI's emphasis may have interacted with these other factors and caused staff to shift their attention to those residents with the greatest care needs and the highest likelihood of decline, including residents with dementia. When attention is so focused, significant reductions in the rates of functional decline are observed, as are reductions in the rate of decline for cognitive performance and incontinence. This shift may have come at the expense of a smaller number of less functionally impaired residents who could have experienced some measure of improvement, but whose improvement was less pronounced after the MDS came into place and shifted facility priorities to those who were at higher risk of functional decline.

In cognitive performance, understanding, and psychosocial well-being, the pattern of changes is somewhat more complex. One sees less attention to improvement among those least in need (i.e., good ADL and good CPS) and those least likely to benefit (i.e., poor ADL and poor CPS). Efforts at decline reduction in these areas may have been focused on those with the cognitive skills necessary to respond to any cognitive or psychosocial intervention.

Assessment and care planning have long been identified as the critical core of improvements of care, as early as in the report of the Institute of Medicine (1986) that engendered OBRA '87. Even if other changes have been observed in the US nursing homes, parallel to the implementation of the RAI, the latter explanation of the better outcomes and quality of care seems to be the most plausible (Phillips et al, 1997).

SUBSCALES OF THE MDS/RAI

Based on the MDS data, several subscales have been developed. Most of these have been validated against golden or at least best standard available. Among these scales are ADL-scales, a cognitive scale (mimicking the MMSE), a social engagement scale, a depression scale (tested against such scales as the Hamilton and the Cornell scales).

MDS-ADL

In order to be able to promote the highest level of functioning among residents, clinical staff must first identify what the resident actually does for himself or herself, noting when assistance is received and clarifying the types of assistance provided (verbal cueing, physical support, etc.). A resident's ADL self-performance may vary from day to day, shift to shift, or within shifts. There are many possible reasons for these variations, including mood, medical condition, relationship issues (e.g., willing to perform for a nurse assistant he or she likes), and medications. An assessment, therefore, should capture the total picture of the resident's ADL self-performance over a longer period of time, not only how the evaluating clinician sees the resident, but how the resident performs on other shifts as well.

The MDS-ADL Summary Scale derived from MDS items has 10 hierarchical categories. The ADL items fall into 3 categories, based on when loss was first noted: Early Loss (dressing and hygiene), Intermediate Loss (transfer, locomotion, and toileting), and Late Loss (bed mobility, eating).

MDS-CPS

In developing the MDS-based Cognitive Performance Scale (CPS) (Morris et al, 1994), the goal was to identify the best system of hierarchical categories that would describe cognitive functional performances. These categories are defined by MDS items, using rules that maximize within-group similarities (and between group dissimilarities) on two cognitive measures: the Mini-Mental Status Examination (Folstein et al, 1975) and the Test for Severe Impairment (Albert and Cohen, 1992).

Seven separate direct measures of cognitive performance were included in the MDS: short- and long-term memory, memory recall or orientation items (four items: recall of season, location of room, identity of staff, and that the resident is in a nursing home), and a single item assessing the ability of the resident to make decisions about activities that are part of daily life (e.g., choosing clothing, setting the daily schedule, using environmental cues, having awareness of one's own strength). The MDS also includes a number of indirect measures of cognitive performance, including an item indicating comatose status, two measures of communication skills, and eight measures of ADL functional performance.

The CPS system that was derived requires only five MDS variables, and uses these items to create a system that moves progressively from relative independence (Level 0) to extreme cognitive impairment (Level 6). Each level is statistically distinct from the others based on the MMSE and TSI cognitive criteria. The five MDS items used in the model are highly reliable with an average interrater reliability of 0.85. Within the CPS system, there are two categories representing relatively intact residents, two categories that represent mild to moderate impairment, and three categories that reflect severe cognitive impairment.

Social engagement

The MDS items measuring psychosocial well-being move beyond a simple counting of social interactions and activity participation and instead focus on residents' engagement with the social world around them. Social engagement includes an ability to take advantage of opportunities for social interaction, limited as they may be in many facilities. Further, it includes an ability to initiate actions that engage residents in the life of the home.

The MDS measure of social engagement is a positive behavioral dimension that is distinct both from negative behaviors such as conflicted relationships and behavior problems, as well as from negative affective states. All MDS items reflecting social engagement are included in the social engagement index. These items are: (1) at ease interacting with others; (2) at ease doing planned or structured activities; (3) at ease doing self-initiated activities; (4) establishes own goals; (5) pursues involvement in the life of the facility; and (6) accepts invitations into most group activities. When summarized into a single scale, these measures of social engagement incorporated in the MDS have been shown to result in a reliable and valid indicator of nursing home residents' involvement in the social and recreational life of the facility. The internal consistency of the six items in the index suggests that they measure a single construct that is correlated with actual participation in the home across three very different types of residents (Mor et al, 1995).

Depression scale

A number of depression assessment batteries which rely on interviews and self-report assessment techniques have been tested in nursing homes. Unfortunately, given the physical, sensory, and cognitive impairments of many nursing home residents, such interview-based assessments can be difficult to conduct and can systematically exclude the more impaired segments of this population. A clear need exists for a screening tool that incorporates daily observations of residents by licensed care staff using a standardized assessment protocol.

In response to this need, a new MDS, a new observation-based instrument to detect depression among nursing home residents has been created. The instrument is derived from 16 mood and behavioral items in the MDS Version 2.0. All MDS mood items have value ranges from zero to two—where zero indicates that the resident did not exhibit the symptom in the last 30 days, one indicates that the resident exhibited the symptom up to five days a week, and two indicates the occurrence of the symptom six or seven days a week. Direct-care staff are instructed to score each item without regard to cause or environment.

The MDS-based depression scale was constructed and validated by comparison with two commonly used measures of depression: the 19-item Cornell Scale (Alexopoulos et al, 1988) and the 17-item Hamilton Depression Rating Scale (Hamilton, 1967).

The resulting MDS Depression Rating Scale (MDS DRS) has a score range of 0–14, and the Cronbach alpha measure of internal consistency for this summary scale is within the acceptable range with a coefficient of 0.75 (Burrows et al, submitted).

Among other scales that are under development are a scale for nutritional assessment, validated against the Mini Nutrition Assessment, MNA, and a scale for the dental state of a resident, validated against the dentist's chart.

RESOURCE UTILIZATION GROUPS, A HEALTH ECONOMICAL TOOL, BASED ON THE MDS

Of all the subscales built into the MDS, the Resource Utilization Groups (RUGs) are the oldest. The RUGs are based on the same assumptions as the Diagnosis Related Groups (DRGs), namely that certain characteristics reduce the statistical variations in resource use between residents or patients (Cooney and Fries, 1985; Fries and Cooney, 1985). The RUGs grouping algorithm, now in its third version (Fries et al, 1994), reduces the variance in resource consumption through an algorithm, comprised of about 1/4 of the MDS items. It is a hierarchical scale with seven levels, based on clinical data. The highest group, that of rehabilitation, uses at an average more resources than the second highest, and so on. Subgrouping is done according to ADLs, depressive symptoms, and the input of certain services. The RUG system also calculates a case-mix index for an individual. For example, a group of persons with a case-mix index of 1.50 uses 50% more resources than the average, while a group with a CMI of 0.75 uses 25% less resources than the average. If a RUG-III computation is done of a nursing home population, either through a full MDS assessment or through a separate RUG-III assessment, we then have a means of comparing true resource input with the anticipated use and in a second step we could get closer to a more equitable resource allocation. The RUG-III system has been validated in several countries, among which are the US, Japan, Sweden, Spain, and the UK (Carpenter et al, 1997).

RUGs and dementia

The RUG system gives us the possibility of analyzing the resource needs of residents over time, between institutions, and between countries.

Dementia patients, as of course many other groups of frail elderly, who have difficulties in making decisions and being understood, need the attention of other persons. To enable a sufficient amount of staff resources, we need reliable methods to allocate and balance resource input not in subjective ways, but as objectively as possible. Therefore, the RUG-III system would have a large impact on true resource allocation, were it used more widely. A recent comparison of Swedish and US residents in nursing homes revealed a vast difference in staff minutes input, particularly of registered nurses, between these two countries, but also when dichotomized between residents with or without cognitive symptoms, Sweden giving a total of 114 minutes per day to cognitively dysfunctional residents compared to 134 minutes cognitively intact ones. In the US, the same figures were 79, and 117 minutes/day respectively. The resource input for registered nurses in Sweden was 18 minutes to those with cognitive dysfunction and 25 minutes to the cognitively intact. In the US, these figures were 4 and 8 minutes, respectively (Ljunggren, 1997). A comparison of US institutions with or without special dementia units has also shown low absolute amounts of resources to demented persons, compared to other residents, but also that the average resource input in a nursing home with a dementia unit is higher than in a nursing home without (Mehr, 1995). Further studies of the impact of these differences on quality of care, mortality, function in many aspects, and so on, are urgently needed. However, the RUG-III system can easily detect discrepancies between true resource input and case-mix, thus enabling a deeper understanding of the care delivered, particularly with the full MDS assessment done.

CONCLUSION

The RAI family of reliable and clinically relevant assessment instruments offers a continuous part of the person's ongoing record, from the home to different kinds of institutions/care levels. Since dementia changes slowly and therefore many actors are involved for long periods of time, we all need reliable patient data, not only for the pure care of the dementia disease but also to screen for other services needed. We also have to screen for the educational needs of the caring teams to enable a care of good quality. Here also, we could get help from the MDS assessments.

Dementia is growing in prevalence, due to the population changes foreseen, which means that the costs of this population will grow. This calls for more studies on cost-effective resource allocation and for this we need reliable case-mix measures, one of which is the RUGs.

ACKNOWLEDGEMENT

Dr Morris's work on this paper was supported in part by Alzheimer's Association Award #Trg-93-022, Assessment outcomes for community based cognitively impaired elderly.

REFERENCES

Albert, M. and Cohen, C. (1992). The test for severe impairment: an instrument for the assessment of patients with severe cognitive dysfunction, *J. Am. Geriatr. Soc.*, **40**, 449–453.

Alexopoulos, G. S., Abrams, R. C., Young, R. C. and Shamoian, C. C. (1988). Cornell scale for depression in dementia, *Biological Psychiatry*, **23**, 271–284.

Burrows, A. B., Morris, J. N., Simon, S. E., Hirdes, J. P. and Phillips, C. (submitted). Development of a MDS-based depression rating scale for use in nursing homes.

Carpenter, G. I., Ikegami, N., Ljunggren, G. and Fries, B. E. (1997). RUG-III and resource allocation, *Age Ageing*, **26**(Suppl. 2), 61–66.

Cooney, L. M. Jr and Fries, B. E. (1985). Validation and use of resource utilization groups as a case-mix measure for long-term care, *Med. Care*, **23**, 123–132.

Folstein, M. F., Fostein, S. E. and McHugh, P. R. (1975). 'Mini-mental state': a practical method for grading the cognitive state of patients for the clinician, *J. Psychiatr. Res.*, **12**, 189–198.

Fries, B. E. and Cooney, L. M. Jr (1985). Resource utilization groups. A patient classification system for long-term care, *Med. Care*, **23**, 110–122.

Fries, B. E., Schneider, D. P., Foley, W. J. et al (1994). Refining a case-mix measure for nursing homes: Resource Utilization Groups (RUG-III), *Med. Care*, **32**(7), 668–685.

Hamilton, M. (1967). Development of a rating scale for primary depressive illness, *British Journal of Social and Clinical Psychology*, **6**, 278–296.

Hansebo, G., Kihlgren, M., Ljunggren, G. and Winblad, B. (forthcoming). Staff view on the Resident Assessment Instrument, RAI/MDS, in nursing homes, and the use of the Cognitive Performance Scale, CPS, in different levels of care. Accepted for publication.

Hawes, C., Mor, V., Phillips, C., Fries, B. E., Morris, J. N., Steele-Friedlob, E., Greene, A. M. and Nennstiel, M. (1997). The OBRA-87 nursing home regulations and implementation of the Resident Assessment Instrument: effects on process quality, *J. Am. Geriatr. Soc.*, **45**, 977–985.

Institute of Medicine (1986). Improving the quality of nursing homes, Washington, DC, National Academy of Sciences Press.

Ljunggren, G. (1997). Quality and resource use in elderly care in Sweden over time in relation to physical and chemical restraints, in K. Iqbal, B. Winblad, T. Nishimura, M. Takeda, and H. M. Wisniewski (Eds), *Alzheimer's Disease: Biology, Diagnosis and Therapeutics*, Chichester, UK, Wiley.

Ljunggren, G., Phillips, C. and Sgadari, A. (1997). Comparisons of restraints use in nursing homes in eight countries, *Age Ageing*, **26**(Suppl. 2), 43–48.

Mehr, D. R. and Fries, B. E. (1995). Resource use on Alzheimer's special care units, *Gerontologist*, **35**(2), 179–184.

Mor, V., Branco, K., Fleishman, J. et al. (1995). The structure of social engagement among nursing home residents, *J. Gerontol. Psychol. Sci.*, **50B**, P1–8.

Morris, J. N., Fries, B. E., Mehr, D. R. et al (1994). MDS cognitive performance scale, *J. Gerontol. Med. Sci.*, **49**, M174–182.

Morris, J. N., Hawes, C., Fries, B. E. et al. (1990). Designing the national resident assessment instrument for nursing homes, *Gerontologist*, **39**, 293–307.

Morris, J. N., Nonemaker, S., Murphy, K. et al. (1997). A commitment to change: revision of HCFA's RAI, *J. Am. Geriatr. Soc.*, **45**, 1011–1016.

Phillips, C. D., Morris, J. N., Hawes, C., Fries, B. E., Mor, V., Nennstiel, M. and Iannacchione, V. (1997). Association of the resident assessment instrument (RAI) with changes in function, cognition and psychosocial status, *J. Am. Geriatr. Soc.*, **45**, 986–993.

Sgadari, A., DuPasquier, J.-N., Morris, J., Jonsson, P., Mor, V., Ljunggren, G. and Fries, B. E. (1997). Establishing the cross-national reliability of the MDS/RAI, *Age Ageing*, **26**(Suppl. 2), 27–30.

2.10 Costs of Diagnostic Procedures

SERGE GAUTHIER

Centre for Studies in Aging, McGill University, Montreal, Canada

INTRODUCTION

An accurate diagnostic assessment is an essential component to the management of dementia, since this is the time when patients are recognized as carrying a specific disorder which will impact their life as well as their families. Associated conditions such as depression, drug misuse or metabolic abnormalities that exaggerate cognitive impairment must be ruled out or treated. This chapter will study the costs associated with this process and highlight the fact that although the human element, for example physician time, is the most important component, it is the least expensive when compared to laboratory costs for blood tests and structural brain imaging. Adequate training of family practitioners in regard to early recognition and diagnosis of dementia will be the most cost-effective approach, and guidelines must be updated on the use of laboratory aids.

METHODS

Published guidelines (see references 1, 2, 3) and recent review articles (see references 4, 5, 6) on the diagnosis of dementia were reviewed. Opinion leaders in industrialized countries (Australia, Canada, France, Israel, Italy, Japan, Switzerland, Unites States of America) with high prevalence and awareness of dementia were surveyed for costs of diagnostic procedures and opinion as to the relevance of tests for use by family practitioners or specialists. All costs were converted to US dollars for ease of comparison, using currency cross rates of 22 August 1997.

RESULTS

Published guidelines and reviews recommend a number of specific tests, summarized in Table 2.10.1. Notable are the *optional* use of head Computer

Health Economics of Dementia. Edited by Anders Wimo, Bengt Jönsson, Göran Karlsson and Bengt Winblad.
© 1998 John Wiley & Sons Ltd.

Table 2.10.1. Recommended laboratory tests for patients suspected of dementia

	ref 1 1991	ref 4 1994	ref 2 1994	ref 5 1995	ref 6 1996
CBC	all	all	all	all	all
Sed rate				all	
TSH	all	all	all	all	all
T4			all		all
Electrolytes	all	all	all	all	all
BUN		all	all	all	all
Creatinine		all	all	all	all
Calcium	all	all	all	all	all
Glycemia	all	all	all		all
ALT			all	all	all
B12		all	all	all	all
Folate		all			
Syphilis serology		all	all	all	all
HIV screen				all	opt
CT head	opt*	all	opt	all	all
MRI brain		opt	opt	opt	opt
SPECT			opt	opt	
PET			opt	opt	
EEG		opt	opt	opt	opt

all: all patients
opt: optional
opt*: optional with specific guidelines

Scanning (CT) in guidelines 1 and 2, whereas emphasis is clearly placed on focused history, physical and mental status examination by primary care practitioners in guideline 3.

The cost of these individual tests was ascertained and is listed in Table 2.10.2 for blood tests and Table 2.10.3 for brain imaging procedures. Costs do not differ greatly for blood tests between the US and other countries, but they do for brain imaging and mean costs have been calculated for non-US versus all countries combined.

The total costs for blood tests based on reference 1 is $61.09, reference 4 is $140.27, reference 2 $143.66, reference 5 is $144.19 and reference 6 $143.66. There is thus a two-fold difference in costs if a more selective approach is used for selection of blood tests based on individual clinical observations (reference 1) rather than a broader screening procedure for haematologic, hormonal, metabolic or infections abnormalities (references 2, 4, 5, 6).

MRI brain imaging technology is twice the cost of uninfused CT and guidelines are needed for its use. SPECT and PET technologies were recognized as experimental or of exceptional use by specialists only. The cost of blood apoE screening was estimated at $65, but its widespread use is not recommended. Detailed neuropsychological assessment cost $2500 in USA and

Table 2.10.2. Cost of blood tests for patients suspected of dementia ($US)

	Aus	Can	Fra	Isr	Ita	Jap	Swi	USA	Mean non-US	Mean all
CBC	10.84	3.60	29.36	21.00	3.95	2.53	26.67	17.50	*14.00*	*14.43*
Sed rate	4.85	1.80	2.94	–	1.97	1.01	4.00	14.75	*2.76*	*4.47*
TSH	19.24	4.32	20.55	27.00	8.51	17.74	20.00	68.75	*16.77*	*23.26*
T4	25.79	4.32	20.55	27.00	9.92	17.74	20.00	12.50	*17.90*	*17.23*
Electrolytes	6.03	4.32	5.87	11.75	4.06	4.56	26.67	17.50	*9.04*	*10.10*
BUN	6.03	1.08	22.02	11.75	1.35	1.52	13.33	15.75	*8.15*	*9.10*
Creatinine	6.03	1.08	8.81	11.75	1.35	1.52	6.67	15.75	*5.31*	*6.62*
Calcium	6.03	1.08	4.40	11.75	1.35	1.52	6.67	26.50	*4.68*	*7.41*
Glycemia	6.03	1.08	2.94	11.75	1.41	1.52	6.67	15.75	*4.49*	*5.89*
ALT	6.03	1.08	5.87	11.75	2.71	2.70	6.67	15.75	*5.26*	*6.57*
B12	15.32	5.76	20.55	24.00	11.39	27.88	15.00	60.75	*17.13*	*22.58*
Folate	15.32	5.76	20.55	24.00	9.92	28.73	15.00	44.00	*17.04*	*20.41*
Syphilis serology	21.83	6.47	5.87	30.00	12.40	5.02	66.67	15.50	*21.18*	*20.47*
HIV screen	7.03	8.63	20.55	21.00	9.58	12.15	55.33	27.00	*19.18*	*20.16*

Aus: Australia   Ita: Italy   Swi: Switzerland
Can: Canada   Isr: Israel   USA: United States of America
Fra: France   Jap: Japan

Table 2.10.3. Cost of brain imaging for patients suspected of dementia ($US)

	Aus	Can	Fra	Isr	Ita	Jap	Swi	USA	Mean non-US	Mean all
CT head no infusion	122	108	147	270	169	68	307	813	*170*	*250*
CT head with infusion	159	108	196	270	197	114	437	1328	*212*	*351*
MRI brain no enhancement	296	306	406	600	338	168	578	1370	*385*	*508*
SPECT	341	226	251	120	260	253	–	1380	*242*	*404*
PET	–	1080	1142	–	1026	–	–	–	*1083*	*1083*

Aus: Australia   Ita: Italy   Swi: Switzerland
Can: Canada   Isr: Israel   USA: United States of America
Fra: France   Jap: Japan

an average of $215 elsewhere. Routine EEG was $335 in USA and an average of $68 elsewhere. Neither of these procedures was recommended for universal use.

The mean cost of blood tests is $127. Head CT scanning adds $250, for a total cost of $377 for the laboratory aids to the diagnosis of dementia.

Costs of visits to family practitioners averaged $45, and those to specialists $90 (mean cost of geriatrician, neurologist and psychiatrist). Since at least two visits are required to the family practitioner, the human element of the diagnosis of dementia costs only $90, to which a consultation may be added in certain cases, for a total of $180. Suggestions were made in guideline 1 as to which patients to refer for consultation.

DISCUSSION

Considering the accelerated aging of our societies and the high prevalence of dementia over age 85, screening for and assessing a large number of individuals for dementia could have a high economic impact. Fortunately, there is now a clear emphasis on focused history, physical and mental status examination by primary care practitioners as the main diagnostic approach (reference 3). Clear guidelines usable by these clinicians are needed in regard to which laboratory tests are needed for all patients suspected of early dementia, who needs uninfused head CT scanning, and who needs to be referred to a consulting specialist.

New issues are being added to the initial diagnostic process such as when to initiate specific treatments for Alzheimer's disease (with cholinesterase inhibitors for instance) and what to do with non-responders, a phenomenon encountered in Parkinson's disease where non-responders to levodopa are usually referred for diagnostic reconsideration. This early treatment phase may thus have to be considered as part of the process and costs of diagnosis of dementia.

The costs used for this study may not be representative of costs in all laboratories within a given country, and there is great variability in patterns or reimbursement for patients. On the other hand the emerging pattern in the diagnosis of dementia is that investment in medical education is the most cost-effective approach, with selective use of laboratory tests based on individualized assessments. Changes may be required in physician reimbursement plans to take into account the time and skill required by the primary care practitioner to take a focused history and perform the required physical and mental status assessments, essential components to the diagnosis of dementia.

CONCLUSION

This attempt at defining the costs of diagnosis of dementia in different countries showed that two-fold differences exist between tests recommended for all patients in some guidelines versus others, and that MRI scanning is twice the cost of CT. There is clearly a need for new consensus guidelines for the primary care practitioner, the health care professional most involved in the diagnosis of dementia.

ACKNOWLEDGEMENTS

The author thanks Drs L. Amaducci, L. Bracco, H. Brodaty, J. Corey-Bloom, F. Forette, A. Homma, A. Korczyn, M. Rossor, and A. von Gunten for their help in collecting the data on costs of diagnostic procedures in their countries.

REFERENCES

1. Organizing Committee, Canadian Consensus Conference on the Assessment of Dementia (1991). Assessing dementia: the Canadian consensus, *Can. Med. Assoc. J.*, **144**, 851.
2. Report of the Quality Standards Subcommittee of the American Academy of Neurology (1994). Practice parameter for diagnosis and evaluation of dementia, *Neurology*, **44**, 2203.
3. US Department of Health and Human Services (1996). *Clinical Practice Guideline, Recognition and Initial Assessment of Alzheimer's Disease and Related Dementias*, Silver Spring, MD: Agency for Health Care Policy and Research Publications.
4. Rossor, M. N. (1994). Management of neurological disorders: dementia, *J. Neurol. Neurosurg. Psychiatry*, **57**, 1451.
5. Corey-Bloom, J., Thal, L. J., Galasko, D. et al (1995). Diagnosis and evaluation of dementia, *Neurology*, **45**, 211.
6. Geldmacher, D. S. and Whitehouse P. (1996). Evaluation of dementia, *N. Engl. J. Med.*, **335**, 330.

2.11 How Will Japan Cope with the Impending Surge of Dementia?

YUMIKO ARAI

National Institute for Longevity Sciences (NILS), Gengo, Obu-shi, Aichi, Japan

NAOKI IKEGAMI

School of Medicine, Keio University, Tokyo, Japan

INTRODUCTION

For patients with dementia, a new era is likely to begin in Japan. Whereas formerly they relied largely on family caregivers and discretionary assistance, from the year 2000, they will have entitlements in the proposed public long-term care insurance, under which ultimate responsibilities will rest with the state (Arai, 1997; Ikegami, 1997). How did this change come about? The underlying factor was the ageing of the population. In 1950, the estimated life expectancy at birth was 50 years in males and 53.9 years in females respectively. In 1994, it had increased up to 76.6 years in males and 83.0 years in females respectively, which are the longest life expectancies in the world (MHW, 1996a). In 1960, the proportion of the aged 65 and over accounted for 6% of the total population in Japan and doubled in 1990, that is 12%; this figure is estimated to double again to 25% by the year 2020 (MHW, 1996a). As shown in Figure 2.11.1, Japan is the most rapidly ageing society in the world (MHW, 1995a).

These demographic trends have resulted in a concomitant increase in the number of the demented elderly. Previous epidemiological studies in Japan have shown that the prevalence of dementia among the aged 65 years or older is 4–6% (MHW, 1995b); the prevalence in the aged 80–84 is shown to be 9–14% and it dramatically increased up to 20–25% in the aged 85 years or older. Given the fact that the elderly population itself is ageing (MHW, 1995a), the number of the demented elderly has been constantly increasing in Japan. For example, the number of the demented elderly in 1991 was 1 million and the number is projected to exceed 3 million in 2025 (MHW, 1995b). This will account for 10% of the elderly population in total.

Health Economics of Dementia. Edited by Anders Wimo, Bengt Jönsson, Göran Karlsson and Bengt Winblad.
© 1998 John Wiley & Sons Ltd.

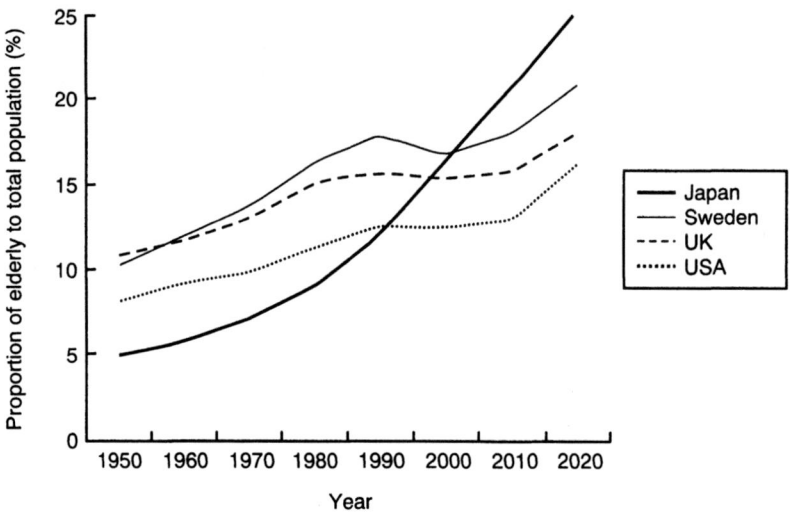

Figure 2.11.1. Actual and projected proportion of the elderly to the total population. *Source*: Institute of Population Problems, Japanese MHW (1995a)

HOME CARE

THE PRESSURE TO PROVIDE INFORMAL CARE

Most of the demented elderly in Japan reside in the community as they do in other developed countries (OECD, 1996). In Japan, it has been reported that 75% of the demented elderly are looked after by their family members whilst the remaining 25% are institutionalized (MHW, 1995b). What makes informal care in Japan unique is two-fold. Firstly, there has been a tremendous social pressure for the family to provide care, particularly by female kinship. This is partly due to Confucianism, in which the virtue of filial piety has been strongly stressed. Secondly, a caregiving role used to be a legal obligation for the eldest son of the family. Before World War II, the Japanese civil law stipulated that the eldest son inherited the assets of the family (Kawabata, 1995); in turn, all the practical responsibility of caring for the parents was placed upon the wife of the eldest son, that is the daughter-in-law.

The government has 'taken advantage of' such a Confucian-influenced norm, which has continued to be influential in Japanese society even after World War II. Indeed, the Prime Minister of Japan in 1979 eloquently proclaimed the establishment of the 'Japanese style welfare', in which self-help, tolerance, and the solidarity of family were emphasized (Campbell, 1992). The government even stressed that the 'European style welfare state' might discourage the prevailing notion of caregiving as a family duty (Kawabata, 1995).

Under these circumstances, it was not surprising that the government was reluctant to provide social services. The development of domiciliary care in Japan has lagged far behind that of the UK or Scandinavian countries. For example, as of 1993, the proportion of elderly people receiving home help accounted for 2% in Japan compared with 13% in the UK and Sweden, and 4% in the US (OECD, 1996).

Moreover, the over-emphasis on family values and self-help at the policy level has enhanced the stigmatization of social services in Japan (Kawabata, 1995). Indeed, there has been a persistent notion that welfare is for those who have slipped out of a 'normal' social network where self-help and/or informal help can be provided. In turn, social services have been targeting their clientele to those who lack social support and have low incomes. For example, it was reported that more than half of those who entered Special Homes for the Aged (SHAs), which is a welfare facility most similar to the nursing home, had less than 400 000 yen (2963 US dollars with 1 dollar equivalent to 135 yen using the 1991 exchange rate) annual income in 1991 (Nogami, 1996); the average annual income per person over 65 years or older was reported to be 1 792 000 yen (13 274 US dollars) in 1992 (MHW, 1994a).

The notion that such services are being provided as a charity, instead of being purchased or offered as a right, has made it difficult to improve the quality. All services are provided by administrative orders after means testing. Payments are made to a municipal welfare office, not to the service agency. Moreover, users are not allowed to choose a specific facility or home help. These conditions may have intimidated the potential users of welfare services, leading to a vicious cycle of stigmatization of social services and little incentive to improve quality. Such stigma attached to the using of social services has limited their accessibility. That is to say, the way in which means tests were conducted has been cumbersome and humiliating (Okamoto, 1996), which has deterred people from even approaching the municipal Social Welfare Office.

THE DEMOGRAPHIC AND SOCIOECONOMIC CHANGES MAKING THE 'JAPANESE STYLE WELFARE STATE' DIFFICULT

The lack of social services for the elderly was not perceived as a major problem until the 1970s. However, due to a rapid increase in the number of the elderly in need, together with changes in the family structure, a paucity of appropriate social services started to draw public attention (Kawabata, 1995; Okamoto, 1996).

Despite this resulting increase in the demand for care, as the nuclear family became the norm, the capacity to provide informal care, on which 'the Japanese style welfare' heavily depended, decreased. As shown in Table 2.11.1, the number of three-generation households, which used to compose 54% of the households of those who are 65 years or older in 1975, decreased dramatically

Table 2.11.1. Changes in household structure

	1955	1992	2000[a]
Number of three-generation households	8 320 000	5 390 000	–
Number of nuclear families	8 600 000	24 320 000	27 950 000
Number of households comprised of a single person	2 040 000	8 970 000	12 180 000
Number of households comprised of a single elderly	260 000	2 250 000	2 910 000
Average number of members per household	4.97	2.99	2.72
Total number of households	18 900 000	41 210 000	46 150 000

[a] The figures in 2000 are projected numbers.

Source: Ministry of Health and Welfare (1994a).

to 35% in 1994. At the same time, the average number of members per household nearly halved (MHW, 1994b). These tendencies are expected to intensify in the year 2000. Already, in some rural areas, the proportion of the elderly over 65 years or older compose over a quarter of the population while that of the elderly living alone or by themselves constitutes a majority.

At the same time, as shown in Figure 2.11.2, the percentage of the elderly who are residing with their children has been continuously decreasing, albeit it is still much higher compared with those of the US or UK (Gerdet, 1995; Ichien, 1996). This implies that the capacity of informal care has been constantly decreasing in Japan.

An increase in the number of the demented elderly and a concomitant decrease in the capacity of informal care have made 'caregivers' burden' a social issue. With increased longevity, many of the daughters-in-law are now in their sixties (MHW, 1994b), some of them requiring care themselves. Yet, because of the above described cultural norms, daughters-in-law and spouses are being forced to take on the burden with little formal or informal support. In such a situation, the informal caregivers are highly distressed (MHW, 1991; Arai et al, 1997). The media have periodically reported stories of exhausted caregivers killing the elderly as well as themselves. A survey conducted in 1994 revealed that a third of caregivers of the frail elderly experienced feelings of hatred towards the elderly (MHW, 1996b).

INSTITUTIONALIZED CARE

AN INADEQUATE SYSTEM FOR TRIAGING THE CARE OF THE DEMENTED ELDERLY

Table 2.11.2 shows the estimated number of the institutionalized demented elderly, obtained from an epidemiological survey conducted by the Ministry of

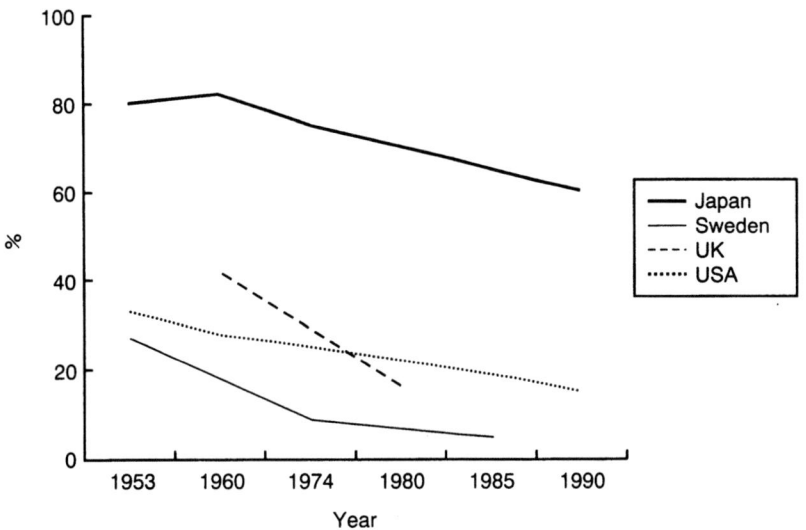

Figure 2.11.2. The percentage of the elderly residing with their children. *Source*: OECD
(1995); Ichien (1996)

Table 2.11.2. Number of institutionalized demented elderly in Japan (1991)

Types of institutions	Number of demented elderly (%)	
General hospitals	60 000	(23.5)
Geriatric hospitals	54 000	(21.2)
Psychiatric hospitals	33 000	(13.0)
Health Facilities for the Elderly (HFEs)	12 000	(4.7)
Subtotal: Health sector	159 000	(62.4)
Special Homes for the Aged (SHAs)	83 000	(32.5)
Homes for the aged	13 000	(5.1)
Subtotal: Welfare sector	96 000	(37.6)
Total	255 000	(100)

Source: Ministry of Health and Welfare (1995b).

Health and Welfare in 1991 (MHW, 1995b). As can be seen from the table,
institutionalized care for the demented elderly has been provided by various
types of facilities both in the health care sector and the welfare sector (MHW,
1995b). In addition to those shown in the table, 4653 demented elderly are
estimated to be hospitalized in 'clinics' (inpatients' facilities with less than 20
beds), based on the prevalence rate in hospitals.

Ideally, the severely demented elderly should have been placed in psychiatric
hospitals, with the less severely demented elderly in welfare facilities. However,
very severe demented cases are often placed in SHAs, which do not have full-

time medical doctors or nurses as they are welfare facilities. Moreover, a lack of clear guidelines as to who should be admitted to each facility has resulted in arbitrary admissions and/or often adverse selections.

For example, Health Facilities for the Elderly (HFEs) were originally developed as intermediate care facilities, where patients can receive approximately 3-month rehabilitation, prior to returning to the community. However, two-fifths of the clients stay in HFEs more than 3 months and about a quarter stay more than 6 months (MHW, 1995c). This indicates that HFEs are not functioning as intermediate care facilities but as LTC facilities. Moreover, a cross-sectional survey has revealed that HFEs tend to have a higher ratio of those requiring relatively little care when compared to hospitals and SHAs (Ikegami et al, 1994).

Moreover, while many hospitals provide long-term care (LTC), and in fact, a good number are *de facto* nursing homes, very few function as assessment units. The national hospital patient survey shows that 46% of the hospital inpatient population is over 65 years or older, and one-third of them have been hospitalized for more than a year (Ikegami et al, 1995). A major problem with hospitals providing LTC care is that, under the fee-for-service payment scheme in the Japanese health care system, the use of drugs and ordering of laboratory tests for LTC patients has led to cost escalation and inappropriate care (Ikegami et al, 1995; Arai et al, 1998). To control this, the government introduced a new scheme in 1990, whereby hospitals with a high proportion of geriatric patients, which meet the prescribed standards of staffing, are allowed to opt out to a new payment scheme with an inclusive *per diem* rate. In 1994, 840 of a total of 1613 hospitals took out this option. However, the introduction of a *per diem* payments scheme, which is not adjusted for case-mix, has led to adverse selection in hospitals (Ikegami et al, 1994).

Another major problem with hospitals providing LTC is that admissions are being made for social reasons, that is 'shakaiteki nyuinn'. This has resulted from the following factors. First, the lack of SHAs has led to long waiting lists, exceeding 2–3 years in Tokyo and large metropolitan areas, which has made it much easier for people to have their relatives admitted to hospitals or HFEs. Second, as already noted, the admission to SHAs involves a cumbersome procedure. Third, families meet less social disapproval in admitting their relatives to health facilities compared to welfare facilities, to which stigma is still attached (Okamoto, 1992). Fourth, there is a financial reason because hospital care is reimbursed through open-ended health insurance compared with the welfare facilities which are financed by the general expenditure budget (Kobayashi, 1993). Fifth, under the inclusive *per diem* payment scheme, admitting 'light care' patients for 'social reasons' could provide a steady source of revenue to hospitals. These factors have led to decisions often being made by 'social' needs rather than 'medical needs', resulting in inappropriate placements. These inappropriate placements can lead to a drain of limited resources (Jackson et al, 1992; Ikegami et al, 1997)

DESIGNATED CARE UNITS FOR THE DEMENTED ELDERLY

To meet the public demand for more appropriate care of the demented elderly, the government responded by establishing specialized care units in 1989 (MHW, 1995b, d). Favourable reimbursement schemes were introduced for geriatric/psychiatric hospitals if they established either (1) a designated treatment unit for the demented elderly; or (2) a designated rehabilitation unit for the demented elderly. The former was designed as a treatment unit for the most severe cases with highly dangerous behavioural disturbances, whose condition is too severe to be treated anywhere else. The latter was designated for the demented elderly who have persistent behavioural problems and require a long period of institutionalized care. Both are required to be staffed by those having necessary expertise for caring for the demented elderly and to provide a relatively large space (6 m^2) for each patient. In addition, MHW made similar arrangements for a designated unit for the demented elderly in HFEs.

However, the following two problems have arisen. First, the number of such designated units is relatively small and geographically unevenly distributed. In 1994, there were only 44 designated treatment units for the demented elderly (2199 beds), 6 designated rehabilitation units for the demented elderly (267 beds) and 59 designated units for the demented elderly in Health Facilities for the Elderly (2540 beds) (MHW, 1995b). These numbers have been far less than the number of the demented elderly who would have required such specialized services. Second, there have been no criteria as to who should be admitted to these designated units. A lack of such criteria has often resulted in inappropriate placements of the elderly.

CHALLENGES

The following are the challenges which Japan faces: (1) rapid ageing of the society; (2) lack of resources for providing long-term care (LTC); (3) lack of any system for targeting limited resources to the demented elderly.

Regarding the first factor, rapid ageing of the society can be regarded as an inevitable result of 'desirable' socioeconomic improvements; therefore, the ageing of the society is a process which cannot be avoided.

To respond to the second challenge, the Japanese government launched a ten-year strategy, 'the Gold Plan', aimed at providing necessary LTC infrastructure, such as home helpers, respite care beds, day services centres, SHAs, HFEs, and visiting nurse stations (MHW, 1992). For example, the number of home helpers was to be increased from 31 405 to 100 000 by the year 2000, the number of respite beds from 4274 to 50 000 and the number of day care centres from 1080 to 10 000. By 1994, the number of home helpers accounted for 59 005, the number of respite beds (24 274) had reached six times as many within the 5 years and the number of day centres (5180) had become five times as many as that of 1989 (OECD, 1996). Initial targets were generally met by 1994. Re-estimation of the needs of the elderly led the government to revise the targets of the schedule in 1995, thereby relaunching the Gold Plan as the 'New Gold Plan' (MHW, 1996c).

In addition, a new public LTC insurance scheme for long-term care ('Kaigo Hoken') was legislated in November 1997, and will be fully implemented from the year 2000 (MHW, 1997). This new LTC insurance, financed by tax revenue and premiums, will pay for institutional and home-based long-term care for those who are 65 years or older, requiring care, and for those over 40 years old suffering from 'age-related' disease. One of the unique aspects of this new LTC lies in the fact that the extent of informal care available to the clients will not be taken into account when the eligibility is determined (Arai, 1997; Ikegami, 1997; MHW, 1997); thus the extent to which formal services will be provided to the clients will be judged purely by their degree of impairment, regardless of available informal care. This is epoch-making in the history of social policy in Japan: the taken-for-granted notion of family caregivers being relied upon as resources for LTC care will be replaced by the social norms set by Nordic countries, which places ultimate responsibilities on the states rather than the caregivers.

However, the requisite for the new system to function is a cadre of health and social service professionals who will assess the eligibility level and determine the care plans. The problem lies in the fact that the education and training of such skills has been long disregarded for doctors and other professionals in Japan (Orimo, 1998). Geriatrics has not been established as a 'proper' discipline in the field of medical science. Of all the 80 medical schools in Japan, only 10 have a geriatric department (Chugai Seiyaku, 1997). Moreover, very few of these geriatric departments serve as geriatric assessment units or focus their research on clinical aspects. Indeed, most of these departments are devoted to biomedical aspects of the ageing process, such as ageing and lipid metabolism. Thus, the responsibility for integrating social and medical care in geriatric care is virtually neglected in geriatric medicine in Japan. Not only geriatrics, but also 'psychogeriatrics' is not properly recognized as a specialty (Arai, 1996). Although all 80 of the medical schools have a department of psychiatry, only 12 of them have declared psychogeriatrics as 'one of their research interests' (Chugai Seiyaku, 1997). Even in these cases, it is biomedical aspects such as the molecular biology of Alzheimer's disease which is stressed.

In the field of nursing, although both geriatric nursing and home care nursing have become compulsory subjects in nursing colleges, the extent to which this has led to real changes remains questionable. Likewise, in the field of social work, it was not until 1987 that social workers became certificated. Up to 1996, 7334 social workers had been registered (MHW, 1996d). Given the number of the clients, the number of qualified social workers is far fewer than needed. Thus, the third challenge facing Japan, that of developing the human resources which can appropriately target the limited resources to the demented elderly, appears to be the most formidable.

CONCLUSIONS

There has been a tremendous increase in the number of demented elderly in Japan. The problems arising from the demographic changes of the rapidly ageing society have been compounded by decreases in the family caring capacity and the fragmented delivery system which has over-emphasized hospital care. The government has revised its former policy of relying on the family for providing LTC and has committed itself to building an infrastructure for a formal care system. These developments would be greatly enhanced if the public LTC insurance is implemented as planned in the year 2000. However, refocusing the training of health and social service professionals to LTC will be essential if Japan wishes to make cost-effective use of its resources.

ACKNOWLEDGEMENTS

The authors would like to thank Dr Robin Fox and Dr Una Maclean for their valuable comments on earlier drafts of this chapter.

REFERENCES

Arai, Y. (1996). Prevalence of dementia in Japan (letter), *Soc. Sci. Med.*, **43**, 1343.

Arai, Y. (1997). Insurance for long-term care planned in Japan, *Lancet*, **350**, 1831.

Arai, Y. and Ikegami, N. (1998). Health care systems in transition: an overview of Japanese health care systems, *J. Public Health Medicine*, **20**(1), 29–33.

Arai, Y., Kudo, K., Hosokawa, T. et al (1997). Reliability and validity of the Japanese version of Zarit Caregiver Burden Interview, *Psychiatry & Clinical Neuroscience*, **51**(5), 281–287.

Campbell, J. (1992). *How Policies Change: the Japanese Government and the Aging Society*, Princeton, NJ, Princeton University Press.

Chugai seiyaku plc (1997). Directory of Researchers in Medical Schools in Japan (Iiku kikann meibo) (in Japanese), Tokyo, Chugai pharmaceutical plc.

Gerdet, S. (1995). Care by families: an overview of trends, in OECD (Eds), *Caring for Frail Elderly*, Paris, OECD.

Ichien, M. (1996). The latest trends of welfare for the elderly: a global perspective (Koureisha fukushi no sekaitekina nagare) (in Japanese), *Popular Medicine*, special issue (25 May), 36–43.

Ikegami, N. (1997). The impending introduction of a public long-term care insurance in Japan and its implication for health care, *JAMA*, **276**, 16, 1310–1314.

Ikegami, N. and Campbell, J. C. (1995). Medical care in Japan, *N. Eng. J. Med.*, **333**(19), 1295–1299.

Ikegami, N., Fries, B. E., Takagi, Y., Ikeda, S. and Ibe, T. (1994). Applying RUG-III in Japanese long-term health care, *Gerontologist*, **34**, 628–639.

Ikegami, N. and Morris, J. N. (1997). Low care cases in Long-Term Care settings: variation among nations, *Age and Ageing*, **26-SZ**, 67–71.

Jackson, M. E., Eichorn, A. and Blackman, D. (1992). Efficacy of nursing home preadmission screening, *Gerontologist*, **32**(32), 51–57.

Kawabata, O. and Association of Welfare and Culture (1995). Lifestyle of the elderly in Japan: a chronological review (Koureisha seikatsu nennpyo) (in Japanese), Tokyo, Japan Editors School.

Kobayashi, Y. R. (1993). Health care financing for the elderly in Japan, *Soc. Sci. Med.*, **37**(3), 343–353.

MHW (1991). Caring for the demented elderly (chihosei roujin soudan manual) (in Japanese), Tokyo, Health and Welfare Statistics Association.

MHW (1992). *Ten-Year Strategy to Promote Health Care and Welfare for the Aged* (Gold Plan), Tokyo MHW.

MHW (1994a). *Graphical Review of Japanese Households: From a Comprehensive 1992 Survey of Living Conditions of the People on Health and Welfare* (Japanese with English abstracts), Tokyo, Health and Welfare Statistics Association.

MHW (1994b). Welfare in the 21st Century (21 seiki fukushi vision) (in Japanese), Tokyo, Daiichihoki.

MHW (1995a). The latest trends of population: Japan and world (jinko no doko: Nihonn to Sekai) (in Japanese), Tokyo, Health and Welfare Statistics Association.

MHW (1995b). Policy guidelines for care of the demented elderly (Chiho rojin taisaku suishin no konngo no houkou) (in Japanese), Tokyo, Chuo hoki shuppann, Tokyo.

MHW (1995c). A profile of health facilities for the elderly (HFEs) (Rojinhokennshisetsu jittai tyosa, Rojinhokennshisetsu houkoku) (in Japanese), Tokyo, Health and Welfare Statistics Association.

MHW (1995d). *Care for the Demented Elderly* (Wagakuni no chiho shikkan taisaku no gennjo to tenbou) (in Japanese), Tokyo, Chuo hoki shuppann.

MHW (Ministry of Health and Welfare) (1996a). The latest trends of vital statistics in Japan (Saikinn no jinnko dotai) (in Japanese), Tokyo, Health and Welfare Statistics Association.

MHW (1996b). White paper on welfare (Kousei hakusho) (in Japanese), Tokyo, Gyosei.

MHW (1996c). *New Gold Plan*, Tokyo, MHW.

MHW (1996d). Trends in welfare (Kokuminn Fukushi no doko) (in Japanese), Tokyo, Health and Welfare Statistics Association.

MHW (1997). White paper on welfare (Kousei Hakusho) (in Japanese), Tokyo, Gyosei.

Nogami, T. (1996). The limitations of welfare provided by administrative orders (Kouteki fukushi service to sochiseido no gennkai) (in Japanese), *Popular Medicine*, special issue (25 May), 72–78.

OECD (1996). Caring for frail elderly people: policies in evolution, Paris, OECD.

Okamoto, Y. (1992). Health care for the elderly in Japan: medicine and welfare in an aging society facing a crisis in long term care, *BMJ*, **305**, 403–405.

Okamoto, Y. (1996). Health and social services for the elderly (Koreika iryo to fukushi) (in Japanese), Tokyo, Iwanami shoten.

Orimo, H. (1998). Training of physicians for long-term care, *Keio J. Med.*, Suppl. 2, A36–A37.

2.12 Drug Costs in Dementia Care

JOHAN FASTBOM and MARIA STELLA T. GIRON

Karolinska Institute, Stockholm, Sweden

INTRODUCTION

Elderly people generally use many drugs, and for several drug groups the use increases further at higher ages (Andersson, 1989; Landahl, 1987; Lindberg et al, 1994). One of the most common drug groups is the psychotropics (Andersson, 1989; Landahl, 1987; Lindberg et al, 1994; Skoog et al, 1993). These are mainly used to treat behavioural symptoms and sleep disturbances (see Taft and Barkin, 1990). However, psychotropic drugs are also prescribed to the elderly for more specific disorders such as depression and dementia.

A few studies have examined drug use in the demented elderly. Although they generally show a lower overall use of drugs compared to the non-demented elderly, they all report a high use of psychotropic drugs (Semla et al, 1995; Taft and Barkin, 1990; Wills et al, 1997; Wolf-Klein et al, 1988). In the light of the increasing number of elderly with dementia in our society, it would be of interest to examine not only the use of drugs but also the drug costs for the demented elderly. There are very few reports about this, and they provide only estimates of the overall cost of drugs (Hay and Ernst, 1987; Huang et al, 1988; Rice et al, 1993, see Wimo et al, 1997b). In these studies drug costs were reported to account for 1–2% of the total direct cost of dementia. This is a small figure, considering the cost of, for example, social service or nursing home care. However, the estimates are based on studies made in the 1980s, and since then a number of new and fairly expensive drugs have been introduced in geriatric care, for example the selective serotonin reuptake inhibitors (SSRI), and the acetylcholine esterase inhibitors used for symptomatic treatment of dementia. Moreover, even though the cost of drugs may be small for society, the economic burden for the individual can be substantial.

In the present study we describe in more detail the costs of different types of drugs in the demented elderly. This was made possible by the use of detailed drug use data from the Kungsholmen Project, an ongoing longitudinal study of ageing, with the emphasis on dementia, in Stockholm, Sweden. Information about drug use and dosage in 224 demented and 457 non-demented elderly aged 80 and older was run together with a computerised drug register supplied

Health Economics of Dementia. Edited by Anders Wimo, Bengt Jönsson, Göran Karlsson and Bengt Winblad.
© 1998 John Wiley & Sons Ltd.

by the National Corporation of Swedish Pharmacies. In the paper we compare the cost of different drug groups in demented and non-demented elderly. In addition, since the level of care has been shown to influence drug use in the elderly, we examine the drug costs for the demented elderly in different types of accommodation, ranging from their own home to institutional care.

MATERIALS AND METHODS

The Kungsholmen Project has been described in detail already (Fratiglioni et al, 1991, 1992, 1997). Briefly, on 1 October 1987 all inhabitants born in 1912 or earlier, registered in the district of Kungsholmen, were invited to participate in the project. Out of the total population of 2368 persons, 1810 (76%) entered the study. Drop-outs were due to death (181), moving out of the district (86) and refusal to participate (291). The drop-outs due to death were older and more often men than the subjects in the studied population. The other drop-outs did not differ from those participating with respect to age and gender. At the start, the mean age of the participants was 81.7 years, ranging from 75 to 101 years. Females accounted for 76% of the population.

The baseline data collection (Phase I) was performed between 1987 and 1989. The elderly were interviewed by one or two nurses who administered a questionnaire including health and social questions. The interview also included questions about current drug use. In this phase the nurses performed a Mini-Mental State Examination (MMSE) in order to screen for possible dementia cases. The dementia diagnoses were subsequently made in a second phase (Phase II) where all the subjects that were screened positive in the MMSE (score $\leq$ 23) together with a random sample matched by age and gender of those screened negative, underwent an additional examination including personal and family interviews performed by a nurse, an extensive clinical examination by a physician, routine laboratory tests, and a neuropsychological test battery. The dementia diagnosis was made using DSM-III-R (American Psychiatric Association, 1987). The diagnostic procedure consisted of the following. A preliminary diagnosis was made after a discussion among the physicians who had examined the persons and the nurses who had performed the social and family interviews, using data from both clinical examination, informants' interviews and available medical records. Then a second preliminary diagnosis for all the subjects was made independently by a specialised clinician who had not participated in the data collection. In the event of agreement, this was the final diagnosis. If there was a disagreement a final diagnosis was made by a senior colleague. Cases fulfilling all the DSM-III-R criteria were diagnosed as having 'definite dementia'. Those who failed to fulfil one of the DSM-III-R criteria for dementia were diagnosed as having 'questionable dementia'. In Phase II, 225 individuals were diagnosed as having dementia, either definite or questionable.

The first follow-up (Phase III) was made 1990–1992. The subjects were interviewed and clinically examined and dementia was diagnosed using the same procedure as in Phase II. Among the 1099 subjects participating in this phase 307 were diagnosed as demented (definite or questionable dementia).

In the present study we have used data from the second follow-up (Phase IV), which was made between 1994 and 1996. The total number of subjects participating in this phase amounted to 683. The interview, clinical examination and dementia diagnosis were made using the same procedure as in Phases II and III. In addition, a detailed interview about drug use was made, using the same protocol as in Phase I.

The dementia diagnosis used in the present study is preliminary, in the sense that it is based only on the second preliminary diagnosis (see description of the diagnostic procedure above). For the sake of simplicity, however, the elderly who got the preliminary diagnosis dementia (226) will be referred to in this paper as demented while those who did not get the diagnosis (457) will be labelled non-demented.

In Phase IV the information about drug use was collected from an interview conducted by a physician. In the majority of cases the interview took place with the subject personally. However, in cases when it was not possible to conduct a full interview with the elderly person, information was obtained from relatives and/or health care personnel. The data concerning medications were based primarily on the subjects' recall. As a guidance all actual prescriptions and medicine packages were collected and discussed. In cases when interviews were carried out with elderly persons in institutions, where medications were administered by health care personnel, the information was based on information from nurses and medical records. All medications that were used at the time of the interview were noted, non-prescription as well as prescription medicines. The name and strength of the medicine, the dosage regimen and the administration form were registered. The data were classified according to the Anatomical Therapeutic Chemical Classification System (ATC) recommended by WHO-Europe (WHO Collaborating Centre for Drug Statistics Methodology, 1990). According to this system drugs are divided into 14 main, or anatomical, groups (labelled A-V). These are further divided into therapeutic subgroups that in turn comprise a number of chemical subgroups. The classification, coding and entering of data into a computer was done by an experienced pharmacist. In Phase IV information about drug use was obtained from all but two participants, bringing the size of the present study population to 681 subjects; 224 demented and 457 non-demented.

In Phase IV the housing was divided into six types, and in this study these are in turn grouped into three levels of care: Level 1 includes own home (either owned or rented); Level 2 includes sheltered accommodation (individual apartments with access to communal facilities and a professional, but not medically skilled, caregiver) and old people's homes; Level 3 includes special care units (accommodation for demented people with common facilities, for example for dining and daily gatherings, with continuous access to nurses and nursing assistants), nursing homes, and geriatric wards.

Drug costs were calculated by running the information obtained from the interviews together with a computerised drug register from the National Corporation of Swedish Pharmacies. The register used in this study was from December 1994. The calculations were made using a computer program according to the following procedure. Each drug of each subject was looked up in the drug register, using a unique drug identification number. Thereafter, a matching preparation and strength was looked up. Among the records in the register that fulfilled these criteria a suitable pack was selected. For tablets or capsules 100-packs (or packs with close to 100 tablets/capsules) were selected. For other preparations, such as mixtures, the largest pack was selected. The price of the packet was divided by the number of units; for example number of tablets/capsules, or number of ml for liquid preparations. The obtained price per unit was then multiplied with the number of units taken daily by the subject. For drugs taken as needed we instead calculated the price per defined daily dose (DDD), that is the average daily dose of a drug when used for their main indication in an average 70 kg adult, as established by WHO (WHO Collaborating Centre for Drug Statistics Methodology, Oslo, Norway), and made the assumption that as needed drugs were taken in an average dose of two DDD per week. For two groups of drugs—namely drugs against hyper-acidity and peptic ulcer, belonging to the main ATC-group alimentary tract and metabolism, and anti-infective drugs—we assumed a limited treatment period of 6 weeks/year and 20 days/year respectively.

The costs are expressed in the Swedish currency (SEK). A transformation to US$ can be made using an exchange rate of 12.60 US$ for 100 SEK (current rate in December 1997). Moreover, the costs are based on current drug prices in December 1994. In order to compensate for price inflation one may adjust the costs using the Swedish drug price index, which showed an average annual increase of 1.6%, 1994–1996 (source National Corporation of Swedish Pharmacies). The results are mainly presented as costs per individual, that is the total cost for a drug or drug group in a group of elderly people, divided by the total number of subjects in that group. Sometimes the cost per user is shown, in which cases it is stated in the text.

The Kungsholmen Project was approved by the ethical committee of the Karolinska Institute. Informed consent was obtained for each participant. If an individual was unable to make an informed decision, a close relative (proxy) consent was requested.

RESULTS

A description of the study population regarding gender, age and types of housing by dementia status is given in Table 2.12.1. The mean age of the

Table 2.12.1. Study population demographics

	Non-demented n = 457	Demented n = 224
Gender		
Men	104	44
Women	353	180
Age groups		
80–84	190	39
85–89	181	97
90–94	70	73
95+	16	15
Housing		
Own home	417	101
Sheltered accommodation	31	17
Old people's home	5	20
Nursing home	3	68
Special care unit	1	17
Geriatric department	0	1

participants was 86.9 years (81–100). The demented elderly were slightly older; 88.6 years compared to 86.1 years for the non-demented.

The drug use was high. Only 5.7% of the non-demented and 6.7% of the demented were non-users. The mean number of drugs per subject was 4.6 (4.4 for the non-demented and 4.8 for the demented elderly). In the whole population costs could be calculated for 2651 of all the 3104 drugs used. In the other instances the cost could not be established, mostly because the participant was uncertain about the drug name or strength, or because of lack of information about DDD which was used for estimating the costs of drugs taken as needed. In the calculations these were treated as missing values, and therefore should not have influenced the costs levels.

In Table 2.12.2 we present the use and the estimated cost of drugs in the main groups of the ATC-system, and compare the elderly diagnosed as demented with those diagnosed as non-demented in our study population. The drug use is presented as the proportion of subjects using at least one drug from the actual drug group. The use of drugs in general was high, both in non-demented and demented elderly. The three most common groups of drugs were: Alimentary tract and metabolism, which includes several therapeutic subgroups, for example the drugs against hyperacidity and peptic ulcer, laxatives, antidiabetic drugs and vitamins; Cardiovascular system, which includes for example cardiac glycosides, organic nitrates, antihypertensive drugs (anti-adrenergic agents, vasodilators and ACE-inhibitors), diuretics and calcium channel blockers; and Nervous system, which includes for example analgesics, antiparkinsonian drugs, neuroleptics, anxiolytics, sedatives-hypnotics and antidepressants.

Since the cost of drugs in a population is determined both by drug costs for each individual and by the use of drugs in the population, we decided to

Table 2.12.2. Use of drugs from the main ATC-groups, and the estimated annual drug cost per individual, in non-demented and demented elderly people

Main ATC-group	Drug use (%)		Cost/year (SEK)	
	Non-dem. n = 457	Dem. n = 224	Non-dem.	Dem.
A Alimentary tract and metabolism	47.0	52.7	320	391
B Blood and blood forming organs	36.3	37.9	182	155
C Cardiovascular system	60.4	56.3	707	541
D Dermatologicals	5.5	3.6	32	11
G Genito urinary system and sex hormones	14.7	12.1	133	99
H Systemic hormonal preparations, excl. sex hormones	14.9	16.5	41	41
J General anti-infectives for systemic use	3.1	4.0	4	13
L Antineoplastic and immunomodulating agents	1.8	1.3	27	76
M Musculo-skeletal system	15.3	13.4	185	142
N Nervous system	58.9	64.7	380	1019
P Antiparasitic products	3.1	1.8	27	19
R Respiratory system	12.9	14.7	328	194
S Sensory organs	13.1	10.3	153	104
V Various	0.4	0	21	–
Total	94.3	93.3	2539	2806

calculate estimates that take both factors into account. In Tables 2.12.2 and 2.12.3 we therefore express the costs as the total cost for a drug or drug group in a group of elderly divided by the total number of subjects in that group. Thus the estimates presented in the tables show the mean cost per individual, regardless of whether they are users or not.

Table 2.12.2 shows that the estimated total cost of drugs was somewhat higher in the demented elderly. Looking separately at the main ATC-groups, there were some clear differences. Most notable was the cost of the nervous system drugs in the demented, which was almost three times higher than in the non-demented. The cost of drugs from the group alimentary tract and metabolism was also higher, while the cost of cardiovascular drug use was lower than in the non-demented.

The high cost of nervous system drugs in both non-demented and demented elderly was mainly represented by the therapeutic subgroups analgesics (including minor analgesics and opioids), neuroleptics, anxiolytics, sedatives-hypnotics, and antidepressants. For analgesics, neuroleptics, anxiolytics and sedatives-hypnotics this was due to a high use (39.4% of non-demented vs 39.3% of demented used analgesics, and 35.2% non-demented vs 45.5% of demented used neuroleptics, anxiolytics or sedatives-hypnotics). However, the doses of these drugs were low. For example, for anxiolytics and sedatives-hypnotics the average dose, expressed as percent of DDD, in those using the drugs regularly was 68% in the non-demented and 61% in the demented. For the neuroleptics the average dose was particularly low: 18% and 14% of DDD respectively.

For antidepressants the costs were more dependent on the price of the drugs. While the overall use of antidepressants was only 5.1% (1.8% in the non-demented and 12% in the demented), the cost of these drugs amounted to 24% of the total cost of nervous system drugs (12% and 33% in non-demented and demented respectively). Among the antidepressants used in the study population 74% were SSRI, representing 85% of the cost of antidepressant drugs. The annual cost per user was estimated as SEK3196 for SSRI, as compared to SEK597 for neuroleptics and SEK310 for anxiolytics and sedatives-hypnotics.

Among the analgesics the use of minor analgesics was on average twice as high as the use of opioids in the study population (28.9% vs 13.4%). On the other hand, the average annual cost per user was twice as high for opioids (SEK701, vs SEK353 for minor analgesics), making the mean cost per individual almost equal for the two drug groups. The main difference between demented and non-demented elderly was a higher use of opioids in the demented (17.0% vs 11.6% in the non-demented).

For the cardiovascular drugs the cost was mainly dependent on the cost of organic nitrates, diuretics and calcium channel blocking agents. To a large extent this was due to a high use of these drugs (on average 19.4% of the study population used cardiac glycosides and 17.3% used organic nitrates). However, for the calcium channel blocking agents the price had more influence. For example the average cost for a user of these drugs was 2.7 times higher (SEK1202) than for a user of diuretics. The lower cost of cardiovascular drugs in the demented elderly was largely explained by a lower use of calcium channel blockers (4.0% vs 14.4% in the non-demented), however a lower use of antihypertensive drugs and beta blocking agents contributed.

In the group alimentary tract and metabolism the high cost was to a large extent due to the cost of laxatives. The use of these drugs was twice as high in the demented elderly (26.8% vs 13.1% in the non-demented), and the cost showed the same difference (SEK161 vs SEK87).

The drug group, among the main ATC-groups, with the highest cost per user was the respiratory system drugs. This was largely due to the high costs of inhalation steroids, which represented about 50% of the total cost of the respiratory drugs. The average annual cost of respiratory drugs for a user was estimated as SEK2056. For the demented the annual cost per user was half of the cost for a non-demented user (SEK1315 vs SEK2487). This was due to a markedly lower use of inhalation steroids in the demented elderly. Instead they showed a higher use of xanthine derivatives and antihistamines. The result was a lower cost of respiratory drugs, despite a higher use, in the demented elderly, as is shown in Table 2.12.2.

Table 2.12.3 shows the use and costs of the main ATC-groups, in demented elderly in different levels of care. Level 1 represents own homes; Level 2,

Table 2.12.3. Use of drugs from the main ATC-groups, and the estimated annual drug cost per individual, in demented elderly people in different levels of care

Main ATC-group	Level 1		Level 2		Level 3	
	Use (%) n = 101	Cost (SEK)	Use (%) n = 37	Cost (SEK)	Use (%) n = 86	Cost (SEK)
A Alimentary tract and metabolism	39.6	278	54.1	382	67.4	527
B Blood and blood forming organs	35.6	151	40.5	140	39.5	166
C Cardiovascular system	55.4	620	54.1	605	58.1	420
D Dermatologicals	0	–	5.4	32[a]	7.0	18
G Genito urinary system and sex hormones	4.0	51	18.9	106	18.6	153
H Systemic hormonal preparations, excl. sex hormones	18.8	48	16.2	36	14.0	36
J General anti-infectives for systemic use	1.0	2[a]	10.8	57	4.7	4
L Antineoplastic and immunomodulating agents	1.0	74[a]	2.7	202[a]	1.2	25[a]
M Musculo-skeletal system	14.9	181	16.2	159	10.5	81
N Nervous system	52.5	452	62.2	1106	80.2	1655
P Antiparasitic products	2.0	26[a]	2.7	36[a]	1.2	5[a]
R Respiratory system	8.9	165	8.1	300	24.4	210
S Sensory organs	7.9	36	16.2	189	10.5	138
V Various	0	–	0	–	0	–
Total	89.1	2083	91.9	3350	98.8	3437

[a] Used by less than three persons.

sheltered accommodation and old people's home; and Level 3, special care units, nursing homes and geriatric wards. The table shows that the estimated total cost of drugs for demented elderly increased with the level of care, being 65% higher in institutionalised subjects (Level 3) compared to those living in their own homes. The increase was mainly owing to an increase in the costs of nervous system drugs, which in turn was largely due to higher use of SSRI (from 4.0% in Level 1 to 15.1% in Level 3), neuroleptics (8.9% to 25.6%), anxiolytics (6.9% to 40.7%), sedatives-hypnotics (19.8% to 32.6%) and opioids (10.9% to 20.9%). Among the demented elderly living in institutions 65% used at least one neuroleptic, anxiolytic or sedative-hypnotic. There was also an increase in the cost of drugs from the group alimentary tract and metabolism, mainly because of an increased use of laxatives (from 9.9% in Level 1 to 46.5% in Level 3). Moreover, there was a decrease in the cost of cardiovascular drugs in Level 3 compared to Levels 1 and 2, mainly owing to a lower use of calcium channel blockers, but also to a lower use of antihypertensives and beta blocking agents.

DISCUSSION

In this study we have tried to estimate in detail the cost of different types of drugs in non-demented and demented elderly people. This was accomplished by using data about drug use and dosage from the participants of the Kungsholmen Project, and combining it with information about the price of individual drug packs, obtained from a computerised drug register supplied by the National Corporation of Swedish Pharmacies. Although previous studies have reported estimates of the overall cost of drugs in elderly people with dementia, we are not aware of any study presenting the costs of individual drugs or drug groups. In addition, our study is population-based, and therefore may provide a good picture of the use of drugs in the elderly.

If we compare the overall drug cost according to our estimations with previous studies and correct for the effects of price inflation (according to the Swedish drug price index the prices have increased around 35% since the middle of the 1980s), our figure is slightly higher than the annual cost reported by Hay and Ernst (1987) for persons with Alzheimer's disease in 1983 (US$244), and considerably lower than the average cost for drug consumption in demented elderly in 1985 (US$370) reported by Huang et al (1988). However, if we relate our estimates to the the average annual cost of care for a demented person (SEK166 200 for the year 1991) reported by Wimo et al (1997a), we find that the drug costs represent about 1.7%, which is in agreement with previous estimations (Hay and Ernst, 1987; Huang et al, 1988; Rice et al, 1993).

In the Kungsholmen Project the aim has been to get information of the actual rather than the prescribed use and doses of drugs. In pharmaco-economical studies this may, however, be considered a disadvantage, since it is the purchased amount that is paid for. Therefore, one may assume that the costs we present are somewhat underestimated, particularly in the group of elderly living in their own homes, although this may be less of a problem in demented elderly who more often have their drugs dispensed and get help with their medication. Another shortcoming of the present study is that the drug use was assessed at a single time point, which means that we do not know if drugs were taken continuously or were sometimes used for a shorter treatment. We have, however, tried to remedy this by restricting the costs of those drugs that are typically used during a limited period, such as the antibiotics. Furthermore, it should also be noted that we have not related the drug use to the time of dementia diagnosis or to the expected survival of a demented elderly person. Thus, our figures should be regarded as estimates of the annual drug costs in a group of demented elderly, but cannot be used to estimate the drug costs specifically associated with the dementia disease.

We found no major difference between the average drug cost in the demented and the non-demented elderly. This is in contrast to the study by Huang et al (1988), where the cost per demented was more than twice as high (US$370 vs US$160 for the non-demented elderly). On the other hand, we found notable differences in some drug groups. The nervous system drugs represented the largest cost in the demented elderly. Looking at different levels of care, the cost of nervous system drugs was seen to dominate even more in institutions, mainly reflecting a higher use of these drugs. The high use of neuroleptics, anxiolytics and sedatives-hypnotics is in line with previous reports showing a high use of psychotropics in the elderly in general (Andersson, 1989; Landahl, 1987; Lindberg et al, 1994; Skoog et al, 1993) and in the demented in particular (Semla et al, 1995; Taft and Barkin, 1990; Wills et al, 1997; Wolf-Klein et al, 1988). However it is remarkable that as many as 65% of the demented elderly living in institutions used one or more drugs from these groups.

Despite the high use of the neuroleptics, anxiolytics and sedatives-hypnotics, antidepressants was the one therapeutic subgroup among the nervous system drugs accounting for the largest proportion of the cost. This was partly due to the fact that most of the antidepressants used were SSRIs, which are more expensive than most other psychotropics, but also due to the low doses of neuroleptics, anxiolytics and sedatives-hypnotics. The doses of neuroleptics were particularly low, the reason being, probably, that they were used primarily for their sedative effects, which are obtained at lower doses than the specific antipsychotic effects (see Andersson, 1989).

We found a high use of SSRI drugs relative to other antidepressants, which is reasonable since they are better tolerated in the elderly (Haider et al, 1993), particularly in the demented who are known to be more sensitive to, for example, anticholinergic effects (see Fastbom et al, 1995). If we compare our results with a previous study from the first phase of the Kungsholmen Project (Fastbom et al, 1995), the use of antidepressants has increased more than three-fold, from 1.4% to 5.1%. It is likely that one important reason for this increase is the introduction of the SSRIs, which were not on the Swedish market at the time of Phase I. Earlier the physicians were probably often reluctant to prescribe antidepressants due to the risk of side-effects, for example those connected to the anticholinergic properties of the tricyclic agents (see Fastbom et al, 1995; Haider et al, 1993).

Even though the use of antidepressants seems to have increased there is reason to believe that there is still an undertreatment of the disorder, considering the reported prevalence of depression in the elderly. In a previous study of the Kungsholmen Project almost 10% (7.7% of the non-demented and 12.4% of the demented elderly) were identified as having a depressive disorder (Forsell et al, 1994). In a study by Cummings et al (1995) in elderly with Alzheimer's disease, 6% met the criteria for a major depressive episode, but at least 30% had symptoms of depression. In addition, there are psychiatric diagnoses in the elderly, other than depression, that may be the subject of treatment with SSRIs, for example anxiety disorders. Thus, there are reasons to expect a future increase in the use of antidepressive drugs in the elderly, which in turn will have a significant effect on the drug costs.

In the present study no one of the demented elderly was using acetylcholine esterase inhibitors, prescribed for the symptomatic treatment of the cognitive dysfunctions in Alzheimer's disease. This may be explained by the fact that the first drug of this type was registered in Sweden in 1995. However, in light of the increasing prevalence of dementia in the ageing population, one may expect an increased use of these drugs, particularly if well-tolerated agents are developed. According to the estimations of Wimo et al (1997) the potential target population for treatment with acetylcholine esterase inhibitors corresponds to about two thirds of the elderly with Alzheimer's disease, or approximately 40% of those with dementia. In addition, these drugs are, at least currently, very costly. In Sweden the cost per DDD is more than three times as expensive as the most common SSRI drugs. Thus, one may expect that the acetylcholine esterase inhibitors will have a major impact on the total drug costs for demented elderly in the future.

Drugs belonging to the group alimentary tract and metabolism also made a considerable contribution to the drug costs in demented elderly, and showed a marked increase by level of care. This was mainly explained by the high use of laxatives. In institutions, these drugs were taken by almost half of the elderly. A similar high use of laxatives has been reported previously in nursing homes (Andersson, 1989; Avorn and Gurwitz, 1995). In our study the use of laxatives appeared to parallel the use of nervous system drugs, and one may speculate if this may be in part explained by the well known constipating effects of the psychotropic drugs and opioids (see Avorn and Gurwitz, 1995).

In contrast to the nervous system drugs, the cost of cardiovascular drugs was lower in the demented elderly, and decreased with institutionalisation. This was mainly attributable to a lower use of the relatively expensive calcium channel blockers. Together with this we observed a lower use of beta blocking agents and antihypertensive drugs, including ACE-inhibitors. This is appropriate, in view of the fact that demented elderly have been reported to often have an impaired blood pressure control (Guo et al, 1996), and therefore may be more sensitive to drugs with blood pressure lowering effects.

The fourth most costly group among the main ATC-groups was the respiratory system drugs. Here the inhalation steroids were by far the most expensive drugs. A notable finding was that the cost of respiratory system drugs was lower, despite a higher use, in the demented than in the non-demented elderly. A closer examination showed that this was mainly due to a markedly lower use of inhalation steroids in the demented elderly. Instead, there was a higher use of the less expensive xanthine derivatives, as well as antihistamines which were probably often used as sedatives-hypnotics.

The lower use of the inhalation steroids, as well as the lower use of calcium channel blockers, beta blocking agents and antihypertensive drugs, is in line with the observation by Wolf-Klein and colleagues (1988). In a study of demented elderly outpatients they found a lower incidence of various diseases along with a lower use of, for example, cardiovascular drugs, and suggested that it could be explained by the fact that the demented elderly are physically more healthy. However, one may argue that this could possibly be due to a survival selection mechanism. As regards our findings, other conceivable explanations could be, for example, difficulties in handling inhalers in the demented elderly. In the case of calcium channel blockers, beta blocking agents and antihypertensive drugs, one reason could be a tendency to be more restrictive with these drugs in the demented elderly due to the above mentioned blood pressure impairment. Finally, it is possible that the lower use of some drugs reflects problems with communications between the demented patient and the caregivers, or a tendency to be less attentive to the demented patient's medical disorders.

In conclusion we have found that the drug costs were somewhat higher in the demented than in the non-demented elderly, although the difference was not marked. There was, however, a considerable increase in the drug costs for the demented by level of care. The dominating group was the nervous system drugs, where the SSRI antidepressants made a large contribution to the cost. Laxatives also accounted for a significant part of the drug cost in the demented elderly, especially in institutions, while the cost of cardiovascular drugs, mainly the calcium channel blockers, was lower. Considering our findings, one may expect a future increase in drug costs in the elderly, particularly in the demented, due to an increased use of SSRIs and acetylcholine esterase inhibitors.

ACKNOWLEDGEMENTS

This study was supported by grants from the National Corporation of Swedish Pharmacies' Fund for Research and Studies in Health Economics and Social Pharmaceutics, the Swedish Council for Social Research, the SHMF Foundation, the Einar Belvén Foundation, and the Municipal Pension Institute. The award (J.F.) of a Riksbankens Jubileumsfond stipendium following a donation by Erik Rönnberg is gratefully acknowledged. We thank all the members of the Kungsholmen Project Study Group for their collaboration. We also wish to thank Mats Wennberg and Marianne Tell at the National Corporation of Swedish Pharmacies for supplying us with their drug register.

REFERENCES

American Psychiatric Association (1987). Diagnostic and Statistical Manual of Mental Disorders, 3rd edn, revised (DSM-III-R). Washington, DC.

Andersson, M. (1989). Drugs prescribed for elderly patients in nursing homes or under medical home care. *Compr. Gerontol.*, **3**(Suppl A+B): 8–15.

Avorn, J. and Gurwitz, J. H. (1995). Drug use in the nursing home. *Ann. Intern. Med.*, **123**: 195–204.

Cummings, J. L., Ross, W., Absher, J. et al (1995). Depressive symptoms in Alzheimer disease: Assessment and determinants. *Alzheimer Dis. Assoc. Disord.*, **9**: 87–93.

Fastbom, J., Claesson, C. B., Cornelius, C. et al (1995). The use of medicines with anticholinergic effects in older people: A population study in an urban area of Sweden. *J. Am. Geriatr. Soc.*, **43**: 1135–1140.

Forsell, Y., Jorm, A. F. and Winblad, B. (1994). Outcome of depression in demented and non-demented elderly: Observations from a three-year follow-up in a community-based study. *Int. J. Ger. Psychiatry*, **9**: 5–10.

Fratiglioni, L., Grut, M., Forsell, Y. et al (1991). Prevalence of Alzheimer's disease and other dementias in an elderly urban population: Relationship with age, sex and education. *Neurology*, **41**: 1886–1892.

Fratiglioni, L., Viitanen, M., Bäckman, L. et al (1992). Occurrence of dementia in advanced age: The study design of the Kungsholmen Project. *Neuroepidemiology*, **11**(Suppl 1): 29–36.

Fratiglioni, L., Viitanen, M., von Strauss, E. et al (1997). Very old women at highest risk of dementia and Alzheimer's disease: Incidence data from the Kungsholmen Project, Stockholm. *Neurology*, **48**: 132–138.

Guidelines for ATC classification (1990). WHO Collaborating Centre for Drug Statistics Methodology, Norway, and Nordic Council on Medicines, Sweden.

Guo, Z., Viitanen, M., Fratiglioni, L. et al (1996). Low blood pressure and dementia in elderly people: the Kungsholmen Project. *Br. Med. J.*, **312**: 805–808.

Haider, A., Miller, D. R. and Staton, R. D. (1993). Use of serotonergic drugs for treating depression in older patients. *Geriatrics*, **48**: 48–51.

Hay, J. W. and Ernst, R. L. (1987). The economic costs of Alzheimer's disease. *Am. J. Public Health*, **77**: 1169–1175.

Huang, L.-F., Cartwright, W. S. and Hu, T.-W. (1988). The economic cost of senile dementia in the United States, 1985. *Public Health Rep.*, **103**: 3–7.

Landahl, S. (1987). Drug treatment in 70–82-year-old persons. A longitudinal study. *Acta Med. Scand.*, **221**: 179–184.

Lindberg, J., Claesson, C. B., Cornelius, C. et al (1994). Medicine use in the elderly: A population study in an urban area of Sweden. *Drug Invest.*, **8**: 241–253.

Rice, D. P., Fox, P. J., Max, W. et al (1993). The economic burden of Alzheimer's disease care. *Health Aff.*, Summer: 164–176.

Semla, T. P., Cohen, D., Freels, S. et al (1995). Psychotropic drug use in relation to psychiatric symptoms in community-living persons with Alzheimer's disease. *Pharmacotherapy*, **15**: 495–501.

Skoog, I., Nilsson, L., Landahl, S. et al (1993). Mental disorders and use of psychotropic drugs in an 85-year-old urban population. *Int. Psychogeriatr.*, **5**: 33–48.
Taft, L. B. and Barkin R. L. (1990). Drug abuse? Use and misuse of psychotropic drugs
in Alzheimer's care. *J. Gerontol. Nurs.*, **16**: 4–10.
Wills, P., Claesson, C. B., Fratiglioni, L. et al (1997). Drug use by demented and non-
demented elderly people. *Age Ageing*, **26**: 383–391.
Wimo, A., Karlsson, G., Nordberg, A. et al (1997). Treatment of Alzheimer's disease
with Tacrine—a cost-analysis model. *Alzheimer Dis. Assoc. Disord.*, **11**: 191–200.
Wimo, A., Karlsson, G., Sandman, P. O. et al (1997a). Cost of illness due to dementia
in Sweden. *Int. J. Geriatr. Psych.*, **12**: 857–861.
Wimo, A., Ljunggren, G. and Winblad, B. (1997b). Costs of dementia and dementia
care: A review. *Int. J. Geriatr. Psych.*, **12**: 841–856.
Wolf-Klein, G. P., Silverstone, F. A., Brod, M. S. et al (1988). Are Alzheimer patients
healthier? *J. Am. Geriatr. Soc.*, **36**: 219–224.

2.13 Costs of Dementia-Specific Care Approaches

ANDERS WIMO
Umeå University, Umeå, Sweden, and Karolinska Institute, Stockholm, Sweden

GUNNAR LJUNGGREN
Karolinska Institute, Stockholm, Sweden

BENGT WINBLAD
Karolinska Institute, Stockholm, Sweden, and Stockholm Gerontology Research Center, Stockholm, Sweden

INTRODUCTION

Although most persons with dementia are cared for in the general care organisation (home care, home nursing care, homes for the aged, nursing homes), there has been a great interest in developing care alternatives that entirely focus on care for demented persons, based on the assumption that demented persons have special care needs. Dementia-specific care can take place in special settings, such as caregiver support at home, day care, intermediate care alternatives or at special units in nursing homes. All these care alternatives have some mutual characteristics: the number of patients in a unit is fairly low, the staff is specially trained in dementia care, the physical care environment is designed for the demented, and care is based on a special care philosophy. There is also a demand that the patients have undergone dementia diagnostic procedures. Such care alternatives have been developed in many countries, such as Special Care Units in the USA, Domus care in the UK and Group Living in Sweden. The major impression is that the quality of care in these settings is of good quality, but economic evaluations are rare. In this 'mini-review' we will present some studies that focus on health economical evaluations of these care alternatives. Many have their origin in local projects and programmes. The scope of these studies is often wide, ranging from studies just including a cost figure without an explanation of how it has been calculated, to complete health economical evaluations, such as CEA or CUA.

Health Economics of Dementia. Edited by Anders Wimo, Bengt Jönsson, Göran Karlsson and Bengt Winblad.
© 1998 John Wiley & Sons Ltd.

METHODS

In this mini-review, all costs are presented as US$ of 1993. The cost comparisons between countries comprise two approaches; firstly a methodological one—how do we compare costs?—and secondly—are there any differences in dementia care costs? Comparisons of costs between countries result in several problems (organisation and financing of care, social structure, taxation level, care and family traditions) and it may be argued that it is easier to compare physical units, such as nursing home days, than costs of nursing home care in different countries. If such comparisons are made transformation of currencies is needed. Currency exchange rates reflect trade between countries rather than purchasing power. By using purchasing power parity (PPP) (OECD, 1995), a better reflection of the purchasing power between countries can be achieved. There may be great discrepancies between exchange rates and PPPs. For instance, in 1992, US$1 corresponded to SEK7.06 and 9.67 by the use of exchange rates and PPPs respectively. In the present survey, foreign currencies are converted to US$ by the use of PPPs. Health care-specific PPPs are under development but this work has methodological problems.

To compare the costs of studies at different points in time, a method of time transformation must be used. The Consumer Price Index (CPI) reflects the change of prices in a whole society, but it does not necessarily reflect the changes in the health care sector. Therefore an index based on expenditure on health for the USA (OECD, 1995, data on file) was used since all costs are expressed in US$. Costs with regard to different caring alternatives are presented as US$/day (i.e. 1/365 part of a year). 1993 was chosen as the year for the presentation because it was possible to calculate valid figures for the PPP transformations, and for the health care expenditure index up to that year.

DAY CARE FOR DEMENTED

Regarding Day Care (DC), two approaches of evaluations can be identified. The first is to analyse the cost of a DC unit, the other is to analyse the costs of the DC patients, using a longitudinal approach. The latter approach therefore also includes costs for other care resources than the DC unit. DC can take place in different settings—in hospitals, apartments, special bungalows—and the number of staff per patient also varies, resulting in different costs. Comparisons are often made with nursing home costs, but since the study populations are often not comparable with respect to the degree of dementia, such an approach may be questionable. For example, there are three papers from the USA in the 1980s presenting uncontrolled results, with great variability of costs (Table 2.13.1). There are four Scandinavian papers with control groups, presenting cost data from the 1980s. The control groups were patients living in their homes at the time of their inclusion. In a Swedish study (Wimo et al,

Table 2.13.1. Costs of day care

Country	Approach	Year	Cost/day	Costs/day US$ 1993	Out of pocket (%)	Controls Cost/day	Controls US$ 1993	Costs of DC vs controls (%)	Ref.
USA	DC unit	1981	US$23	48	70				Sands & Suzuki (1983)
USA	DC unit	1983	US$35	62	71				Kays & Szpak (1983)
USA	DC unit	1984	US$77	128	91				Panella et al (1984)
Sweden	Long.	1985	SEK269	53		SEK199	40	135	Wimo et al (1990)
Sweden	Long.	1987	SEK473	80		SEK546	92	87	Wimo et al (1994a)
			SEK619	105[a]		SEK661	112	94	Wimo el al (1994a)
Sweden	Long.	1987	SEK466	79		SEK534	90	87	Wimo et al (1994b)
Norway	Long.	1989	NOK330	42		NOK383	49	86	Engedal (1989)

DC unit = costs of a DC unit, Long. = longitudinal analysis

[a] hotel costs also included

1990), where the patients were their own controls during the period previous to DC, care was more expensive in DC. In two other Swedish studies (Wimo et al, 1994a, b), where waiting list patients were used as controls, DC was cheaper. In a Norwegian study (Engedal, 1989), where a randomised design was used, the costs were lower in absolute figures compared to the Swedish studies, but the relation between the DC group and the controls was the same, 86%.

In two of the Swedish papers, a CEA-approach was used. In the first paper (Wimo et al, 1990), the cost of a 'year of well-being' was US$7537 for the patients and US$6887 for the family members. In the second study (Wimo et al, 1994a), the costs and utility values of a day care group were not significantly better than a control group (although the trend was in that direction) and the study did not confirm the cost-effectiveness of day care.

INTERMEDIATE CARE ALTERNATIVES: GROUP LIVING, RESIDENTIAL CARE

Group Living (GL, Group Dwellings, Group Homes, Collective Living; in Swedish 'Gruppboende') for demented people is a care alternative which was developed in Sweden during the 1980s. GL units are located in flats or houses, but sometimes as one part of a home for the aged, or in a nursing home. They are staffed around the clock and six to nine patients live together. The main purpose is to offer community, supervision and a natural life situation without the characteristics of an institution. Economic evaluations are sparse, all published papers cover only short periods, 12 months or less (Table 2.13.2). A comparison with nursing home care is appropriate only if the demented must stay at nursing homes because GL is not available. The cost of GL in Sweden is about 40–80% of nursing home costs. In a paper from Sweden (Wimo et al, 1994b), the costs of dementia care in different care alternatives were compared with the decline in cognitive function and ADL capacity and behavioural disturbances. The costs increased considerably in home care and in a day care group, parallel to the progression of dementia, but not in GL. When the MMSE score was lower than 11–13 points, GL was cheaper than home care. In another Swedish study (Wimo et al, 1995a), GL costs vs three comparison alternatives were analysed; GL costs were 68% of nursing home costs, 91% of the costs of the home care group and 81% of a mixed comparison alternative (i.e. GL was cheaper in all comparison alternatives).

In this study, a Cost Utility Analysis was also performed, where QALYs were calculated, based on a Markov model (see Chapter 2.3 in this book) of the expected period of survival (Wimo et al, 1995a). The costs were lower and the number of QALYs were greater for the group living residents in comparison with demented people in home care and nursing home care. It was therefore concluded that the cost/QALY was <0 (the comparisons were restricted to dementia care).

Table 2.13.2. Costs of intermediate care alternatives such as group living and residential care (UK)

Country	Year	Costs/day	Costs/day US$ 1993	Out of pocket (%)	Nursing home cost	Nursing home cost US$ 1993	Out of pocket (%)	Group Living % of nursing home costs	Ref.
Sweden	1985	SEK472	94		605	120		78	Wimo et al (1991)
Sweden	1985	SEK338	72	18	837	166	5	40	Annerstedt (1993)
Sweden	1987	SEK612	104	13	900	152	6	68	Wimo et al (1994b)
Sweden	1987	SEK541	92		788	133		69	Wimo et al (1995a)
Sweden	1992	SEK986	123						Svensson et al (1996)
USA	1985?	US$43	68		566	112		60	OTA (1988), Sands (1986)
USA	1985?	US$565	103		566	112		92	OTA (1988), Sands (1986)
UK	1993?	£34–51	53–80		£48	75		70–106	Knapp (1995), Kavanagh et al (1993)

Staff costs amounted to approximately 80% of the costs in Svensson et al's (1996) study of Group Living. Johansson (1990) has in an overview article estimated the costs of GL to be about 60–70% of nursing home costs.

In the UK, the concept of Domus care comprises registered mental health nursing homes where residents live in a purpose-built facility with their own room. Costs of a Domus care unit with demented residents were higher than the costs of private or voluntary nursing homes in the UK (Beecham et al, 1993; Knapp, 1995).

Some cost reports of 'residential care for dementia patients', sometimes called 'boarding home care' in the USA, indicate similar costs to GL in Sweden, 60% (low nursing load) to 92% (high nursing load) of nursing home costs (OTA, 1988; Sands and Belman, 1986).

SPECIAL CARE UNITS

In the USA, special care units for dementia patients (SCU) have been a focus of great interest. The SCU concept is broad, but care is provided in nursing homes or similar settings. In 1988, the Office of Technology Assessment Task Force (OTA) stated that these programmes were controversial and that studies on costs were urgently needed (OTA, 1988). It was estimated that the costs were US$5–10 more per day than at conventional nursing homes. In a paper in the special issue of *Alzheimer's Disease and Associated Disorders* regarding SCUs, some principles for cost evaluations were presented (Holmes et al, 1994), but no cost figures. In one study, which did not measure the basic costs of care, it was found that the annual cost for medication, radiology, laboratory service and treatment (catheterisation, tracheal suctioning, etc.) was US$1477 lower in SCUs than in traditional nursing home care (Volicer et al, 1994).

Costs of fever management (Hurley et al, 1993) were studied on a small sample of SCU patients with dementia as compared to nursing home patients. In a randomised trial, Rovner et al (1996) found that even if a special intervention programme including, *inter alia*, a day programme within the nursing home reduced behavioural disturbances, costs were not reduced during a 6-month follow up.

CAREGIVER SUPPORT PROGRAMMES

In an Australian study, Brodaty et al (1991) evaluated a training programme for dementia carers. They concluded that the programme resulted in an annual saving of US$2160. Drummond et al (1992) focused in a randomised CUA on the effects of a support programme on the caregivers, which consisted of caregiver support nurses who helped the caregivers to enhance their competence and coping capacity. The incremental cost was about US$17 000/ QALY gained.

In another randomised evaluation, Weinberger et al (1993) longitudinally studied the effects of a social intervention programme in terms of resource utilisation and cost. The intervention consisted of extensive contacts between a social worker and the families, which led to an individualised service plan. The programme was not significantly cheaper than the controls.

DISCUSSION

Randomised studies are rare. Often the costs of a particular care unit/care alternative or care strategy are evaluated, and compared with other care alternatives, but the allocation to the different alternatives is seldom done randomly. Long-term studies of different aspects of dementia care are difficult for many practical reasons (e.g. because of complicated care organisation which makes it difficult to keep research teams and research plans constant over time, and mortality and drop-out rates are high). Nevertheless, prospective longitudinal studies with a health-economic approach, where both total costs and costs of different care alternatives are studied, are needed. Many studies only cover 3–6 months, which is a short time perspective since the expected survival period from early to severe dementia is 7–10 years or more. An alternative is to use modelling, such as Markov models (Sonnenberg and Beck, 1993). Population-based studies, such as the Kungsholmen Project in Sweden and the Canadian Study of Health and Aging (CSHA), are also necessary to get basic information of how the dementia population is distributed in the care organisation in relation to type and severity of dementia, social network, symptomatology and so on. Without such basic data, any discussions of the links between efficacy from an intervention and effectiveness in clinical practice are very difficult.

The care alternatives presented in this mini-review cover a wide spectrum of dementia care and therefore the results (both in terms of costs and outcome) cannot be compared directly. With respect to all the methodological considerations, it seems that specially designed programmes for the demented and their caregivers have positive effects in terms of a variety of outcome measures, while the results regarding costs are more difficult to judge. If a cost-consequence approach is used, many of the special designs programmes are not significantly more expensive but they are better in terms of outcome, and therefore it may be concluded that these programmes are cost-effective.

However, the variety of care alternatives illustrates that dementia care today not only consists of 'home care' or/and 'institutional care' and this aspect should be included in evaluations of dementia care. 'Nursing home postponement' or 'institutionalisation postponement' are concepts that are used as outcomes in evaluation of dementia care, but the availability of different care alternatives today shows that the dichotomous split in 'institutional care' and 'home care' is too rough.

It is also important to stress the importance of outcome measurements. Studies with a complete health economical evaluation (CEA, CUA, CBA) are rare and studies just presenting cost figures or cost comparisons give limited information about the advantages of a particular care alternative. However, the number of important outcomes is great, which the outcome section in this book (Part 3) illustrates, and therefore a variety of complete health economical evaluations must be used.

ACKNOWLEDGEMENTS

This paper is based on a review published in *Int. J. Geriatr. Psychiatr.*: Wimo, A., Ljunggren, G. and Winblad, B. Costs due to dementia and dementia care—a review. *Int. J. Geriatr. Psychiatr.*, 1997, **12**: 841–856.

REFERENCES

Annerstedt, L. (1993). Development and consequences of group living in Sweden. A new model of care for the demented elderly. *Soc. Sci. Med.*, **37**, 1529–1538.

Beecham, J., Cambridge, P., Hallam, A. and Knapp, M. (1993). The costs of domus care. *Int. J. Geriatr. Psychiat.*, **8**, 827–831.

Brodaty, H. and Peters, K. E. (1991). Cost effectiveness of a training programme for dementia carers. *Int. Psychogeriatr.*, **3**, 11–22.

Drummond, M. F., Mohide, E. A., Tew, M., Streiner, D. L., Pringle, D. M. and Gilbert, J. R. (1992). Economic evaluation of a support programme for caregivers of demented elderly. *Int. J. Technol. Assess. Health Care*, **7**, 209–219.

Engedal, K. (1989). Day care for demented patients in general nursing homes. Effects on admission to institutions and mental capacity. *Scand. J. Prim. Health Care*, **7**, 161–166.

Holmes, D., Ory, M. and Teresi, J. (Eds) (1994). Special dementia care: research, policy, and practice issues. *Alzheimer. Dis. Assoc. Disord.*, **8** (suppl. 1).

Hurley, A. C., Vilicer, B., Mahoney, M. and Volicer, L. (1993). Palliative fever management in Alzheimer patients: quality plus fiscal responsibility. *Adv. Nurs. Sci.*, **16**, 21–32.

Johansson, L. (1990). Group dwellings for dementia patients a new care alternative. *Ageing International*, **17**, 35–37.

Kavanagh, S., Schneider, J., Knapp, M. R. J., Beecham, J. and Netten, A. (1993). Elderly people with cognitive impairment: costing possible changes in the balance of care. *Health. Soc. Care. Commun.*, **2**, 69–80.

Keys, B. and Szpak, G. (1983). Day care for Alzheimer's disease, profile of one programme. *Postgraduate Medicine*, **73**, 245–250.

Knapp, M., Cambridge, P., Thomason, C., Beecham, J., Allen, C. and Darton, R. (1994). Residential care as an alternative to long-stay hospital: a cost-effectiveness evaluation of two pilot projects. *Int. J. Geriatr. Psychiat.*, **9**, 297–304.

Knapp, M. (1995). Resource scarcity chasing scarce resources: health economics and geriatric psychiatry. *Int. J. Geriatr. Psychiat.*, **10**, 821–829.

OECD Health Data/ECO-Sante-OCDE (1995). (datafile), Paris, France.

Office of Technology Assessment Task Force (OTA) (1988). *Confronting Alzheimer's Disease and Other Dementias*. Philadelphia, PA, Science Information Center.

Panella, J. J., Lilliston, B. A., Brush D. and McDowell, F. H. (1984). Day care for dementia patients: an analysis of a four-year programme. *J. Am. Geriatr. Soc.*, **32**, 883–886.

Rovner, B. W., Steele, C. D., Shmuely, Y. and Folstein, M. F. (1996). A randomized trial of dementia care in nursing homes. *J. Am. Geriatr. Soc.*, **44**, 7–13.

Sands, D. and Belman, J. (1986). Evaluation of a 24-hour care system for Alzheimer's and related disorders. Contract report prepared for the Office of Technology Assessment, US Congress.

Sands, D. and Suzuki, T. (1983). Adult day care for Alzheimer's patients and their families. *Gerontologist*, **23**, 21–23.

Sonnenberg, F. A. and Beck, J. R. (1993). Markov models in decision making: a practical guide. *Med. Decis. Making*, **13**, 322–338.

Svensson, M., Edebalk, P. G. and Persson, U. (1996). Group Living for elderly patients with dementia—a cost analysis. *Health Policy*, **38**, 83–100.

Volicer, L., Collard, A., Hurley, A., Bishop, C., Kern, D. and Karon, S. (1994). Impact of special care unit for patients with advanced Alzheimer's disease on patient's discomfort and costs. *J. Am. Geriatr. Soc.*, **42**, 597–603.

Weinberger, M., Gold, D. T., Divine, G. W., Cowper, P. A., Hodgson, L. G., Schreiner, P. and George, L. K. (1993). Social interventions for caregivers of patients with dementia. Impact on health care utilisation and expenditures. *J. Am. Geriatr. Soc.*, **41**, 153–156.

Wimo, A., Wallin, J. O., Lundgren, K. et al (1990). Impact of day care on dementia patients—costs, well-being and relatives' views. *Fam. Pract.*, **4**, 279–287.

Wimo, A., Wallin, J. O., Lundgren, K., Rönnbäck, E., Asplund, K., Mattsson, B. and Krakau, I. (1991). Group Living, an alternative for dementia patients. A cost analysis. *Int. J. Geriatr. Psychiat.*, **6**, 21–29.

Wimo, A., Mattsson, B., Krakau, I., Eriksson, T. and Nelvig, A. (1994a). Cost-effectiveness analysis of dementia day care for patients with dementia disorders. *Health Econ.*, **3**, 395–404.

Wimo, A., Mattsson, B., Krakau, I., Eriksson, T. and Nelvig, A. (1994b). The impact of different levels of cognitive decline and work load on costs of dementia care at different caring levels. *Int. J. Geriatr. Psychiat.*, **9**, 479–489.

Wimo, A., Eriksson, T., Mattsson, B., Krakau, I., Nelvig, A. and Karlsson, G. (1995a). Cost-utility analysis of Group Living in dementia care. *Int. J. Technol. Assess. Health Care*, **11**, 49–65.

3 Outcome Measurements

3.1 Test Scores in Clinical Trials vs Performance in Real Life: Can Clinical Global Assessments Bridge the Gap?

RACHELLE SMITH DOODY
Baylor College of Medicine, Houston, Texas

INTRODUCTION

The purpose of outcome measures in clinical trials for anti-dementia drugs is two-fold: to demonstrate statistically significant improvements due to drug treatment for the registration dossier, and to convince prospective users that the drug is beneficial. The prospective users in this case are prescribing physicians. Patients and their families will likely not be convinced one way or the other until they have actually tried the medication.

The discrepancies between economics, research, clinical practice, and patient experience do not begin after drug approval. Perceptions of dementia itself, and its impact on human lives, differ from the time a disease is perceived. Usually, patients and their families are eventually educated to a medical model of dementia, and this model helps them to accept the diagnosis, assess the results of interventions, and plan for the future. This medical model casts the patient's behaviors into categories, such as cognitive disturbances, behavioral disturbances, and deficits in basic and complex activities of daily living. For treatment and research purposes, the medical approach further parses these categories into finer behaviors, such as memory function, language ability, visuospatial ability, and so on. Assessments are then refined into primary and secondary outcome measures, with some attention to the cultural environment in which the trials will take place because researchers, regulators, and future prescribers have faith in the measures that are most familiar to them. Increasingly, outcome measures also include an attempt to quantify the cost-savings attributable to a drug, although this process often puts a dollar figure on phenomena that are not thought of in economic terms by patients and their caregivers (e.g. caregiver time, caregiver medical utilization).

Health Economics of Dementia. Edited by Anders Wimo, Bengt Jönsson, Göran Karlsson and Bengt Winblad.
© 1998 John Wiley & Sons Ltd.

This chapter will focus on Alzheimer's Disease (AD) as the most common and most illustrative form of dementia. We will begin with a review of the phenomenology of AD, first from the patient and caregiver perspective, and then as it is structured by standardized assessment measures. The purpose of this section is to identify potential real life changes that should occur as a result of drug treatment, but are not necessarily achieved or assessed in clinical trials. We will then examine some of the common outcome measures used in recent AD drug trials, and point out ways in which the study results utilizing these measures differ from ideal evidence that such drugs are useful in real life. Finally, we will review the concept of Clinical Global Impressions and the feasibility of using this type of outcome measure to (partially) bridge the gap between the patient's and caregiver's experience, clinical practice, and the outcome of clinical anti-dementia trials.

PATIENT AND CAREGIVER EXPERIENCE OF AD: THE ALZHEIMER'S DISEASE VOICES PROJECT

It is difficult to know precisely how AD affects the lives of patients and their families. The information provided to health professionals is selected, biased by the reporter's acumen and point of view, and sometimes shaped by what the informant thinks he/she is supposed to say. The best information about the impact of AD on real lives would, therefore, likely come from interviews conducted shortly after the diagnosis and before the patient and caregiver have had their perceptions shaped by their medical care. We therefore conducted a pilot study called Alzheimer's Disease Voices in which we interviewed 20 AD patients and 20 caregivers shortly after diagnosis with questions designed to gauge the impact of the disease up until the point of diagnosis. All patients met NINCDS-ADRDA criteria for Probable AD (McKhann et al, 1984) and we invited consecutive patients seen in our Alzheimer's Disease Center to participate until 20 were enrolled, along with their caregivers. We asked the patient and caregiver the same 12 questions (Table 3.1.1) worded appropriately according to whether the patient or caregiver was being interviewed. The demographic characteristics of our patients and caregivers are shown in Table 3.1.2.

Several of the questions asked in this study are pertinent to the issue of what symptoms (as perceived by patients and their families) should be the targets for AD drugs. Thematic analysis of the answers to questions 1, 5, 7, and 8 are summarized in Table 3.1.3. A patient or caregiver might have mentioned more than one category of response in response to a question. Although a significant number of patients denied the diagnosis or impact of AD on their lives (question 1), the majority mentioned memory loss, word finding difficulty, or other problems with verbal expression. Those who denied or minimized the condition emphasized what they *could do*, while those who acknowledged it

Table 3.1.1. AD voices: interview project questions (patient version)

[a]1. What is it like having AD? How did it begin? What's happening now?
2. When you found out you had AD, did you know very much about it? How did you know about AD?
3. Is AD different than you thought it was going to be? How so?
4. How have friends reacted to you and your having AD? How do strangers react? Any problems?
[a]5. What do you think is different or wrong in your thinking and memory?
6. Do you have trouble finding the right words? What's that like?
[a]7. Are there other difficulties that you think might be due to the AD?
[a]8. Do you have good days and bad days? What makes the difference? How do you spend your day?
9. How are you and those close to you getting along?
10. What has your experience with the health care professionals been like since all this started?
11. Apart from AD, what would you most like to change about your present circumstances?
12. Do you have any questions you'd like to ask me, or anything you would like to add?

[a] Questions analyzed in the current chapter.

Table 3.1.2. Patient and caregiver characteristics

	Patients (N=20)	Caregivers[a] (N=20)
Age	70 (8.6)	64 (4.0)
Education	14 years (2.2)	13 years (3.1)
Gender (% female)	60%	55%
MMSE	21 (5.5)	N/A

Mean (standard deviations in parentheses)
[a] 9 = male spouses; 7 = female spouses; 4 = female children

emphasized what they *could not do*. In contrast to the patient's anosagnosia or focus on memory and language problems, most of the caregivers mentioned frustration or other difficulty in their lives as a result of the patient's condition. They also enumerated specific disturbances (Table 3.1.4), in much more detail than the patients, and there was a lot of variability in their responses. The responses are grouped together loosely by theme for convenience, although caregivers did not tend to group them. In response to question 5 (what is actually wrong with the patient's thinking?), most patients and caregivers mentioned memory and language abilities, but several of each also mentioned the loss of speed of mental or physical processes. Caregivers tended to make general statements about the patients' thought processes (muddled, loses train of thought, problems making decisions, etc.) while the patients did not. In response to question 7, the patients seldom offered additional examples of problems due to AD, but if they did, they mentioned additional activities of daily living that they were having problems with, such as mechanical abilities,

Table 3.1.3. Thematic analysis of responses to interview questions

	Patients (N=20)	Caregivers (N=20)
Question 1	Denial, minimizing (6) Mentioned memory loss (13) Could not answer (1)	Denial, minimizing (3) Mentioned frustration or difficulty of life (15) Used analogy of caring for child (2)
Question 5	Described memory problem (11) Described language problem (4) Mentioned physical/mental speed (3)	Described memory problem (6) Described language problem (7) Mentioned physical/mental speed (3) Mentioned general aspects of intellectual function (5)
Question 7	Denied other difficulties (13) Mentioned other problems (4) (with ADLs e.g. driving)	Denied other difficulties (14) Mentioned other problems (6) (with ADLs e.g. driving) Other: non-cognitive, general, legal issues, etc. (9)
Question 8	Denied good/bad days (7) Agreed good/bad days (13) Supplied reason (11)	Denied good/bad days (3) Agreed good/bad days (17) Supplied reason (11)

Number of patients/caregivers giving response in parentheses.

Table 3.1.4. Caregiver-reported symptoms of AD: AD voices project

Memory loss	Word finding problems
Repeating	Poor comprehension
Losing things	Stuttering
Hiding things	Slowness—mental
Frustration—Caregiver	Slowness—physical
Frustration—Patient	Getting lost
Moodiness	Trouble recognizing family
Irritability	Shoulder spasms
Delusions	Loss of the following: analytic ability, independence,
Hallucinations	cooking, cleaning, ability to follow sequences, job
Increased sexuality	performance, game playing, reading, mechanical ability

driving, and household chores. Caregivers frequently mentioned additional activities of daily living (especially driving) but also general capacities and other consequences of the AD diagnosis, like the distasteful job of designating Power of Attorney. In response to question 8, most patients and caregivers reported that there were good days and bad days, and both commonly linked these to whether or not there were structured activities (linked to good days) and to the tenor of interpersonal relationships (linked to bad days).

We examined the responses to each question provided by each patient/ caregiver pair in order to look for patterns which might suggest a lack of insight on the part of the patients or other systematic bias on the part of patients or caregivers. We found that there was little overall agreement in patient and caregiver responses: On question 1, patients were often unaware of their difficulties or actively denied them; on question 5, patient and caregiver responses agreed on memory and language manifestations (in about half the pairs) but most other observations did not agree; on question 7, under-reporting by patients again resulted in little agreement; on question 8, the overall answer as to whether or not there were fluctuations usually agreed, but the reasons given agreed in only three cases.

Of course this is just a pilot study with a small number of families representing the many millions who are affected worldwide. Even so, the opportunity to hear from these individuals who had experience with AD even before they knew the diagnosis provides us with some insight into potential patient and caregiver expectations. Clearly, the major target for symptomatic benefit is memory loss, followed by dysnomia. Families offer the most detailed observations when reporting changes in performance of actual activities in life, activities which may fail for more than one reason (e.g. driving) and which may be difficult to categorize on a psychometric assessment (e.g. ability to follow sequences). If our patients' responses are representative, the caregiver's mood, the quality of his/her relationship with the patient, and the extent to which patients are involved in structured activities may impact performance to the point where these variables would have to be controlled in the randomization process for clinical trials. Further, we should not expect agreement between caregiver ratings and patient ratings in clinical trials. Let us now examine the outcomes used in recent trials, and return to these issues later.

OUTCOME MEASURES USED IN ANTI-DEMENTIA DRUG TRIALS

As we have seen, patients seldom come to medical attention complaining of: impaired word list learning, temporal disorientation, trouble with copying intersecting pentagons, and so on. Nor do they necessarily complain of these phenomena in lay terms, at least not spontaneously, although they often endorse such difficulties when directly asked. The face validity of our AD outcome measures is usually derived by comparison to established clinical staging measures, such as the Mini-Mental Status Examination (Folstein et al, 1975) or Global Deterioration Scale (Reisberg et al, 1982), rather than comparison to direct reports of patients and caregivers. Although this practice has been consistently applied and has worked well, it means that our measures are good at capturing those aspects of the disease that we deemed important in designing the staging measures in the first place. These measures do have limitations, in comparison to more comprehensive assessments (Feher et al, 1992) and in comparison to real life experience.

Table 3.1.5. Anti-dementia trials outcome measures (does not include global change measures)

Staging measures	Mini-Mental Status Examination (MMSE) Global Deterioration Scale (GDS) Clinical Dementia Rating (CDR) Clinician's Interview-Based Impression Severity Scale (CIBIS)
Psychometric measures	Alzheimer's Disease Assessment Scale—Cognitive subscale (ADAS-cog) Syndrom Kurz Test (SKT) Digit-Symbol Substitution Test of Wechsler Adult Intelligence Scale-Revised (DSS-WAIS-R)
Behavioral measures	Neuropsychiatric Inventory (NPI) Alzheimer's Disease Symptomatology Scale (unpublished) BEHAVE-AD Consortium to Establish a Registry for Alzheimer's Disease—Behavior Rating Scale for Dementia (CERAD-BRSD)

Activities of daily living	Activities of Daily Living
	  Physical Self-Maintenance Scale (PSMS)
	  Instrumental Activities of Daily Living (IADL)
	Blessed Activities of Daily Living Scale
	Alzheimer's Disease Cooperative Study Unit—Activities of Daily Living Inventory (ADCSU-ADL)
	Alzheimer's Disease Functional Assessment and Change Scale (ADFACS) (unpublished)
	Interview for Deterioration in Daily Living Activities in Dementia (IDDD)
	Nurnberger-Alters-Beobachtungsskala (NAB)
	Nurses' Observation Scale for Geriatric Patients (NOSGER)
	Disabilities in Alzheimer's Disease Scale (DAD)

Other	Quality of Life Scale Caregiver Burden Scale Dependence Scale

Table 3.1.5 summarizes outcome measures utilized in recent anti-dementia drug trials. The table is organized into staging measures, psychometric measures, behavioral measures, measures of activities of daily living, and miscellaneous measures. The table includes only measures that are available in English, and it does not include global change measures which are shown in Table 3.1.6. The published measures are listed in the reference section. One of the challenges to dementia drug development is the fact that clinicians learn to use particular measures as they study and treat AD in their own settings. Part of the face validity of an instrument therefore comes from the clinicians' own experience with its use. Since it is clear that literally translated measures are not equivalent or interchangeable between populations, considerable attention

must be paid to the selection of measures for multinational studies (Amaducci et al, 1997).

The outcome measures listed in Table 3.1.5 are, in most instances, well-designed, validated for use in AD populations, and successful for assessing changes in natural history studies as well as in treatment trials. Still, group changes on these measures do not necessarily mean that individual patients have experienced remission of their unique symptom profiles. These measures can demonstrate efficacy without demonstrating improvement on memory, word finding or other language skills, problems that our pilot study would suggest are central to the negative impact of AD on patients and their families. Finally, the difficulties of assessing large populations at multiple intervals, populations who live uncontrolled lives and experience natural fluctuations in the subjective experience of their disease, often lead to results that are difficult to interpret.

OUTCOME MEASURES FOR THE TACRINE STUDIES

Several published studies support the clinical benefits of tacrine for patients with Alzheimer's Disease (Davis et al, 1992; Farlow et al, 1992; Knapp et al, 1994; Knopman et al, 1996). The first three studies show benefits based upon statistically significant differences between tacrine-treated patients and placebo-treated patients at the endpoint of each study, and the fourth study uses a survival analysis to show that those patients who tolerate high doses of tacrine take longer to reach nursing home placement than those who remain on placebo. All of these studies passed the standards of rigorous peer review, and two were pivotal studies used to gain FDA approval. Yet, although they clearly support the benefits of tacrine, they are not easy to translate into clinical situations. The first study (Davis et al, 1992) showed benefits on the ADAScog (Rosen et al, 1984) Instrumental Activities of Daily Living (Lawton and Brody, 1969), and Progressive Deterioration Scale (PDS) (DeJong, 1989), but not on the unstructured CGIC form of the clinician's global assessment (Guy, 1979) or on the Mini-Mental Status Examination (MMSE) (Folstein et al, 1975). The second study (Farlow et al, 1992) showed benefits on the ADAScog and CGIC, but not on the MMSE, caregiver version of the CGIC, or PDS. The third study (Knapp et al, 1994) showed benefits for some patients on the ADAScog, CGIC, a Final Clinical Consensus Assessment, Global Deterioration Scale (Reisberg et al, 1982), caregiver-CGIC, PDS, and MMSE. Clearly, benefits of the drug were not uniformly demonstrated across studies, even when the same rating scales were used, and the reasons for this remain obscure. The temporal sequence of statistically significant results for these measures also varied across studies (i.e. number of weeks it took to see a response, and which weeks were statistically significant during the study) and within studies it varied depending upon which assessment measures were examined (i.e. benefits might be seen for one measure at a certain assessment, but not for another). Although such findings are not unusual in clinical trials, they make it difficult to choose an assessment tool or interval of assessment that best determines whether or not a drug is working. This difficulty is compounded by the fact that for most of the outcome measures the difference between drug-treated and placebo-treated patients was primarily accounted for by less worsening in the drug-treated group compared to placebo, rather than by actual improvements on the scales, and by the fact that the actual mean differences between the groups on all of the outcome measures were quite small. *Post-hoc* analyses of the data (unpublished) have not supported a specific effect of tacrine on memory performance or on any other particular aspect of cognition. No particular language assessment was used, but most of the tests given to patients were highly dependent upon language skills.

A fourth tacrine study (Knopman et al, 1997) used the dataset from one of the earlier studies as well as data from the open label phase to see if tacrine use could delay the time to nursing home placement and/or death. The results indicate that nursing home placement may be delayed for those who tolerate high dose (160 mg/day) tacrine. Yet the relationship between nursing home placement and disease progression is not clear, and it is likely that factors such as active study participation have an independent influence on families who are making such decisions, so that time to nursing home placement does not necessarily reflect drug effects.

OUTCOME MEASURES IN THE DONEPEZIL STUDIES

Analysis of outcome measures in the Donepezil studies yields findings that are similar in some respects. The ADAScog and Alzheimer's Disease Cooperative Study Unit version of the CIBIC (ADCSU-CGIC) (Schneider et al, 1997) statistically differentiated drug and placebo-treated groups at endpoint in two studies (Rogers et al, 1998; Rogers et al, in press; donepezil package insert). The data for the longer study were more consistent in that the ADAScog, CIBIC, and MMSE were statistically better in drug-treated patients from week 12 until the study endpoint (week 24), but the Clinical Dementia Rating—Sum of the Boxes (CDR-SB) (Hughes et al, 1982) was not significant until week 16. The Quality of Life Measure (QOL) (Blau, 1977) did not support drug efficacy (Rogers et al, 1998). In a shorter study (Rogers et al, in press), the ADAScog was positive at week 3, week 9, and endpoint (week 12), while the CIBIC was positive at week 9 and endpoint only, and the MMSE was only positive at week 9. The CDR-SB and QOL measures did not support efficacy. Again, the statistically significant differences were due to small absolute value differences, and they were more related to diminution of decline in the treated patients relative to placebo patients, rather than to improvements over baseline. *Post hoc* analyses of these studies did not reveal a specific effect on memory, language, or any cognitive area examined (unpublished). Like the tacrine data, these group mean data do not answer important questions about individual patient responses, such as 'Does improvement on one of the measures correlate at each time point with improvement on the other measures?' These answers would make it considerably easier to devise a monitoring strategy to assess drug response.

OUTCOMES IN THE SELEGILINE–TOCOPHEROL STUDY

Time is a concept that most non-demented individuals can relate to. So analyses that purport to show time savings could prove more useful than those showing small differences on psychometric test measures, although individuals will vary in their beliefs about how much time constitutes a significant time saving. The double-blind, placebo-controlled study that compared selegiline and tocopherol (vitamin E)—individually and combined—to placebo assessed the ability of these treatments to slow the time to the development of clinical markers of progression (Sano et al, 1997). The preselected endpoints indicating progression were: death, institutionalization, loss of two out of three basic activities of daily living (i.e. eating, grooming, using the toilet), or conversion from moderate to severe dementia as defined by an increase in the Clinical Dementia Rating Scale from 2 to 3 (Hughes et al, 1982). Unfortunately, the randomization was not completely successful and there was a trend for MMSE scores to be highest in the placebo group and lowest in the tocopherol group. When Cox regression analysis was performed to assess the likelihood that treatment status affected the time to reaching the endpoints, there was initially no treatment effect for any of the therapies. But when baseline MMSE differences were controlled statistically, there was a treatment effect for all three therapies compared to placebo. The treatment effect was not present for any of the individual endpoints: it was only present when comparing the ability of the drug treated groups to delay any of the three endpoints, compared to placebo. The best effect was seen for vitamin E alone, which was associated with a 230 day (approximately 7.5 month) delay in reaching any of the combined endpoints. Clinically, and in taking care of patients, there are big differences between death, nursing home placement, loss of self-care, and global worsening. So it is difficult to relate the study findings to benefits which might be visible to the caregiver or treating physician since the effect demonstrated was delay of a combined endpoint, rather than of the individual ones. Perhaps the most concrete endpoint, the loss of two out of three basic ADLs, is the easiest to relate to. But factors other than dementia, such as physical illnesses affecting mobility, may play a role in this loss, and the interventions had no effect on this outcome in isolation. Although they were not primary outcome measures, cognitive and functional tests were performed (ADAScog, MMSE, Blessed ADLs, Dependence scale, and Behavior Rating Scale for Dementia), and the data show that drug treatment did not affect the progression of cognitive loss as assessed by these measures. Selegiline and tocopherol appear to have been beneficial to patients, but there are no data to translate those benefits into the kinds of concerns raised by patients and caregivers in our AD Voices project.

To conclude this section of the discussion, we have seen that statistically significant results are not always internally consistent (within or across studies) and not always easy to relate to the caregiving circumstance (such as combined endpoints in relation to the patient's specific disabilities). Drugs may show benefit while failing to change the symptoms most commonly cited as impactful by patients and caregivers. Assessment of therapeutic benefits by economic analyses has been proposed as an alternative or addition to these other methodologies. Although such analyses will make it easier for societies to allocate their resources, such analyses will be difficult to relate to the caregiving circumstance as well. Perhaps the best compromise for the present time includes an 'objective' demonstration of benefit utilizing psychometric, staging, behavioral or ADL scales, with or without an economic analysis, coupled with a clinician's global measure assessing the relevance of the testing and economic data to the clinical circumstance.

CLINICIAN'S GLOBAL IMPRESSIONS

Global assessments are holistic, impressionistic, interview-based assessments that lead to an impression about how a patient is doing. The global arises out of the tradition of clinical practice, where clinicians are free to examine patients using whatever techniques are best suited to the patient and the question at hand. Although they have been used for many years in psycho-pharmacological research, global change measures have undergone an evolution in recent years. The initial approach was to leave all procedures unspecified, and to mark the clinician's final assessment on a seven point Likert-type scale indicating no change (4), degrees of improvement (3–1) or degrees of worsening (5–7) (Guy, 1979). This global, called the Clinician's Interview-based Impression of Change (CGIC), left the details of the assessment, including whether or not to interview the caregiver, up to the clinician and ensured little uniformity to the assessment. It also provided no baseline reference point, except the clinician's own memory, for use at later assessments. This CGIC type of global was used in an early tacrine study, and it did not yield a positive treatment result (Davis et al, 1992). Over time, particularly when the FDA suggested that a positive global measure would be necessary in addition to a psychometric measure to prove an anti-dementia claim, the global became more structured. A later tacrine study used a structured questionnaire at baseline and suggested that the clinician return to this assessment at later points, although there were no guidelines for these later assessments (Knapp et al, 1994). This global, a version of the Clinician's Interview-Based Impression of Change (CIBIC), was performed without caregiver input in some studies, but caregiver input was added in later studies (CIBIC-plus). The

Table 3.1.6. Global change measures

Unstructured	Clinician's Interview-Based Impression of Change Scale (Guy)
Semi-structured	Parke-Davis Clinician's Interview-Based Impression (only baseline structured)
	Alzheimer's Disease Cooperative Study Unit—Clinician's Interview-Based Impression of Change (ADCSU-CGIC)
Structured	NYU Global

terms CIBIC-plus and CIBIC are generic terms which indicate global assessments performed with or without caregiver input, respectively, and the Parke-Davis adaptation represents only one version (Knapp et al, 1994). The Alzheimer's Disease Cooperative Study Unit developed a global (Schneider et al, 1997) after first interviewing experienced clinicians about what they thought was important (Olin et al, 1996). An adapted form of this global was successfully used in the donepezil approval studies and continues to be used worldwide. Another approach to the global was developed at NYU and has been used in the global ENA studies (unpublished). These recent versions of global change assessments developed approaches to ensure the comprehensive assessment of cognition, behavior, and functioning in a clinical setting, by a clinician who was blinded to psychometric test scores. Both the ADCSU and NYU versions incorporated information obtained from caregivers, and both are therefore versions of the CIBIC-plus. Current global change measures are summarized in Table 3.1.6.

In contrast to the psychometric measures and other performance scales discussed above, global assessments do not simply assess the patient's and caregiver's experience according to predefined categories. Globals begin with discussion, which allows the patient and caregiver to share their observations, even if they do not know what category these observations belong to. The degree of structure built into the global instrument varies, which has sometimes been a point of controversy: for example should clinicians make up the questions as they go according to guidelines (ADCSU-CGIC) or should they ask the same specific questions to each patient and caregiver (NYU global)? If the clinician has more freedom, there is more of a chance to customize the instrument to the patient's level of functioning, and experienced clinicians can more effectively use their skills. The more structured approach with pre-specified questions ensures more inter-examiner consistency, but it suffers the danger of becoming a psychometric instrument rather than a true global. Because these recent globals all include information derived from the caregiver as well as patient reports and direct observations of the patient, they afford the possibility of integrating these sources of information. ADCSU data suggest that this process is significant and, in some ways, predictable: clinicians tend to

Table 3.1.7. Proposed Clinician's Global Impression of Change Scale anchor points[a]

☐ 1 Marked Improvement; definite improvement in more than one domain
☐ 2 Moderate Improvement; definite improvement in one domain or small improvements in more than one domain
☐ 3 Minimal Improvement; small improvements in one domain
☐ 4 No Change; no significant improvement or worsening
☐ 5 Minimal Worsening; slight worsening in one domain
☐ 6 Moderate Worsening; definite worsening in one domain or slight worsening in more than one domain
☐ 7 Marked Worsening; definite worsening in more than one domain

[a] For use with the ADCSU-CGIC, which specifies domains in the interview questionnaire.

rate patients as worse after talking to the caregiver, regardless of the order of the interviews (Schneider et al, 1997).

Global assessments can take individual patient and caregiver experience into account, generating an individualized patient profile. They therefore add a measure of real life validity to claims of drug efficacy. Yet, because globals are still scored on the original seven point Likert-type scale devised by Guy, it is difficult to rate the numerical degree of improvement reported on a mean group global score to a patient's life experience. One author has proposed anchor point descriptions that relate degrees of change on the CGIC scale to patient functional independence (Knopman et al, 1994). This approach could privilege 'functional improvements,' which are difficult to define and undervalue cognitive or behavioral benefits. Another approach, applicable to the ADCSU instrument, might be to specify the *scope* of patient changes in the anchor points (Table 3.1.7): *minimal improvement/worsening* would reflect small changes in one domain, *moderate improvement/worsening* would indicate definitely significant changes in one domain or small changes in more than one domain, and *marked improvement/worsening* would describe definitely significant change in more than one domain. Domains in the ADCSU-CGIC include memory, language ability, orientation, praxis, mood, abnormal behaviors, IADLs, basic ADLs, and so on. Small change in a domain would be presumed to be clinically significant, although small changes might also be consistent with fluctuating performance, and it is not always possible for a clinician to separate these possibilities. These proposed anchor points would make it easier to translate results obtained on the CGIC scale to practice settings, and they would not constrain the examiner by specific formulas, or require the clinician to make value judgments regarding the impact of a change on patient independence.

Clearly, global change measures aid the assessment of clinical efficacy and help to bridge the gap between study performance measures and Alzheimer's disease as it is experienced by patients and their caregivers. Limitations include the fact that they are performed in an artificial setting (made worse by study protocol procedures such as videotaping), and that they take place at an arbitrary interval, which must somehow average out normal fluctuations in the patient's performance. The sensitivity of a global is also a direct reflection of the skills/experience of the examiner, which means that only experienced clinicians should perform them. Even with anchor points, it is difficult to analyze the clinical significance of numerical scores on the CGIC scale, especially when looking at group mean data.

CONCLUSION

This chapter has explored some of the current outcome measures used in clinical anti-dementia trials and contrasted them with concerns of clinicians, patients and their families. Beginning with their experience prior to diagnosis, patients and caregivers have a different set of priorities and a different view of AD. Although the major symptoms, memory loss and language problems, are universally acknowledged in the lay and medical formulations of AD, currently available drugs do not necessarily improve these symptoms. And the typical inconsistencies within and across studies make it difficult to choose precise measures or intervals to assess medication response in clinical practice.

Although it is unlikely that one measurement tool will be developed to solve these problems, the use of a clinical global at least helps to bring the patient and caregiver voices into the assessment. Without directly asking either to assess change (as their responses are not likely to agree), globals allow the clinician to test hypotheses about change based upon these interviews against actual, individualized patient assessments. The translatability of the final global score might be improved upon by, for example, specifying anchor point descriptions, but the global is not likely to stand alone as a demonstration of drug effect. Given the problems of assessment discussed in this and other chapters, a combination of outcome measures remains necessary, but a well-selected global should be central among them.

REFERENCES

Amaducci, L., Baldereschi, M., Chandra, V., Doody, R. S., Khatchatuvian, Z. and Antuono, P. (1997). The clinical diagnosis and staging of Alzheimer's disease: cultural issues, *Alzheimer's Disease and Associated Disorders*, **11**(3), 19–21.

Aricept (donepezil hydrochloride tablets) (1996). US Package Insert, Eisai Inc, New Jersey.

Blau, T. H. (1977). Quality of life, social indicators and criteria of change, *Professional Psychology*, **8**, 464–473.

Blessed, G., Tomlinson, B. E. and Roth, M. (1968). The association between quantitative measures of dementia and senile change in the cerebral gray matter of elderly subjects, *British Journal of Psychiatry*, **114**, 797–811.

Cummings, J. L., Mega, M., Gray, K., Rosenberg-Thompson, S., Carusi, D. A. and

Gornbein, J. (1994). The Neuropsychiatric Inventory: comprehensive assessment of psychopathology in dementia, *Neurology*, **44**, 2308–2314.

Davis, K. L., Thal, L. J., Gamzu, E., Davis, C. S., Woolson, R. F., Gracon, S. I. et al (1992). Tacrine in patients with Alzheimer's disease: a double-blind, placebo-controlled multi-center study, *New England Journal of Medicine*, **327**(18), 1253–1259.

DeJong, R., Osterlund, O. W. and Roy, G. W. (1989). Measurement of quality-of-life changes in patients with Alzheimer's disease, *Clinical Therapy*, **11**, 545–554.

Erzigkeit, H. (1986). SKT: Ein Kurztest zur Erfassung von Gedachtnis- und Aufmerksamkeitsstorungen, Beltz Test GmbH, Weinheim.

Farlow, M., Gracon, S. I., Hershey, L. A., Lewis, K. W., Sadowsky, C. H. and Dolan-Ureno, J. (1992). A controlled trial of tacrine in Alzheimer's disease, *Journal of the American Medical Association*, **268**(18), 2523–2529.

Feher, E., Mahurin, R., Doody, R. S., Cooke, N., Sims, J. and Pirozzolo, F. (1992). Establishing the limits of the Mini-Mental State: examination of subtests, *Archives of Neurology*, **49**, 877–892.

Folstein, M. F., Folstein, S. E. and McHugh, P. R. (1975). 'Mini-Mental State': a practical method for grading the cognitive state of patients for the clinician, *Journal of Psychiatry Research*, **12**, 189–198.

Galasko, D., Bennett, D., Sano, M., Ernesto, C., Thomas, R., Grundman, M., Ferris, S. and The ADCS (1997). An inventory to assess activities of daily living for clinical trials in Alzheimer's disease, *Alzheimer's Disease and Associated Disorders*, **11**(2), S33–S39.

Gelinas, I. (1995). Disability assessment in dementia of the Alzheimer's type, in Ph.D. Thesis, School of Physical and Occupational Therapy, McGill University, Montreal.

Guy, W. (1979). Clinical Global Impressions (CGI), in *ECDEU Assessment Manual for Psychopharmacology* (US Department of Health and Human Services, Public Health Service, Alcohol Drug Abuse and Mental Health Administration, NIMH, Psychopharmacology Research Branch, pp. 218–222, Rockville, MD.

Hughes, C. P., Berg, L., Danziger, W. L., Coben, L. A. and Martin, R. L. (1982). A new clinical scale for the staging of dementia, *British Journal of Psychiatry*, **140**, 566–572.

Knapp, M. J., Knopman, D. S., Solomon, P. R., Pendlebury, W. W., Davis, C. S. and Gracon, S. I. (1994). A 30-week randomized controlled trial of high-dose tacrine in patients with Alzheimer's disease, *Journal of the American Medical Association*, **271**(13), 985–991.

Knopman, D. S., Knapp, M. J., Gracon, S. I. and Davis, C. S. (1994). The Clinician Interview-Based Impression (CIBI): a clinician's global change rating scale in Alzheimer's disease, *Neurology*, **44**(12), 2315–2321.

Knopman, D., Schneider, L., Davis, K., Talwalker, S., Smith, F., Hoover, T., Gracon, S. and The Tacrine Study Group (1996). Long-term tacrine (cognex) treatment: effects on nursing home placement and mortality, *Neurology*, **47**(1), 166–177.

Lawton, M. P. and Brody, E. M. (1969). Assessment of older people: self-maintaining and instrumental activities of daily living, *Gerontologist*, **9**, 179–186.

McKhann, G., Drachman, D., Folstein, M., Katzman, R., Price, D. and Stadlan, E. M. (1984). Clinical diagnosis of Alzheimer's disease: report of the NINCDS-ADRDA work group under the auspices of the Department of Health and Human Services Task Force on Alzheimer's disease, *Neurology*, **34**, 939–944.

Mohs, R. C., Knopman, D., Petersen, R. C., Ferris, S. H., Ernesto, C., Grundman, M. et al and The ADCS (1997). Development of cognitive instruments for use in clinical trials of antidementia drugs: additions to the Alzheimer's disease Assessment Scale that broaden its scope, *Alzheimer's Disease and Associated Disorders*, **11**(2), S13–S21.

Olin, J., Schneider, L., Doody, R. S., Clark, C., Ferris, S., Morris, J. et al (1996).

Evaluating global change in Alzheimer's disease: identifying consensus, *Journal of Geriatric Psychiatry and Neurology*, **9**(4), 176–180.

Oswald, W. D. and Fleischmann, U. M. (1986). Nurnberger Altersinventar NAI, Nurnberg, Universitat Erlangen-Nurnberg.

Pearlin, L. I., Mullan, J. T., Semple, S. J. and Skaff, M. M. (1990). Caregiving and the stress process: an overview of concepts and their measures, *Gerontologist*, **30**(5), 583–594.

Reisberg, B. (1996). Behavioral pathology in Alzheimer's disease (BEHAVE-AD) rating scale, *International Psychogeriatrics*, **8**, 301–308.

Reisberg, B., Ferris, S. H., de Leon, M. J. and Crook, T. (1982). The global deterioration scale for assessment of primary degenerative dementia, *American Journal of Psychiatry*, **139**(9), 1136–1139.

Rogers, S. L., Farlow, M. R., Doody, R. S., Mohs, R. C., Friedhoff, L. T. and The Donepezil Study Group (1998). A 24-week, double-blind, placebo-controlled trial of donepezil in patients with Alzheimer's disease, *Neurology*, **50**, 136–145.

Rogers, S., Doody, R. S., Mohs, R., Friedhoff, L. and The Donepezil Study Group (1998). Donepezil improves cognition and global function in Alzheimer's disease: a 15-week, double-blind, placebo-controlled study, *Archives of Internal Medicine* (in press).

Rosen, W. G., Mohs, R. C. and Davis, K. L. (1984). A new rating scale for Alzheimer's disease, *American Journal of Psychiatry*, **141**(11), 1356–1364.

Sano, M., Ernesto, C., Thomas, R., Klauber, M., Schafer, K., Grundman, M. and The Alzheimer's Disease Cooperative Study (1997). A controlled trial of selegiline and alpha-tocopherol, or both as treatment for Alzheimer disease, *New England Journal of Medicine*, **336**, 1216–1222.

Schneider, L., Olin, J., Doody, R. S., Morris, J., Reisberg, B., Schmitt, F. et al (1997). Validity and reliability of the ADCSU clinical global impression of change (ADCS-CGIC), *Alzheimer's Disease and Associated Disorders*, **11**(2), 522–532.

Spiegel, R. (1991). A new behavioral assessment scale for geriatric out- and in-patients: the NOSGER (Nurses' Observation Scale for Geriatric Patients), *Journal of the American Geriatric Society*, **39**(4), 339–347.

Stern, Y., Albert, S. M., Sano, M. et al (1994). Assessing patient dependence in Alzheimer's disease, *Journal of Gerontology, Biological Science, and Medical Science*, **49**, M216–M222.

Tariot, P. N. (1995). The Behavior Rating Scale for Dementia of the CERAD, The Behavioral Pathology Committee of the CERAD, *American Journal of Psychiatry*, **152**(9), 1349–1357.

Teunisse, S., Derix, M. M. and van Crevel, H. (1991). Assessing the severity of dementia: patient and caregiver, *Archives of Neurology*, **48**, 274–277.

Wechsler, D. (1981). *Wechsler Adult Intelligence Scale-Revised*, The Psychological Corporation, Harcourt Brace Jovanovich.

3.2   Severity Scales

BARRY REISBERG, EMILE FRANSSEN, LIDUIN SOUREN,
SUNNIE KENOWSKI and STEFANIE AUER
*Zachary and Elizabeth M. Fisher Alzheimer's Disease Education and
Resources Program at the New York University Medical Center, USA*

Severity scales have been demonstrated to be very robust and useful measures
of dementia in general and Alzheimer's disease, the major cause of dementing
disorder, in particular. This chapter will focus upon severity scales in dementia
and the economic import of these measures. Particular scales will be utilized as
illustrative models. These models, with appropriate adaptations, could be
applied to other situations or measures.

ALZHEIMER'S DEMENTIA: SEVERITY SCALES

An illustration of the course of Alzheimer's disease (AD) as it is presently
understood is provided in Figure 3.2.1. As can be seen in Figure 3.2.1, the
course of AD can be described in terms of various measures. For example in
terms of global severity measures, the Clinical Dementia Rating (CDR) (Berg,
1984, 1988) and the Global Deterioration Scale (GDS) (Reisberg et al, 1982,
1988a) have both come into wide usage. However, CDR staging for severe AD
remains undecided upon. Furthermore, CDR staging is generally somewhat
less detailed than the seven stage GDS. Therefore, in describing the economic
import of severity scales, this chapter will focus upon the GDS stages. Figure
3.2.1 provides the information necessary for translating the information
discussed into other severity assessment modalities.

   The GDS stages of the severity of AD are part of a staging system known as
the GDS staging system (Reisberg et al, 1993). An important element of this
staging system is the Functional Assessment Staging (FAST staging) procedure
(Reisberg, 1988). The FAST, as well as the other elements of the GDS staging
system, is enumerated so as to be optimally concordant with the corresponding
GDS stages. The relationship between the FAST functional severity measures
and the GDS stages is illustrated in Figure 3.2.1.

   Mental status and psychometric assessments are other modalities for assessing the severity of AD and other dementias. As can be seen in Figure 3.2.1, a

Health Economics of Dementia. Edited by Anders Wimo, Bengt Jönsson, Göran Karlsson and Bengt Winblad.
© 1998 John Wiley & Sons Ltd.

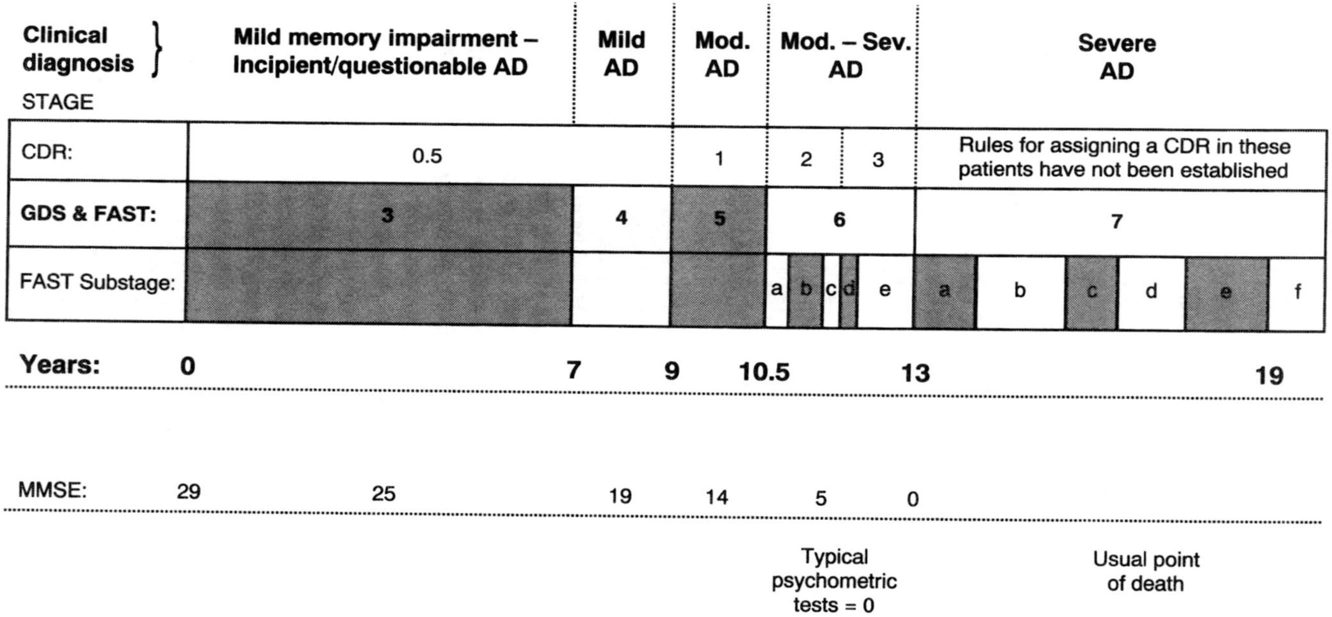

Clinical diagnosis STAGE	Mild memory impairment – Incipient/questionable AD	Mild AD	Mod. AD	Mod. – Sev. AD		Severe AD
CDR:	0.5		1	2	3	Rules for assigning a CDR in these patients have not been established
GDS & FAST:	3	4	5	6		7
FAST Substage:				a b c d e		a b c d e f
Years:	0	7	9	10.5	13	19
MMSE:	29	25	19	14	5	0

Typical psychometric tests = 0

Usual point of death

Figure 3.2.1. Typical time course of Alzheimer's disease (AD). CDR, Clinical Dementia Rating; GDS, Global Deterioration Scale; FAST, Functional Assessment Staging Measure; MMSE, Mini-Mental State Examination. *Source:* data and figure adapted from Reisberg et al, The stage specific temporal course of Alzheimer's disease: functional and behavioral concomitants based upon cross-sectional and longitudinal observation. *Prog. Clin. Biol. Res,* 1989, **317,** 23–41. Functional descriptors are based upon published CDR, GDS, and FAST criteria. Diagnostic categorizations and temporal durations are based upon current knowledge derived from longitudinal studies of the respective instruments (e.g., Berg et al, 1984, 1988; Flicker et al, 1991, 1993a, 1993b; Reisberg et al, 1996a, 1996b). Figure compiled by Barry Reisberg, M.D.

disadvantage of these mental status and psychometric assessments from the standpoint of the description of the economic factors in dementia is the bottoming out of these measures in the final seven to ten years of the potential time course of the duration of AD. Mental status and psychometric assessments are also strongly influenced by education, occupation, cultural factors, the version utilized, practice effects, and other factors (Ganguli et al, 1990; Molloy et al, 1991; Murden et al, 1991; Uhlmann and Larson, 1991; Tombaugh and McIntyre, 1992; Frisoni et al, 1993; Weiss et al, 1995; Tangalos et al, 1996; Reisberg et al, 1997a, b). For these reasons and others, the primary description of the economic impact of severity measures in AD will focus on the GDS/ FAST staging system. However, concordant descriptions for the Mini-Mental State Examination (MMSE) (Folstein et al, 1975) and other assessment modalities are available, have been published, and will be referred to (see Figure 3.2.1 and Reisberg et al, 1988b, 1992; Auer et al, 1994).

The global progression of normal aging and AD as described by the Global Deterioration Scale (GDS) is shown in Table 3.2.1. The corresponding functional progression of AD as described by the Functional Assessment Staging (FAST) procedure is shown in Table 3.2.2. For ease of interpretation, approximate MMSE scores corresponding to each of the GDS stages are shown in Table 3.2.1. Table 3.2.2 provides current information regarding the mean duration of each of the functional stages in AD subjects in which the disease is not complicated by comorbidities which can result in a more rapid course.

It should be noted that the GDS and the FAST, which is derived from the GDS, have been enumerated to be optimally concordant and furthermore a 0.9 correlation coefficient between these measures has been observed. Consequently, the GDS and FAST stages are closely related. Therefore, the MMSE score information provided in Table 3.2.1 for the GDS stages can be applied to the corresponding FAST stages and the time course information shown in Table 3.2.2 for the FAST stages can be applied to the corresponding GDS stages. Furthermore, both the GDS and the FAST have been demonstrated to be reliable, valid, and useful, in the assessment of AD (e.g. Gottlieb et al, 1988; Foster et al, 1988; Reisberg et al, 1989a; Dura et al, 1990; Hartmaier et al, 1994; Reisberg et al, 1988b; Overall et al, 1990; Reisberg et al, 1996a; Sclan and Reisberg, 1992; Auer et al, 1994; Bobinski et al, 1995, 1997; Reisberg et al, 1996b). Because of its global properties, the management corollaries of the GDS stages in AD patients who are free of concomitant significant comorbidity can be, and have been, described (Table 3.2.3) (Reisberg, 1984).

Clearly, the economic impact of AD is in part a product of the management needs of the AD patient at each stage, the duration of each stage of AD and the total duration of the disease until the point of demise, and the epidemiologic distribution of AD in the population. The basis for these calculations is largely contained in the brief information provided in the preceding discussion. However, an additional factor which must be considered before a calculation

Table 3.2.1. Global Deterioration Scale for age-associated cognitive decline and Alzheimer's disease[a]

GDS stage	Clinical characteristics	Diagnosis	Approximate mean MMSE[b,c,d]
1	No subjective complaints of memory deficit. No memory deficit evident on clinical interview	Normal	29–30
2	Subjective complaints of memory deficit, most frequently in following areas: (a) forgetting where one has placed familiar objects (b) forgetting names one formerly knew well No objective evidence of memory deficit on clinical interview No objective deficit in employment or social situations Appropriate concern with respect to symptomatology	Normal aged forgetfulness	29
3	Earliest clear-cut deficits Manifestations in more than one of the following areas: (a) patient may have gotten lost when traveling to an unfamiliar location (b) co-workers become aware of patient's relatively poor performance (c) word and/or name finding deficit become evident to intimates (d) patient may read a passage or book and retain relatively little material (e) patient may demonstrate decreased facility remembering names upon introduction to new people (f) patient may have lost or misplaced an object of value (g) concentration deficit may be evident on clinical testing Objective evidence of memory deficit obtained only with an intensive interview Decreased performance in demanding employment and social settings Denial begins to become manifest in patient Mild to moderate anxiety frequently accompanies symptoms	Mild cognitive impairment	25

| 4 | Mild Alzheimer's disease | 20 | Clear-cut deficit on careful clinical interview
Deficit manifest in following areas:
(a) decreased knowledge of current and recent events
(b) may exhibit some deficit in memory of personal history
(c) concentration deficit elicited on serial subtractions
(d) decreased ability to travel, handle finances, etc.
Frequently no deficit in following areas:
(a) orientation to time and place
(b) recognition of familiar persons and faces
(c) ability to travel to familiar locations
Inability to perform complex tasks
Denial is dominant defense mechanism
Flattening of affect and withdrawal from challenging situations |
| 5 | Moderate Alzheimer's disease | 14 | Patient can no longer survive without some assistance
Patient is unable during interview to recall a major relevant aspect of current life, e.g.,
(a) his or her address or telephone number of many years
(b) the names of close family members (such as grandchildren)
(c) the name of the high school or college from which he or she graduated
Frequently some disorientation to time (date, day of the week, season, etc.) or to place
An educated person may have difficulty counting backward from 40 by 4s or from 20 by 2s
Persons at this stage retain knowledge of many major facts regarding themselves and others
They invariably know their own names and generally know their spouse's and children's names
They require no assistance with toileting or eating but may have difficulty choosing the proper clothing to wear |

continued overleaf

Table 3.2.1. (*continued*)

GDS stage	Clinical characteristics	Diagnosis	Approximate mean MMSE[b,c,d]
6	May occasionally forget the name of the spouse upon whom they are entirely dependent for survival Will be largely unaware of all recent events and experiences in their lives Retain some knowledge of their surroundings; the year, the season, etc. May have difficulty counting by 1s from 10 backward and sometimes forward from 1 to 10 Will require some assistance with activities of daily living: (a) may become incontinent (b) will require travel assistance but occasionally will be able to travel to familiar locations Diurnal rhythm frequently disturbed Almost always recalls own name Frequently continues to be able to distinguish familiar from unfamiliar persons Personality and emotional changes occur. These are variable and include: (a) delusional behavior, e.g., patient may accuse spouse of being an imposter; may talk to imaginary figures in the environment or to own reflection in the mirror (b) obsessive symptoms, e.g., person may continually repeat simple cleaning activities (c) anxiety symptoms, agitation, and even previously nonexistent violent behavior may occur (d) cognitive abulia, i.e., loss of willpower because an individual cannot carry a thought long enough to determine a purposeful course of action	Moderately severe Alzheimer's disease	5

| 7 | All verbal abilities are lost over the course of this stage | Severe Alzheimer's disease | 0 |

Early in this stage words and phrases are spoken, but speech is very circumscribed

Later there is no speech at all—only unintelligible verbalizations

Incontinent; requires assistance toileting and feeding

Basic psychomotor skills (e.g., ability to walk) are lost with the progression of this stage

The brain appears to no longer be able to tell the body what to do

Generalized and cortical neurological signs and symptoms are frequently present

Note. MMSE = Mini-Mental State Exam.

[a] Source: Reisberg, B., Ferris, S. H., de Leon, M. J. and Crook, T., Am. J. Psychiat., 1982; 139, 1136–1139.
[b] Source: Folstein, M. F., Folstein, S. E., McHugh, P. R., J. Psychiatry Res., 1975; 12, 189–198.
[c] Source: Reisberg, B., Ferris, S. H., de Leon, M. J. et al, Drug Dev. Res., 1988; 15, 101–114.
[d] Source: Auer, S. R., Sclan, S. G., Yaffee, R. A. and Reisberg, B., JAGS, 1994; 42, 1266–1272.

Table 3.2.2. Functional Assessment Staging (FAST)[a] in aging and progressive Alzheimer's disease (AD) and time course of functional loss[b]

FAST stage[c]	Clinical characteristics	Level of functional incapacity	Clinical diagnosis	Estimated duration of FAST stage or substage in AD[d]
1	No difficulty, either subjectively or objectively	No deficit	Normal adult	
2	Complains of forgetting location of objects. Subjective work difficulties	Subjective forgetting	Normal aged forgetfulness	
3	Decreased job functioning evident to co-workers. Difficulty in traveling to new locations. Decreased organizational capacity[e]	Executive functioning	Mild cognitive impairment	7 years
4	Decreased ability to perform complex tasks (e.g., planning dinner for guests), handling personal finances (e.g., forgetting to pay bills), difficulty marketing etc.[e]	Instrumental activities of daily living	Mild Alzheimer's disease	2 years
5	Requires assistance in choosing proper clothing to wear for the day, season, or occasion (e.g., patient may wear the same clothing repeatedly, unless supervised)[e]	Incipient basic activities of daily living	Moderate Alzheimer's disease	18 months
6	(a) Improperly putting on clothes without assistance or cuing (e.g., may put street clothes on over night clothes, or put shoes on wrong feet, or have difficulty buttoning clothing) occasionally, or more frequently, over the past weeks[e]	Deficient basic activities of daily living	Moderately severe Alzheimer's disease	5 months
	(b) Unable to bathe properly (e.g., difficulty adjusting bath-water temperature), occasionally or more frequently over the past weeks[e]	Deficient basic activities of daily living		5 months
	(c) Inability to handle mechanics of toileting (e.g., forgets to flush the toilet, does not wipe properly or properly dispose of toilet tissue) occasionally or more frequently over the past weeks[e]	Deficient basic activities of daily living		5 months

(d)	Urinary incontinence (occasionally or more frequently over the past weeks)[e]	Incipient incontinence	4 months
(e)	Fecal incontinence (occasionally or more frequently over the past weeks)[e]	Incipient incontinence	10 months
7 (a)	Ability to speak limited to approximately a half a dozen intelligible different words or fewer, in the course of an average day or in response to queries in the course of an interview	Semiverbal	Severe Alzheimer's disease 12 months
(b)	Speech ability limited to the use of a single intelligible word in an average day or in response to queries in the course of an interview (the person may repeat the word over and over)	Semiverbal	18 months
(c)	Ambulatory ability lost (cannot walk without personal assistance)	Nonambulatory	12 months
(d)	Cannot sit up without assistance (e.g., the individual will fall over if there are no lateral rests [arms] on the chair)	Immobile	12 months
(e)	Loss of the ability to smile	Immobile	18 months
(f)	Loss of ability to hold up head independently	Immobile	12 months or longer

[a] *Source:* Reisberg, B., *Psychopharmacology Bulletin*, 1988; **24**, 653–659.
[b] *Source:* Adapted from Reisberg, B., *Geriatrics*, 1986; **41**(4), 30–46.
[c] The stage is the highest consecutive incapacity level.
[d] In subjects without other complicating illnesses who survive and progress to the subsequent deterioration stage.
[e] Scored primarily on the basis of information obtained from a knowledgeable informant and/or caregiver.

Table 3.2.3. Management needs in normal aging and of the Alzheimer's patient (AD)[a]

Global deterioration and FAST stage of aging and AD	Diagnosis	Management needs of aged and AD patients
1	Normal	None
2	Normal aged forgetfulness	None
3	Mild cognitive impairment	None
4	Mild Alzheimer's disease	Independent survival still attainable
5	Moderate Alzheimer's disease	Patient can no longer survive in the community without part-time assistance
6	Moderately severe Alzheimer's disease	Patient requires full time supervision
7	Severe Alzheimer's disease	Patient requires continuous care

[a] *Source*: Adapted from Reisberg, Franssen, Souren et al, *Journal of Neural Transmission*, in press.

of the economic impact of AD can be initiated is the care needs of the AD patient.

As distinct from management, care needs can be defined in this context as the environment necessary for the optimal psychologic and physical functioning of the AD patient. An appreciation of these care needs in AD is enhanced by a recognition of the developmental age (DA) corresponding to each stage of AD (Reisberg et al, 1998b). Research has indicated the relevance of developmental (ontogenic) parallels of AD in terms of cognitive, functional, behavioral, neurologic, physiologic, and neuroanatomic changes (de Ajuriaguerra and Tissot, 1975; Cole et al, 1983; Sclan et al, 1990; Auer et al, 1994; Reisberg et al, 1986, 1990, 1998a; Franssen et al, 1991, 1993, 1997; Prichep et al, 1994; McGeer et al, 1990; Braak and Braak, 1996; Reisberg et al, 1998b). Because of these striking parallels, each stage of AD can be described in terms of a corresponding DA. This correspondence is best illustrated by reference to the functional progression of AD as described by the FAST staging procedure. This functional progression of deterioration in AD, described with the FAST, is a precise reversal of the order of acquisition of the same functions in normal development (Table 3.2.4). Consequently, it is possible to describe each FAST stage of AD in terms of a corresponding DA. Because the developmental parallel also extends to cognition and other modalities, the DA equivalence applies to the global staging of AD as well as the FAST staging.

The DA model of AD has clear limitations. For example, AD patients do not undergo a DA analogous parallel physical regression and the care needs of the AD patient are based in part on the AD patient's physical size and

Table 3.2.4. Functional stages in normal human development and Alzheimer's disease[a,b]

Developmental age	Acquired abilities in DA	Lost abilities in AD	Alzheimer stage
12+ years	Hold a job	Hold a job	3—INCIPIENT
8–12 years	Handle simple finances	Handle simple finances	4—MILD
5–7 years	Select proper clothing	Select proper clothing	5—MODERATE
5 years	Put on clothes unaided	Put on clothes unaided	6—MODERATELY SEVERE
4 years	Shower unaided	Shower unaided	
4 years	Toilet unaided	Toilet unaided	
3–4½ years	Control urine	Control urine	
2–3 years	Control bowels	Control bowels	
15 months	Speak 5–6 words	Speak 5–6 words	7—SEVERE
1 year	Speak 1 word	Speak 1 word	
1 year	Walk	Walk	
6–10 months	Sit up	Sit up	
2–4 months	Smile	Smile	
1–3 months	Hold up head	Hold up head	

Note. DA = developmental age; AD = Alzheimer's disease.
[a] *Source:* Reisberg B., Dementia: a systematic approach to identifying reversible causes. *Geriatrics*, 1986, **41**(4), 30–46.
[b] *Source:* Reisberg, B., Functional Assessment Staging (FAST). *Psychopharmacology Bulletin*, 1988, **24**, 653–659.

strength. Nevertheless, because care requirements are primarily the product of cognitive, and cognition-based functional needs, and because these parallels are relatively precise in AD and normal human development, the DA of AD can inform the care requirements at each stage of AD and will be referenced in describing these care needs.

Apart from the salient factors in management and care already alluded to, additional physical changes and disabilities occur in AD which have considerable impact. Among the most salient of these additional factors are progressive rigidity and the occurrence of physical deformities known as contractures. The occurrence of these major disabilities with the progression of AD is illustrated in Figures 3.2.2 and 3.2.3.

ECONOMIC IMPACT OF THE STAGES OF AD

The economic impact of each stage of AD can be summarized based upon the patient's capacity, consequent management needs and care requirements and additional disabilities associated with the disease. A brief summary of these factors referenced to the GDS staging system follows.

Stage 1:   No cognitive or functional decline.
             Diagnosis: Normal.
             Prognosis: Excellent.
             Economic Impact: Not applicable.

Stage 2:   Subjective cognitive and functional decline only. No objective evidence of deficit with assessment procedures currently in routine use.
             Diagnosis: Normal aging.
             Prognosis: Generally benign.
             Economic Impact: These subjective complaints do not interfere with occupational or social functioning. They can generally be treated with reassurance regarding the generally benign outcome of subjects with these subjective complaints over intervals of many years (Flicker et al, 1993a). However, persons with these subjective complaints do endeavor to seek out treatments. In part because there are no therapies of proven efficacy for this condition, the nature of the treatment sought is very variable. This variability includes national and cultural differences, among others. The particular treatments sought also change relatively rapidly from year to year. Substances which have been, or are presently, widely used for this condition in various nations include gingko biloba plant derivatives, ergoloid mesylates, piracetam, choline, lecithin, multivitamins, antioxidants, and numerous other substances. Since a majority of elderly persons in the community appear to manifest these subjective complaints of deficit (Lowenthal et al, 1967; Sluss et al, 1980; Lane and

Snowden, 1989), the economic costs of these nostrums and medications are considerable. One indication of the magnitude of these costs is that these substances are some of the most widely used medications taken including all age groups and all disease categories.

Stage 3:   Subtle cognitive and cognition-related deficit generally of sufficient magnitude to interfere with complex occupational and social tasks.

Diagnosis: Mild cognitive impairment.

Prognosis: Benign in a significant proportion of subjects; further deterioration in perhaps a majority of subjects over a follow-up interval of approximately two to four years (Flicker et al, 1991; Reisberg and Kluger, 1998).

Economic Impact: The primary economic impact of these symptoms is probably related to decreased performance in employment settings. In some instances this may result in early retirement. Other persons become less active in social settings. It should be noted that persons at this stage remain competent both legally and socially despite decrements in capacities.

The pharmacologic costs described for patients in the previous stage, including both prescription and nonprescription substances, are applicable in this stage as well. In addition, anxiety, depression, or other behavioral symptoms which are present in many of these patients, are sometimes treated pharmacologically, adding to medication costs.

A major economic cost at this stage which is easily overlooked is the interaction of the morbidity associated with mild cognitive impairment with other medical conditions in these generally elderly persons. For example, mild cognitive impairment greatly increases the predisposition to delirium in response to concomitant stressors, such as anesthesia, surgery, and various medications.

A final calculation of the economic impact of this condition must take into consideration the prevalence of this condition which is probably somewhat greater than the prevalence of AD.

Stage 4:   Manifest cognitive and cognition-related deficit generally of sufficient magnitude to interfere with instrumental activities of daily life such as the ability to manage personal finances, to prepare meals for guests, and the ability to market properly.

Diagnosis: Mild Alzheimer's disease.

Prognosis: The diagnosis of Alzheimer's disease, a progressive degenerative disorder, can be reliably arrived at from the beginning of this stage. This stage lasts approximately two years in AD patients who are free of significant comorbidity (Reisberg et al, 1996a).

Economic Impact: The primary economic impact is the inability to perform appropriately or accurately in a complex occupational setting, such as a professional role. It should be noted that for various reasons including, notably, the desire to maintain the dignity of an adult role, persons at this stage will frequently prefer to continue in their occupational setting. In these cases, a concerned colleague or family member has frequently begun to shoulder many of the patient's former responsibilities. To the extent that this is not the case, job performance and productivity generally decline.

In community settings, persons at this stage may begin to forget to pay their rent or other bills in a correct or timely fashion, or develop other financial management problems. If the mild AD patient continues to reside with their spouse or other concerned family members, then these family members generally begin to assume increasing responsibilities for financial management and oversight. If the patient continues to reside or act on their own, then the fiduciary responsibility of those in contact with the patient becomes increasingly important. At the simplest level, it is desirable that the patient maintain as much independence as possible and, for example, market independently. However, it is the responsibility of the personnel at the grocery or supermarket not to swindle the patient.

This fiduciary responsibility also extends to more complex financial transactions. For example, persons at this stage frequently continue to sign checks. This is desirable in service of the patient's dignity. If one, to some extent prematurely, denied the patient this ability, the patient might become very angry and this in turn might trigger a series of events, such as the necessity for psychotropic medication. This scenario might be clearly deleterious to the health and well-being of the patient. However, persons at this stage are clearly more susceptible to undue influence and fraud because of their decreased cognition and the decreased judgement which is a necessary corollary of the decreased cognition.

The legal aspects and ramifications of AD at this stage have been discussed previously in depth (Reisberg et al, 1985). In summary, when patients are residing independently in the community, a guardian may be necessary to husband the patient's assets to maintain community residence. When there is a spouse or other trustworthy relative or companion, it is desirable that the trusted and trustworthy person have power of attorney. That person should ideally cosign significant transactions of diverse nature including consents to participate in research projects. Persons at this stage are no longer capable of judiciously assessing simultaneously the nature and extent of their property, and the natural objects of their bounty, and achieving a judicious distribution based upon these simultaneous assessments. Consequently, persons at this stage of mild AD are no longer competent to execute a will in the absence of appropriate fiduciary assistance, or very simple and straightforward decisions in this regard. Since persons at this stage frequently appear superficially competent in the absence of an appropriate neuropsychiatric evaluation, problems frequently develop in this regard. An attorney, or friend, or physician, who sees the patient might note that they 'look fine', seem to be their 'normal selves', and appear to know what they are doing. However, an examination and evaluation in which appropriate questions are posed invariably reveals the deficits of mild AD. Consequently, there are many cases in which the last wills and testaments of these patients are ultimately contested and should be overturned.

Other economic consequences develop when persons in this stage of mild AD continue to perform in sensitive occupational settings in which their competence is assumed and not questioned. For example, one judge at this stage continued to adjudicate cases and his attorney daughter assisted in writing up the opinions. Once the diagnosis was made, this patient retired. However, clearly, an informed economic analysis must take into consideration the fact that many patients with AD are not diagnosed in this stage at all.

Also important for an economic analysis in this stage is an understanding of retained capacity. Patients at this stage can still survive independently in community settings if they obtain appropriate financial assistance and if there is not sufficient comorbidity to further compromise their capacities. Also, persons at this stage who are otherwise healthy, and whose FAST level is 4 or less, can still continue to drive an automobile. Consequently, the major ostensible economic consequence for many housewives at this stage is less efficient preparation of meals for family gatherings.

The DA at this stage of AD is approximately 8 to 12 years. In this context, the patient's residual capacities and limitations can be clearly appreciated. Just as an 8 to 12 year old might conceivably survive in a community setting if assistance were provided with managing finances, paying the rent, and so on, the same is true of the mild AD patient. Just as we consider an 8 to 12 year old a minor, who is perhaps able to handle money, but not competent to sign contracts, the same limitations apply to the AD patient at this stage.

The DA of this stage, that is stage 4 or mild AD, can also inform the care needs of the AD patient. As already noted, many patients at this stage choose to continue in their former occupations. Despite decreased performance, this is frequently a therapeutic choice for the patient. An artist may no longer be able to conceptualize or realize works of the same vision or complexity, but may still be able to produce drawings or sculptures of which they can remain proud. Equally importantly, even if no new works are produced, they can claim to be active and working and productive, and derive satisfaction from these claims. A musician may continue to play an instrument, although they may have had to retire from professional performances. One man, an opera singer, did give a successful performance at this stage.

Particularly for those who have had to retire from their former occupations, therapy for the AD patient at this stage includes guiding the patient into new activities. Physical activities are frequently ideal. For example, one professor of dance could no longer teach choreography, she would, however, participate in dancercize classes. Activities which are not complex, such as swimming, should be encouraged.

For certain persons at this stage, particularly those with a bias towards introspection and psychotherapy, early stage support groups are very useful. One woman at this stage went so far as to speak to professional audiences about her experiences with AD. This experience once again made her the expert on her topic. She stated, 'You begin to think that Alzheimer's disease is an achievement'. Although there were also many darker, more anxiety provoking, and less optimistic aspects to this woman's experiences, this ability to turn the adversity of AD into a new or neutral experience is what is sought in the care of the AD patient at this stage. Ideally, the economics of AD should factor in these optimal care goals.

The medication costs described for the previous stages largely apply to patients with mild AD. Additionally, various AD specific medications, such as cholinesterase inhibitors, are likely to be prescribed. The issues associated with comorbidity increase at this stage. These patients are even more prone to develop delirium and behavioral symptoms in response to stressors than patients at the previous stage. Similarly, physical limitations become magnified by cognitive losses.

Stage 5:   Major cognitive deficits which are generally of sufficient magnitude to cause incipient deficits with basic activities of daily life. The classic incipient activity of daily life deficit in this stage is decreased ability to choose the proper clothing to wear for the season and the occasion.

Diagnosis: Moderate Alzheimer's disease.

Prognosis: This stage lasts approximately one-and-a-half years in AD patients who are free of significant comorbidity.

Economic Impact: Persons at this stage can no longer survive independently in community settings. Consequently, the economic impact includes physical care needs as well the loss of occupational skills.

Even at this stage, persons who have the choice sometimes cling to their now increasingly nominal occupations, from which they may continue to derive dignity. For example, one 82 year old woman, a psychologist and psychoanalyst who was at this stage globally, but who functionally had some additional disability, and hence required 24 hour per day home care assistance, still maintained her final psychoanalytic patient. As further indication of her still strong professional identity was the sentence she chose to write as part of the MMSE, that is, 'I am interested to know what this Dr is trying to learn from his questions to me'. Her score on the MMSE was 16.

Other persons at this stage continue, with varying success, to cling to roles as physicians, dentists, business owners, and so on. One scientist reported that he continued to supervise the nuclear reactor at a major university. Perhaps a complete economic analysis of the costs of this stage should include not only loss of occupational productivity, but also the errors and lost opportunities which result for those who continue in occupational roles.

Persons at this stage who reside independently in the community frequently are preyed upon. For example, one physician discovered that intruders were living in her father's apartment. Other patients at this stage who live alone in the community become fearful, angry, and suspicious.

When a spouse or other family caregiver is present, no further assistance is frequently necessary for persons at this stage. Indeed, because of the affront to their dignity, patients will often become angry if there is an effort to provide them with further help, which the patient feels they do not need. However, a day care center is a useful option for many patients at this stage. If there is excess physical disability, then additional personal caregiver assistance, apart from the spouse or other family member's support, may be necessary.

The legal aspects of this stage are interesting and important. Clearly, without appropriate fiduciary assistance, persons at this stage are not competent to sign sophisticated contracts and these persons lack testamentary capacity. The DA of this stage is approximately 5 to 7 years of age and this provides an indication of the capacity in these contractual and testamentary matters. However, interestingly, for various reasons, persons at this stage occasionally marry. Sometimes the new relationship fits the circumstances. For example one woman remained sociable, warm, physically attractive and enjoyed dancing, despite her decreased cognitive capacities. She met a man at a dance who was older and more physically disabled, and somewhat less sociable than herself. However, his memory was excellent. As a couple, they complemented each other. They married with the approval of their family and physicians. The union lasted briefly. However, for a time, it bought satisfaction to the newly weds.

Over the course of FAST stage 5, that is, between the point where patients have difficulties with instrumental activities of daily life and when the patient loses the ability to put on their clothing properly, AD patients lose the ability to drive. Naturally, physical or mental excess disability can compromise driving skills sooner. Generally, patients voluntarily discontinue operating an automobile or the family or society intervenes at the appropriate time and tragic accidents are virtually unknown.

Naturally, the medication costs and the increased tendency to delirium, which applied to persons in the previous stage, apply to this fifth stage as well. These medication costs and disability costs probably are somewhat greater in stage 5 than stage 4.

Stage 6: Cognitive deficits of sufficient magnitude to interfere with basic activities of daily life. Basic life activities which are increasingly compromised at this stage include the ability to dress, bathe and toilet.

Diagnosis: Moderately severe Alzheimer's disease.

Prognosis: This stage lasts approximately two-and-a-half years in AD patients who are free of significant comorbidity.

Economic Impact: Persons at this stage require continuous assistance or supervision. The economic impact at this stage includes the absolute absence of a useful role for the patient and major care needs which compromise the family caregiver's productivity and at some point generally necessitate additional paid professional assistance. Medication costs become even more extensive at this stage and costs of other health supplies become increasingly relevant.

Persons at this stage can no longer successfully pretend to function in an adult employment setting. However, interestingly, patients may still get some satisfaction from mimicking their former adult role. For example, one 81 year old woman at this stage who had incipient urinary incontinence (GDS stage 6, FAST stage 6d) stayed behind a cash register for four-and-a-half hours. Previously, this patient had worked behind a cash register when she had been less impaired and prior to the onset of her AD. Now at stage 6 of AD, she made numerous errors but derived satisfaction from endeavoring to assist and handling money. When things slowed down, she said, 'There's nothing for me to do right now, we might as well go home', just as she would have done when she was healthy.

At the beginning of this stage, many family members who are devoted prefer to care for the patient themselves, independently. These family members are generally devoted retired spouses. Even these devoted retired spouses, who are in the best position to manage the patient, will generally prefer, or need, additional assistance as this stage progresses. This additional assistance is generally in the form of a home health aide. By the end of this stage, 24 hour per day home health assistance is desirable for most patients. Even at night, most late stage 6 patients require observation to prevent anxieties regarding being unattended, for assistance in toileting to minimize or eliminate actual episodes of incontinence, and to prevent falling. Despite all of this assistance, institutionalization generally becomes a consideration by the end of the sixth stage. The major proximate causes of institutionalization are incontinence and behavioral disturbances.

When the caregiver is a child rather than a spouse, full-time professional care is generally desirable from the onset of the sixth stage so that the adult child can continue to function in their employment setting and care for the patient. When no concerned family members are available to coordinate and supervise the patient's care then institutionalization is frequently necessary even at the onset of the sixth stage and even in the absence of concomitant morbidity.

Emotional changes become very important at this stage. Behavioral disturbances are greater in magnitude at this stage than at any other stage of AD (Reisberg et al, 1989b; Sclan et al, 1996; Reisberg et al, 1992). Few patients, if any, are entirely free of emotional disturbances. The magnitude of these disturbances appears to be the product of both psychological factors and endogenous (neurochemical) pathology. The patient's environment and the quantity and quality of the care provided are salient factors influencing the magnitude of psychologic disturbance in the patient. A patient who is insecure regarding the constancy or quality of their care is more likely to have greater emotional disturbances. A patient who is temporarily left alone will generally manifest greater anxieties. A patient who has reason from past experience to distrust their caregiver is more likely to manifest the delusion that people are stealing things. A patient who is not toileted properly or cleaned properly is likely to become agitated, angry or violent.

An understanding of the developmental age of the AD patient is fundamental for an appreciation of the patient's management needs, emotional reactions, and care requirements.

The DA of stage 6 AD is approximately 2 to 5 years of age. A stage 6 AD patient requires approximately the same amount of care as a 2 to 5 year old, hence the need for full-time help. If one leaves a stage 6 AD patient alone, similar anxieties are expressed by a stage 6 AD patient as might be expressed by a 2 to 5 year old child who is left alone.

Many of the other behavioral disturbances of the AD patient are also readily understood through an appreciation of the DA (Reisberg et al, 1998a, b). For example, the so-called delusions of the AD patient are actually transient and not firmly held, and, consequently, very similar to fantasies which occur in children at the corresponding DA. Similarly, so called catastrophic reactions in AD patients are virtually identical to symptoms which are termed 'temper tantrums' in children at the corresponding DA. Just as children who are raised in less supportive, more stressful environments will have more behavioral symptoms, AD patients who are cared for in less supportive, more stressful environments will exhibit more behavioral disturbances. Just as the most pathologic behavioral disturbances, such as biting, spitting, and scratching, are exhibited most frequently in children who are raised in deprived or pathologic settings, such as institutions, these same symptoms are seen frequently in AD patients in institutional settings, but are quite infrequently noted in patients receiving community-based care.

The DA of the AD patient is particularly useful for achieving an understanding of the patient's care needs. A stage 6 AD patient cannot decide upon and choose their activities any more than a 2 to 5 year old child. Consequently, just as a child who is not provided with directed activity might run back and forth, a stage 6 AD patient who is not provided with activity might pace back and forth. The kinds of activities which are appropriate for a stage 6 AD patient are similar to those which are appropriate for a child at the corresponding DA, that is, 2 to 5 years. One major caveat is that if an AD patient perceives an activity as 'childish', they will become angry and insulted by the activity. However, it should be noted that children also become insulted by activities they consider 'baby like'.

In day care settings, these activity principles are generally followed for the stage 6 AD patient, who has stories read to them, fills in coloring books, sings simple songs, and so on. These activities are very similar to those in a nursery school or kindergarten. Unfortunately, few professional caregivers in home settings provide these kinds of activities.

Therefore, the economic costs of stage 6 AD can be summarized as: (1) absolute loss of previous economic productivity on the part of the patient; (2) costs of supervision by family and professional caregivers, including institutionalization in some cases; (3) costs of minimizing emotional disturbances with quality care and the provision of optimal patient dignity; (4) costs of providing proper activities for the patient; (5) medication costs, including medications for behavioral disturbances; and (6) costs of excess disability, in interaction with other comorbidities common in these aged patients.

Stage 7:   Cognitive and functional deficits of sufficient magnitude to require continuous care. Patients are doubly incontinent and speech is severely limited, then lost entirely. Motor capacities, including ambulation, become increasingly compromised.

Diagnosis: Severe Alzheimer's disease.

Prognosis: Patients die at all points in the course of this stage. Death results from both identifiable causes and nonspecific causes. Prominent among identifiable proximate causes of demise are aspiration pneumonia and other forms of pneumonia, which are responsible for approximately half of deaths. Infected decubital ulcerations and infectious conditions are responsible for many of the remaining deaths. Patients with AD also die of strokes and other common causes of death in the elderly, such as cancer. In some cases, patients appear to die of no identifiable cause other than AD.

The mean duration of this stage until demise is approximately 2 to 3 years. However, patients who survive into the final substage of AD survive for 7 years and, potentially, longer survival is possible.

Economic Impact: Persons at this stage require continuous care. The quality and availability of this care directly and immediately affect the patient's physical and emotional health. In North America, Europe and in other highly industrialized nations, care in this stage is generally provided in institutional settings, such as nursing homes. Costs of care in these settings are considerable and average approximately $40 000 per patient, per annum, in the United States at the present time. A third of the United States nursing home population, approximately 500 000 Americans, appear to be in this stage (German et al, 1985; Gurland et al, 1992; Teresi et al, 1994). This latter figure, it should be noted, includes persons with AD, persons with AD accompanied by other conditions, and some persons with other dementing disorders. Since AD accounts for the great majority of these cases as the major contributory factor, it is probably reasonable to estimate that the direct institutional costs of care for AD patients in this stage alone in the United States are approximately $20 billion. It must be emphasized that the quality of care received by these patients in the nursing home settings is far from ideal. Consequently, these costs in many ways represent simply the expense of keeping these patients alive, with a quality of life ranging from deplorable suffering to equanimity, but rarely extending to optimal functioning.

Some patients in this final seventh stage continue to be cared for in the community. The quality of community-based care is very variable. Fortunately, there appear to be a few patients who receive relatively good care in community-based settings. This community-based care is generally provided both by family members and professionals.

There are dramatic examples of the neglect and absence of attention to patients at this stage. One example of the absence of attention to the cognitive needs of these patients is that only recently was it demonstrated that these patients can still think and that the magnitude of their residual cognitive capacities can be measured and, hopefully, someday optimized (Auer et al, 1994). Under the present circumstances, these patients, tragically, frequently suffer in silence. Since they cannot speak, patients are frequently treated as if they cannot think, and there is frequently indifference to the suffering of a person who 'cannot speak up for themselves'. In an effort to communicate, some patients begin to scream or cry out semi-intelligibly or unintelligibly. The institutional response to these cries for help is frequently sedating and tranquilizing medication which further compromises the residual cognitive and physical capacities of these patients.

Physical capacities of patients in this final seventh stage of severe AD are readily dramatically compromised. Virtually all patients in this stage manifest rigidity upon movement of the major joints, such as the elbow, wrists or knee (Franssen et al, 1991, 1993) (Figure 3.2.2). This rigidity is most probably the result of both endogenous and exogenous factors.

The endogenous factors include the brain changes which are occurring in the AD patient, such as compromised neuronal function. These brain changes predispose to rigidity as a result of decreased central nervous system inhibition of the spinal reflex arc.

Exogenous factors which predispose to rigidity include decrements in physical activity as a result of decreased cognitive capacities. Because of decreased cognition, patients at this stage can no longer guide their own activities. Consequently, an activity or physical therapy program is necessary even for the maintenance of such basic skills as walking. More complex skills, such as dressing, bathing, brushing teeth, and eating with silverware, are no longer initiated by the patient spontaneously, even in the early part of the seventh stage. Unless these basic psychomotor skills are practiced and the patient is continuously retrained, these skills are rapidly lost. The result is a cascading pattern of decreased psychomotor stimulation and decreased movement. The decreased movement further increases rigidity of the joints.

The end result of this increasing rigidity and physical immobility is physical deformities known as contractures (Figure 3.2.3). Approximately 40% of patients in the semi-verbal early portion of severe AD were found to manifest

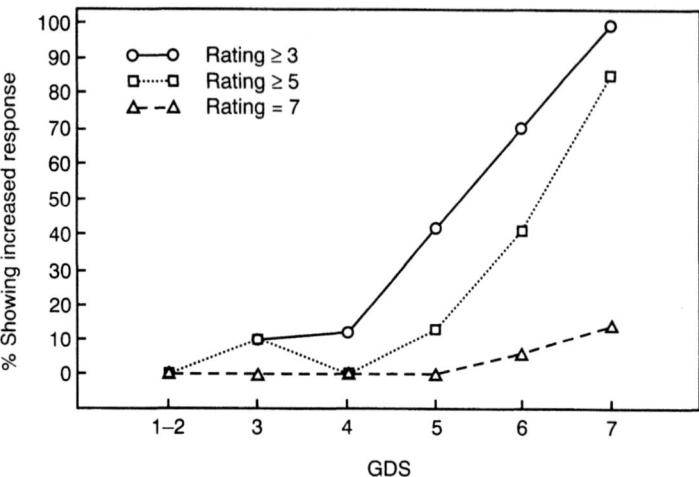

Figure 3.2.2. Percentage of subjects with increased paratonic rigidity in normal aging and AD of progressively increasing severity. The graph depicts the percentages of subjects showing paratonia as a function of the Global Deterioration Scale (GDS) stage, using three different ratings of activity. Paratonic rigidity, defined as stiffening of a limb in response to contact with the examiner's hand and an involuntary resistance to passive changes in position and posture, was graded according to the amount of passive force necessary to elicit it. A rating of 1 denotes an absence of paratonic rigidity, whereas a rating of 7 indicates that minimal passive force is required for elicitation of the sequence. Further detail regarding the scoring procedure can be found in Franssen (1993). *Source*: data and figure are from Franssen, Reisberg, Kluger et al, *Archives of Neurology*, 1991; **48**, 148–154

these deformities (Souren et al, 1995). In nonambulatory, FAST stage 7c AD patients who were followed in this longitudinal study, contractures were noted in half of patients. Immobile patients in the final stage 7 substages (FAST stages 7d to 7f) virtually invariably manifested contractures. It should be noted that contractures in this study of Souren et al (1995) were defined as loss of 50% or more of the ability to move a major joint (that is, the shoulder, elbow, wrist, hip, knee or ankle). Importantly, in more than two-thirds of patients with contractures, these deformities affected all four extremities.

Contractures themselves predispose to further disabilities. For example, the presence of contracture renders movement of the affected joint painful and results in greatly increased care needs for these patients who can no longer move themselves. Expressions of pain on the part of the patient may produce screaming, which readily disrupts the institutional environment. Also, the patient's cries of pain may result in the prescription of medications such as neuroleptics, which may increase the tendency to immobility and even further disability. Contractures also enormously predispose to decubital ulcerations in

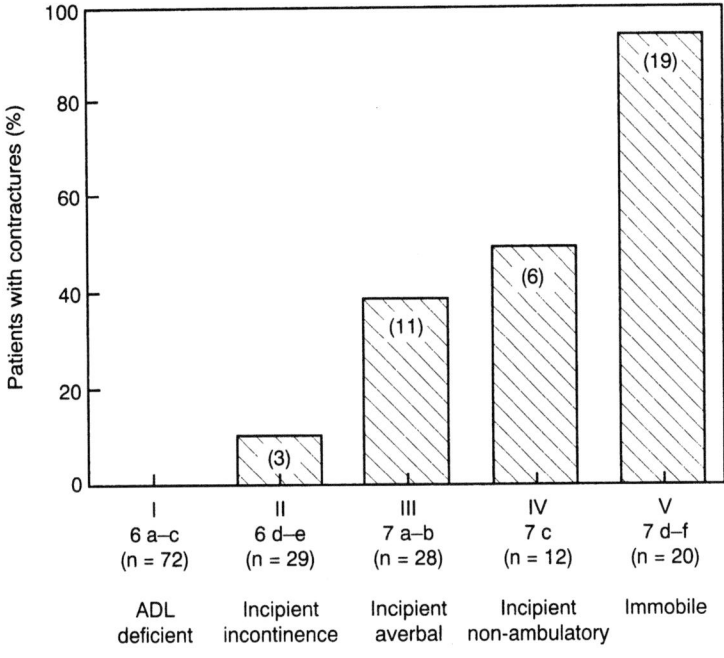

Figure 3.2.3. Percentages of Patients with Contractures in Stage 6 and Stage 7 AD. All subjects fulfilled criteria for probable AD. FAST (Functional Assessment Staging [Reisberg, 1988]) categories are as follows: I. ADL (activities of daily life) deficient, 6a, b and c; II, incipient incontinence, 6d and e; III, incipient nonverbal, 7a and b; IV, incipient nonambulatory, 7c; and V, immobile, 7d, e and f. The numbers in parentheses indicate the number of patients with contractures in the functional categories. The significance of change in the prevalence of contractures from the preceding functional categories is as follows: between functional categories I and II: $p < 0.01$; between functional categories II and III: $p < 0.05$; between functional categories III and IV: not significant; and between functional categories IV and V: $p < 0.01$. Across the five functional categories, there are significant differences in the proportions of patients with contractures ($X^2 = 88.4$, df = 4, $p < 0.001$). The prevalence of contractures was highly correlated with FAST staging levels ($r = 0.70$, $p < 0.001$). *Source*: data and figure are adapted from Souren, Franssen, and Reisberg, *Journal of the American Geriatrics Society*, 1995; **43**, 650–655

patients and joints which are increasingly immobile. The ulcerations in turn predispose to infections.

The alternative to the terrible scenario of physical disability just described, which appears to presently occur in approximately half of all stage 7 patients, roughly a quarter-of-a-million persons in the United States alone, is a proper program of physical and activity therapy, and retraining and optimal maintenance of basic psychomotor skills. Naturally, both scenarios in the stage 7 AD patient are expensive. The stage 7 AD patient who is neglected develops disabilities, deformities, infections and other complications which increase the costs of care. The patient who receives necessary physical care also has a calculable economic cost of care. Clearly, however, the human costs in terms of suffering are much less for the patient who receives proper physical training and care.

Although some stage 7 patients receive basic physical therapy, which includes some effort to encourage the patients to move, retraining, which is necessary for the maintenance of optimal psychomotor capacity, is received by only a privileged few patients in the world at the present time. This involves modeling, encouraging, assisting, and explicating basic activities on a constant basis. For example, the patient must be shown how to hold a fork, reminded how to chew, reminded how to behave at the table, and so on. These activities must be encouraged and explicated in an emotionally supportive manner. Patient successes must be celebrated and rewarded. Exercising these skills appears to be necessary for both physical and mental health. Failure to exercise these skills results not only in the rigidity, contractures and resulting agitation, which have been noted, but also in the loss of such basic capacities as the ability to chew and to swallow.

Patients in this final seventh stage require mental and emotional stimulation in addition to physical stimulation. An understanding of these needs is readily appreciated if consideration is given to the developmental age.

The DA of the stage 7 AD patient corresponds to infancy, that is, birth to approximately 2 years of age. A stage 7 AD patient requires approximately the same amount of mental, emotional and physical stimulation and care as an infant.

Of course, a basic element in good infant care is love. This love must be expressed physically, emotionally, and verbally. If an infant does not receive this love and they are healthy, they will cry out. If one continues to deprive the infant, they develop an anaclitic depression marked by withdrawal, or, in some cases, a failure to thrive syndrome, marked additionally by a refusal to take sustenance and, consequently, to survive. Patients with AD in stage 7 develop similar kinds of reactions. If they are not given the love and attention which they require, then they withdraw. If they continue to be deprived of love and attention, then this withdrawal becomes increasingly pathological. Some AD patients develop what is also termed in AD a failure to thrive syndrome, in which they refuse sustenance and, unless a nasogastric tube is inserted, the patient succumbs.

Just as in infants, it is necessary for love to be expressed both verbally and physically, the same is true for the AD patient who must receive physical expressions of love, such as being held and kissed. Social attention is also important. A healthy infant is frequently made the 'center of attention' and their every move and accomplishment is a source of delight and even celebration. The same kind of attention is necessary for the stage 7 AD patient. They need to be greeted, they need to be given attention, they need to frequently be the center of attention, and their accomplishments need to be celebrated.

It must be noted that these recommendations for optimal care are vastly divergent from current reality. In most institutional settings, physical expressions of love are prohibited, in some cases being seen as tantamount to assault. Generally, stage 7 patients are not only not celebrated socially, these patients are virtually entirely ignored.

The DA of the stage 7 AD patient also provides a guide to the kinds of activities which are appropriate and useful for these patients. For example, just as a 1 to 2 year old child will enjoy simple ball toss games, an early stage 7 AD patient will enjoy, and benefit from, simple ball toss games. Just as a 1 to 2 year old child may enjoy music, being taken for walks, being dressed up nicely and kept clean, and playing with simple toys, such as a talking animal, the same kind of activities are enjoyed by the stage 7a and 7b AD patient. Various modifications in activities are necessary for the AD patient. For example, AD patients are physically much larger and stronger than infants. Clearly, an informed economic analysis of the costs of AD must take into consideration the costs of these necessary activities.

The DA of the AD patient in stage 7 also provides an indication of basic management needs. For example, like infants, stage 7 AD patients are doubly incontinent. Like small children, continence in stage 7a and 7b semi-verbal AD patients can be, to some extent, supported and maintained by techniques such as modeling, running of water, and frequent toileting. To the extent that continence is not maintained, patients must be cleaned. If they are not kept clean then urine or feces will produce skin irritation, infections, and so on. Clearly, the costs of maintenance of continence and cleanliness are an important consideration in stage 7.

If stage 7 AD patients are provided with the emotional, physical, and management support which is both optimal and, in a human sense, necessary, then the patient is capable of providing a similar human reward for those who care for them and love them. These mutual human rewards are very similar to those which accrue from the care of an infant or 1 to 2 year old child. For example, even though the infant or child may not be able to respond verbally, a loving parent can 'confide' with a child and derive emotional support from the child's acquiescence. The same kind of tacit emotional support is provided by the cared-for and beloved stage 7 AD patient.

The stage 7 AD patient can also provide more explicit empathy and support for their caregivers. For example, an 84 year old stage 7 AD patient receiving excellent community-based care was taken to see her ailing husband in the hospital. When her husband received an injection from the nurse and started to scream, empathetically, his wife with stage 7b AD also started to scream.

In summary, an informed economic analysis of stage 7 AD should consider not only basic management needs but also the costs of maintaining the patients' emotional, social, and physical health. Such an analysis should also consider not only the patient's loss of productivity and care needs, but also the emotional rewards which those who care for the patient derive from the patient's continued life and existence.

OTHER DEMENTING DISORDERS

The economic analysis which has been described for AD applies, to a greater or lesser extent, to other dementing disorders. For example, cerebrovascular dementia generally presents in a very similar manner to AD and the stages are generally identifiable in accordance with the progression of AD. The primary difference between cerebrovascular dementia and AD is that cerebrovascular dementia appears to proceed more rapidly than AD. When significant focal cerebrovascular deficits are present, then the stages of cerebrovascular dementia may present with excess morbidity in comparison with AD.

Some dementias, such as dementia associated with normal pressure hydrocephalus (NPH), or dementia associated with Creutzfeldt–Jakob Disease (CJD) or other transmissible spongiform encephalopathies (prion diseases), do proceed in a more or less different manner than AD. For example, in NPH, gait disturbances and incontinence generally antedate cognitive disturbances and will result in special management needs. However, current research is demonstrating that hydrocephalus is frequently a complication of AD with these special clinical features due to the excess ventricular cerebrospinal fluid accumulation.

CJD sometimes presents with a clinical picture much like AD, although the time course is different and more variable. Sometimes CJD presents with gait disturbances or sensory disturbances, which add to morbidity.

Despite examples of variability, and despite the acknowledged variability in temporal course of dementia depending upon etiology, a remarkable aspect of the dementias is the extent to which they frequently follow a similar clinical path, despite divergent etiologies. For example, a 23 year old man with recently diagnosed spinocerebellar ataxia type 1 (with a 44 substitution on chromosome 6 on genetic testing) and a 7 year history of mental illness, presented with dementia. Although the time course of this man's evolution of dementia pathology was greatly truncated in comparison with the temporal course of dementia in AD, cross-sectionally the dementia appeared to be very similar to the dementia of AD. On the FAST, this 23 year old man was 7a ordinal. Consequently, as per the course of functional loss in AD described in Table 3.2.2, he was unable to attend school (specifically his university classes) (FAST stage 3), was unable to handle complex daily life activities (FAST stage 4), unable to pick out his clothing (FAST stage 5), unable to put on his clothing without assistance (FAST stage 6a), unable to bathe without assistance (FAST stage 6b), unable to toilet properly (he wouldn't always wipe himself properly)

(FAST stage 6c), and he was incontinent of urine and feces (FAST stages 6d and 6e). Furthermore, his speech ability was limited during the course of three hours of evaluation on two separate occasions to two words, which he used repeatedly, 'scared . . . scared' and 'stop' (FAST stage 7b). The patient's FAST score was 7a ordinal. Consequently he did not, at the time of evaluation, have any of the deficits occurring in FAST stages 7b to 7f. Therefore, he could still walk, despite the presence of ataxia. Also, he could still sit up, smile, and hold up his head. In summary, his FAST presentation was very similar to that seen in uncomplicated AD. Cross-sectionally, this case of spinocerebellar ataxia with dementia in this 23 year old man also fits the AD phenotypic pattern in that scores on the Brief Cognitive Rating Scale (BCRS) axes, which are enumerated to be optimally concordant with the FAST in AD patients (Reisberg et al, 1983; Reisberg et al, 1992, 1993, 1996b), were all seven for BCRS Axes I through IV. His score on the BCRS praxis axis, which assesses the ability to draw figures and does not require verbal skills (Reisberg et al, 1990), was also seven, indicating the optimal concordance anticipated for an AD patient in this area. In summary, this dementia, very different from AD in its origins and occurring in a young adult, followed a clinical course very similar to AD. This similarity is often noted in dementing disorders. The reasons for the observed similarity are no doubt due to a common neuropathologic etiopathogenic pathway in diverse dementing disorders. Economically, these observations imply that analyses which are applicable for the stages of AD can frequently be applied to other dementing conditions of non-AD etiology.

CONCLUSION

The evolution of dementing disorder has profound economic consequences which vary enormously depending upon the stage (severity level). Economic consequences can be described for each stage of the dementia of AD. These economic consequences must be placed in the context of optimal care requirements. These economic analyses for AD can, to a greater or lesser extent, be applied to other dementias of diverse etiology.

ACKNOWLEDGEMENT

Supported by the Zachary and Elizabeth M. Fisher Medical Foundation and USDHHS grants AG03051 and AG08051.

REFERENCES

Auer, S. R., Sclan, S. G., Yaffee, R. A. and Reisberg, B. (1994). The neglected half of Alzheimer disease: Cognitive and functional concomitants of severe dementia. *JAGS*, **42**, 1266–1272.

Berg, L. (1984). Clinical dementia rating. *Brit. J. Psychiatry*, **145**, 339.

Berg, L., Danziger, W. L., Storandt, M., Coben, L. A., Gado, M., Hughes, C. P., Knesevich, J. W. and Botwinick, J. (1984). Predictive features in mild senile dementia of the Alzheimer type. *Neurology*, **34**, 563–569.

Berg, L. (1988). Clinical dementia rating (CDR). *Psychopharmacology Bulletin*, **24**, 637–639.

Berg, L., Miller, J. P., Storandt, M., Duchek, J., Morris, J. C., Rubin, E. H., Burke, W. J. and Coben, L. A. (1988). Mild senile dementia of the Alzheimer type: 2. Longitudinal assessment. *Ann. Neurol.*, **23**, 477–484.

Bobinski, M., Wegiel, J., Wisniewski, H. M., Tarnawski, M., Reisberg, B., Mlodzik, B., de Leon, M. J. and Miller, D. C. (1995). Atrophy of hippocampal formation subdivisions correlates with stage and duration of Alzheimer disease. *Dementia*, **6**, 205–210.

Bobinski, M., Wegiel, J., Tarnawski, M., Reisberg, B., de Leon, M. J., Miller, D. C. and Wisniewski, H. M. (1997). Relationships between regional neuronal loss and neurofibrillary changes in the hippocampal formation and duration and severity of Alzheimer disease. *J. Neuropath. Exp. Neurol.*, **56**, 414–420.

Braak, H. and Braak, E. (1996). Development of Alzheimer-related neurofibrillary changes in the neocortex inversely recapitulates cortical myelogenesis. *Acta Neuropathol.*, **92**, 197–201.

Cole, M. G., Dastoor, D. P. and Koszycki, D. (1983). The hierarchic dementia scale. *Journal of Clinical Experimental and Gerontology*, **5**, 219–234.

de Ajuriaguerra, J. and Tissot, R. (1975). Some aspects of language in various forms of senile dementia: Comparisons with language in childhood. In E. H. Lennenberg and E. Lennenberg (Eds), *Foundations of Language Development (Vol. 1)*, New York: Academic Press.

Dura, J. R., Haywood-Niler, E. and Kiecolt-Glaser, J. K. (1990). Spousal caregivers of persons with Alzheimer's and Parkinson's disease dementia: a preliminary comparison. *Gerontologist*, **30**, 332–336.

Flicker, C., Ferris, S. H. and Reisberg, B. (1991). Mild cognitive impairment in the elderly: predictors of dementia. *Neurology*, **41**, 1006–1009.

Flicker, C., Ferris, S. H. and Reisberg, B. (1993a). A longitudinal study of cognitive function in elderly persons with subjective memory complaints. *JAGS*, **41**, 1029–1032.

Flicker, C., Ferris, S. H. and Reisberg, B. (1993b). A two-year longitudinal study of cognitive function in normal aging and Alzheimer's disease. *J. Geriat. Psychiat. Neurol.*, **6**, 84–96.

Folstein, M. F., Folstein, S. E. and McHugh, P. R. (1975). Mini-mental state: A practical method for grading the cognitive state of patients for the clinician. *J. Psychiat. Res.*, **12**, 189–198.

Foster, J. R., Sclan, S., Welkowitz, J., Boksay, I. and Seeland, I. (1988). Psychiatric assessment in medical long-term care facilities: Reliability of commonly used rating scales. *Int. J. Geriat. Psychiat.*, **3**, 229–233.

Franssen, E. H., Reisberg, B., Kluger, A., Sinaiko, E. and Boja, C. (1991). Cognition-independent neurologic symptoms in normal aging and probable Alzheimer's disease. *Arch. Neurol.*, **48**, 148–154.

Franssen, E. H. (1993). Neurologic signs in ageing and dementia. In A. Burns (Ed.), *Aging and Dementia, A Methodological Approach*, pp. 144–174. London: Edward Arnold.

Franssen, E. H., Kluger, A., Torossian, C. L. and Reisberg, B. (1993). The neurologic syndrome of severe Alzheimer's disease: Relationship to functional decline. *Arch. Neurol.*, **50**, 1029–1039.

Franssen, E. H., Souren, L. E. M., Torossian, C. L. and Reisberg, B. (1997). Utility of developmental reflexes in the differential diagnosis and prognosis of incontinence in Alzheimer disease. *J. Geriat. Psychiat. Neurol.*, **10**, 22–28.

Frisoni, G. B., Rozzini, R., Bianchetti, A. and Trabucchi, M. (1993). Principal lifetime occupation and MMSE score in elderly persons. *Journal of Gerontology: Social Sciences*, **48**, S310–S314.

Ganguli, M., Ratcliff, G., Huff, J., Belle, S., Kancel, M. J., Fischer, L. and Kuller, L. H. (1990). Serial sevens versus world backwards: A comparison of the two measures of attention from the MMSE. *J. Geriat. Psychiat. Neurol.*, **3**, 203–207.

German, P. S., Shapiro, S. and Kramer, M. (1985). Nursing home study of the Eastern Baltimore epidemiological catchment area study. In M. S. Harper and B. Lebowitz (Eds), *Mental Illness in Nursing Homes: Agenda for Research*, Washington, DC, NIMH.

Gottlieb, G. L., Gur, R. E. and Gur, R. C. (1988). Reliability of psychiatric scales in patients with dementia of the Alzheimer type. *Am. J. Psychiat.*, **45**, 857–859.

Gurland, B. J., Wilder, D. E., Cross, P., Teresi, J. A. and Barrett, V. W. (1992). Screening scales for dementia: Toward a reconciliation of conflicting cross-cultural findings. *Int. J. Geriat. Psychiat.*, **9**, 105–113.

Hartmaier, S. L., Sloan, P. D., Guess, H. A. and Koch, G. G. (1994). The MDS Cognition Scale: A valid instrument for identifying and staging nursing home residents with dementia using the Minimum Data Set. *JAGS*, **42**, 1173–1179.

Lane, F. and Snowdon, J. (1989). Memory and dementia: A longitudinal survey of suburban elderly. In P. Lovibond and P. Wilson (Eds), *Clinical and Abnormal Psychology*, pp. 365–376. North-Holland: Elsevier Science.

Lowenthal, P. M., Berkman, P. L., Buehler, J. A., Pierce, R. C., Robinson, B. C. and Trier, M. L. (1967). *Aging and Mental Disorder in San Francisco: A Social Psychiatric Study*, San Francisco, Jossey Bass.

McGeer, P. L., McGeer, E. G., Akiyama, H., Itagaki, S., Harrop, R. and Peppard, R. (1990). Neuronal degeneration and memory loss in Alzheimer's disease and aging. *Exp. Brain Res.*, Suppl. **21**, 411–426.

Molloy, D. W., Alemayehu, E. and Roberts, R. (1991). Reliability of a standardized mini-mental state examination compared with the traditional mini-mental state examination. *Am. J. Psychiat.*, **148**, 102–105.

Murden, R. A., McRae, T. D., Kaner, S. and Bucknam, M. E. (1991). Mini-mental state exam scores vary with education in blacks and whites. *JAGS*, **39**, 149–155.

Overall, J. E., Scott, J., Rhoades, H. M. and Lesser, J. (1990). Empirical scaling of the stages of cognitive decline in senile dementia. *J. Geriat. Psychiat. Neurol.*, **3**, 212–220.

Prichep, L. S., John, E. R., Ferris, S. H., Reisberg, B., Alper, K., Almas, M. and Cancro, R. (1994). Quantitative EEG correlates of cognitive deterioration in the elderly. *Neurobiology of Aging*, **15**, 85–90.

Reisberg, B., Ferris, S. H., de Leon, M. J. and Crook, T. (1982). The global deterioration scale for assessment of primary degenerative dementia. *Am. J. Psychiat.*, **139**, 1136–1139.

Reisberg, B., Schneck, M. K., Ferris, S. H., Schwartz, G. E. and de Leon, M. J. (1983). The brief cognitive rating scale (BCRS): Findings in primary degenerative dementia (PDD). *Psychopharmacology Bulletin*, **19**, 47–50.

Reisberg, B. (1984). Stages of cognitive decline. *American Journal of Nursing*, **84**, 225–228.

Reisberg, B., Gordon, B., McCarthy, M., Ferris, S. H. and de Leon, M. J. (1985). Insight and denial accompanying progressive cognitive decline in normal aging and Alzheimer's disease. In B. Stanley (Ed.), *Geriatric Psychiatry: Ethical and Legal Issues*, pp. 37–79. Washington, DC, American Psychiatric Press.

Reisberg, B., Ferris, S. H. and Franssen, E. H. (1986). Functional degenerative stages in dementia of the Alzheimer's type appear to reverse normal human development. In C. Shagass et al (Eds), *Biological Psychiatry 1985, Vol. 7*, pp. 1319–1321. New York: Elsevier Science.

Reisberg, B. (1988). Functional assessment staging (FAST). *Psychopharmacology Bulletin*, **24**, 653–659.

Reisberg, B., Ferris, S. H., de Leon, M. J. and Crook, T. (1988a). The Global Deterioration Scale (GDS). *Psychopharmacology Bulletin*, **24**, 661–663.

Reisberg, B., Ferris, S. H., de Leon, M. J., Sinaiko, E., Franssen, E. H., Kluger, A., Mir, P., Borenstein, J., George, A. E., Shulman, E., Steinberg, G. and Cohen, J. (1988b). Stage-specific behavioral, cognitive, and in vivo changes in community residing subjects with age-associated memory impairment (AAMI) and primary degenerative dementia of the Alzheimer type. *Drug Dev. Res.*, **15**, 101–114.

Reisberg, B., Ferris, S. H., Steinberg, G., Shulman, E., de Leon, M. J. and Sinaiko, E. (1989a). Longitudinal study of dementia patients and aged controls: An approach to methodologic issues. In M. P. Lawton and A. R. Herzog (Eds), *Special Research Methods for Gerontology*, pp. 195–231. Amityville (NY), Baywood Publishers.

Reisberg, B., Franssen, E. H., Sclan, S. G., Kluger, A. and Ferris, S. H. (1989b). Stage specific incidence of potentially remediable behavioral symptoms in aging and Alzheimer's disease: A study of 120 patients using the BEHAVE-AD. *Bull. of Clin. Neurosci.*, **54**, 95–112.

Reisberg, B., Pattschull-Furlan, A., Franssen, E. H., Sclan, S., Kluger, A., Dingcong, L. and Ferris, S. H. (1990). Cognition-related functional, praxis and feeding changes in CNS aging and Alzheimer's disease and their developmental analogies. In K. Beyreuther and G. Schettler (Eds), *Molecular Mechanisms of Aging*, pp. 18–40. Berlin, Springer-Verlag.

Reisberg, B., Ferris, S. H., Torossian, C. L., Kluger, A. and Monteiro, I. (1992). Pharmacologic treatment of Alzheimer's disease: A methodologic critique based upon current knowledge of symptomatology and relevance for drug trials. *Int. Psychogeriat.*, **4** (Suppl. 1), 9–42.

Reisberg, B., Sclan, S. G., Franssen, E. H., de Leon, M. J., Kluger, A., Torossian, C. L., Shulman, E., Steinberg, G., Monteiro, I., McRae, T., Boksay, I., Mackell, J. A. and Ferris, S. H. (1993). Clinical stages of normal aging and Alzheimer's disease: The GDS staging system. *Neurosci. Res. Communications*, **13** (Suppl. 1), 551–554.

Reisberg, B., Ferris, S. H., Franssen, E. H., Shulman, E., Monteiro, I., Sclan, S. G., Steinberg, G., Kluger, A., Torossian, C. L., de Leon, M. J. and Laska, E. (1996a). Mortality and temporal course of probable Alzheimer's disease: A five-year prospective study. *Int. Psychogeriat.*, **8**, 291–311.

Reisberg, B., Franssen, E. H., Bobinski, M., Auer, S. R., Monteiro, I., Boksay, I., Wegiel, J., Shulman, E., Steinberg, G., Souren, L., Kluger, A., Torossian, C. L., Sinaiko, E., Wisniewski, H. M. and Ferris, S. H. (1996b). Overview of methodologic issues for pharmacologic trials in mild, moderate, and severe Alzheimer's disease. *Int. Psychogeriat.*, **8**, 159–193.

Reisberg, B., Auer, S. R., Monteiro, I., Franssen, E. and Kenowsky, S. (1998a). A rational psychological approach to the treatment of behavioral disturbances and symptomatology in Alzheimer's disease (AD) based upon recognition of the developmental age (DA). *International Academy for Biomedical and Drug Research*, **13**, 102–109.

Reisberg, B., Burns, A., Brodaty, H., Eastwood, R., Rossor, M., Sartorius, N. and Winblad, B. (1997a). Diagnosis of Alzheimer's disease: Report of an International Psychogeriatric Association Special Meeting Work Group Under the Cosponsorship of Alzheimer's Disease International, the European Federation of Neurological Societies, the World Health Organization, and the World Psychiatric Association. *Int. Psychogeriat.*, **9** (Suppl. 1), 11–38.

Reisberg, B., Schneider, L., Doody, R., Anand, R., Feldman, H., Haraguchi, H., Kumar, R., Lucca, U., Mangone, C. A., Mohr, E., Morris, J. C., Rogers, S. and Sawada, T. (1997b). Clinical global measures of dementia: position paper from the International Working Group on Harmonization of Dementia Drug Guidelines. *Alzheimer Disease and Associated Disorders*, **11** (Suppl. 3), 8–18.

Reisberg, B., Franssen, E. H., Souren, L. E. M., Auer, S. and Kenowsky, S. (1998b). Progression of Alzheimer's Disease: Variability and consistency: Ontogenic models, their applicability and relevance. *J. Neural. Transm.*, In Press.

Reisberg, B. and Kluger, A. (1998). Assessing the progression of dementia: Diagnostic considerations. In C. Salzman (Ed.), *Clinical Geriatric Psychopharmacology*, 3rd edn., pp. 432–462. Baltimore: Williams and Wilkins.

Sclan, S. G., Foster, J. R., Reisberg, B., Franssen, E. H. and Welkowitz, J. (1990). Application of Piagetian measures of cognition in severe Alzheimer's disease. *Psychiatric Journal of the University of Ottawa*, **15**, 221–226.

Sclan, S. G., Saillon, A., Franssen, E. H., Hugonot-Diener, L. and Reisberg, B. (1996). The Behavioral Pathology in Alzheimer's Disease Rating Scale (BEHAVE-AD): Reliability and analysis of symptom category scores. *Int. J. Geriat. Psychiat.*, **11**, 819–830.

Sclan, S. G. and Reisberg, B. (1992). Functional assessment staging (FAST) in Alzheimer's disease: Reliability, validity and ordinality. *Int. Psychogeriat.*, **4** (Suppl. 1), 55–69.

Sluss, T. K., Rabins, P. and Gruenberg, E. M. (1980). Memory complaints in community residing men. *Gerontologist (Part II)*, **20**, 201 (Abstract).

Souren, L. E. M., Franssen, E. M. and Reisberg, B. (1995). Contractures and loss of function in patients with Alzheimer's disease. *JAGS*, **43**, 650–655.

Tangalos, E. G., Smith, G. E., Ivnik, R. J., Petersen, R. C., Kokmen, E., Kurland, L. T., Offord, K. P. and Parisi, J. E. (1996). The Mini-Mental State Examination in general medical practice: Clinical utility and acceptance. *Mayo Clinic Proceedings*, **71**, 829–837.

Teresi, J. A., Lawton, M. P., Ory, M. and Holmes, D. (1994). Measurement issues in chronic care populations: dementia special care. *Alz. Dis. Assoc. Dis.*, **8**, S144–S183.

Tombaugh, T. N. and McIntyre, N. J. (1992). The Mini-Mental State Examination: A comprehensive review. *JAGS*, **40**, 922–935.

Uhlmann, R. F. and Larson, E. B. (1991). Effect of education on the Mini-Mental State Examination as a screening test for dementia. *JAGS*, **39**, 876–880.

Weiss, B. D., Reed, R., Kligman, E. W. and Abyad, A. (1995). Literacy and performance on the Mini-Mental State Examination. *JAGS*, **43**, 807–810.

3.3 Measuring QALYs in Dementia

PETER J. NEUMANN
Harvard School of Public Health, Boston, MA, USA

RICHARD C. HERMANN
Cambridge Hospital, Cambridge, and Harvard Medical School, Boston, MA, USA

MILTON C. WEINSTEIN
Harvard School of Public Health, Boston, MA, USA

INTRODUCTION

While it has become increasingly common for cost-effectiveness analyses (CEAs) in health and medicine to measure effectiveness in terms of quality-adjusted life-years (QALYs) gained, there has been little applied work in the area of dementia. This chapter explores issues raised in such applications. The first section provides some background on the QALY concept and the debate over appropriate estimation techniques. The second section discusses key challenges in applying QALYs in the context of dementia. The chapter concludes with an example drawn from a recent study.

QALYS AS A MEASURE OF HEALTH BENEFITS

THE QALY CONCEPT

One way to assess the health effectiveness of a treatment for dementia is with an instrument such as the Mini-Mental State Exam (MMSE), which measures cognitive aspects of mental functioning (Folstein et al, 1975). For example, analysts could assess a new drug for Alzheimer's disease by comparing changes in MMSE scores for patients on treatment versus no treatment. The advantage of using a scale such as the MMSE is that it focuses on a dimension of primary interest—cognitive functioning—and is familiar to the clinicians who treat AD patients.

One limitation of such a scale is that it does not capture the impact of the drug on a person's quality of life or overall well-being. A second drawback is

Health Economics of Dementia. Edited by Anders Wimo, Bengt Jönsson, Göran Karlsson and Bengt Winblad.
© 1998 John Wiley & Sons Ltd.

that it does not permit comparisons of treatments for dementia with interventions for other medical conditions. Conceivably, both of these objectives could be accomplished by using a 'generic' health-status instrument, such as the Short Form (SF)-36 (Ware and Sherbourne, 1992), which measures a range of health attributes, including physical and role functioning, bodily pain, and mental health, and is designed for use across diverse illnesses and populations.

But while useful in discriminating levels of health status among groups and in detecting changes in health status over time (Revicki and Kaplan, 1993), the numeric scores of health status scales do not necessarily reflect the values that people attach to different health outcomes. Measuring these values is essential in determining how to allocate resources efficiently—that is, how to provide more health outcomes that people desire and fewer that they do not (Gold et al, 1996).

QALYs are useful as a measure of health benefit because they capture both quantity- and quality-of-life effects, because they reflect individual values for different health outcomes, and because they permit comparisons across diverse interventions. The QALY approach depicts life as a series of 'quality-weighted' health states, where the quality weights reflect the desirability of living in each state. A higher weight reflects a more preferred state; generally, a health state is rated on a scale in which a weight of 0.0 corresponds to death and a weight of 1.0 corresponds to 'good health' or 'best attainable health.' The quality weight for each state is multiplied by the time spent in the state; these products are summed to obtain the total number of QALYs.

The advantage of using QALYs in cost-effectiveness analyses[1] for societal resource allocation decisions has been recognized in recommendations of the US Panel on Cost-Effectiveness in Health and Medicine (Weinstein et al, 1996), in guidelines for the economic evaluation of pharmaceuticals in both Australia and Canada (Henry, 1992; Ministry of Health, 1992), and in the large and growing number of studies in the medical literature for interventions as diverse as cardiovascular treatment, cancer, and AIDS (Neumann et al, 1997a).

Alternatives to QALYs, including disability-adjusted life-years (DALY) (Murray, 1994) and healthy-years equivalents (HYE) (Mehrez and Gafni, 1989), have been proposed, though both have limitations. DALYs may be criticized because the weightings of health states are based on economic productivity rather than social preferences, and HYEs are not practical because they require independent valuations of all possible health scenarios rather than individual health states (Johannesson et al, 1993).

METHODOLOGICAL ISSUES

Over the years, researchers have debated the appropriate techniques for estimating QALYs. One issue concerns the relation between quality-of-life weights based on direct, holistic utility assessment versus weights based on prespecified health-state classification systems. Under the direct, holistic utility assessment, patients are asked a time trade-off, standard gamble, or rating scale question in which their current health state is placed on a 0–1 scale between perfect health (1.0) and death (0.0).

Standard gamble and time trade-off methods involve asking respondents to value health states (e.g., a state with mild chest pain and limited ambulation) by considering explicitly how much they would be willing to sacrifice—in terms of risk of death or of time living in good health—in order to avoid being in the state. In the standard gamble approach, respondents are asked to weigh a choice between continuing life in the health state under consideration, or selecting a gamble in which the possible outcomes are full health and death (Torrance, 1986). The probabilities in the gamble are altered until the respondents are indifferent between the gamble and continued life in the given health state; the expected value of the gamble at this point is the utility for the health state. In the time trade-off approach, respondents are asked to trade-off life-years in a health state for a shorter life span in a state of perfect health (Torrance et al, 1972). The rating scales involve asking respondents to rate the strength of their preferences on either a visual analogue (e.g., 10 cm linear) scale or a numerical (e.g., 0–100) scale.

In contrast, the idea behind health-state classification systems is that patients can be classified, based on clinical information, into appropriate strata, each of which reflects a unique combination of dimensions and levels of severity. For example, patients with Alzheimer's disease would be assigned, based on their clinical profiles, into relevant cells of the classification system. The patient—or an observer, who is likely to be a clinician or a family member—would complete a questionnaire that asks about the patient's functioning on the domains of the system such as self-care, ambulation, and cognition. Once the individual is 'mapped' into the system, previously obtained preferences of individuals in the community for various cells of the system would be used for the quality weights.[2] An illustration of the process is presented in Figure 3.3.1.

Health-state classification systems may be generic or disease-specific. Examples of generic systems for which preference weights have been obtained include the Health Utilities Index developed at McMaster University (Torrance, 1986; Feeny et al, 1995; Torrance et al, 1995), the Quality of Well-Being Scale developed at the University of California, San Diego (Kaplan et al, 1989) and the EuroQol (EuroQoL Group, 1990). Though they differ in terms of how they define the relevant domains or attributes of health, as well as the level of severity within each domain, the systems are designed to be comprehensive and general enough to apply to many different types of treatments and conditions. For example, the EuroQol system uses five attributes of health—mobility, self-care, usual activities, pain/discomfort, anxiety/depression—at three levels of severity for each, resulting in 243 (3^5) health states. The Health Utilities Index Mark III contains eight dimensions: vision, hearing, speech, emotion, pain, ambulation, dexterity, and cognition. The

362

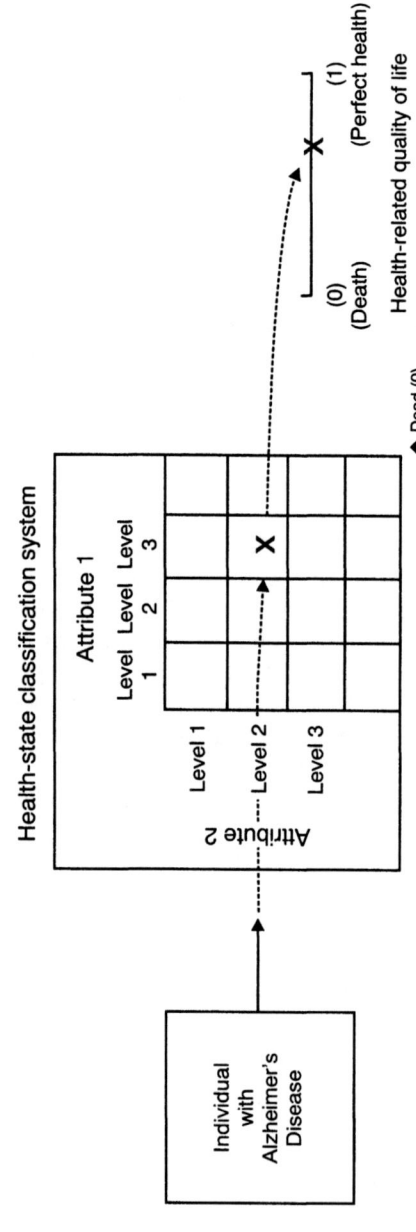

Step 1: Individual with AD is assigned, based on their clinical condition, to a cell in the health-state classification system

Step 2: The cell is mapped to a preference score, based on previously-obtained preference weights

Figure 3.3.1. Assigning preferences to health stakes for individuals with Alzheimer's disease. *Source:* adapted from Gold, M. R., Siegel, J. E., Russell, L. B. and Weinstein, M. C (1996). *Cost-effectiveness in Health and Medicine.* New York, Oxford University Press

cognition dimension in turn is comprised of six levels of severity, encompassing the most important combinations of *memory* (1—able to remember most things; 2—somewhat forgetful; 3—very forgetful; and 4—unable to remember anything at all), and *thinking* (1—able to think clearly and solve day-to-day problems; 2—have a little difficulty when trying to think and solve day-to-day problems; 3—have some difficulty when trying to think and solve day-to-day problems; 4—have great difficulty when trying to think and solve day-to-day problems; and 5—unable to think or solve day-to-day problems).

Disease-specific classification systems define health states explicitly to capture the dimensions of health relevant to a particular condition or treatment. An example is the Quality-adjusted Time Without Symptoms or Toxicity (Q-TWiST), a cancer-specific classification system, which describes health states based on whether a patient has treatment toxicity, symptoms of the disease, neither, or both (Gelber and Goldhirsch, 1986; Goldhirsch et al, 1989).

A second methodological issue in the estimation of QALYs pertains to the question of whose preferences should form the basis for the quality weights. One option is to use patient preferences, since they reflect the values of the individuals affected most directly by clinical decisions. A common and convenient practice has been to use the preferences of the study investigators themselves, or the preferences of clinicians, under the rationale that these individuals represent the most informed decision makers by virtue of their medical expertise (Neumann et al, 1997a). Another alternative is to use a representative sample of the population. The argument for this approach is that societal resource allocation decisions should be made by appealing to population-based 'community' values.

Other methodological issues concern the appropriate measurement technique (that is, standard gamble, time trade-off, or rating scale method) for constructing the quality weights, and whether to quality-adjust life-years added as a result of an intervention.

RECOMMENDATIONS FOR PRACTICE

One guide to currently recommended practices for estimating QALYs comes from the US Panel on Cost-Effectiveness in Health and Medicine, which was charged with 'assessing the state of the science of the field, and with providing recommendations for the conduct of studies in order to improve their quality and encourage their comparability' (Gold et al, 1996). Among other recommendations, the Panel proposed the use of a 'reference case,' or standard set of methodologic practices that an analyst would seek to follow in a cost-effectiveness analysis (CEA) if results from different studies are to be compared. The Panel recommends that reference case cost-effectiveness analyses use QALYs as their measure of health effectiveness.

In terms of selecting a health-state classification system, the Panel recommends that the system should reflect the domains important for the particular problem under consideration. If the CEA is intended for use in a reference case, the system used should be a generic one, or be calibrated in such a way that it is capable of being compared with a generic system.

For the source of preferences, the Panel recommends that community weights for health states are most appropriate for use in a reference case analysis, and that weights should be collected from a representative sample of the general population. The Panel argues that a consistent set of community weights for health conditions and health states, used across studies intended to assist in resource allocation decisions, would significantly improve the comparability of analyses.

In terms of valuing health states, the Panel recommends that quality weights should be preference-based (that is, they should reflect people's values for being in the states). Furthermore, the Panel advocates that if results are based upon measurement techniques such as rating scales, they should be compared with results obtained using trade-off methods such as the time trade-off or standard gamble approaches.

Finally, the Panel notes that the health-related quality of life of those whose lives have been saved or extended by a health intervention may be influenced by age, gender, race, or socioeconomic status, and recommends that sensitivity analysis should be conducted to indicate explicitly how the analysis is affected by these characteristics.

In practice, few studies in the literature have adhered to these recommendations, and it remains to be seen whether practice will change. A recent study of 86 original cost-effectiveness analyses, published between 1975 and 1995, which used QALYs as their measure of effectiveness, found extensive variation in the manner in which researchers have estimated QALYs (Neumann et al, 1997a). Only 20% of the studies followed the Panel's recommendation to use a preexisting generic system (e.g., Health Utilities Index); 21% complied with the Panel's recommendation to use community-based weights; and 40% used a formal measurement technique (e.g., time trade-off method). The lack of uniformity in methodology for QALY valuation raises questions regarding the usefulness of previous studies for policy makers.

APPLYING QALYs IN THE CONTEXT OF DEMENTIA

Conceptualizing and measuring health-related quality of life in the context of dementia raises a number of challenges. Researchers have questioned, for example, whether intact cognitive ability is necessary for happiness and emotional well-being (Whitehouse and Rabins, 1992).

Estimating QALYs in accordance with the standard recommendations of the Panel on Cost-Effectiveness in Health and Medicine raises several specific challenges. One involves the sensitivity of generic health-state classification systems to the changes characteristic of dementia (DeJong et al, 1989;

Neumann et al, 1997b). For example, some generic health status scales contain a 'physical functioning' attribute, though simply being able to function physically is not the same as being able to perform activities of self-care (Revicki and Kaplan, 1993). Other dementia-specific attributes that may be ill-captured by generic scales include: one's ability to participate in enjoyable activities; one's ability to perform household tasks; the degree of frustration or confusion; the extent to which a person can leave their immediate neighborhood and travel on public transportation; and one's ability to function in social settings (DeJong et al, 1989; Stewart et al, 1994). It may also be important to capture changes attributable to setting of care—for example, residence in a nursing home may cause feelings of depersonalization, lack of autonomy, and social distance from friends and family (Stewart et al, 1996). More research is needed to assess the ability of existing generic instruments to measure health-related quality of life in demented populations, and perhaps to develop disease-specific instruments if necessary.

A second challenge relates to the elicitation of information. Obtaining information from individuals with dementia can be extremely difficult given patients' cognitive and behavioral problems (Teresi et al, 1994; Brod and Stewart, 1994; Stewart et al, 1996). Direct utility assessment may be impossible, given the complex nature of the task—which is difficult even for many individuals without cognitive impairments. Symptoms that accompany dementia such as depression can exacerbate this problem (Teri and Logsdon, 1995).

While some patients with early to moderate dementia might be capable of responding to limited questions (Stewart et al, 1996), the use of proxy respondents may be necessary in analyses of QALYs in dementia. However, proxy respondents—who are typically caregivers of patients—often have their own shortcomings. For one, caregivers themselves may be elderly and chronically ill. Moreover, proxy respondents generally tend to rate disability higher than do patients (Magaziner et al, 1988; Epstein et al, 1989), though the magnitude and nature of bias depends on a variety of factors, such as the type of caregiver, the rater's skill and knowledge of the resident, and the thoroughness of the assessment (DeJong et al, 1989; Teresi et al, 1994; Stewart et al, 1996). More research to validate the use of proxy respondents in dementia is needed.

AN EXAMPLE

A recent cost-effectiveness analysis of a new treatment for Alzheimer's disease (Neumann et al, 1997c) illustrates some of the problems and opportunities involved in estimating QALYs in the context of dementia. The objective of this analysis was to estimate the incremental cost per QALY gained associated with the use of a new drug for Alzheimer's disease, donepezil, in treating mild or moderate Alzheimer's disease patients compared to the option of no treatment. The study involved the development of a Markov model to characterize AD in terms of progression through different health states (mild, moderate or severe AD) and residential settings (community or nursing home). As cohorts of patients with and without the drug cycle through the model, they accrue costs and quality-of-life weights associated with each stage and setting for each cycle, providing the basis for calculating the incremental cost per QALY gained.

Because preference-weighted measures were not included in the original randomized clinical trial of the drug (Rogers et al, 1998), the study relied upon a companion, cross-sectional study of 528 caregivers of Alzheimer's disease patients, stratified by disease stage (mild, moderate, and severe, based on CDR staging), and setting of care (community and nursing home) to obtain the utility weights. The 528 patients included 201 mild, 175 moderate, and 142 severe; of these 354 were cared for in community settings and 164 in nursing homes.

In the cross-sectional study, the study investigators administered the Health Utilities Index Mark II (HUI:2) along with a battery of other instruments (Leon, 1996). The HUI:2 was chosen because it provides a means of obtaining community-based preference weights in accordance with the Panel recommendations (Weinstein et al, 1996) for reference case analyses, and because weights are based on the standard gamble. Another advantage of the HUI:2 is that, unlike other preference-weighted, health-status classification systems (e.g., EuroQol), the HUI:2 contains cognition as a separate attribute, which may make it more sensitive to changes in Alzheimer's disease stage. The HUI:3 could not be used for this study because its weights had not been finalized at the time.

Due to limitations in patients' abilities to respond to questions themselves, primary caregivers (in most cases the spouse or adult child of the patient) were asked to complete the HUI:2 questionnaire as proxy respondents. These caregivers were also asked to assess separately their own health, under the hypothesis that caregivers' own health-related quality of life might be influenced by patient disease stage and setting. The responses of the questionnaire were then converted into preference weights using the HUI Mark II multi-attribute utility function (Torrance et al, 1995).

Table 3.3.1 shows the weights obtained from the cross-sectional study for AD patients and caregivers. The weights suggest that patient values are sensitive to Alzheimer's disease stages and settings of care. On the other hand, caregiver preferences appear to be insensitive to the stage and setting of the patient, which may reflect the fact that the health-related quality of life of caregivers is the result of complex factors that are not well-captured by the attributes of the HUI or not well-reflected in the aggregated scores.

There are a number of limitations associated with the exercise. First, the HUI has not been validated for use in Alzheimer's disease. Second, since the data were not collected as part of the clinical trial itself, it is unclear how the drug itself affects health-related quality of life, or how health-related

Table 3.3.1. Estimates of quality-of-life weights across
Alzheimer's disease stages and settings of care

Stage/Setting	Quality-of-life weights	
	Patients	Caregivers
Mild AD		
Community	0.68	0.86
Nursing Home	0.71	0.86
Moderate AD		
Community	0.54	0.86
Nursing Home	0.48	0.88
Severe AD		
Community	0.37	0.86
Nursing Home	0.31	0.88

Source: Neumann, P. J., Kuntz, K. M., Hermann, R. C., Duff, S.,
Leon, J., Schaffler, P. A., Goldman, P., and Weinstein, M. C., The Cost
Effectiveness of Donepezil in the Treatment of Mild or Moderate
Alzheimer's Disease. Presentation at the Annual Meeting of the Society
for Medical Decision Making, Houston, October 1997.

quality of life changes with disease progression for individual patients. A
related problem is that the variability in the preference weights across disease
stages and settings in the cross-sectional study could reflect other comorbid
conditions apart from dementia. As noted above, the use of proxy respondents
in the cross-sectional study is also potentially problematic. Research to explore
these data in greater detail is ongoing.

CONCLUSIONS

QALYs provide a potentially valuable means of capturing health-related
quality of life and survival effects in a single aggregated score. But while there
has been a dramatic increase in the performance and publication of cost-
effectiveness analyses using QALYs in recent years, the methods used have
varied widely, raising questions about the usefulness of the information to
policy makers for societal resource allocation decisions. The comparability and
utility of future cost-effectiveness analyses would be enhanced if analysts use
standardized methods across studies.

Estimating QALYs in the context of dementia presents some unique challenges given the cognitive impairments of patients. But the possibility of using
QALYs in dementia exists: one way to obtain preference weights for patients is
for clinicians or caregivers to assign them into prespecified health-state classification systems for which community preferences have already been obtained.
Such an approach would be consistent with recommendations of leaders in the
field to use community-based preference weights for cost-effectiveness analyses
using QALYs. In addition, this method avoids the problem of eliciting

preferences from demented individuals themselves. Researchers might also assess the preferences of their caregivers, since these individuals may be substantially affected by patients' conditions. The usefulness and validity of these techniques should be investigated in the years ahead.

ACKNOWLEDGEMENT

Segments of this chapter have been adapted from Neumann et al (1997a) and Neumann et al (1997b).

NOTES

1 Some authors refer to cost-effectiveness analyses that use QALYs as their measure of effectiveness as 'cost-utility' analyses (e.g., Drummond et al, 1987). In this paper, we follow the practice of the US Panel on Cost-Effectiveness in Health and Medicine to describe such studies using the more generic term, cost-effectiveness analyses (Gold et al, 1996).
2 The time trade-off, standard gamble or rating scale approach has been used as the means of obtaining the community-based weights.

REFERENCES

Brod, M. and Stewart, A. L. (1994). Quality of life in persons with dementia: a theoretical framework. *Gerontologist*, **34**, 47.

DeJong, R., Osterlund, O. W. and Roy, G. W. (1989). Measurement of quality-of-life changes in patients with Alzheimer's Disease. *Clinical Therapeutics*, **11**, 545–554.

Drummond, M. F., Stoddart, G. L. and Torrance, G. W. (1987). *Methods for the Economic Evaluation of Health Care Programmes*. Oxford, UK, Oxford University Press.

Epstein, A. M., Hall, J. A., Tognetti, J. et al (1989). Using proxies to evaluate quality of life: can they provide valid information about patients' health status and satisfaction with medical care? *Medical Care*, **27**(suppl), S91–S98.

EuroQol Group (1990). EuroQol: a new facility for the measurement of health-related quality of life. *Health Policy*, **16**, 199–208.

Feeny, D., Furlong, W., Boyle, M. and Torrance, G. W. (1995). Multi-attribute health status classification systems: Health Utilities Index. *PharmacoEconomics*, **7**(6), 490–502.

Folstein, M. F., Folstein, S. E. and McHugh, P. R. (1975). Mini-Mental State: A practical method for grading the cognitive state of patients for the clinician. *J. Psychiat. Res.*, **12**, 189–198.

Gelber, R. D. and Goldhirsch, A. (1986). A new endpoint for the assessment of adjuvant therapy in postmenopausal women with operable breast cancer. *J. Clin. Oncol.*, **4**, 1772–1779.

Gold, M. R., Siegel, J. E., Russell, L. B. and Weinstein, M. C. (Eds) (1996). *Cost-effectiveness in Health and Medicine*. New York, Oxford University Press.

Goldhirsch, A., Gelber, R. D., Simes, R. J. et al (1989). Costs and benefits of adjuvant therapy in breast cancer: A quality-adjusted survival analysis. *J. Clin. Oncol.*, **7**, 36–44.

Henry, D. (1992). Economic analysis as an aid to subsidization decision: the development of Australian guidelines for pharmaceuticals. *PharmacoEconomics*, **1**, 54–67.

Johannesson, M., Pliskin, J. S. and Weinstein, M. C. (1993). Are healthy-years equivalents an improvement over quality-adjusted life-years? *Medical Decision Making*, **13**, 281–286.

Kaplan, R. M., Anderson, J. P., Wu, A. W., Matthews, W. C., Kozin, F. and Orenstein, D. (1989). The Quality of Well-Being Scale: applications in AIDS, Cystic Fibrosis, and arthritis. *Med. Care*, **27**(3 Suppl), S27–S43.

Leon, J. (1996). *A Proposal for a Cross-Sectional Outcomes Research Study of Individuals with Alzheimer's Disease*, Project HOPE Center for Health Affairs, Bethesda, MD, June.

Magaziner, J., Simonsick, E. M., Kashner, T. M. and Hebel, J. R. (1988). Patient-proxy response comparability on measures of patient health and functional status. *J. Clin. Epidemiol.*, **41**(11), 1065–1074.

Mehrez, A. and Gafni, A. (1989). Quality-adjusted life-years, utility theory, and healthy years equivalents. *Medical Decision Making*, **9**, 142–149.

Ministry of Health, Drug Programs Branch, Toronto, Canada (1992). *Memorandum Subject: Status Report on Ontario's Draft Guidelines for Economic Analysis of Drugs*, May 7.

Murray, C. J. L. (1994). Quantifying the burden of disease: the technical basis for disability-adjusted life-years. *Bulletin of the World Health Organization*, **72**(3), 429–445.

Neumann, P. J., Zinner, D. E. and Wright, J. C. (1997a). Are methods for estimating QALYs in cost-effectiveness analyses improving? *Medical Decision Making*, **17**, 402–408.

Neumann, P. J., Hermann, R. C., Berenbaum, P. A. and Weinstein, M. C. (1997b). Methods of cost-effectiveness analysis in the assessment of new drugs for Alzheimer's disease. *Psychiatric Services*, **48**, 1440–1444.

Neumann, P. J., Kuntz, K. M., Hermann, R. C., Duff, S., Leon, J., Berenbaum, P. A., Goldman, P. and Weinstein, M. C. (1997c). The Cost Effectiveness of Donepezil in the Treatment of Mild or Moderate Alzheimer's Disease. Abstract. *Medical Decision Making*, **17**, 532.

Revicki, D. A. and Kaplan, R. M. (1993). Relationship between psychometric and utility-based approaches to the measurement of health-related quality of life. *Quality of Life Research*, **2**, 477–487.

Rogers, S. L., Farlow, M. R., Mohs, R., Friedhoff, L. T. and Donepezil Study Group (1998). A 24-week, double-blind, placebo-controlled trial of donepezil in patients with Alzheimer's disease. *Neurology* (in press).

Stewart, A. L. and King, A. C. (1994). Conceptualizing and measuring quality of life in older populations. In R. P. Abeles, H. C. Gift and M. G. Ory (Eds), *Aging and Quality of Life*. New York, Springer.

Stewart, A. L., Sherbourne, C. D. and Brod, M. (1996). Measuring health-related quality of life in older and demented populations. In *Quality of Life and Pharmacoeconomics in Clinical Trials*, B. Spilker (Ed.), 2nd edn, pp. 819–830, Philadelphia, Lippencott-Raven.

Teresi, J., Lawton, M. P., Ory, M. and Holmes, D. (1994). Measurement issues in chronic care populations: dementia special care. *Alzheimer Disease and Associated Disorders*, **8**(suppl 1), S144–S183.

Teri, L. and Logsdon, R. G. (1995). Methodologic issues regarding outcome measures for clinical drug trials of psychiatric complications in dementia. *Journal of Geriatric Psychiatry and Neurology*, **8**(suppl 1), S8–S17.

Torrance, G. W. (1986). Measurement of health state utilities for economic appraisal. *J. Health Econ.*, **5**, 1–30.

Torrance, G. W., Thomas, W. H. and Sackett, D. L. (1972). A utility maximation model for evaluation of health programs. *Health Services Research*, **7**, 118–133.

Torrance, G. W., Furlong, W., Feeny, D. and Boyle, M. (1995). Multi-attribute preference functions: Health Utilities Index. *PharmacoEconomics*, **7**(6), 503–520.

Ware, J. E. and Sherbourne, C. D. (1992). The MOS 36-item short form health survey (SF-36): I. Conceptual Framework and Item Selection. *Med. Care*, **30**(6), 473–483.

Weinstein, M. C., Siegel, J. E., Gold, M. R., Kamlet, M. S., Russell, L. B. for the Panel on Cost-Effectiveness in Health and Medicine (1996). Recommendations of the Panel on Cost-effectiveness in Health and Medicine. *JAMA*, **276**(15), 1253–1258.

Whitehouse, P. J. and Rabins, P. V. (1992). Quality of life and dementia. *Alzheimer Disease and Associated Disorders*, **6**, 135–137.

3.4 Assessing ADL/IADL in Persons with Dementia

LOUISE NYGÅRD

Huddinge University Hospital, Huddinge and Karolinska Institute, Stockholm, Sweden

THE CONCEPTS OF ADL/IADL

Activities of daily living (ADL) and instrumental activities of daily living (IADL) are two widely used concepts in different areas of medical and human science, and the scope and the definitions of the concepts therefore also vary greatly both in the literature and in practical use. For example, most activities that are performed by humans in a society may be considered to be ADL/IADL, since they occur in our daily lives. However, although leisure, vocational, religious and sexual activities are part of many peoples' daily lives, they are not generally considered to be ADL/IADL activities and usually not included in such assessment scales (Törnquist, 1995).

Certain aspects of ADL/IADLs are also often included in global *functional scales* (see for example Reisberg et al, 1996). However, such scales are not intended to measure ADL/IADL ability *per se*, but to describe and identify stages of disease severity. Another related concept is *functional health*, which also explicitly or implicitly may include ADL/IADL, although conceptualized differently. For example, in a study by Willis (1996) *everyday cognitive competence* is defined as 'the ability to perform adequately those cognitively complex tasks of daily living considered essential for living on one's own in society' (p. 595). Obviously, aspects of ADL/IADL are considered important enough to be present in most attempts to access human function, although in different conceptualizations.

In most health care praxis, the concept ADL is often used as incorporating self-care activities of daily living, such as toileting, dressing, eating, grooming, ambulating and bathing. These self-care activities are also sometimes referred to as personal or physical activities of daily living, PADL. The concept of IADL is often used for complex activities, including items such as shopping, food preparation, housekeeping, and use of private or public transportation. The distinction between PADL and IADL was first introduced by Lawton and

Health Economics of Dementia. Edited by Anders Wimo, Bengt Jönsson, Göran Karlsson and Bengt Winblad.
© 1998 John Wiley & Sons Ltd.

Brody (1969), and has been commonly accepted for more than a decade (Törnquist, 1995). As will be obvious in this chapter, different scales include different ADL/IADL tasks and items. Moreover, different scales attempt to measure ADL/IADL in different modalities, such as dependency or safety, and for different reasons, as will be further discussed. I will hereafter generally use the general concept of ADL/IADL, except when referring to authors who use other specified concepts.

ASSESSING ADL/IADL IN PERSONS WITH DEMENTIA

Although dementing diseases are first and foremost considered to cause cognitive impairment, it is also obvious that they cause limitations to a person's ADL/IADL ability. While most health care professionals would agree so far, the conceptions of the ADL/IADL limitations may vary between professionals, as may both the descriptions and the assessment techniques of the manifestations of the disease in the afflicted persons' daily lives. Consequently, there are also many different reasons for assessing ADL/IADL and many different opinions of what might cause disability in ADL/IADL among persons with dementia. This chapter will cover these issues without any claim to represent a current consensus. Rather, the aim will be to present examples of how these issues may be viewed in our contemporary body of knowledge, and to discuss them. Finally, the chapter will also provide a short reflection on the actual assumption that meaningful human activity may be scientifically objectified and measured in terms of mathematical symbols.

ADL/IADL LIMITATIONS DURING DEMENTIA PROGRESSION

Descriptions of the progressive decline in ADL/IADL in dementia must be undertaken with great caution, since there seems to be significant variability in both the rate and severity of the decline (Bennet and Knopmann, 1994). However, several studies indicate that a dementing disease first affects the person's ability to carry out the most complex activities. At the onset of the disease, the person, if not yet retired, often first experiences changes in vocational capacity (Reisberg et al, 1996; Robinson et al, 1997). The early phase of dementia also often impacts on the person's social activity (DeJong et al, 1989).

Many studies suggest that the ability to perform IADLs generally is affected earlier than self-care ADLs (Galasko et al, 1991; Green et al, 1993; Juva et al, 1994; Loewenstein and Rupert, 1995; Poon, 1994; Stern et al, 1990). Certain IADL activities also seem to be impaired very early on in the disease progression and could therefore be used as dementia indicators in screening surveys: for example telephone use, use of transport, handling medication intake, budget management (Barberger-Gateau et al, 1993) and preparing a letter for mailing (Loewenstein et al, 1995).

However, there seem to be more discrepancies in the declining profile regarding self-care ADLs than IADLs in general among persons with dementia (Juva et al, 1994). Reisberg et al (1996) showed evidence of need for assistance in choosing proper attire when dressing before need for assistance in dressing, bathing and mechanisms of toileting in the moderately severe to severe stages of dementia. In a study of object use in self-care ADLs among persons with moderate to severe dementia, the ability to use a spoon and fork in eating seemed to be better preserved than the ability to use a comb (Borell et al, 1993). In the final stages of the disease, loss of continence, communication skills, and motor movements occurs (Reisberg et al, 1996; Woods, 1991). While the decline may show great individual discrepancies, the needs for assistance and support in ADL/IADL increase with the progression of the disease.

WHAT CAUSES ADL/IADL LIMITATIONS AMONG PERSONS WITH DEMENTIA AND WHY ASSESS ADL/IADL?

Since dementing diseases are regarded primarily as cognitive diseases of the brain, one would expect that the limitations in ADL/IADL ability should also be directly related to the cognitive impairment. While many studies have shown evidence of significant relationships between cognition or mental capacity and ADL/IADL ability (see for example Aske, 1990; Hill et al, 1995; Loewenstein et al, 1992; Nygård, 1996; Reed et al, 1989), no known study has explained the variability in ADL/IADL ability with cognition to a higher degree than 50% (Nygård, 1996). Therefore, multifactorial explanations of the cause of ADL/IADL disability in persons with dementia seem inevitable, and there are many suggestions of what might affect the ability to carry out daily activities.

Apraxia or dyspraxia, as well as agnosia, are common symptoms in dementia that might cause functional disability (APA, 1995; Kramer and Duffy, 1996). Memory impairment might directly impact on activity performance, as for example when a person forgets to do something or forgets that a task has already been completed (Woods, 1991). Further, sequencing failures and lapses of judgment may cause ADL/IADL problems, as for example when misjudging the need for a bath or having problems in sequencing the steps and actions needed to complete an activity (Woods, 1991). Declining ability to sequence and plan an activity has recently been included as a dementia criterion in the DSM-IV (APA, 1995). Volition is another important source of influence on activity performance (Kielhofner, 1995; Woods, 1991). Additionally, the person with dementia might have additional physical impairments which impact on the ADL/IADL ability, and the familiarity of the environment might affect the person's performance (Woods, 1991; Nygård, 1996).

Other factors that might have influence on the ADL/IADL performance are the person's compensational efforts (Nygård and Borell, 1995), the individual meaning of the experienced decline in ability (Nygård et al, 1995), age (Zanetti et al, 1993), the degree of assistance from a caregiver, neuropsychological heterogeneity, insight into the disease, psychiatric symptoms, co-morbidity, pre-morbid personality, education, occupation, and psycho-relational environment (Zanetti et al, 1995).

When confronted with the multiplicity of factors that might impact on the result of ADL/IADL assessment in persons with dementia, this area of human life certainly reveals its complexity in forming inevitable aspects of any person's life. The recommendation is therefore to do one's best to tap the area of ADL/IADL in a manner relevant to the purpose of one's practice or research. This is also a strong recommendation for any therapeutic trial in dementia, expressed as follows by Woods (1991):

> The major implication for therapeutic trials of the multifactorial influences on ADL function in people with dementia is that therapeutic effects on one important factor (e.g. memory or judgment) may be obscured by limitations imposed by other factors (e.g. volition or environment). The effects of these interacting variables must be carefully considered in deciding how best to evaluate change in self-care ability in any particular study. (Woods, 1991, p. 73)

When discussing what is clinically meaningful interference in Alzheimer's disease (AD) progression, Phelps (1995) also clearly stated that 'To the patient, this [meaningful interference] might mean continuing to function independently, maintaining his/her autonomy, with preservations of competence' (p. 877). Recently, Lawton (1996) explicitly made a connection between ADL/IADL and quality of life as follows: 'Quality of life for the AD patient is defined broadly as personal competence in the physical and cognitive realms, absence of distress, presence of positive states, social engagement, and meaningful activity involvement' (Lawton, 1996, p. 95).

Mohs (1995) concluded that 'Drug studies will require some combination of ADLs plus IADL measures, unless one has a very homogeneous group of patients' (p. 869). Rubenstein et al (1984) also suggested three important reasons for determining ADL/IADL status among geriatric patients. First, ADL/IADL assessment is a major determinator both of whether a person can live independently and of the kind of assistance needed. Second, ADL/IADL assessments are necessary for the definition of specific goals in rehabilitation or other forms of therapy, and third, as an outcome measure of interventions (Rubenstein et al, 1984). It is also imperative to acknowledge the health economy consequences of dependency in ADL/IADL, since persons in need of ADL/IADL assistance require caring resources that influence the costs of care.

Increased needs for supervision and care in everyday life have also been identified as more important predictors of institutionalization than the severity of dementia (Wimo et al, 1992).

It has also been recommended that assessment of ADL/IADLs should be part of a multiple outcome measurement battery in studies assessing the impact of interventions in dementia (Montgomery, 1996). While ADL/IADL assessment is important in any therapeutic program or research trial, several issues of measurement must be considered when going into assessment of ADL/IADL.

ISSUES OF MEASUREMENT

DIFFERENT RATIONALES FOR ASSESSING ADL/IADL ABILITY IN DEMENTIA

When choosing a scale for assessing ADL/IADL ability, one of the most important issues is the rationale for the assessment. While ADL/IADL scales traditionally were developed to measure the construct of independence, as suggested by Katz et al (1963), they have been widely used by scholars to assess many other constructs as, for example, safety, functional impairment, functional performance, functional health, need for health services (Porter, 1995; Törnquist, 1995). Furthermore, assessment of ADL/IADL as an outcome measure in pharmacological studies might require other scale features than assessment of ADL/IADL with the purpose of deciding level of services or as a guide for providing/evaluating individual support or care. For example, in a pharmacological trial, the focus in outcome evaluation might be on overall ADL/IADL functioning, while an assessment to decide level of care has a focus on dependency. In contrast, an evaluation of ADL/IADL support needs to give detailed information about the assessed person's quality, safety, and independence in different ADL/IADL tasks. Consequently, careful consideration of what one actually wants to assess is called for.

When considering any assessment, there are several scale properties that need attention. Of course, any instrument's reliability and validity have to be established and demonstrated. Additionally, the scale construct, the levels of function, the unidimensionality, the scoring system, the method of assessment, the differences between raters and ecologies need special concern in relation to the rationale for assessment.

SCALE CONSTRUCTS

If a scale is used to detect possible changes in ADL/IADL it should be sensitive enough to expose even marginal changes. While scales defined by small increments are more sensitive, global scales allow for assessment over a broader range of ability. On the other hand, the increments between global task categories tend to be large, which results in insensitivity in detecting small or modest improvements in function (Fisher, 1992). Woods (1991, p. 74) described this as 'a function both of the number of items in each area of function and the size of the steps between rating points' and called it 'a trade-off with the reliability of the scale'. The more sensitive a test is to small changes, the less reliable it may become, since scoring systems including many different scaling steps are often unclear and can be interpreted differently by different raters (Eakin, 1989). While the sensitivity increases by the number of items, the number of items is also connected to the method of assessment. For example, if the scale is developed to be a proxy-report with a family caregiver, it will also be important to retain the informant's goodwill and cooperation, and a large number of items might be a disadvantage (Woods, 1991).

LEVELS OF FUNCTION

Another related issue of concern is the level of function: the assessment's target level of function must be appropriate to the population being studied. While self-care ADL might be an appropriate target level for assessment among persons with moderate to severe dementia, the outcome investigation among persons in the early or mild stages of dementia needs to tap IADL tasks to avoid ceiling effects. This has also been underscored by Poon as follows: 'the paradox of employing ADL scales for early detection (and when the treatment effect size is small) is that *when the highest level of measurement sensitivity is needed, ADL scale sensitivity is at its lowest*' (Poon, 1994, pp. 172–173).

UNIDIMENSIONALITY

Unidimensionality is a somewhat controversial issue in ADL/IADL assessment discussions, but it should be noted that many existing ADL/IADL scales lack considerations of dimensionality. For example, sphincter and bladder control belongs to another functional dimension than eating and grooming. When such different dimensions of human function are conceptualized as unidimensional, the validity of assessment could be questioned (Törnquist, 1995).

SUMMED SCORES

Moreover, ordinal scores from different dimensions of function are often added to a total score (Fisher, 1992). Such summing procedures have been criticized for lack of meaningfulness, because two persons with totally different scoring profiles may receive an equal total sum representing the ADL/IADL function, while their ability, independence or quality of performance actually may differ greatly (Fisher, 1992; Törnquist, 1995).

The very procedure of adding ordinal scores has also been criticized because it means misinterpreting ordinal counts as being representative of equal interval, quantitative units (Fisher, 1992; Wright and Linacre, 1989). In fact, most ADL/IADL scales provide ordinal data, which also may limit the scientific use of ADL/IADL assessment in outcome studies. The importance of developing and using ADL/IADL scales that provide interval data, instead of interpreting and using ordinal data as if they were interval, is hereby emphasized.

METHOD OF ASSESSMENT

One of the most often discussed issues in ADL/IADL assessment is the method of assessment. While self/proxy reports are convenient, time-effective and easily administered, observational performance evaluations have advantages in both validity and reliability. Among persons with dementia, self-reports in particular have been questioned because of the risk of overestimation of their own ability and the declining awareness of their ADL/IADL problems (Barberger-Gateau et al, 1993; Rubenstein et al, 1984). Proxy-reports by caregivers or relatives also imply a risk of bias, since the person's ability may be underestimated for several reasons: the caregiver may be overburdened, overprotective, or simply assume that certain disabilities exist (Mangone et al, 1993; Rubenstein et al, 1984). Many scales may also be difficult to administer for family caregivers and place high demands on clarity to ensure reliability (Woods, 1991). Additionally, there may be personal relationships between the caregiver and the assessed person that might impact on the report, unknown to the researcher.

While performance observations are more time-consuming and imply the presence of an observing rater, they are often suggested to be superior in avoiding the bias effects described above (Fisher, 1992; Rubenstein et al, 1984).

RATER STRICTNESS

An issue related to the sensitivity, the reliability and to the method of assessment is the difference in strictness between raters. While raters tend to stay stable over time, strictness differs between individual raters (Lunz and Stahl, 1990). Consequently, scales that use a scoring system for the ADL/IADL items may have shortcomings in inter-rater reliability, since the raters' judgment of the quality of the person's performance tends to affect the score: lenient raters award performance while stricter raters are more severe. Therefore, rater training and calibration are important procedures to counteract such bias effects (Fisher, 1992).

ECOLOGICAL VALIDITY

Ecological validity is undoubtedly a very important issue in assessment of ADL/IADLs. Given that the physical and social environments affect the performance of ADL/IADL, any assessment should seek the highest possible natural ecology to ensure validity. This is especially important when observational assessments are used (Woods, 1991). For example, if a person is asked to perform an IADL task in a hospital setting, it is important that the task is relevant and familiar to the person, and that the environment is arranged to be as similar to the person's home environment as possible. Similarly, in order to have valid assessment results, it is important to observe the whole process of carrying out a real-life task (Fisher, 1997). To observe a person who is asked to demonstrate how to use a fork without connection to a real meal situation, for example, is not sufficiently valid, and from such an assessment situation the person's ability to eat cannot be evaluated.

A few studies have investigated the impact of the environment on ADL/IADL performance among persons with dementia. Nygård et al (1994) found no group differences but significant individual differences in a comparison of IADL ability in home and clinic settings among 19 persons with suspected dementia. Bédard et al (1995) found no significant ADL/IADL differences between home and clinic in a sample of 24 older adults with cognitive impairment. In contrast, Borell et al (1994) found great differences in activity performance between a day care hospital and own homes among cases of dementia. Since the research concerning the ecological impact on ADL/IADL performance in dementia is very limited, further research is called for to clarify the issue of ecological validity.

SOME ADL/IADL SCALES OFTEN USED IN DEMENTIA

THE LAWTON AND BRODY SCALE

One of the most commonly used ADL/IADL scales in dementia research is Lawton and Brody's scale (1969) for assessing older people (Mohs, 1995). In an overview of assessment scales used in evaluations of the efficacy of drug interventions on ADL/IADL ability, the Lawton and Brody scale was used in 12 out of 19 studies (Oakley and Sunderland, 1997). In studies comparing cognitive functioning and ADL/IADL in persons with dementia, Lawton and Brody's scale has also been frequently used (see for example Zanetti et al, 1993).

Further examples of the use of this scale are as follows: to compare the reliability of assessing the outcome of clinical trials in home versus clinic environments among cognitively impaired elderly (Bédard et al, 1995); to investigate the relationship between temporal adaptation and ADL/IADL functioning in persons with AD (Venable and Mitchell, 1991); and in comparisons between caregivers' feelings of burden and the cognitive, behavioral, and functional (ADL/IADL) impairment of persons with dementia (Mangone et al, 1993).

The Lawton and Brody assessment scale is composed of two parts: the Physical self-maintenance scale, and the Instrumental activities of daily living scale. In the PADL scale, six tasks are included: toileting, feeding, dressing, grooming, physical ambulation and bathing. In the IADL scale, the following tasks are included: ability to use the telephone, shopping, food preparation, housekeeping, laundry, mode of transportation, responsibility for own medication, and ability to handle finances. Each of these tasks is assessed for independence using an ordinal scale ranging from 1 to 5 (PADL), and from 1 to 3, 4 or 5 (IADL). For example, grooming is defined as 'neatness, hair, hands, face, clothing'. A score of 1 is assigned for 'Always neatly dressed, well-groomed, without assistance', and a score of 5 is assigned for 'Actively negates all efforts of others to maintain grooming' (Lawton and Brody, 1969, p. 189). The ordinal scores are summed for PADL and IADL respectively, and higher scores represent lower functioning.

The Lawton and Brody assessment can be based on the patient's self-report but more often it is based on the report by family members or caregivers. Lawton and Brody concluded that the scale demonstrated practical utility in several areas: it provides early, brief and objective assessment; it is an aid in formulation, implementation and evaluation of treatment plan, as well as an aid in the casework process. Further, it has utility in the teaching, training and planning of facilities and services, according to Lawton and Brody (1969).

The Lawton and Brody scale has been criticized for gender bias in favor of females, because it overestimates tasks traditionally performed by females. The IADL tasks have also been challenged for lack of meaning across cultures (Oakley and Sunderland, 1997). The scale is an ordinal-level tool, which sums individual task scores to an overall ADL or IADL score. This has been criticized by, for example, Wright and Linacre (1989) and Fisher (1992), as discussed above.

The global scope of the scale may also result in lack of sensitivity in detecting small but significant changes in ADL/IADL ability (Oakley and Sunderland, 1997). Finally, the assessment method based on self-report or caregivers' reports has been challenged concerning the risk of inaccuracy and possible bias (Rubenstein et al, 1984).

In conclusion, the Lawton and Brody scale is widely used, since it taps important areas of ADL and IADL and a wide range of ability levels, and because it is based on self- or caregiver reports and is therefore easily and quickly administered. However, its value may be questioned for cohesive meaning across culture and gender, for scoring system, and for method of assessment.

THE KATZ ADL-INDEX

One of the most internationally well known assessments of ADL is probably the hierarchical ADL-index developed by Katz et al (1963). However, the Katz ADL-index is also widely used in dementia research, as for example in studies comparing mental status and ADL ability (Aske, 1990; Hill et al, 1995; Zanetti et al, 1993) and in efforts to predict burden in dementia care (Grafström et al, 1994). The Katz ADL-index assesses dependence in bathing, dressing, going to the toilet, transferring, continence, and feeding. The hierarchical assessment results in an overall grading of the patient's dependence from A (independent in all activities) to G (dependent in all six activities).

The Katz ADL-index may be considered useful as a screening for need of services, since it is well known and easily administered by any health professional, but it is less useful in detecting quality of ADL ability or the nature of the support needed. The Katz ADL-index, like other global scales, also tends to be insensitive to smaller increments of change because the increments of challenge between the tasks and the levels are large (Fisher, 1992). Because of its focus on self-care ADL, the original Katz ADL-index is less useful among persons with mild dementia, and consequently less useful in many pharmacological trials. In summary, the Katz ADL-index may be insensitive and therefore less useful as an outcome measure.

THE FUNCTIONAL INDEPENDENCE MEASURE, FIM

The FIM was developed to be a tool for outcome evaluation of rehabilitation (Keith et al, 1987). It is an internationally accepted assessment to be used by different health care professionals, who score a person's ADL/IADL performance based on observations and knowledge of the person.

The FIM is divided into two subscales: a motor scale for basic self-care activities, sphincter management, mobility, and locomotion, and a social/cognition scale for comprehension, expression, social interaction, problem solving and memory. The scales separate the motor and cognition aspects of performance, rather than summing up performance scores from different dimensions of human behavior. Furthermore, the FIM raw scores are converted to linear measures based on the Rasch measurement model (Heinemann et al, 1991) which transforms ordinal raw scores to interval scores. For these two reasons, the FIM seems to be well suited as an outcome measure in evaluative studies in dementia.

However, when it was used as an outcome measure in a drug study (Petracca et al, 1996), no significant effects were found on FIM scores. The sensitivity of the FIM needs to be further investigated among persons with dementia, since insensitivity in evaluating the functional ability of high-motor-functioning persons with dementia has been suggested as a problem (Robinson, 1994). Furthermore, the FIM scale might not separate performance deficits caused by motor impairment from those caused by cognitive impairment: 'It was clear that some subjects had a low FIM motor score because their cognitive impairments impacted on their ability to be independent in self-care activities, regardless of the fact that they had the physical or motor capacity to independently perform the task' (Robinson, 1994, p. 63).

In conclusion, the FIM has good measurement qualities and is well known and accepted, but it may lack sufficient sensitivity and ability to distinguish between different aspects of ADL/IADL disability.

THE DIRECT ASSESSMENT OF FUNCTIONAL STATUS, DAFS

Loewenstein et al (1989) developed a direct assessment of functional status, DAFS, for use among persons with AD. DAFS incorporates both ADL and IADL represented by different functional domains as follows: time orientation, communication abilities (telephone skills, preparing a letter for mailing, taking a telephone message), transportation, financial skills (identifying currency, counting currency, high order financial abilities), shopping skills, eating skills, and dressing and grooming skills.

Loewenstein et al (1989) recommended that the assessment should be based on observations, and a specified ordinal scoring system is used. Each correct item under the subscales of time orientation, shopping, grooming and eating is scored as 2 points, but as 1 point in the other subscales (Loewenstein et al, 1989). This means that the ability is weighted in relation to each subscale's functional domain, which has been criticized as an arbitrary procedure (Eakin, 1989; Törnquist, 1995). Further, the DAFS scales claim to directly assess functional skill by observation to provide ecologically valid assessment (Loewenstein and Rupert, 1995). However, the claim for ecological validity may be challenged. For example, the eating scale is scored based on the following: 'The patient was given eating utensils and was then required to pour water into a glass, demonstrate how to drink from a cup, and to properly use a fork, spoon, and knife' (Loewenstein et al, 1989, p. 116). Thus, the scale constructors assume that the ability to eat is equivalent to the ability to demonstrate how to use cutlery in a contrived test situation.

In summary, the DAFS taps important areas of ADL/IADL and uses observation as method of assessment, but may be criticized for summing up weighted ordinal scores and for questionable ecological validity in observations.

THE ASSESSMENT OF MOTOR AND PROCESS SKILLS, AMPS

The AMPS is an internationally and cross-culturally standardized performance evaluation of ADL/IADL, which can be used for all age groups, given that the person is motivated to perform ADL/IADL tasks (Bernspång and Fisher, 1995; Fisher, 1997). The person being evaluated is observed doing individually and culturally relevant tasks. Simultaneously, the ability to perform ADL/IADL tasks and the motor and process skill components underpinning the performance are evaluated.

In the AMPS, the quality of performance is measured in terms of the effectiveness, efficiency, independence, and safety of component actions involved in the task performance. After observation, the occupational therapist scores the performance on 16 motor and 20 process skill items using a 4-point ordinal scale, ranging from deficient to competent. By using the Rasch measurement model, the ordinal scoring data are converted to interval ability measures that are adjusted to account for task challenge and rater leniency (Fisher, 1993, 1994; Fisher et al, 1994). The AMPS is testfree, which means that it is possible to estimate a person's position along a common unidimensional continuum of increasing ADL/IADL ability independent of which of the 63 AMPS ADL/IADL tasks a person undertakes (Fisher, 1997).

The AMPS has been used in several studies among persons with dementia, for example in a drug intervention outcome study where significant drug effects were detected (Oakley and Sunderland, 1997), in a comparison of IADL performance in clinical versus home settings (Nygård et al, 1994), and in comparisons of cognitive performance and IADL (Doble et al, 1997; Nygård, 1996; Robinson, 1994).

In conclusion, the AMPS has good scaling qualities and a range to detect even small changes in ability. Since it is an occupational therapy instrument, other health care professionals are excluded from education in and use of the instrument. Thus, while it seems promising as an outcome measure because of its measurement properties, a research team without an AMPS-trained occupational therapist cannot use it.

In this chapter, only a few of all the ADL/IADL assessment scales that are tested for validity and reliability and used in the area of dementia have been presented in summary. For the health care professional interested in these aspects of assessment, I will emphasize that there are indeed many assessment scales for ADL/IADL out there. When choosing one of those, the assessment purpose must be the rule of thumb. If I, for example, want to assess ADL/IADL to predict needs and costs of care, the choice of assessment instrument should be made based on this purpose. Again, in other words: 'Before a functional measure is chosen, a thorough consideration of what the measure is going to be used for should be made' (Avlund, 1997; p. 170).

IDEAL ASSESSMENT—IN RELATION TO PURPOSE

The only way of considering what would be the perfect ADL/IADL scale must also, of course, be in relation to the purpose of the assessment. To give a perspective, I will however try to state some of the most important aspects and properties of an ideal ADL/IADL assessment.

The ideal ADL/IADL assessment would be broad enough in range to be useful for persons with both mild and severe dementia. It would also be testfree and allow for choice, so that each person could do the most relevant task with regard to ability, habits, motivation, environment and disease symptoms. This means that many ADL and IADL tasks would be included. To allow for comparison between different tasks, the differences in task difficulty must be accounted for, which would require use of a Rasch measurement model.

Considering that some outcome evaluation studies need to rely on information given by caregivers or family members, it would also be an advantage if this ideal ADL/IADL scale could offer a choice between being taken as an observational tool and as a self/proxy report. If two such versions of the assessment could be compared at all, this would certainly also require the use of Rasch analysis to account for differences.

To be useful in many different kinds of outcome studies, the scale would need to provide an overall ability measure, which would have to be sensitive enough to detect even small changes, although not based on summed ordinal scores. The assessment dimension needs to consider both ability, dependence and quality of performance in the skill components underpinning overall ADL/IADL performance. Additionally, the quality or frequency of assistance/ support needed would provide useful information. For example, in an outcome study of an ADL/IADL intervention program in a dementia day care centre, Josephsson et al (1995) found that assessment of frequency of support in occupations showed up as an informative parallel to intervention-related gains of ADL/IADL ability in some subjects.

Considering the different rationales and needs when assessing ADL/IADL, it would probably not be wise to include all these qualities in a single assessment, since such a tool would be hard to administer. ADL/IADL ability seems to be such a complex area of human functioning that we have to recognize the need for highly specialized assessment scales and exclusive training of professional raters, as well as brief and simple scales to be used by non-professionals.

CAN MEANINGFUL ACTIVITY AND ILLNESS EXPERIENCES BE MEASURED?

In summing up this chapter, a few moments will be spent on the basic question of whether such a multidimensional and complex aspect of human life as ADL/IADL ability really can be captured in sufficient depth by a strict assessment approach.

If we take a closer look at the epistemological underpinnings of assessment in the area of human behavior, we discover that the original idea of evaluative measurement emanates from the Galilean tradition of natural objective science

(Karlsson, 1993). By applying mathematics to pure nature, Galileo began the tradition of the natural sciences, implying a belief in the possibility of obtaining exact and objective knowledge about all aspects of nature, including human beings and their actions and behavior (Karlsson, 1993). In the process of seeking access by measurement to natural phenomena such as ADL ability, the first step involves an abstraction of the object for measurement. For example, a transformation of a complex set of actions within the context of daily life to an abstract operationalization, 'dressing', is undertaken. The second step involves the application of measurement, that is, an element of judging the operationalization takes place, by implementing a set of symbols or numbers on the performance outcome. This second step involves the actual quantification.

These two steps also raise two problems in all formalized ADL assessments: *what?* and *how?* The what-question concerns what actually is assessed, for example: what is ability? The how-question pertains to how this measurement or assessment is obtained, for example: how can ability be measured? (Törnquist, 1995). It has been recommended that the concept of *measurement* should only be used when the assessment scale is based on *units of like meaning*, for example: minutes, meters, ability measures (Short-DeGraff and Fisher, 1993; Fisher, 1993). If, for example, the ability to dress is measured in minutes, this does not imply measurement based on units of like meaning because minutes measure time, not dressing ability. Therefore, in the area of ADL/IADL, the concept of evaluation or, synonymously, assessment should be used rather than measurement because most tests of human behavior do not assess by units of like meaning; that is, they are not measurements (Fisher, 1993; Short-DeGraff and Fisher, 1993).

The core of the critical question as to whether ADL/IADL ability can be fully ascertained by measurement or assessment lies in the actual assumption that human behavior in everyday life situations is equal to the objects of reality that were measured by the original Galilean tradition. Is it really possible to obtain the same type of objective and exact knowledge about a disabled person's ability in and experiences of attending to, for example, his or her personal hygiene as about the properties of a mineral? And, if not, how far away from understanding the afflicted persons' experiences of increased ability can we go, still claiming to validly assess ADL/IADL ability by objective assessment or measurement?

Finally, let me conclude this chapter by emphasizing the importance of theoretical awareness. When we use an ADL/IADL instrument, we also need to be aware of the theoretical framework to which our assessment may be connected. Any assessment is at risk of being highly invalid if not related to a theoretical frame that helps us to understand and interpret the collected data (Avlund, 1997). This issue of theory also reflects the question stated above: to what extent can human ability in complex life situations be measured, since any person's ability could be understood and explained from several different viewpoints? In terms of needs and health care costs it is also highly important to be able to interpret the data from an ADL/IADL assessment, since the interpretations will result in decisions about interventions which will affect the costs of care. For cost-effective intervention, the person's ability, efficiency, dependency and safety in ADL/IADL need to be correctly understood and interpreted from a reliable and valid method of assessment.

REFERENCES

American Psychiatric Association (1995). *Diagnostic and Statistical Manual of Mental Disorders*, 4th edn (DSM-IV). Washington, DC, Author.

Aske, D. (1990). The correlation between Mini-Mental State Examination scores and Katz ADL Status among dementia patients. *Rehabilitation Nursing*, 15, 140–146.

Avlund, K. (1997). Methodological challenges in measurements of functional ability in gerontological research. A review. *Aging: Clinical and Experimental Research*, 9, 164–174.

Barberger-Gateau, P., Dartigues, J-F. and Letenneur, L. (1993). Four instrumental activities of daily living score as a predictor of one-year incident dementia. *Age and Ageing*, 22, 457–463.

Bédard, M., Molloy, D. W., Standish, T., Guyatt, G. H., D'Souza, J., Mondadori, C. and Darzins, P. J. (1995). Clinical trials in cognitively impaired older adults: Home versus clinic assessments. *Journal of the American Geriatric Society*, 43, 1127–1130.

Bennet, D. A. and Knopman, D. S. (1994). Alzheimer's disease: A comprehensive approach to patient management. *Geriatrics*, 49, 20–26.

Bernspång, B. and Fisher, A. G. (1995). Validation of the Assessment of Motor and Process Skills for use in Sweden. *Scandinavian Journal of Occupational Therapy*, 2, 3–9.

Borell, L., Gustavsson, A., Sandman, P. O. and Kielhofner, G. (1994). Occupational programming in a day hospital for patients with dementia. *Occupational Therapy Journal of Research*, 14, 219–238.

Borell, L., Rönnberg, L. and Sandman, P. O. (1993). The ability to use familiar objects among patients with Alzheimer's disease. *Occupational Therapy Journal of Research*, 13.

DeJong, R., Osterlund, O. and Roy, G. (1989). Measurement and the quality-of-life changes in patients with Alzheimer's disease. *Clinical Therapeutics*, 11, 545–554.

Doble, S. E., Fisk, J. D., MacPherson, K. M., Fisher, A. G. and Rockwood, K. (1997). Measuring functional competence in older perons with Alzheimer's disease. *International Psychogeriatrics*, 9, 25–38.

Eakin, P. (1989). Problems with assessments of activities of daily living. *British Journal of Occupational Therapy*, 52, 50–54.

Fisher, A. G. (1992). The foundation—Functional measures, Part 2: Selecting the right test, minimizing the limitations. *American Journal of Occupational Therapy*, 46, 278–281.

Fisher, A. G. (1993). The assessment of IADL motor skills: An application of many-faceted Rasch Analysis. *American Journal of Occupational Therapy*, 47, 319–338.

Fisher, A. G. (1994). Development of functional assessment that adjusts ability measures for task simplicity and rater leniency. In M. Wilson (Ed.), *Objective Measurement: Theory into Practice* (Vol. 2). Norwood, NJ, Ablex.

Fisher, A. G. (1997). *Assessment of Motor and Process Skills*, 2nd edn. Test manual,

Department of Occupational Therapy, Colorado State University. Fort Collins, CO, Three Star Press.

Fisher, A. G., Bryze, K. A., Granger, C. V., Haley, S. M., Hamilton, B. B., Heinemann, A. W., Puderbaugh, J. K., Linacre, J. M., Ludlow, L. H., McCabe, M. A. and Wright, B. D. (1994). Applications of Rasch analysis to the development of functional assessments. *International Journal of Educational Research*, **21**, 579–593.

Galasko, D., Corey-Bloom, J. and Thal, L. J. (1991). Monitoring progression in Alzheimer's disease. *Journal of the American Geriatric Society*, **39**, 932–941.

Grafström, M., Fratiglioni, L. and Winblad, B. (1994). Caring for an elderly person. Predictors of burden in dementia care. *International Journal of Geriatric Psychiatry*, **9**.

Green, C. R., Mohs, R. C., Schmeidler, J., Aryan, M. and Davis, K. L. (1993). Functional decline in Alzheimer's disease: A longitudinal study. *Journal of the American Geriatric Society*, **41**, 654–661.

Heinemann, A. W., Hamilton, B. B., Granger, C. V., Wright, B. D., Linacre, J. M. et al (1991). *Rating Scale Analysis of Functional Assessment Measures*. Rehabilitation Institute of Chicago, Chicago.

Hill, R. D., Bäckman, L. and Fratiglioni, L. (1995). Determinants of functional abilities in dementia. *Journal of American Geriatrics Society*, **43**, 1092–1097.

Josephsson, S., Bäckman, L., Borell, L., Nygård, L. and Bernspång, B. (1995). Effectiveness of an intervention to improve occupational performance in dementia. *Occupational Therapy Journal of Research*, **15**, 36–51.

Juva, K., Sulkava, R., Erkinjuntti, T., Ylikoski, R., Valvanne, J. and Tilvis, R. (1994). Staging the severity of dementia: comparison of clinical (CDR, DSM-III-R), functional (ADL, IADL) and cognitive (MMSE) scales. *Acta Neurologica Scandinavia*, **90**, 293–298.

Karlsson, G. (1993). *Psychological Qualitative Research from a Phenomenological Perspective*. Stockholm, Almqvist & Wiksell International.

Katz, S., Ford, A. B., Moskowitz, R. W., Jackson, B. A. and Jaffee, M. W. (1963). The index of ADL: A standardized measure of biological and psychosocial function. *JAMA*, **185**, 914–919.

Keith, R. A., Granger, C. V., Hamilton, B. B. and Sherwin, F. S. (1987). The Functional Independence Measure: A new tool for rehabilitation. In N. G. Eisenberg and R. C. Grzzesiak (Eds), *Advances in Clinical Rehabilitation*. New York, Springer.

Kielhofner, G. (1995). *A Model of Human Occupation: Theory and Application*, 2nd edn. Baltimore, Williams and Wilkins.

Kramer, J. H. and Duffy, J. M. (1996). Aphasia, apraxia and agnosia in the diagnosis of dementia. *Dementia*, **7**, 23–26.

Lawton, M. P. (1996). Behavioral problems and interventions in Alzheimer's disease: Research needs. *International Psychogeriatrics*, **8**, 95–98.

Lawton, M. P. and Brody, E. M. (1969). Assessment of older people: Self-maintaining and instrumental activities of daily living. *Gerontologist*, **9**, 179–186.

Loewenstein, D. A., Amigo, E., Duara, R., Guterman, A., Hurwitz, D., Berkowitz, N., Wilkie, F., Weinberg, G., Black, B., Gittelman, B. and Eisdorfer, C. (1989). A new scale for the assessment of functional status in Alzheimer's disease and related disorders. *Journal of Gerontology: Psychological Sciences*, **44**, 114–121.

Loewenstein, D. A., Duara, R., Rupert, M. P., Aruelles, T., Lapinski, K. J. and Eisdorfer, C. (1995). Deterioration of functional capacities in Alzheimer's disease after a 1-year period. *International Psychogeriatrics*, **7**, 495–503.

Loewenstein, D. A. and Rupert, M. P. (1995). Staging functional impairment in dementia using performance-based measures: A preliminary analysis. *Journal of Mental Health and Aging*, 1, 47–56.

Loewenstein, D. A., Rupert, M. P., Berkowitz-Zimmer, N., Guterman, A., Morgan, R. and Heyden, S. (1992). Neuropsychological test performance and prediction of functional capacities in dementia. *Behavior, Health and Aging*, 2, 149–158.

Lunz, M. E. and Stahl, J. A. (1990). Judge consistency and severity across grading periods. *Evaluation of the Health Professions*, 13, 425–444.

Mangone, C. A., Sanguinetti, R. M., Baumann, P. D., Gonzales, R. C., Pereyra, S., Bozzola, F. G., Gorelick, P. B. and Sica, R. E. P. (1993). Influence of feelings of burden on the caregiver's perception of the patient's functional status. *Dementia*, 4, 283–293.

Mohs, R. C. (1995). Methodological aspects of evaluating effects of AD progression. *Neurobiology of Aging*, 16, 867–870.

Montgomery, R. J. V. (1996). Group overviews. Measuring outcome in Alzheimer's disease. *International Psychogeriatrics*, 8, 13–16.

Nygård, L. (1996). Everyday life with dementia. Aspects of assessing and understanding the experiences and consequences of living with dementia. Doctoral thesis, Department of Clinical Neuroscience and Family Medicine, Division of Geriatrics, Karolinska Institute, Stockholm.

Nygård, L., Bernspång, B., Fisher, A. and Winblad, B. (1994). Comparing motor and process ability of persons with suspected dementia in home and clinic settings. *American Journal of Occupational Therapy*, 48, 689–696.

Nygård, L. and Borell, L. (1995). Daily living with dementia—two cases. *Scandinavian Journal of Occupational Therapy*, 2, 24–33.

Nygård, L., Borell, L. and Gustavsson, A. (1995). Managing images of occupational self in early stage dementia. *Scandinavian Journal of Occupational Therapy*, 2, 129–137.

Oakley, F. and Sunderland, T. (1997). The assessment of motor and process skills as a measure of IADL functioning in pharmacological studies of people with Alzheimer's disease: A pilot study. *International Psychogeriatrics*, 9, 197–206.

Petracca, G., Teson, A., Chemerinski, E., Leiguarda and Starkstein, S. E. (1996). A double-blind placebo-controlled study of clomipramine in depressed patients with Alzheimer's disease. *Journal of Neuropsychiatry and Clinical Neurosciences*, 8, 270–275.

Phelps, C. H. (1995). Clinically meaningful interference in AD progression. *Neurobiology of Aging*, 16(6), 877–878.

Poon, L. W. (1994). On the paradox of improving sensitivity of ADL scales for the detection of behavioral changes in early dementia. *International Psychogeriatrics*, 6, 171–177.

Porter, E. J. (1995). A phenomenological alternative to the 'ADL research tradition'. *Journal of Aging and Health*, 7, 24–45.

Reed, B. R., Jagust, W. J. and Seab, J. P. (1989). Mental status as a predictor of daily function in progressive dementia. *Gerontologist*, 29, 804–807.

Reisberg, B., Franssen, E. H., Bobinski, M., Auer, S., Monteiro, I., Boksay, I., Wegiel, J., Schulman, E., Steinberg, G., Souren, L., Kluger, A., Torossian, C., Sinaliko, E., Wisniewski, H. M. and Ferris, S. H. (1996). Overview of methodological issues for pharmacological trials in mild, moderate and severe Alzheimer's disease. *International Psychogeriatrics*, 8(2), 159–193.

Robinson, P., Ekman, S-L., Meleis, A., Winblad, B. and Wahlund, L-O. (1997). Suffering in silence: The experience of early memory loss. *Health Care in Later Life*, 2, 107–120.

Robinson, S. (1994). Functional and cognitive assessment in dementia. Master's thesis, University of Bath, England.

Rubenstein, Z., Schairer, C., Wieland, G. D. and Kane, R. (1984). Systematic biases in functional status assessment of elderly adults: Effects of different data sources. *Journal of Gerontology*, **39**, 686–691.

Short-DeGraff, M. and Fisher, A. G. (1993). A proposal for diverse research methods and a common research language. *American Journal of Occupational Therapy*, **47**, 295–297.

Stern, Y., Hesdorffer, D., Sano, M. and Mayeux, R. (1990). Measurement and prediction of functional capacity in Alzheimer's disease. *Neurology*, **40**, 8–14.

Törnquist, K. (1995). *Att fastställa och mäta förmåga till dagliga livets aktiviteter (ADL). En kritisk granskning av ADL-instrument och arbetsterapipraxis.* In Swedish. (Verifying and measuring the ability to perform activities of daily living (ADL)—A critical examination of ADL instruments and the practice of occupational therapy.) Doctoral thesis, University of Göteborg, Department of Social Work.

Venable, S. D. and Mitchell, M. M. (1991). Temporal adaptation and performance of daily living activities in persons with Alzheimer's disease. *Physical and Occupational Therapy in Geriatrics*, **9**, 31–51.

Willis, S. L. (1996). Everyday cognitive competence in elderly persons: Conceptual issues and empirical findings. *Gerontologist*, **36**(5), 595–601.

Wimo, A., Gustavsson, L. and Mattson, B. (1992). Predictive validity of factors influencing the institutionalization of elderly people with psycho-geriatric disorders. *Scandinavian Journal of Primary Health Care*, **10**, 65–71.

Woods, R. T. (1991). Activities of daily living in dementia. In C. G. Gottfries, R. Levy, G. Clincke and L. Tritsmans (Eds), *Diagnostic and Therapeutic Assessments in Alzheimer's disease*. Petersfield, Wrightson Biomedical Publishing.

Wright, B. D. and Linacre, J. M. (1989). Observations are always ordinal: Measurements, however, must be interval. *Archives of Physical Medicine and Rehabilitation*, **70**, 857–860.

Zanetti, O., Bianchetti, A., Frisoni, G. B., Rozzini, R. and Trabucchi, M. (1993). Determinants of disability in Alzheimer's disease. *International Journal of Geriatric Psychiatry*, **8**, 581–586.

Zanetti, O., Bianchetti, A. and Trabucchi, M. (1995). The puzzle of functional status in mild and moderate Alzheimer's disease: Self-report, family report and performance-based assessment. *Gerontologist*, **35**, 148.

3.5 Assessment of Cognitive Functioning

OVE ALMKVIST

Huddinge University Hospital, Huddinge, Sweden

This chapter will briefly present the concept of cognition as well as different aspects of cognition. Next some of the most frequently used methods for assessment of cognition are presented covering screening instruments, observational scales, short neuropsychological tests, and a glimpse of a comprehensive neuropsychological testing. Finally, these methods are commented upon by pointing out some of the advantages and disadvantages associated with the use of these methods.

CONCEPT OF COGNITION

Cognition (Latin: cognoscere = to know) refers to all aspects of perceiving, attending, thinking, remembering, language comprehension and communication, control of actions, and motor performance. The different aspects of cognition may be assessed by choosing tasks in which a certain cognitive aspect dominates. When the subject is working with a task, the evaluation, observation, and judgment of task performance is used to learn about possible deficits of cognitive function. This information may indicate the functional status of the brain, assuming certain brain–behavior relationships. Given the result of performance for cognitive functions, these data may aid to diagnose, predict future outcome, evaluate treatment effects, help in guidance and counseling with relatives and others with dementia patients.

Alzheimer's disease and other dementia disorders are characterized by a decline of mental function but also by a specific sequence of decline in various aspects of cognitive function. Although dementia development concerns various aspects of cognition, these aspects are not changed in parallel, but to a large extent independently from each other. It has been found that the decline in AD occurs in three statistically independent domains: memory, language, and visuospatial ability. It has also been found that the decline in AD occurs

Health Economics of Dementia. Edited by Anders Wimo, Bengt Jönsson, Göran Karlsson and Bengt Winblad.
© 1998 John Wiley & Sons Ltd.

in a specific sequence (Almkvist, 1996): in the very early stage, only memory functioning is impaired, whereas other cognitive functions remain essentially intact. In the early stage, when a clinical diagnosis is possible, other cognitive functions, for instance verbal and visuospatial functions, are affected in addition to further deterioration of memory. In later stages of AD, motor functioning may be involved in the disease process. The information matrix on time and degree of decline in various aspects of cognitive function may be very useful in learning about type of disease, degree of disease progression, and providing guidance for societal authorities in finding appropriate care, housing, and support for the patient.

The earliest, and the predominant, sign of dementia development is an impairment in *episodic memory*, that is the memory of specific events related to a specific time, location, and situation—often referred to as 'recent memory' and denoting information acquired at a specific recent occasion. Later during the course of dementia development, 'remote memories' are lost, that is the memory of well-learned items, including the patient's general fund of knowledge, acquired early in life before the dementia development started, referred to as *semantic memory*. *Short-term memory*, verbal or non-verbal, refers to a capacity-limited immediate memory store used to hold material recalled without distraction within a number of seconds after the presentation of the material. This store seems to be relatively intact in the early disease process. *Procedural memory*, or skill memory, denotes the memory of motor habits, which is preserved to a large extent in AD, but impaired very early on in, for instance, Parkinson's disease. *Implicit and explicit memory* are related to the conscious and unconscious awareness of learning and retrieval. Interestingly, explicit learning and retrieval may be impaired in early AD, but implicit memory may be spared until the later stages.

Language deficits are common in the mild stage of AD in terms of anomia, decrease of word fluency, and marked impairment of complex verbal comprehension, although verbal skills such as articulation and use of syntax may be relatively intact. That is, semantics seem to be more affected than syntax. Late stage AD is characterized by severely and globally deteriorated communicative skill. Finally only non-speech utterances remain.

Executive functions denote complex mental operations involved in planning, organizing and evaluating performance, controlling actual performance, as well as the adaptation of skills to present task demands. This complex of operations is thought of as a supervisory system for all other mental activity, which may be particularly associated with frontal lobe regions. Most forms of dementia show a malfunctioning of the executive functions early on during the disease process.

Visuospatial abilities are concerned with orientation in space of the body and the surrounding environment. Dysfunctioning in this domain is apparent in moderate dementia, when people get lost, are unable to operate complex machinery, and have difficulties in drawing and copying.

Attention is thought of as a mechanism that reduces the overwhelming influx of sensory and internal stimulation, makes it possible to focus and sustain on some specific part of the stimulation, and is responsible for the shift between different stimulations. The three components of attention are subserved by different brain regions and they are also differentially impaired during the disease process.

Perception is not primarily affected in most dementia syndromes. Dementia due to cerebrovascular disease may be an exception.

Motor performance is not primarily affected in most dementia syndromes. Dementia due to cerebrovascular disease or Parkinson's or Huntington's disease may be an exception.

Very often cognition is assessed positively in terms of a *global measure* such as intelligence (e.g., full-scale intelligence quotient, FSIQ, of the WAIS-R battery), intellectual ability, mental capacity, or reversed in terms of degree of cognitive deterioration, severity of dementia, or stage of dementia. The problem with these measures is primarily associated with the composition of the global score. The measure is a summary score, but the summary of what? Different measures summarize cognition in different ways, and the specific composition has to be known in order to make proper use of the score (see below, MMSE).

It should be pointed out that cognitive function does not operate in isolation from personality, emotions, motivation, and biological drives. These factors are particularly important in assessing dementia vs depression or other affective syndromes. Therefore, a functional assessment of dementia should include not only an assessment of cognitive function, but also an evaluation of affective status or behavior (see below, Chapter 3.7).

ASSESSMENT OF COGNITION

There are several types of assessment of cognition differing in comprehensiveness (detail, length, and diversity of cognitive domains), in psychometric properties (reliability, validity, sensitivity, specificity, existence of norms, etc.), and in informativeness (single global vs many specified measures, internationally known or not). Typically, the individual is presented with a *task*, that is the individual is instructed what to do with some material. The result of the task performance is observed and scored numerically. When the task is standardized and evaluated in relation to reference groups, the task has become a *test*. Task performance, behavior, emotional reactions, attitudes, language, verbal responses to questions and so on may also be observed or rated in order to design *observation* forms or *rating scales*. Ratings can be performed by the patient him-/herself or by other persons. Obviously, only a few assessment methods can be described here. The most frequently used methods are briefly presented.

SCREENING INSTRUMENTS

MMSE, the Mini-Mental Status Examination score (MMSE; Folstein et al, 1975), was developed to gauge the degree of cognitive impairment and to document change of cognitive status in clinical settings and in epidemiological research. It is well known worldwide and has been translated into a number of languages. The original version of MMSE is a non-standardized, informally presented, 11-item set of simple tasks (orientation to time, orientation to place, registration of three words, attention and calculation, recall, language, and visual construction), summarizing to a global score with a maximum of 30 points. It can be administered in 5–10 minutes, and it can be used after some training by a diversity of medical personnel. In epidemiology, the cut-off of 23/24 is usually utilized as the border between dementia and normal performance. Its reliability was judged to be satisfactory (Tombaugh and McIntyre, 1992). Validity was high for sensitivity in moderate to severe dementia, but less good for mild dementia, mainly because of its sensitivity to variations in age, education, and cultural background (Tombaugh and McIntyre, 1992). There are some minor ambiguities in MMSE, for instance with the use of spelling WORLD backwards and counting backwards from 7, the highest score of the two tasks should be used. Similarly, the county and the street where the subject lives should be asked for rather than the county and the street of the testing location.

The positive and negative features of MMSE are listed below:

+ high test-retest reliability
+ may be used for staging
− high rate of false positives in low education, blacks, etc.
− low discrimination of normal aging to very mild dementia
− low discrimination of moderate to severe dementia
− no patterning of deficits in varying cognitive domains
− predominance of verbal items, visuospatial abilities are poorly evaluated
− some ambiguities exist, which can be overcome

There are a number of other screening tests that give a global measure of cognitive function by employing a short assessment. Among these instruments are the Dementia Rating Scale (DRS; Mattis, 1988), the Information-Memory-Concentration test (IMC; Blessed et al, 1968), and the Short Portable Mental Status Questionnaire (SPMSQ; Pfeiffer, 1975) as well as a number of modifications of the MMSE. None of these screening instruments have attained the distribution of MMSE or have been documented to be markedly more efficient than the MMSE for assessment of cognitive functioning (Christensen et al, 1991).

OBSERVATION SCALES

CDR, the Clinical Dementia Rating scale (CDR; Hughes et al, 1982; Morris, 1993), is a global staging measure in five levels (0 = no impairment, 0.5 = questionable dementia, 1 = mild dementia, 2 = moderate dementia, and 3 = severe dementia) commonly employed in clinical settings and treatment trials. Based on a semi-structured interview with the patient and an informant, CDR assesses the magnitude of cognitive impairment in six domains: concentration, memory, orientation, judgment and problem solving, community affairs, home and hobbies, and personal care. Its reliability has been established (Burke et al, 1988). Its validity is proven against autopsy data (Morris et al, 1988).

The merits and drawbacks of CDR are listed below:

+ high test-retest reliability and validity
+ designed for staging, therefore useful over a wide range of cognitive decline
− low discrimination of total range because only five categories are used
− no patterning of deficits in varying cognitive domains

BCRS, the Brief Cognitive Rating Scale (BCRS; Reisberg et al, 1983; Reisberg and Ferris, 1988), is a global staging measure commonly employed in clinical settings and treatment trials. The BCRS assesses the magnitude of cognitive impairment based on information regarding five items: concentration, recent memory, past memory, orientation and self-care. Items are scored in seven steps after a structured interview conducted in the presence of a caretaker.

The primary advantages and drawbacks with the BCRS are listed below:

+ designed for a brief assessment of cognitive status
− documentation on reliability, validity, etc. is lacking
− no patterning of deficits in varying cognitive domains

GDS, the Global Deterioration Scale (GDS; Reisberg et al, 1982), includes the entire continuum from normal aging and senescent forgetfulness to stages of dementia, which is divided into seven clinically identifiable stages (no, very mild, mild, moderate, moderately severe, severe, and very severe cognitive decline). These stages are assumed to describe the sequence in dementia development, although clinical practice may not confirm this. The data collection is based on a semi-structured interview with the patient and/or the carer in eleven domains: attention and concentration, recent memory, past memory, orientation, self-care, speech, psychomotor function, mood, behavior, praxis, and calculation. Occasionally, the integration of information from the eleven domains may prove difficult. The GDS scores correlated significantly with psychometric measures (Reisberg et al, 1989). Furthermore, the relationships between GDS scores and neuroimaging data such as ventricular dilation and sulcal enlargement are relatively good (Reisberg et al, 1982).

The merits and drawbacks of GDS are listed below:

+ high test-retest reliability and validity
+ designed for staging, therefore useful over a wide range of cognitive decline
+ good clinical applicability, relatively little influenced by educational/ sociocultural background
− low discrimination of total range because only seven categories are used
− no patterning of deficits in varying cognitive domains

GBS, the Gottfries, Bråne, Gullberg and Steen scale (1982; GBS), assesses motor function (6 items), intellectual disturbance (11 items), emotional disturbance (3 items), and typical dementia symptoms (6 items) in a seven-point scale for each item after observation of the patient's behavior in the ward. The scale is easy to use after a short period of training for unskilled personnel. Its reliability and validity have been established (Gottfries et al, 1982). The GBS scale has been translated into a large number of languages.

Below, the GBS scale is evaluated in terms of positive and negative features:

+ high test-retest reliability and validity
+ good clinical applicability, relatively little influenced by educational/ sociocultural background
+ applicable from mild to severe dementia
+ easy to use and rapid assessment for ward personnel
− not applicable for borderline or very mild dementia
− low discrimination of total range because only seven categories are used
− no patterning of deficits in varying cognitive domains

SHORT NEUROPSYCHOLOGICAL TESTS

ADAS, the Alzheimer's Disease Assessment Scale (ADAS; Rosen et al, 1984), was designed to measure the severity of the most important symptoms associated with AD. ADAS is divided into two parts, a cognitive part (ADAS-Cog) and a non-cognitive part, which may be used separately. The ADAS-Cog makes use of performance tests, tapping orientation, memory, praxis, drawing, and anomia as well as observations of language ability. The non-cognitive part assesses behavior such as tremor, pacing, motor activity and psychiatric problems in terms of behavioral ratings by observing the patient or interviewing a reliable informant. The reliability of the ADAS is very high, both in terms of interrater reliability and test-retest reliability (Rosen et al, 1984). Its validity has also been reported to be high (Rosen et al, 1984). However, the

ADAS-Cog is not very sensitive to the distinction between normal aging and very mild dementia, because of the fact that ceiling effects occur.

The major strengths and weaknesses of the ADAS-Cog are listed below:

+ the principal symptoms of AD are assessed
+ high reliability and validity
+ no timing of task performance
− not useful for very mild dementia
− not useful for severe dementia
− patterning of impairment is not pronounced

CAMCOG is one part of a comprehensive dementia investigation protocol, the Cambridge Mental Disorder of the Elderly Examination (CAMDEX; Roth et al, 1986; Huppert et al, 1995), which was designed for epidemiological research. It comprises three parts: a structured clinical interview with the patient, a structured clinical interview with an informant to obtain information on the patient's present state, past history and family history, and a range cognitive test (CAMCOG; Huppert et al, 1995). In addition to the MMSE, the CAMCOG battery consists of eight subscales on orientation, language, memory, praxis, attention, abstract thinking, perception, and calculation. There is an overall measure of cognitive function as well as scores for specific cognitive domains. The maximum summary score is 106 and a cut-off 79/80 is recommended for differentiation of dementia and normal aging (Roth et al, 1986). For interrater reliability the sensitivity and specificity of CAMCOG are high (Roth et al, 1986).

The merits and drawbacks of CAMCOG are summarized below:

+ high test-retest reliability and validity
+ discrimination of very mild dementia is possible to some extent
+ patterning of deficits in varying cognitive domains is possible
+ good distribution properties
− sensitive for socio-demographic variables (age, sex, education, and social class)
− somewhat time-consuming

CERAD, the Consortium to Establish a Registry for Alzheimer's Disease (CERAD et al, 1989), was developed to detect and stage dementia disease in epidemiological research and in clinical settings. It includes the MMSE and six other neuropsychological tests (verbal fluency, an abridged version of the Boston naming test, word list learning in three trials, constructional praxis, word list delayed recall, and word list recognition). It is administered in 20–30 minutes by a non-psychologist. The interrater agreement is substantial, the test-retest reliability is high, and its longitudinal validity has been established

(Welsh et al, 1994). Its clinical applicability is largely improved by the publication of norms for ages between 50 and 90 (Welsh et al, 1994). The best predictor of dementia has been found to be the difference score between delayed recall and learning (Welsh et al, 1994), which was relatively unaffected by influences of age, gender, and level of education.

The pro and con features of CERAD are listed below:

+   high test-retest reliability and validity
−   poor discrimination between dementia and normal aging
−   the influence of demographic variables on single measures
−   poor patterning of deficits in varying cognitive domains
−   predominance of verbal items, visuospatial abilities are poorly evaluated

To assess the cognitive status of severely demented individuals, specially designed instruments are needed. One example of these is the Severe Cognitive Impairment Profile (SCIP; Saxton et al, 1993), which appears to be a reliable and valid instrument (Peavy et al, 1996).

CANTAB, the Cambridge Neuropsychological Test Automated Battery (CANTAB; Robbins et al, 1994), represents a new type of assessment method that exploits computers to aid in the presentation of task, evaluation of performance, and interpretation of results. The battery includes a task used for non-human primates, for instance, pattern recognition, simultaneous and delayed matching-to-sample, paired associate learning, spatial working memory, and reaction time. A principal component analysis revealed four components, the first equated with learning and memory performance, a second factor was related to speed of performance, a third to executive functioning, and a fourth to visual perception. These components remained consistent across age groups. The CANTAB has been demonstrated to have a high level of reliability and validity (Robbins et al, 1994). It is not, however, the only computerized cognitive assessment system (see Braconnier et al, 1981).

The primary advantages and disadvantages of computerized testing are listed below:

+   rigorous standardization of presentation and recording
+   enables ease of assessment by use of computers
+   high level of reliability and validity
+   ties up with non-human primate research on learning and memory
+   relatively low sensitivity for age variation
+   enables patterning of cognitive components
−   difficulty in presenting certain forms of material and difficulty in using verbal responses
−   necessity of using a keyboard/mouse or other technical equipment

Table 3.5.1. A profile of cognitive functioning expressed as standardized scores in early Alzheimer's disease

Function	Test	Raw score	Norm	Profile (Z) −2	−1	0	+1	+2
Cognition	WAIS-R	79 iq	2	.	*	.	.	.
	MMSE	26 p	wr	.	.	*	.	.
Verbal	Similarities	9 p	2	.	*	.	.	.
	Boston Naming	58 p	7	.	.	.	*	.
	FAS word fluency	30 p	3	.	*	.	.	.
Spatial	Block Design	12 p	1	*	.	.	.	.
	Rey–Osterrieth Copy	32 p	2	.	*	.	.	.
Memory	Digit Span Forward	5.0 p	3	.	*	.	.	.
	Corsi Span	4.4 p	3	.	*	.	.	.
	Rey AVLT	21 p	1	*	.	.	.	.
	Rey–Osterrieth Retention	1 p	1	*	.	.	.	.
Attention	Digit Symbol	15 c	1	*	.	.	.	.
	Trail-Making, part A	36 s	6	.	.	.	*	.
	Trail-Making, part B	162 s	1	*	.	.	.	.
Motor	Finger-Tapping: right	70 p	8	.	.	.	.	*
	Finger-Tapping: left	68 p	7	.	.	.	*	.

wr = without remarks c = number correct
iq = intelligence quotient s = seconds
p = points

COMPREHENSIVE NEUROPSYCHOLOGICAL TESTING

The comprehensive assessment of cognitive functioning covers general intellectual ability, executive functions, language and communication, visuospatial functions, and various aspects of memory, attention, sensory and motor performance, which are usually presented in standardized scores and summarized as a profile, see below. Usually several tests are used within each cognitive domain. Accounts of some of the possible tests can be found in textbooks of neuropsychological assessment (see Lezak, 1995). The examination requires a minimum of a skilled psychology assistant for conducting the tests and scoring, and a neuropsychologist for interpretation of the results. The high costs of manpower in comparison to other methods of cognitive assessment have to be evaluated in relation to the precision and richness of data obtained. However, a detailed account of neuropsychological testing deserves a book of its own. Consequently we can give only a brief example in the form of a case report of early Alzheimer's disease, including a summary of the neuropsychological report (Table 3.5.1).

Case story—early Alzheimer's disease

This case was a married man, aged 54, with two children, who had had years of formal education, and was previously a skilled worker in a printing office, and an artist and a carpenter in his spare time, but at the time of investigation was unemployed due to reorganization of the company. He was referred to the hospital because of chest pain, but the cause of this was identified. He had a massive heredity of dementia, several individuals having developed dementia with an early onset between 50 and 60 years of age. There was no illness in his previous life history. No drug abuse. No psychiatric symptoms. Currently, he himself reported perfect health, he denied any problems with memory (he had always been easily distracted), spatial orientation or any other cognitive function. The electrocardiogram was normal. On magnetic resonance tomography, some small white matter was observed and bilateral hyperintensities in addition to normal ventricles, sulci, and gyri. The hippocampus was normal at visual inspection. A single photon emission tomography showed somewhat lower perfusion in the left versus the right hemisphere, but otherwise a normal perfusion pattern. The electroencephalogram was pathological, episodes of focal abnormality of the left frontotemporal region were found, but the background activity was quite normal. The neurological status was unremarkable. Laboratory tests were normal. The neuropsychological report said that personal relations were adequate, more specifically he was cooperative ('for the sake of science') when examined. The premorbid cognition was judged to be average. His current general cognition was below average according to the Wechsler Adult Intelligence Scale—Revised (WAIS-R). Good results were obtained in confrontation naming (the Boston Naming test), but they were below average in verbal abstraction as indicated by the Similarities test (WAIS-R). Verbal fluency (the FAS test) demonstrated a borderline performance. Visuospatial functions were clearly below average (remember that the patient was an artist as a hobby) according to the Rey–Osterrieth Copy task and the Block Design test (WAIS-R). Primary memory was at the lower normal limit for verbal and visuospatial material (Digit Span Forward and Corsi block Tapping Span). Most markedly, the episodic memory was impaired both for verbal and for visuospatial material (intrusion errors were frequent). The psychomotor performance was clearly below average (Digit Symbol and Trail-Making). Finger motor performance was superior, no assymmetry was observed (right-handed). The progression was obvious in most cognitive functions during a 3.5 year period, illustrated below on the Rey–Osterrieth Copy test (see Figure 3.5.1). The diagnosis was early Alzheimer's disease, because episodic memory and some other cognitive functions showed clear deficits which were clearly below the premorbid level of functioning. In addition, the EEG indicated a possible brain disease and no other reason could be found for symptoms and progression apart from AD.

The primary advantages and disadvantages of a comprehensive neuropsychological assessment are listed below:

+ high reliability and validity
+ well-known worldwide tests may be used

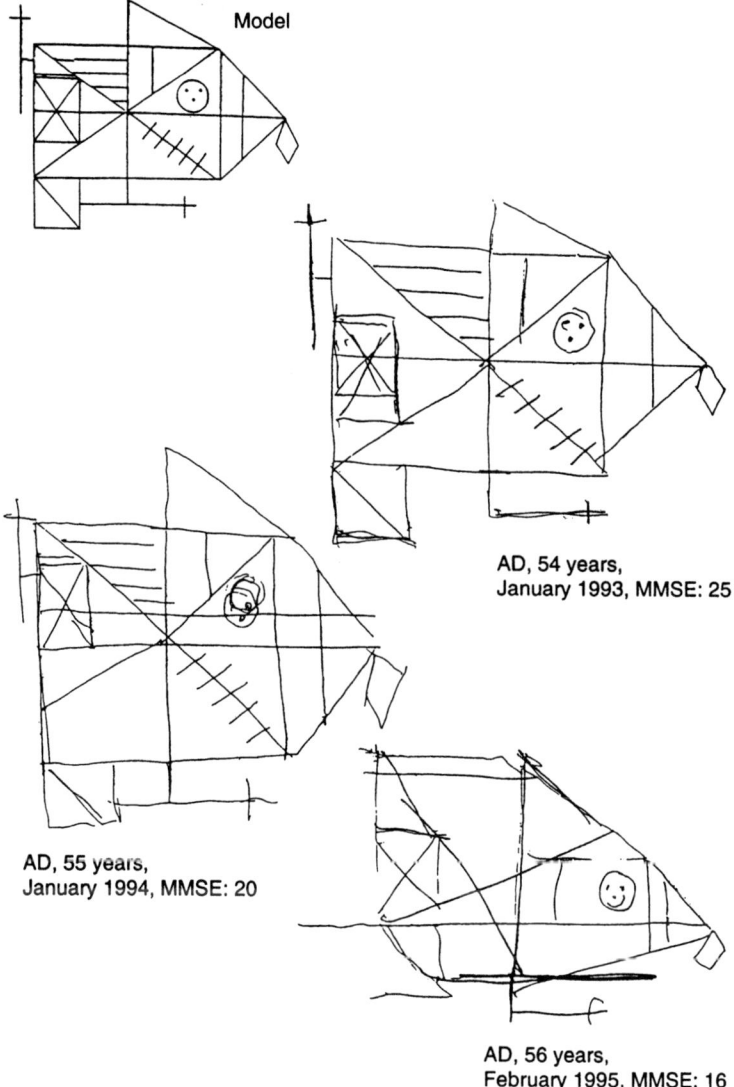

Figure 3.5.1. Performance on the Rey–Osterrieth Copy test on three annual examinations for a patient with early Alzheimer's disease

+ low rate of false positives in low education, blacks, etc., because premorbid functioning is taken into account
+ discrimination between normal aging and very mild dementia is possible
+ patterning of deficits in varying cognitive domains
+ well suited for research purposes

- low discrimination of moderate to severe dementia
- high costs in terms of manpower and time
- a neuropsychologist is required for analysis
- no worldwide consensus battery of neuropsychological tests exists

COMMENT

The requirements for a cognitive assessment are: comprehensive coverage of cognitive domains; reliability and validity; appropriate difficulty for the population intended; opportunity for repeated assessment; internal distribution; a balance between the demands of time and richness of information.

The brief methods of cognitive assessment discussed in this chapter have a number of merits compared to a full and comprehensive neuropsychological assessment. The costs are relatively low, the assessment requires less time, the administration requires less training, the information is satisfactory for detection of moderate dementia vs normal aging. Weaknesses include the shortage of information, which makes separation between very mild dementia and normal aging very difficult, also the differential diagnosis may be difficult, and for research purposes the scaling properties may lack precision.

The reliability and validity of the methods mentioned are satisfactory with regard to mild and moderate dementia. Most methods lack validity for the differentiation of very mild dementia from normal aging. There is also a lack of methods for grading severe dementia. The international distribution of methods may be improved by trying to standardize the procedures for diagnosis, differential diagnosis, prognosis of long-term outcome, prognosis of societal support and care, as well as treatment evaluation. International authorities may take the initial measures to improve the standardization of assessment procedures and possibly arrive at a consensus of methods to use for assessment of cognitive function. International authorities may also take the initial measures to begin developing methods that are still required (e.g., methods for assessing premorbid level of functioning, procedural memory, and executive function; Almkvist et al, 1996) as well as the development of reference data.

SUMMARY

To be successful in the diagnosis, the prognosis, the evaluation of treatment and so on, it is important to have access to reliable and valid assessment methods. However, the issue of methods for assessing cognitive function is not sufficiently developed, because internationally agreed-upon methods are lacking, and because methods are not available for the assessment of certain cognitive functions (e.g., procedural memory, complex executive functions, premorbid level of functioning; see Almkvist et al, 1996).

For the time being, it is recommended that a screening instrument—MMSE—is used to assess global cognitive function in addition to a short test of cognitive function to learn about the patterning of cognitive functions—ADAS, or CERAD, or CAMCOG. For staging, CDR or GDS may be used. For a comprehensive neuropsychological assessment, the battery used at the local specialist unit has to be used while we await a consensus battery to be agreed upon by an international forum.

REFERENCES

Almkvist, O. (1996). Neuropsychological features of early Alzheimer's disease: Preclinical and clinical stages. *Acta. Neurol. Scand.*, **165**(Suppl), 63–71.

Almkvist, O., Bråne, G. and Johanson, A. (1996). Neuropsychological assessment of dementia: State of the art. *Acta. Neurol. Scand.*, **168**(Suppl), 45–49.

Blessed, G., Tomlinson, B. E. and Roth, M. (1968). The association between quantitative measures of dementia and the senile change in the cerebral grey matter of elderly subjects. *Br. J. Psychiatry*, **114**, 797–811.

Braconnier, R. J., DeVitt, D. R. and Cole, J. O. (1981). Evaluation of drug efficacy in dementia: a computerized cognitive assessment system. *Psychopharmacol. Bull.*, **17**, 4–6.

Burke, W. J., Miller, P., Rubin, E. H. et al (1988). Reliability of the Washington University Clinical Dementia Rating. *Arch. Neurol.*, **54**, 3–32.

Christensen, H., Hadzi-Pavlovic, D. and Jacomb, P. (1991). The psychometric differentiation of dementia from normal aging: a meta-analysis. *Psychological Assessment: Journal of Consulting and Clinical Psychology*, **3**, 147–155.

Folstein, M. F., Folstein, S. E. and McHugh, P. R. (1975). 'Mini-Mental State'. A practical method for grading the cognitive state of patients for the clinician. *J. Psychiatr. Res.*, **12**, 189–198.

Gottfries, C. G., Bråne, G., Gullberg, B. and Steen, G. (1982). A new rating scale for dementia syndromes. *Arch. Gerontol. Geriatr.*, **1**, 311–330.

Hughes, C. P., Berg, L., Danziger, W. L., Coben, L. A. and Martin R. L. (1982). A new clinical scale for the staging of dementia. *Brit. J. Psychiat.*, **140**, 566–572.

Huppert, F. A., Brayne, C., Gill, C., Paykel, E. S. and Beardsall, L. (1995). CAMCOG—a concise neuropsychological test to assist dementia diagnosis: sociodemographic determinants in an elderly population sample. *Brit. J. Clin. Psychol.*, **34**, 529–541.

Lezak, M. D. (1995). *Neuropsychological Assessment* (third edn). New York, Oxford University Press.

Mattis, S. (1988). *Dementia Rating Scale: Professional Manual*. Odessa, FL, Psychological Assessment Resources.

Morris, J. C. (1993). The Clinical Dementia Rating (CDR): Current version and scoring rules. *Neurology*, **43**, 2412–2414.

Morris, J. C., Heyman, A., Mohs, R. C. et al (1989). The Consortium to Establish a Registry for Alzheimer's Disease (CERAD). Part I. Clinical and neuropsychological assessment of Alzheimer's disease. *Neurology*, **39**, 1159–1165.

Morris, J. C., McKeel, D. W., Fulling, K. et al (1988). Validation of clinical diagnostic criteria for Alzheimer's disease. *Ann. Neurol.*, **24**, 17–22.

Peavy, G. M., Salmon, D. P., Rice, V. A. et al (1996). Neuropsychological assessment of severely demented elderly. *Arch. Neurol.*, **53**, 367–372.

Pfeiffer, E. J. (1975). A Short Portable Mental Status Questionnaire for the assessment of organic brain deficits in elderly patients. *J. Am. Ger. Soc.*, **23**, 433–441.

Reisberg, B., Schneck, M. K., Ferris, S. H., Schwartz, G. E. and deLeon, M. J. (1983). The Brief Cognitive Rating Scale (BCRS): Findings in primary degenerative dementia (PDD). *Psychopharmacol. Bull.*, **19**, 47–50.

Reisberg, B. and Ferris, S. H. (1988). Brief Cognitive Rating Scale (BCRS): Findings in primary degenerative dementia (PDD). *Psychopharmacol. Bull.*, **24**, 629–636.

Reisberg, B., Ferris, S. H., deLeon, M. J. and Crook, T. (1982). The Global Deterioration Scale (GDS) for assessment of primary degenerative dementia. *Am. J. Psychiat.*, **139**, 1136–1139.

Reisberg, B., Ferris, S. H., Kluger, A. et al (1989). Symptomatic changes in CNS aging and dementia of the Alzheimer type: cross-sectional, temporal, and remedial concomitants. In Bergener and Reisberg (Eds), *Diagnosis and Treatment of Senile Dementia.*, pp. 193–223. Berlin, Springer-Verlag.

Robbins, T. W., James, M., Owen, A. M., Sahakian, B. J., McInnes, L. and Rabbitt, P. (1994). Cambridge neuropsychological automated battery (CANTAB): A factor analytic study of a large sample of normal elderly volunteers. *Dementia*, **5**, 266–281.

Rosen, W. G., Mohs, R. C. and Davis, K. L. (1984). A new rating scale for Alzheimer's disease. *Am. J. Psychiatry*, **141**, 1356–1364.

Roth, M., Tyme, E., Mountjoy, Q., Huppert, F. A., Hendrie, H., Verma, S. and Goddard, R. (1986). CAMDEX: A standard instrument for the diagnosis of mental disorder in the elderly with special reference for early detection of dementia. *Brit. J. Psychiatry*, **149**, 698–709.

Saxton, J., McGonigle, K. L., Swihart, A. A. and Boller, F. (1993). *The Severe Impairment Battery*. Bury St Edmunds, UK, Thames Valley Test Co.

Tombaugh, T. N. and McIntyre, N. J. (1992). The Mini-Mental State Examination: A comprehensive review. *J. Am. Geriatr. Soc.*, **40**, 922–935.

Wechsler, D. (1955). *Manual for the Wechsler Adult Intelligence Scale*. New York, Psychological Corporation.

Welsh, K. A., Butters, N., Hughes, J. P., Mohs, R. C. and Heyman, A. (1992). Detection and staging of dementia in Alzheimer's disease: use of the neuropsychological measures developed for The Consortium to Establish a Registry for Alzheimer's Disease (CERAD). *Arch. Neurol.*, **49**, 448–452.

Welsh, K. A., Butters, N., Mohs, R. C., Beekly, D., Edland, S., Fillenbaum, G. and Heyman, A. (1994). The Consortium to Establish a Registry for Alzheimer's Disease (CERAD). Part V. A normative study of the neuropsychological battery. *Neurology*, **44**, 609–614.

3.6 Measurements of Quality of Life in Dementia

PETER WHITEHOUSE

Case Western Reserve University, Cleveland, OH, USA

INTRODUCTION

The term quality of life (QOL) has become quality-of-life or perhaps qualityoflife. In other words, the phrase rolls off the tongue as if a single word or at least concept. The links between quality and life are so intimate that Katz (personal communication) referring to Pirsig can barely imagine life without quality (Pirsig, 1991). In many areas of health and other human activities improving QOL has been the dominant goal (Birren et al, 1991; Spilker, 1996). Despite the work of some pioneers (Lawton, 1994, 1997; Teri and Logsdon, 1991; DeJong et al, 1989) building on work in other fields (Katz, 1987) the concept of quality of life has not received adequate attention in the study of dementia, although this is now changing (Howard and Rockwood, 1994; Hollister and Gruber, 1996; Albert et al, 1996).

In an editorial in 1992, we said 'more and more we are coming to recognize that quality of life is not an isolated concept to be included as one of many measurements of the benefits of our care but rather it is the central goal of our professional activity driving the organization of both our clinical and research efforts' (Whitehouse and Rabins, 1992). In this chapter we will provide a conceptual framework for considering QOL, discuss QOL assessment in patients and caregivers of individuals affected by dementia, consider linkages to the field of pharmacoeconomics and conclude by discussing the incorporation of QOL in future research and care programs for dementia.

Prior to proceeding with this plan, let us consider why the study of QOL has been ignored in the field of dementia research and why it is now achieving some additional prominence. Scientists, clinicians and caregivers alike have focused excessively on the cognitive problems in Alzheimer's disease (AD). The core symptoms are considered problems with memory, attention, language, praxis and perception. The focus on cognitive symptoms has precluded serious consideration of the noncognitive symptoms such as agitation, depression, psychosis, wandering and other activity disturbances (Mendez et al, 1990). It is

Health Economics of Dementia. Edited by Anders Wimo, Bengt Jönsson, Göran Karlsson and Bengt Winblad.
© 1998 John Wiley & Sons Ltd.

these symptoms that have been neglected that are major contributors to the impairment of QOL. A patient who becomes only cognitively impaired but not disturbed by psychiatric symptoms may in fact not have a dramatically impaired QOL and may be a minimal burden on the caregiver. As insight and executive function are lost, the individuals themselves may be less tormented by the progressive loss of cognitive impairment (Patterson et al, 1996). Yet a patient who suspects a loved one of theft, curses and hits, and wanders all night, will not have a good QOL for themselves or their caregivers.

The focus on cognition also created a sense that there is no point in asking the patient about their QOL. If an individual cannot remember what they did the day before, cannot judge whether one activity is better than another, does not perceive the visual world accurately and cannot communicate their values and preferences, then they may clearly be limited in their ability to discuss their own QOL. As we will see later, the concept of QOL incorporates many subjective features. Thus, a disease that alters the subject's own ability to report their experience will limit assessment of QOL. However, this limitation is not absolute. Once investigators began to recognize that one could get reliable and valid information by asking patients about their own QOL, they removed a critical block to further investigation (Brod and Stewart, 1996; Logsdon et al, submitted). Thus, the focus on cognitive symptoms ignored other aspects of the phenomenology of the disease that impair QOL and created an environment in which investigators frequently did not study the patient's own preferences.

Of late, renewed attention has been paid to the assessment of behavioral symptoms and of activities of daily living (ADL) (Patterson et al, 1996; Gauthier et al, 1997) or functions that are important components of QOL (Whitehouse et al, 1997). Many instruments have been developed to assess cognition and relative consensus exists concerning the characteristics of desirable tests. A relatively short list could be offered that would include so-called standard instruments in the field (Ferris et al, 1997). For the assessment of behavior and ADLs the situation is quite different. In the initial studies of noncognitive symptoms and function in dementia, scales developed for assessing patients who were cognitively intact were used, for example the BPRS in the assessment of behavior symptoms. Now there has been a relatively rapid evolution of instruments to assess noncognitive symptoms including for example the BEHAVE-AD, the Consortium to Establish a Registry for Alzheimer's Disease (CERAD), Behavior Rating Scale for Dementia (BRSD) and the Neuropsychiatric Inventory (NPI) (reviewed in Homma et al, 1997; Weiner et al, 1996). So too in the area of function we have moved from using generic scales to those designed to assess patients with dementia such as the DADS, the NIA ADL Scale and the Cleveland ADL Scale (reviewed in Gauthier et al, 1997). The study of QOL in dementia can build on the developments of these disease-specific approaches to assessing behavior and function.

Another reason that QOL has not received much attention in the study of dementia has to do with the reaction of different groups of scientists, clinicians and public officials to the term. QOL is like the proverbial elephant surrounded by the seven blind men attempting to understand it as a holistic concept but being unable to do so. To some QOL cannot be defined and to others it is a term of no substance used by marketing agents that obscures consumers' ability to make health care choices. However, QOL can be defined both conceptually and operationally as discussed below and the misuse of the concept in the past does not imply that we should abandon the concept but rather that we should be wary about its application in different spheres of activity.

QOL is also receiving more attention because of its tie to outcomes research (Maslow and Whitehouse, 1997). A major force in both the health care market and other markets for products and services is the need to demonstrate that purchased services contribute to a positive outcome. Education is another area of service where the focus is increasingly on the value of the learning to the student consumer. Universities are being asked to demonstrate objective outcomes of their educational programs to students, parents, and employers. As a result, medical education is reeling under the pressure of outcomes orientation on both the health and education sides. Thus, outcomes research and evidence-based approaches are becoming dominant in scientific, educational, and clinical arenas.

Outcome measures are increasingly being demanded at a system- or population-level rather than just as individual patient outcomes. Interventions are likely to be considered more worthwhile (by payers for example) if they have positive effects on the community. Thus, in drug development we are moving beyond requiring efficacy for antidementia drugs to effectiveness (i.e. moving from a positive effect of a drug in carefully selected individual patients to a broader impact on populations of patients likely to be treated in a clinical setting). Moreover, we are recognizing that the drugs that only improve cognition and do not have an effect on function are less desirable than those with demonstrable broader effect. QOL assessment offers the opportunity to look at populations and patient outcomes. Improving QOL is a more profound effect than just improving paper and pencil tests of cognition or clinicians' impressions of change. This focus on QOL has also been driven by the fact that some medications have significant toxicities and so QOL offers a way of assessing the balance between positive and negative drug effects. Finally, in the United States particularly, an increasingly strong consumer focus has occurred in healthcare. QOL has become one of the rallying concepts for the consumer movement.

More generally we can ask why QOL has become such a dominant focus in health care and other areas of human life. This question could be an opportunity for great discussion and speculation. In health care we have done relatively well in terms of the goals of *quantity* in both years of life and numbers of people on the planet. As we recognize increasingly restricted resources, we are perhaps naturally (and rather belatedly) focusing on the *quality* of our time and life on this planet rather than purely the number of people and number of years. Thus, as the population of the world grows and we continue to extend individual life expectancy in many other countries, it is likely that focus on QOL will become even more evident. Hopefully QOL will be intimately tied to a deeper appreciation of our dependency and inter-relationships with our environment and fellow living creatures.

The continued growth of concerns about ethical aspects of health care will also foster considerations of QOL. Already discussions of abortion, *in-vitro* fertilization, transplants, end-of-life care and countless other biomedical ethical issues are replete with references to QOL concerns. Our own personal sense of our QOL is intimately connected with our values and hence to ethics. Bio-medical ethics, as a field, has been in existence for 25 years. The original coinage of the term bioethics was by Van Rensselaer Potter, elaborated in a book called *Bioethics: A Bridge to the Future* (1971). Such a view of bioethics as deeply and globally tied to environmental ethics and ecology will likely be a guiding ethic for QOL considerations in the future.

CONCEPTUAL FRAMEWORK

It has become the norm to start off a discussion of the concept of QOL by saying that there is no universally accepted definition. QOL is an abstract term and multiple definitions may be expected. However, there is considerable agreement about what forms the components of QOL. Both face and content validity of an assessment instrument can be judged by examining the domains of QOL that are captured. For clinicians the issue of the breadth of the concept of QOL has led to consideration of the concept of health-related QOL. Although this term is widely used, how it narrows the definition of QOL is unclear. The scope of health-related QOL depends on one's definition of health. If one considers the World Health Organization definition of 1948 as psychosocial well-being and not just the absence of disease then there seems to be little that is precluded from health-related QOL (see Szabo, 1996). One domain that is particularly challenging is the spiritual or religious side of QOL that is often excluded for health-related QOL. Perhaps financial status should be excluded from health-related QOL considerations. Yet these exclusions would seem to be unwise as a caregiver or patient's spiritual beliefs, religious traditions and financial well-being contribute strongly to the state of their health. Excluding these factors for health-related QOL might, in fact, be leaving out variables that have the strongest effect on preventing disease and enhancing psychosocial well-being. Thus, if a broad definition of health is considered, then there seems to be little difference between health-related QOL and general quality of life.

Perhaps Lawton (1997) offered the most widely used definition in the dementia field of QOL. He says QOL is the evaluation by both subjective and social normative criteria of the behavioral and environmental situation of the person. Lawton has proposed a model that is represented by a four-part overlapping ven diagram. The components in the model include objective environment, behavioral competence, psychosocial well-being and perceived QOL. Behavioral competence includes activities of daily living, cognitive performance and social behavior. Environment can be assessed objectively by measuring the amount of space and opportunities for both privacy and social interaction. The subjective components, psychosocial well-being and perceived QOL, are perhaps less easy to differentiate. Clearly, however, the subjective components are important because individuals with the same objective behavioral competencies and environment may perceive their QOL to be quite different. One can image a quadriplegic schizophrenic who is impoverished and living in a marginal long-term care institute who still values the quality of his or her life highly. Research has clearly shown that depression or a person's emotional status more generally is an important component in their assessment of their own subjective well-being (Albert et al, 1996).

The list of objectively assessable components of QOL is large and includes cognitive abilities, mental health, living arrangements, social relationships, financial well-being and spirituality or religion. Each of these components can be evaluated subjectively by the person being assessed as well as objectively by defining attributes of the person's behavioral repertoire or environmental situation. However, from the foregoing discussion and list of components it is clear that the assessment of QOL ideally requires input from the individual being assessed, that is, self-rating as well as objective measures of their situation. Until recently relatively few instruments were developed to assess QOL of patients with dementia although this is now changing rather rapidly.

ASSESSMENT OF QOL IN DEMENTIA

When considering assessment of QOL in dementia one is faced immediately with the fact that the disease affects a number of individuals in addition to the patient. Hence, it is appropriate to consider the assessment of QOL in both the affected individual and their caregivers, usually family members or professional staff (Stuckey et al, 1996). Thus we will separate our discussion and assessment of QOL and dementia to the patient and to the caregiver. We should make note here, however, that dementia affects the QOL of other individuals more distant from the primary caregiving team. First, there are many times secondary caregivers who may be affected in a less profound and consistent fashion than those who are the primary caregivers (i.e., sons and daughters in different cities or staff on other floors of a long-term care facility). Second, and this foreshadows our discussion of cost utility analysis later on, resources used to provide care for patients with dementia affect the QOL of individuals with other diseases and other social needs. There is an opportunity cost associated with investing in research and clinical care in dementia. Thus, it is reasonable to claim that practically everybody's QOL is affected by the rapidly growing problem of dementia around the world in one way or another.

ASSESSMENT OF PATIENT QUALITY OF LIFE

As mentioned above, a variety of instruments are available to assess certain components of QOL in dementia. The area of assessment of cognition is most well developed followed by noncognitive or psychiatric symptoms and finally by some new efforts to assess ADLs. The efforts to assess ADLs reveal that function in dementia is clearly affected by the patient's cognitive state. Executive functions strongly associated with activities in the front parts of the cortex are perhaps the most critical to cognitive abilities that affect function (Patterson et al, 1996). Executive functions include the motivation and the ability to set goals and to monitor whether the goals are achieved. Thus in some sense executive functions are one's own supervisor or caregiver. A patient with profound frontal lobe difficulties may become apathetic and lose initiative, requiring another individual to provide step by step advice about task completion. Moreover, patients damaged frontally may also show social disinhibition and loss of control of affect that are distressing to both patients and caregivers. Thus it is clear that the severity and pattern of an individual's cognitive disabilities will dramatically affect the QOL of the individual and his loved ones.

Three approaches have been used to assess QOL of the patient: (1) observer ratings of patient behavior, (2) proxy informants concerning the patients QOL and (3) most recently self-ratings of the patient concerning their QOL. It is likely that more approaches and instruments will emerge that cannot be covered here (Kerner et al, 1995).

Observer measures

Any clinician or family member observing an individual with dementia can make some reasonable interpretations of QOL based on objectively assessed behavior. A patient who is screaming or wandering and showing physiological signs of anxiety would be judged as not enjoying a high QOL at the moment. Much of the research on direct observation has been done in nursing homes (Lawton et al, 1994). Lawton and associates have developed the Philadelphia Geriatric Affect Scale and new approaches are being developed that use computerization to assess behavior. Most of these approaches are direct observation and can be very time-consuming. The rater is asked to directly observe the patient and record certain behaviors. Displays of affect can be also assessed although this represents a higher level of interpretation than just observing whether the patient is wandering or vocalizing. One of the first published uses of affect observation was a distress index (Hurley et al, 1992). More recently Cornelia Beck has expanded on the original Lawton scale to develop the Observed Displays of Affect Scale (Beck, unpublished). This scale requests that the observer examines facial display, for example eye contact and smiles, vocalizations, including the speech content and nonspeech utterances, movements and posture, including nonverbal communication and activity. The patient is observed for ten minutes and the numbers of occurrences are assessed. Such observation measures require some degree of interpretation in order to connect to assessment of QOL.

Caregiver ratings of Quality of Life

A second approach to assessment of QOL in patients is to ask other individuals to rate the QOL of the patient. The problem here is that a caregiver or some individual must fill out a rating scale as if they were the patient (Logsdon et al, submitted; Rabins and Kasper, 1997). However, the patient's behavior affects the QOL of the caregiver and consequently may affect their assessment of the patient. One of the first scales developed using this approach was the Pleasant Event Schedule in AD (Teri and Logsdon, 1991). A family caregiver, ideally working along with the patient to fill out the form, rates 53 items. The focus of this instrument is on positive events and an assessment is made of the frequency of performance at these pleasant events. One of the problems of this approach is the type of pleasant events to consider as individuals live in different settings and different activities may or may not be available. More recently, activity participation has been assessed using the HFCA-Uniform Minimum Data Set (MDS), a federally mandated resident assessment process. This has led to development of a Social Engagement Index, which can be used to assess the patient's participation in a variety of activities that affect QOL. Recently, Logsdon et al (submitted) have developed a rating scale which includes opportunities for family and the person to assess QOL. They found reasonable reliability for the instrument for both patients and caregivers separately as well as validity in terms of the relationship between the two raters. They found the depressive symptoms were the best predictor of QOL scale scores.

An instrument, which was also developed early in the field, was developed for clinical drug trials (DeJong et al, 1989). This scale, called the Progressive Deterioration Scale, contains 27 items, which were developed from in-depth interviews with caregivers. Most of the items however related to activities of daily living; thus, this scale is heavily focused on function.

Recently Albert et al (1996) have looked at the relationship between activities and affect. This study included rating of patients' participation and enjoyment of certain non-ADL activities as well as an assessment by facial and body expressions of positive and negative affects. They found that activity frequency was linearly related to severity of disease and that high QOL defined by a combination of frequent activity and positive affect was evident in about a quarter of their sample. Functional and cognitive status independently predict QOL with patient education predicting some activity patterns. The authors conclude, 'while the subjective world of the demented patient is not directly assessable, readily observable behaviors offer a basis for assessing quality of life.' Although this is important pioneering work, we should point out that the subjective world is not directly accessible in any individual whether demented or not.

Self-ratings by demented patients of Quality of Life

For the reasons discussed above, only recently have individuals assessed whether patients can reliably self-report their own sense of QOL. Interestingly, an early instrument developed by Blau (1977) was incorporated in studies of donepezil (a cholinesterase approved for the treatment of AD). The Blau instrument asked patients to assess life quality in domains relating to working, leisure, eating, sleeping, social contact, earning, parenting, loving, environment and self-acceptance. Thus this instrument extends beyond activities of daily living to social relationships and subjective states. Although as yet unpublished, the preliminary data suggest that donepezil at least in some studies had a positive effect on self-ratings of QOL. This instrument was not specifically designed for use with demented patients however.

A specific project to assess the abilities of patients to self-rate QOL has been developed by Drs Meryl Brod and Anita Stewart (Brod and Stewart, 1996). These investigators conducted a two-phase study in which they refined the concept of QOL in demented populations and then developed an instrument for use by patients in assessing their own QOL. The expert panel confirmed that assessment of QOL in demented patients is not futile. There was considerable consensus around the domains to be assessed. They found relatively low correlation between proxy and subject reports as had been reported previously in the literature, but found that patients with a Mini-Mental State Exam score as low as 12 could reliably fill out a self-rating form. Their instrument includes mechanisms to assess reliability and employs a simple response set. Their domains include physical functioning, daily activities, mobility, social functioning, subjective well-being and psychological self-concept. Thus, it appears that self-rating for patients with dementia, at least into the moderate stages of the disease, can be accomplished reliably and with good content validity.

CAREGIVERS

Both family member and professional caregivers have their QOL affected by the dementing illness. Numerous national and international projects have developed ways of assessing the impact of Alzheimer's disease on caregivers. The concept of caregiver burden has evolved in the field of dementia to focus on the impact of caregiving on individuals caring for patients with chronic disease (Deimling et al, 1989; Stuckey et al, 1996). In addition to assessing specific affects of the disease, attempts have been made to assess QOL of caregivers without specific reference to their caregiving situation. Since caregivers are likely to be intellectually unimpaired, any appropriate approaches to assess QOL in nondemented subjects can be used.

In our center we have developed a two-faceted approach to assess the impact of the disease on caregivers. The first is to assess the impact of caregiving itself, including both the negative and positive aspects, and the second is to assess caregiver QOL. This approach has been adopted by the National Institute of Aging Cooperative Study for use in clinical drug trials.

Our approach to assessing the caregiver experience includes measuring impact on physical health, relationship with the affected individual, overall assessment of burden and finances, as well as use of formal and informal services, including steps taken to learn about particular services.

The assessment of caregiver QOL is not tied to the caregiving experience but includes physical health, the use of a list of adjectives to assess affect, social relationships, overall QOL, and positive experiences. The purpose of combining these two approaches is to understand the interrelationships between patient characteristics, caregiver characteristics, and the caregivers' response to the illness and general QOL (Stuckey et al, 1996). Collecting information about the costs of care and health care utilization in parallel will allow us to understand the relationship among patient and caregiver variables and the impact on the health care system.

RELATIONSHIPS BETWEEN QUALITY OF LIFE AND PHARMACOECONOMICS

Pharmacoeconomics is a new area of study that has emerged in the 1990s from concerns about the relative effectiveness and costs of different medications (Spilker, 1996; Bootman et al, 1996; Ernst and Hay, 1994; Henke, 1994). Some recent attention has been paid to chronic diseases, particularly to the study of dementia (Hu et al, 1987; Huang et al, 1988; Lubeck et al, 1994). Yet, there is much work to be done on assessing cost, developing models for health service utilization and understanding ways of assessing the impact of interventions on individuals, families and society (Aronson, 1997; Lane, 1987; Gunderson, 1996; Wilson and Cleary, 1995).

As mentioned above, studies of tacrine, the first drug approved for Alzheimer's disease in the United States and in some other countries, and donepezil, the second drug, have included assessments of QOL (DeJong et al, 1989). These were not considered part of measurements obtained for regulatory approval purposes but have been included both on an experimental basis and perhaps to attempt to impact pricing of drugs.

The direct involvement of QOL in pharmacoeconomics involves cost-utility studies (Hay and Ernst, 1997; Ernst et al, 1997; Max, 1996). There are two basic forms of cost-effectiveness analysis, cost benefit and cost utility. In cost benefit, the cost of an intervention is compared with the costs that are estimated to be saved by using the intervention. Thus both the numerator and the denominator involve dollars or some other currency. In cost-utility studies, QOL appears as the denominator as utility weights to be compared with costs in the numerator. These utility weights account for preferences for particular outcomes that are often represented in units called Quality Adjusted Life Years (QALYs). A variety of ways of calculating utility weights have been used including magnitude estimation, time trade-off and standard gamble (Berzon et al, 1996). Unfortunately, comparisons between these different methods may not give consistent or even similar patterns of results. Moreover, only recently have attempts been made to develop standard approaches to conducting cost-utility analysis (Gold et al, 1996).

We are also trying to develop pharmacoeconomic models that incorporate QOL. Dr Marian Patterson, a neuropsychologist, is considering which patient variables contribute to a caregiver's desire to institutionalize the patient. This model depends on the assessment of executive functions as described above. This set of higher cognitive abilities includes goal setting, planning, organization and self-monitoring. The Patterson model also considers functional disability and impairment of activities of daily living. The concept of desire to use services was developed for use in clinical intervention trials when enough patients and time may not be included in the design to allow a large number of transition events, for example, from home to nursing home. In the model the desire to use services is measured by asking caregivers how many steps they have taken to approach a particular service. For example, before placing a patient in a nursing home, the caregiver needs to find out what is a nursing home, which nursing homes are available, what is required for admission and perhaps make a visit and place the patient on a waiting list. All of these occur before placement occurs and can be used as a measure of the likelihood that a patient will be actually admitted in the future.

Dr Smyth and her colleagues in our center have developed a model that elaborates the variables that affect caregiver burden and QOL (Stuckey et al, 1996). Thus, the emphasis in the Smyth model is on the characteristics of the caregiver and in the Patterson model the emphasis is on the patient characteristics reflecting the relative disciplines of the individuals involved. However, we will eventually develop a comprehensive model, which includes patient and caregiver characteristics to predict both QOL and service utilization.

FUTURE ISSUES

The importance of QOL in dementia will likely grow in the future. A number of issues will affect this development that relate to general trends in the health care system. As mentioned above, these are likely to contribute to an emphasis on outcomes research and evidence-based medicine. Thus, whether the intervention is a special care unit in a nursing home or a new drug, demonstration of positive affects of a broader nature on populations of patients will likely be expected, if not by regulatory bodies, by payers. Although it is unlikely that QOL measures will be included in decisions about regulatory approval of a drug, it is likely that managed care organizations and national governments will take into account evidence of positive impact on QOL for either the inclusion of drugs on formularies or pricing.

Major changes in health care systems around the world are continuing largely as a result of the impact of the aging of the world's population. Dementia represents one of the major feared illnesses of the elderly and a major force driving change. A number of different types of dementia-specific care programs have developed around the world, including community-based respite, integrated managed care, and special care units for long-term institutionalized care. In the US a Medicare demonstration project was designed to study effects of case management on patients with dementia and their families. It continues to be difficult in community demonstrations to demonstrate an effect of such case-management approaches. The literature on special care units is also unclear as to whether there is an impact and if so, what the impact is of these units. There is no uniform definition about what is a special care unit. They include programs with entirely new buildings, with different staffing and models of care to minimal shifts in existing bed usage and service pattern. However, attempts to demonstrate that these provide an improved level of care for patients' families or professional caregivers have been rather unsuccessful.

In the future integration of acute and chronic care will likely occur. The National Chronic Care Consortium is developing several models for integration of care models, finance and information systems to bridge between the acute world of the hospital and the world of the community and institutional long-term care. In such attempts to demonstrate that such integrated programs are beneficial to society, measuring impact on the QOL patients' families and caregivers will likely be an important component.

An additional factor that will be important in future studies of QOL is the globalization of dementia and the appreciation of cultural diversity both between countries and within countries. Certainly cultural beliefs play an important role in defining aspects of QOL. For example, some cultures may value social relationships and family ties more than others that may emphasize the value of privacy and individual freedom. Thus, as we conduct intervention studies across national boundaries or within countries and try to assess QOL, sensitivity to cultural variables will be critical (Whitehouse et al, 1997).

An area of QOL often ignored in scientific studies is the dimension of religion and spirituality. Changes are occurring in traditional religions as well as the development of new sources of spiritual belief. Studies have shown that spiritual beliefs do affect health. One would expect that these effects could operate through conceptions of what QOL is and how one should achieve it. Thus it seems impossible to ignore spirituality and religious beliefs as a part of the assessment of QOL.

One could extend this argument to ask whether a science of QOL is possible or whether scientific approach risks distorting the subject of the inquiry. Certainly it is possible to study QOL scientifically as we have attempted to demonstrate above. Equally, there are aspects of QOL which are subjective, ineffable, and spiritual. The assessment of QOL necessarily involves a discussion of values. These are areas in which scientific inquiry is either incompetent or unsure, thus it is likely that the scientific study of QOL leads us to some fundamental issues at the heart of how much of any social problem scientific analysis can capture its full richness and complexity (and therefore likely or not to provide a technological fix).

Finally, we should recognize that the study of QOL should inform some serious public policy discussions. The health of the world will be an increasingly important and difficult problem because of the growing numbers of individuals and the ravages of poverty and environmental pollution. How can the world support a growing number of older people with birth rates in many countries shrinking? What should be the relative priorities for research among different diseases, for example AIDS and Alzheimer's disease? One of the advantages of the study of QOL, particularly with a technique such as cost-utility analysis, is that it allows comparisons amongst diseases. One can compare an intervention in AIDS with one in Alzheimer's disease and ask what is the relative magnitude of effect of one intervention versus another. If we examine stage-specific issues of QOL of dementia (as we should) then what do we say about the value of interventions that slow the progression of disease in a patient who can no longer recognize their spouse of 50 years or feed him or herself? Thus a focus on QOL will lead us into difficult topics concerning the relative allocation of resources to research and clinical care in dementia as well as to the allocation of resources of different stages for the disease. However, these are important topics that we will inevitably need to address more fully as our population ages and health care systems are increasingly strained. It is better that we add a richer understanding of QOL in dementia to this discussion of the links between science and social and individual values. Yet we must realize that the study of QOL is not a panacea. QOL (or the perceived lack thereof) could be used to justify inhumane and unjust changes in our caring (or lack thereof) for each other on this fragile planet.

REFERENCES

Albert, S. M., Del Castillo-Castaneda, C., Sano, M., Jacobs, D. M., Marder, K., Bell, K., Bylsma, F., Lafleche, G., Brandt, J., Albert, M. and Stern, Y. (1996). Quality of life in patients with Alzheimer's disease as reported by patient proxies, *J. Amer. Geria.*, **44**, 1342–1347.

Aronson, S. M. (1997). Cost-effectiveness and quality of life in psychosis: the pharmacoeconomics of risperidone, *Clin. Ther.*, **19**(1), 139–147, discussion 126–127.

Beck C. (unpublished, 1996). Observable Displays of Affect Scale.

Berzon, R. A., Mauskopf, J. A. and Simeon G. P. (1996). Choosing a health profile (descriptive) and/or a patient-preference (utility) measure for a clinical trial. *Quality of Life and Pharmacoeconomics in Clinical Trials*, 2nd edn, pp. 375–378, Philadelphia, Lippincott-Raven.

Birren, J. E., Lubben, J. E., Rowe, C. J. and Deutchman, D. E. (1991). *The Concept and Measurement of Quality of Life in the Frail Elderly*, New York, Academic Press.

Blau, T. H. (1977). Quality of life, social indicators and criteria of change, *Professional Psychology*, **11**, 464–473.

Bootman, J. L., Townsend, R. J. and McGhan, W. F. (1996). *Principles of Pharmacoeconomics*, 2nd edn, Cincinnati, Harvey Whitney Books.

Brod, M. and Stewart, A. (1996). Quality of life in dementia: conceptualization and measurement. Final report to the Alzheimer's Association.

Deimling, G. T., Bass, D. M., Townsend, A. L. and Noelker, L. S. (1989). Care-related stress: A comparison of spouse and adult-child caregivers in shared and separate households, *J. Aging Health*, **1**, 76–82.

DeJong, R., Osterlund, O. W. and Roy, G. W. (1989). Measurement of quality of life changes in patients with Alzheimer's disease, *Clinical Therapeutics*, **11**(4), 545–554.

Ernst, R. L. and Hay, J. W. (1994). The U.S. economic and social costs of Alzheimer's disease revisited, *Am. J. Public Health*, **84**, 1261–1264.

Ernst, R. L., Hay, J. W., Fenn, C., Tinklenberg, J. and Yesavage, J. A. (1997). Cognitive function and the costs of Alzheimer disease: an exploratory study, *Arch. Neurol.*, **54**, 687–693.

Ferris, S. H., Lucca, U., Mohs, R., Dubois, B., Wesnes, K., Hellmut, E., Geldmacher, D. and Bodick, N. (1997). Objective psychometric tests in clinical trials of dementia drugs: position paper from the International Working Group on Harmonization of Dementia Drug Guidelines, *Alzheim. Disea. Assoc. Disord.*, **11**(Suppl 3), 34–37.

Gauthier, S., Bodick, N., Erzigkeit, E., Feldman, H., Geldmacher, D. S., Huff, J., Mohs, R., Orgogozo, J.-M. and Rogers, S. (1997). Activities of Daily Living as outcome measure in clinical trials of dementia drugs: position paper from the International Working Group on Harmonization of Dementia Drug Guidelines, *Alzheim. Disea. Assoc. Disord.*, **11**(Suppl 3), 6–7.

Gold, M. R., Siegel, J. E., Russell, L. B. and Weinstein, M. C. (Eds) (1996). *Cost-Effectiveness in Health and Medicine*. New York, Oxford University Press.

Gunderson, C. H. (1996). The impact of new pharmaceutical agents on the cost of neurologic care, *Neurology*, **45**, 569–572.

Hay, J. W. and Ernst, R. L. (1997). Economic research on Alzheimer's disease: A review of the literature, *Alzheim. Disea. Assoc. Disord.*, **11**(Suppl 6), 135–145.

Henke, C. J. (1994). The costs of Alzheimer's disease and its treatment, *Am. J. Public Health*, **84**, 1261.

Hollister, L. and Gruber, N. (1996). Drug treatment of Alzheimer's disease. Effects on caregiver burden and patient quality of life, *Drugs in Aging*, **8**(1), 47–55.

Homma, A., Brodaty, H., Bruno, G., Cummings, J. L., Gilman, S., Gracon, S. and McKeith, I. G. (1997). Clinical trials of treatment for noncognitive symptoms of dementia: position paper from the International Working Group on Harmonization of Dementia Drug Guidelines, *Alzheim. Disea. Assoc. Disord.*, **11**(Suppl 3), 54–55.

Howard, K. and Rockwood, K. (1994). Quality of life in Alzheimer's disease, *Dementia*, **6**, 113–116.

Hu, T., Huang, L. and Cartwright, W. S. (1987). Evaluation of the costs of caring for the senile demented elderly: A pilot study, *Gerontologist*, **26**, 158–163.

Huang, L., Cartwright, W. S. and Hu, T. (1988). The economic cost of senile dementia in the United States, *Public Health Rep.*, **103**, 3–7.

Hurley, A. C., Volicer, B. J., Hanarahan, P. A., Houde, S. and Volicer, L. (1992). The assessment of discomfort in advanced Alzheimer's patients, *Res. Nurs. Health*, **15**, 369–377.

Katz, S. (1987). The Science of Quality of Life, *J. Chron. Dis.*, **6**, 459–463.

Kerner, D. N., Patterson, T. L. and Kaplan, R. M. (1995). Validity of the Quality of Well-Being Scale for patients with Alzheimer's disease, *Annual Meeting Supplement Posters D035-D038*. S171:D037.

Lane, D. A. (1987). Utility, decision and quality of life, *J. Chron. Dis.*, **40**(6), 585–591.

Lawton, M. P. (1994). Quality of life in Alzheimer's disease, *Alzheim. Disea. Assoc. Disord.*, **8**(3), 138–150.

Lawton, M. P. (1997). Assessing quality of life, *Alzheim. Disea. Assoc. Disord.*, **11**(Suppl 6), 91–99.

Lawton, M. P., van Haitsma, K. and Klapper, J. (1994). A balanced stimulation and retreat program for a special care dementia unit, *Alzheim. Disea. Assoc. Disord.*, **8**(Suppl 1), S133–S138.

Logsdon, R. G., Gibbons, L. E., McCurry, S. M. and Teri, L. (submitted). Quality of life in Alzheimer's disease: patient and caregiver reports.

Lubeck, D. P., Mazonson, P. D. and Bowe, T. (1994). Potential effect of tacrine on expenditures for Alzheimer's disease, *Pharmacoeconomics*, **7**, 130–138.

Maslow, K. and Whitehouse, P. (1997). Defining and measuring outcomes in Alzheimer disease: Conference findings, *Alzheim. Disea. Assoc. Disord.*, **11**(Suppl 6), 186–195.

Max, W. (1996). The cost of Alzheimer's disease. Will drug treatment ease the burden? *Pharmacoeconomics*, **9**(1), 5–10.

Mendez, M. F., Martin, R. J., Smith, K. A. and Whitehouse, P. J. (1990). Psychiatric symptoms in Alzheimer's disease, *J. Neuropsych. Clin. Neurosci.*, **2**, 228–233.

Patterson, M. B., Mack, J. L., Geldmacher, D. S. and Whitehouse, P. J. (1996). Executive functions and Alzheimer's disease problems and prospects, *Euro. J. Neur.*, **3**, 5–15.

Pirsig, R. M. (1991). *Lila: an inquiry into Morals*. New York, Bantam.

Potter, V. R. (1971). *Bioethics: Bridge to the Future*. Englewood Cliffs, NJ, Prentice-Hall.

Rabins, P. V. and Kasper, J. D. (1997). Measuring quality of life in dementia: conceptual and practical issues, *Alzheim. Disea. Assoc. Disord.*, **11**(Suppl 6), 100–104.

Spilker, B. (1996). Adopting higher standards for quality of life trials. *Quality of life and Pharmacoeconomics in Clinical Trials*, 2nd edn, pp. 57–58, Philadelphia, Lippincott-Raven.

Stuckey, J. C., Neundorfer, M. M. and Smyth, K. A. (1996). Burden and well-being: the same coin or related currency? *Gerontologist*, **36**, 686–693.

Szabo, S. (on behalf of the WHOQOL Group) (1996). The World Health Organization Quality of Life (WHOQOL) Assessment Instrument, *Quality of Life and Pharmacoeconomics in Clinical Trials*, 2nd edn, pp. 355–362, Philadelphia, Lippincott-Raven.

Teri, L. and Logsdon, R. G. (1991). Identifying pleasant activities for Alzheimer's disease patients: The Pleasant Events Schedule-AD, *Gerontologist*, **31**(10), 124–127.

Weiner, M. F., Koss, E., Wild, K. V., Folks, D. G., Tariot, P., Luszczynska, H. and Whitehouse, P. J. (1996). Measures of psychiatric symptoms in Alzheimer patients: a review, *Alzheim. Disea. Assoc. Disord.*, **10**(1), 20–30.

Whitehouse, P. J. and Rabins, P. V. (1992). Quality of life and dementia, *Alzheim. Disea. Assoc. Disord.*, **6**(3), 135–137.

Whitehouse, P. J., Orgogozo, J.-M., Becker, R. E., Gauthier, S., Pontecorvo, M., Erzigkeit, H., Rogers, S., Mohs, R. C., Bodick, N., Bruno, G. and Dal-Bianco, P. (1997). Quality of life assessment: Role in dementia drug development, *Alzheim. Disea. Assoc. Disord.*, **11**(3), 56–60.

Wilson, I. B. and Cleary, P. D. (1995). Linking clinical variables with health-related quality of life: A conceptual model of patient outcomes, *J. Amer. Med. Assoc.*, **273**(1), 59–65.

3.7 Assessment of Behavioral and Psychiatric Symptoms in Patients with Dementia Disorders

STURE ERIKSSON
Umeå University, Umeå, Sweden

ANDERS WIMO
Karolinska Institute, Stockholm, Sweden

INTRODUCTION

Patients with dementia disorders show two main groups of symptoms. The first is the obligate cognitive decline, characterized by memory as well as other cognitive disturbances such as disorientation in space and time, reduced logical thinking, impaired language function and visuospatial disturbances. The second group of symptoms is often referred to as complications, non-cognitive behavioral disturbances, disruptive behavior, secondary symptoms, psychic or psychiatric symptoms in dementia. A Consensus Group has suggested the term behavioral and psychological signs and symptoms in dementia (Finkel et al, 1996). This group of symptoms includes a wide spectrum such as delusions and paranoid symptoms, hallucinations, disturbances in motor activities, including wandering, repetitive motor activities (cognitive abulia) and inadequate activities. This group also comprises verbal and physical agitation and aggressiveness, refusal behavior, sleep disturbances, depressive symptoms and various patterns of anxiety.

SYMPTOMS

One form of delusional ideation in dementia is confabulations, including ideas such as 'people stealing things', 'this house is not my house' or 'my spouse is an imposter'. These confabulations may be rather easy to divert temporarily and they are often not stable, that is, the symptoms occur only part of the day. Examples of paranoic psychotic symptoms are ideas of a conspiracy to put the

Health Economics of Dementia. Edited by Anders Wimo, Bengt Jönsson, Göran Karlsson and Bengt Winblad.
© 1998 John Wiley & Sons Ltd.

patient in hospital or that the spouse is unfaithful. Paranoic ideas are firmly held and impervious to any evidence to the contrary. It is important to separate delusions from illusions. The latter means that the patient misinterprets sensory input. Spaghetti may be worms and shadows may be real things. Illusions are usually regarded as a part of the cognitive symptoms and not as delusions. Hallucinations mean the patient experiences sensations without any real basis, such as visual, auditory, olfactory and haptic forms. The latter means that the patients have a sense of something touching the body, such as small insects.

Wandering without any purpose or goal is a well known behavior among demented patients. Cognitive abula consists of a meaningless repetition, such as repetition of a question but also a repeated motoric activity like going-up-and-down movements, or hammering on the table.

Inadequate behavior involves inappropriate activities such as hiding things, eating flowers and using waste baskets as toilets. Aggression and agitation may be verbal or physical, but the predominant group of symptoms are fending movements, particularly during nursing activities. Disturbances in sleep are common in dementia. There is a variety in such disturbances, from slight insomnia problems to a totally inverted diurnal rhythm.

Depression occurring in dementia is seldom of the classical melancholic type if the patient has not previously suffered from this type of depression. Instead, dysthymic conditions dominate with symptoms of anxiety, apathy and agitation. Anxiety linked to expectations (real or unreal, known or unknown) is usual as well as phobic anxiety, linked to a fear of being left alone.

EPIDEMIOLOGY OF BEHAVIORAL AND PSYCHIATRIC SYMPTOMS IN DEMENTIA

Most patients with dementia develop some kind of behavioral and psychiatric symptoms. In a study by Mega et al (1996), only 16% did not present any such symptoms. However, there is a great span in the prevalence figures, due to a number of factors, such as diagnostic criteria for dementia, different types of dementia, sampling technique, study design, setting and presence or absence of medication. The variation seems to be greater in the community than in nursing homes (Ritchie, 1996) and there are also differences between countries (Homma, 1996). In general, the frequency of psychiatric symptoms peaks in the middle phase of dementia, and not in the early or late stages (Ferris and Mackell, 1997; Reisberg et al, 1992, 1996). Reisberg et al (1991) also found that 24–48% of a community sample of persons with Alzheimer's disease presented symptoms such as agitation, violent behavior and verbal outbursts. Of demented patients entering nursing home care 40% had symptoms of depression, delirium and delusions (Rovner et al, 1990). A review by Flint (1991) indicated that the prevalence of delusions in Alzheimer's disease ranges from 15–56% and in Vascular dementia (VD) from 27–60%. Burns et al (1990) reported delusions in 30% and hallucinations in 30% of patients with Alzheimer's disease. The presence of delusional symptoms has also been associated with a more rapid cognitive (Mayeux et al, 1975) but not functional (Stern et al, 1987) decline. There is a variety in the prevalence figures of depression, in most studies around 20–30% (Reifler et al, 1986; Skoog, 1993) but both lower (5–10%) (Brodaty and Luscombe, 1996) as well as higher figures have been presented (Mega et al, 1996). Anxiety varies in frequency, according to the degree of dementia, between about 20–80% (Reisberg et al, 1989; Mega et al, 1996).

INTERPRETATION OF BEHAVIOR

Symptoms which we regard as 'behavioral disturbances' must in some way be interpreted in the clinical situation. The symptoms should be given an explanation, leading to a strategy for treatment. However, analysis of behavioral disturbances often needs a multifactorial approach. A logical approach is to use the organ, person and social levels as a structure for interpretation. At the organ level the focus of interest is on the diseased brain, at the personal levels the focus is on effects on the whole person and thus most on functional decline, and at the social level most interest is on the effects and interactions with the environment and other people. Another approach is to link the symptomatology to an acute confusial state, which may be added as a complication to dementia. Another model is based on a theory of emotional instability caused by deficiencies in the serotoninergic system (Whitford, 1986; Gottfries, 1990) causing anxiety, agitation, aggressiveness and depression. The premorbid profile of the personality also influences how a demented person will react in different situations (Hamel et al, 1990). The brain damage itself, with loss of synapses and neurons, probably also causes behavioral manifestations which we regard as 'disturbances' (Cummings, 1997a). It is also important to search for somatic complications, such as fractures, urinary retention, constipation, pain, before different types of treatment are carried out (Nygaard, 1991).

ECONOMIC IMPACT

The occurrence of behavioral and psychiatric symptoms in dementia is in many cases a great cause of suffering, both for the patients and for their caregivers, which itself is a challenge for anyone engaged in dementia care and research. However, these symptoms also have a great economic impact. The process of institutionalization of the demented is multifactorial, where many factors such as behavior, comorbidity, relationships and caregiver burden interact in a complex way (Clipp and George, 1986; Potter, 1993; Wright,

1994; Mittelman et al, 1996), but psychiatric symptoms are obviously very important reasons for institutionalization (Stern et al, 1987; Nygaard, 1991; Wimo et al, 1992; Brodaty and Luscombe, 1996). Psychiatric symptoms are therefore of great interest when the economic impact of dementia is discussed. Since institutional care in all its forms comprises the major body of the costs of dementia care (Wimo et al, 1997) and psychiatric symptoms at least partly and sometimes to a great extent are treatable, all kinds of intervention activities (non-pharmacologic as well as pharmacologic) dealing with psychiatric symptoms are of great significance. Assessments of psychiatric symptoms should therefore be almost a mandatory part of any intervention study where health economic aspects are included.

ASSESSMENTS

Assessment of psychiatric symptoms and behavior in dementia has during recent years been the focus of various comprehensive presentations (e.g. Medical Products Agency and The Norwegian Medicines Control Authority, 1995; Finkel, 1996a, b; Cummings, 1997), because of the great impact such symptoms have on the outcome of care. There are several scales assessing different psychiatric symptoms in dementia and there is also debate among researchers in this field regarding several methodological issues (e.g. which dimensions of psychiatric symptoms should be included in a scale and whether the frequency or the severity or both should be assessed) (Finkel and Cooler, 1996).

Some scales focus on the whole pattern of symptomatology in dementia, such as ADAS (Rosen et al, 1984) and GBS (Gottfries et al, 1982), while some are designed to cover certain groups of symptoms, such as cognitive symptoms, behavioral and psychiatric symptoms and symptoms of functional decline. In this chapter we will briefly present three frequently used scales which focus on behavioral and psychiatric symptoms in dementia, but with different approaches: the BEHAVE-AD assesses the severity of symptoms, the NPI assesses both frequency and severity while the CMAI assesses the frequency of symptoms and it also has a more narrow approach since it focuses on different aspects of one dimension of behavior, agitation.

BEHAVE-AD

BEHAVE-AD (Reisberg et al, 1989) is a rating scale assessing most non-cognitive symptoms in Alzheimer's disease. BEHAVE-AD consists of 25 items in seven groups, assessing the severity (in four levels: 0–3) of symptoms (Table 3.7.1). There is also a global rating including on how the behavior affects the caregiver. The rating in BEHAVE-AD is based on reports from the caregiver and takes up to 45 minutes to administer but takes a considerably shorter time

Table 3.7.1. Dimensions in the BEHAVE-AD

Delusions and paranoic symptoms
Hallucinations
Disturbed motor patterns
Aggressiveness and agitation
Diurnal rhythm disturbances
Affective symptoms
Anxiety and phobias

Table 3.7.2. Dimensions in the NPI

Delusions
Hallucinations
Dysphoria
Anxiety
Agitation/aggression
Apathy
Euphoria
Disinhibition
Irritability/lability
Aberrant motor activity

if the report is given by an experienced caregiver in a hospital setting. It can also be used as a measurement of the effects of behavior on caregivers (Kluger and Ferris, 1991). Various tests have shown that BEHAVE-AD is reliable and valid (Reisberg et al, 1996).

NEUROPSYCHIATRIC INVENTORY (NPI)

The Neuropsychiatric Inventory, NPI (Cummings et al, 1994), includes assessments of ten dimensions of behavioral disturbances in dementia (Table 3.7.2). Both the frequency and the severity of the behavioral dimensions are assessed. Every dimension has a screening question with 7–9 follow-up questions regarding symptoms in detail if the answer to the screening question is yes. Tests regarding interrater and intrarater reliability as well as concurrent and content validity have shown that the instrument is reliable and valid. The results can be presented both for the subscales (dimensions) and as a global score. It takes about 7–10 minutes for an experienced clinician to administer the scale by interviewing the caregiver.

COHEN-MANSFIELD AGITATION INVENTORY (CMAI)

The CMAI (Cohen-Mansfield et al, 1989) consists of items describing various aspects of agitated behavior. There are different versions of the CMAI but the original version consists of 29 items (Table 3.7.3). Each item in the CMAI

Table 3.7.3. Items in the CMAI (long version)

Aimless wandering	Trying to get to a different place
Inappropriate dressing/undressing	Intentional falling
Spitting	Complaining
Cursing/verbal aggression	Negativism
Constant requests for attention/help	Eating inappropriate substances
Repeated sentences/questions	Hurting self or others
Hitting	Handling things inappropriately
Kicking	Hiding things
Grabbing	Hoarding things
Pushing	Tearing things
Throwing things	Repetitious mannerism
Making strange noises	Verbal sexual advances
Screaming	Physical sexual advances
Biting	General restlessness
Scratching	

assesses the frequency of symptoms during the last two weeks in a 7-point way (1 = never, 7 = several times an hour). CMAI can be administered by the caregivers themselves or through interviews. Even if the scale was originally developed for nursing home patients, there are also other versions for different purposes, for example a 37-item version for community-based use.

CONCLUSION

Psychiatric symptoms of demented patients are heavy predictors of institutionalization and caregiver burden and these symptoms also result in suffering for the patients themselves. However, these conditions are also potentially treatable and therefore are assessments of great importance in any intervention in dementia care.

REFERENCES

Brodaty, H. and Luscombe, G. (1996). Depression in persons with dementia. *Int. Psychogeriatr.*, **8**(4), 609–622.

Burns, A., Jacoby, R. and Levy, R. (1990). Psychiatric phenomena in Alzheimer's disease II: disorders of perception. *Br. J. Psychiatr.*, **157**, 76–81.

Clipp, E. J. and George, L. K. (1986). Predictors of institutionalization among caregivers of patients with Alzheimer's Disease. *J. Am. Geriatr. Soc.*, **34**, 493–498.

Cohen-Mansfield, J., Marx, M. S. and Rosenthal, A. S. (1989). A description of agitation in a nursing home. *J. Gerontol. (Medical Sciences)*, **44**, M77–M84.

Cummings, J. L. (Ed.) (1997a). Alzheimer Disease Therapy. Behavior as an efficacy outcome. *Alzheimer Dis. Assoc. Disord.*, **11** (suppl 4).

Cummings, J. L. (1997b). Changes in neuropsychiatric symptoms as outcome measures in clinical trials with cholinergic therapies for Alzheimer Disease. *Alzheimer Dis. Assoc. Disord.*, **11** (suppl 4), 1–9.

Cummings, J. L., Mega, M., Gray, K., Rosenberg-Thompson, S., Carusi, D. A. and Gornbein, J. (1994). The Neuropsychiatric Inventory: Comprehensive assessment of psychopathology in dementia. *Neurology*, **44**, 2308–2314.

Eriksson, S. (1995). Pharmacological treatment of psychiatric symptoms in patients with dementia disorders. In Medical Products Agency (Sweden) and The Norwegian Medicines Control Authority. Treatment of mental conditions in patients with dementia. Medical Products Agency, Stockholm, Sweden.

Ferris, S. H. and Mackell, J. A. (1997). Behavioral outcomes in clinical trials for Alzheimer's disease. *Alzheimer Dis. Assoc. Disord.*, **11** (suppl 4), 10–15.

Finkel, S. I. (Ed.) (1996a). Research Methodologic issues in evaluating behavioral disturbances in dementia. *Int. Psychogeriatr.*, **8** (suppl 2).

Finkel, S. I. (Ed.) (1996b). Research Methodologic issues in evaluating behavioral disturbances in dementia. *Int. Psychogeriatr.*, **8** (suppl 3).

Finkel, S. I. and Cooler, C. (1996). Clinical experiences and Methodological challenges in conducting clinical trials on the behavioral disturbances of dementia. *Int. Psychogeriatr.*, **8** (suppl 2), 151–163.

Finkel, S. I., Costa e Silva, J., Cohen, G. et al (1996). Consensus statement. Behavioral and psychological signs and symptoms of dementia. A consensus statement on current knowledge and implications for research and treatment. *Int. Psychogeriatr.*, **8**(3), 497–500.

Flint, A. J. (1991). Delusion in dementia: A review. *Journal of Neuropsychiatry*, **3**, 121–128.

Gottfries, C. G. (1990). Disturbance of the 5-hydroxytryptamine metabolism in brains from patients with Alzheimer's dementia. *J. Neural Transm.*, **30** (suppl), 33–43.

Gottfries, C. G, Bråne, G., Gullberg et al (1982). A new rating scale for dementia symptoms. *Arch. Gerontol. Geriat.*, **1**, 311–330.

Hamel, M., Gold, D. P., Andres, D. et al (1990). Predictors and consequences of aggressive behavior by community based dementia patients. *Gerontologist*, **30**, 206–211.

Homma, A. (1996). Parameters considered in multinational clinical drug trials. *Int. Psychogeriatr.*, **8**(2), 165–167.

Kluger, A. and Ferris, S. H. (1991). Scales for the assessment of Alzheimer's disease. *Psychiatr. Clin. North. Am.*, **14**, 309–327.

Maycux, R., Stern, Y. and Sano, M. (1975). Psychosis in patients with dementia of the Alzheimer type. *Ann. Neurol.*, **257** (suppl), 8–35.

Medical Products Agency (Sweden) and The Norwegian Medicines Control Authority (1995). Treatment of mental conditions in patients with dementia. Medical Products Agency, Stockholm, Sweden.

Mega, M., Cummings, J. L., Fiorello, T. et al (1996). The spectrum of behavioral changes in Alzheimer's disease. *Neurology*, **46**, 130–135.

Mittelman, M. S., Ferris, S. H., Shulman, E. et al (1996). A family intervention to delay nursing home placement of patients with Alzheimer's disease. *JAMA*, **276**, 1725–1731.

Nygaard, H. A. (1991). Who cares for the caregiver? Factors exerting influence on nursing home admissions of demented elderly. *Scand. J. Caring Sci.*, **5**, 156–162.

Potter, J. F. (1993). Comprehensive geriatric assessment in the outpatient setting: population characteristics and factors influencing outcome. *Exp. Gerontol.*, **28**, 447–457.

Reifler, B. V., Larson, E., Teri, L. et al (1986). Dementia of the Alzheimer's type and depression. *J. Am. Geriatr. Soc.*, **34**, 855–859.

Reisberg, B., Franssen, E., Sclan, S. G. et al (1989). Stage specific incidence of potentially remediable behavioral symptoms in aging and Alzheimer's disease: a study of 120 patients using the BEHAVE-AD. *Bull. Clin. Neurosci.*, **54**, 95–112.

Reisberg, B., Borenstein, J., Salob, S. P. et al (1991). Behavioral symptoms in Alzheimer's disease: Phenomenology and treatment. *J. Clin. Psychiatry*, **48** (suppl), 9–15.

Reisberg, B., Ferris, S. H., Torossian, C. et al (1992). Pharmacological treatment of Alzheimer's disease: a methodological critique based upon current knowledge of symptomatology and relevance of drug trials. *Int. Psychogeriatr.*, **4** (suppl 1), 9–42.

Reisberg, B., Auer, S. R., Monteiro, I., Boksay, I. and Sclan, S. G. (1996). Behavioral disturbances of dementia: an overview of phenomenology and methodologic concerns. *Int. Psychogeriatr.*, **8** (suppl 2), 169–180; discussion 181–182.

Ritchie, K. (1996). Behavioral disturbances of dementia in ambulatory care settings. *Int. Psychogeriatr.*, **8** (suppl 3), 439–442.

Rosen, W. G., Mohs, R. C. and Davis, K. L. (1984). A new rating scale for Alzheimer's Disease. *Am. J. Psychiatry*, **14**, 1356–1364.

Rovner, B. W., German, P. S., Broadhead, J. et al (1990). The prevalence and management of dementia and other psychiatric disorders in nursing homes. *Int. Psychogeriatrics*, **2**, 13–24.

Skoog, I. (1993). The prevalence of psychotic, depressive and anxiety syndromes in demented and non-demented 85-year-olds. *Int. J. Geriatr. Psychiatr.*, **8**, 247–253.

Steele, C., Rovner, B., Chase, G. A. et al (1990). Psychiatric symptoms and nursing home placement of patients with Alzheimer's Disease. *Am. J. Psychiatry*, **147**(8), 1049–1051.

Stern, Y., Mayeux, R., Sano, M. et al (1987). Predictors of disease course in patients with probable Alzheimer's disease. *Neurology*, **37**, 1649–1653.

Whitford, G. M. (1986). Alzheimer's disease and serotonin: a review. *Neuropsychology*, **15**, 133–142.

Wimo, A., Mattsson, B. and Gustafsson, L. (1992). Predictive validity of factors influencing the institutionalization of elderly people with psycho-geriatric disorders. *Scand. J. Prim. Health Care*, **10**, 185–191.

Wimo, A., Ljunggren, G. and Winblad, B. (1997). Costs of dementia and dementia care—a review. *Int. J. Geriatr. Psychiatr.*, **12**, 841–856.

Wright, L. K. (1994). Alzheimer's disease afflicted spouses who remain at home: Can human dialectics explain the findings? *Soc. Sci. Med.*, **38**, 1037–1046.

3.8 Instruments to Measure the Family Caregiver Burden

MARGARETA GRAFSTRÖM
Karolinska Institute and Stockholm Gerontology Research Center, Stockholm, Sweden

P. O. SANDMAN
University of Umeå, Umeå, Sweden

When a family is stricken by an illness like Alzheimer's disease it is necessary to take care of the patient as well as his/her family. From the literature we know that the family is often very involved and the experience of being a caregiver has been fully described. Living together with a demented person will affect the caregiver physically and psychologically as well as socially.

Isolation in the role as a family member, the need for constant supervision with little or no support from others, a reduction in ordinary personal or social activities, and conflicting multiple role demands are some of the issues described in studies of the demented elderly and their family members (Haley et al, 1987; Cohen and Eisdorfer, 1988; Pruchno and Potanshnik, 1989; Rankin, 1990).

The experience of being a caregiver to a demented patient will differ from individual to individual. There is no exact, objective method for assessing stress related to the caregiving situation. Vulnerability to stress, the relationship to the demented person, and the caregiver's personality, health and degree of social and spiritual support dictate the nature of the relationships in the individual experience of stress. It is important to understand that the caregiver could react in many different ways and that their reactions could change during the course of the disease. For example, one caregiver may experience the caregiving situation as a challenge which calls for spirit and drive, while another person may react to a similar situation with anxiety, guilt or depression (Pearlin et al, 1990).

In the main, there are two different points of departure when studying relatives' experiences of being caregivers. The first strategy has been to use instruments with the specific purpose of measuring the experience of burden in relation to the demented elderly. Another strategy has been to use instruments established for other purposes than gauging the family caregiver burden,

Health Economics of Dementia. Edited by Anders Wimo, Bengt Jönsson, Göran Karlsson and Bengt Winblad.
© 1998 John Wiley & Sons Ltd.

for example instruments measuring anxiety, health, depression, the family member's interrelationship, economy and social network. The first strategy was aimed at measuring the burden in a global perspective, while the second strategy focuses on more specific factors in the caregiver's situation.

When reviewing the literature one can see a need for studies where caregivers to demented patients are compared to relatives of non-demented patients. For this purpose instruments developed specifically to measure the burden related to dementia and caregiving are not suitable since the control group may not have had experience either of a demented person or of a caregiving situation. In that case it may be better to use instruments focusing on more specific stressors.

THE CONCEPTS OF BURDEN AND STRESS

Burden has been a key concept in research on family caregiving. The concept has been an 'umbrella' that can take on a number of different meanings. However, there is little clarity about the content and scope of the concept 'burden'. One well-known definition is: 'Caregiver burden is the physical, psychological or emotional, social and financial problems that can be experienced by family members caring for impaired older adults' (George and Gwyther, 1986, p. 253).

However, not all caregivers to the demented elderly are necessarily stressed. What is stressful for one caregiver may not be for another. Burden is likely to be a multivariate phenomenon, and is related to many care-recipient and caregiver variables. For that reason, burden has been broadly defined and differentially measured. The concept has been operationally defined in different ways by different researchers. The fact that burden is defined and measured in so many ways makes cross-study comparisons difficult.

As a result of the range of definitions researchers have divided the concept 'burden' into two components: subjective and objective (Thompson and Doll, 1982). Subjective burden is defined as the subjective experience related to the elderly patient's specific impairment. Objective measures of burden include the impact caregiving has on family relationships, social activities, health or employment changes (Poulshock and Diemling, 1984). Here we will describe some of the measures used in research on AD-caregivers' burden.

The Burden Interview (BI) (Zarit et al, 1980; Zarit and Zarit, 1987) is a 22-item self-report inventory that examines burden associated with functional/behavioral impairment and the home care situation. The interview is based on clinical reports and previous studies. Items in their interview cover five areas: health, psychological well-being, finances, social life and the relationship between the caregiver and the impaired person. A 5-point scale (ranging from never to nearly always present) is used. As BI is focused on consequences of caregiving it is often complemented by the Memory and Behavior Problems

Checklist (Zarit and Zarit, 1987), which measures both the problems of the impaired elder and the perceptions of these demands as stressful for the caregiver. This 30-item checklist is scored on two grids, one to measure the frequency of the behavior, and the other to measure caregiver reactions. Together these two scales assess care-recipient-centered problems, and offer a complete picture of the problems of the impaired elder and the caregiver's responses to the problems, making it possible to separate and evaluate prevalence of experience and caregiver distress. The scoring of the BI and Behavior Problems Checklist together assesses both the subjective and the objective burden.

Another instrument for assessing both subjective and objective burden is the *Caregiver Social Impact Scale* (Poulshock and Deimling, 1984). This is a model in which burden plays a central role between the elder's impairment on the one hand, and the impact that caregiving has on the life of the caregiver and the family on the other hand. Elder impairment was represented by the number of activities of daily living with which the elder required assistance, and three mental impairment indicators—sociability, disruptive behavior and cognitive incapacity—which were all based on the caregiver's responses to questions about the degree to which the specific impairment upset them or created a problem for them. The variable impact is operationalized as disruption of family life (job conflict, finances, interpersonal relationship) and restriction of activity. In this model it is stated that similarly to burden, impact is a multidimensional concept, which needs to be redefined as a limited number of dimensions that describe the different kinds of impact that caregivers experience. The two impact items in the measure were negative impact on elder-caregiver family versus caregiver social activity restriction. Analysis of this model highlights the need to apply the concept of burden to subjective interpretations by caregivers of the elderly's impairments (Poulshock and Deimling, 1984).

Major changes and unexpected daily problems are two types of stressors, often leading to chronic stress (Lazarus and Folkman, 1984, p. 13). Daily troubles occurring in the routine in the care of a demented elderly person give rise to everyday problems which have to be solved. It is important that these less dramatic, but still stressful experiences, arising from the role as a caregiver, must also be regarded as stressors. To measure these items, the *Caregiver Hassles Scale* (CHS) was developed as a global measure of day-to-day demands of caregiving (Kinney and Stephens, 1989). This instrument yields information about the occurrence and degree of hassle in the daily care of an elderly person with AD but does not assess subjective burden in relation to them. It consists of 110 items, reflecting a variety of potential hassles that might have occurred during the previous week of caregiving. Five rationally derived categories of potential caregiving stressors were represented, including hassles associated with assisting the care-recipient with basic activities of daily living (ADL), the care-recipient's cognitive status and behavior, and practical aspects of the caregiving and caregiver support network. The caregiver indicates along a 5-point scale, ranging from not at all to extremely, how distressed they were by each symptom during the previous week (Kinney and Stephens, 1989). This restriction to occurrences during the past week may be reflected as a weakness, as some tasks are time-limited, whereas other items may be experienced over a longer period.

The Caregiver Burden Inventory (CBI) (Novak and Guest, 1989) is a multidimensional measure of caregiver burden. To construct a caregiver burden inventory, caregivers were interviewed in their own homes using a questionnaire with open-ended and fixed choice questions dealing with caregiver burden. Burden items were identified and selected after a principal component factor analysis. The factors derived were: time dependence (e.g. 'my care-receiver needs my help to perform many daily tasks'), developmental burden (e.g. 'I feel that I am missing out on life', 'I wish I could escape from this situation'), physical burden (e.g. 'I'm not getting enough sleep, my health has suffered'), social burden (e.g. 'I don't get along with other family members as well as I used to'), and emotional burden ('I feel embarrassed about my care-receiver's behavior'). Responses to each item range from 0 (not at all) to 4 (very descriptive). As with the BI (Zarit et al, 1980), the items include both affective responses and task-related sources of burden, mixing subjective and objective burden (Vitaliano et al, 1991a). Summarizing burden scores masks underlying sources of burden (George and Gwyther, 1986) and may make it difficult to follow the change of burden items longitudinally. The authors therefore constructed a Caregiver Burden Profile. This can be used as a comprehensive measure of burden within both the clinical and the research field (Vitaliano et al, 1991a).

The screen for *Caregiver Burden* (SCB) is a 25-item measure designed to assess objective and subjective burden among caregivers of spouses with AD (Vitaliano et al, 1991a). The SCB is used to target potentially distressing experiences. Caregivers were asked to name the most upsetting caregiver experience in their lives. The most frequently cited stressors were translated into structured items, which tap several domains, such as recipient behaviors, disruptions in family and social life and caregiver affective responses. Scoring on the SCB yields both objective (prevalence count of potentially negative experiences) and subjective burden (appraised distress in relation to each experience). The SCB does not measure the full domain of caregiver experiences, but rather those that are related to burden. The authors stress that a more accurate definition of subjective and objective burden would be 'appraisal of distress from experiences' instead of subjective burden, and 'prevalence of experiences' instead of objective burden. The authors have stated that because the CBI lacks subscales, it may best be used as a rapid screening measure (Vitaliano et al, 1991b). In three separate studies it was reported that changes in objective and subjective burden over time are explained by changes in care-recipient functioning and caregiver distress (Vitaliano et al, 1991b).

CONCLUSION

There is no exact, objective method for assessing stress in the caregiving situation. In the measures presented above, caring for a demented elderly person is mostly reflected as a heavy burden and a tremendous challenge, but burden may also be looked upon as an opportunity to fulfil a sense of obligation to a spouse or a parent. Being a close relative to an elderly demented person may also have positive outcomes, such as a feeling of success or satisfaction in meeting the demands as a challenge. A challenge that has characteristics similar to threat but also involves the opportunity for gain and growth (Lazarus and Folkman, 1984, pp. 32–35; Sällström, 1994). The caregiving situation may provide an opportunity for finding inner growth and meaning in life. Lawton et al (1989) suggest that researchers should focus on relationships between burden, mastery and satisfaction, as positive appraisals are associated with the satisfaction of caring for a loved one with dementia and a broader rubric than burden.

REFERENCES

Cohen, D. and Eisdorfer, C. (1988). Depression in family members caring for a relative with Alzheimer's disease. *J. Am. Geriatr. Soc.*, **36**, 885–889.

George, L. and Gwyther, L. P. (1986). Caregiver well-being: A multidimensional examination of family caregivers of demented adults. *Gerontologist*, **6**, 253–259.

Haley, W. E., Levine, E. G., Brown, S. L., Berry, J. W. and Hughes, G. H. (1987). Psychological, social and health consequences of caring for a relative with senile dementia. *J. Am. Geriatr. Soc.*, **35**, 405–411.

Kinney, J. and Stephens, M. A. (1989). Caregiving Hassles Scale: Assessing the daily hassles of caring for a family member with dementia. *Gerontologist*, **29**, 328–332.

Lawton, M. P., Kleban, M. H., Moss, M., Rovine, M. and Glicksman, A. (1989). Measuring caregiver appraisal. *Journal of Gerontology*, **44**, 61–67.

Lazarus, R. S. and Folkman, S. (1984). *Stress, Appraisal and Coping*. New York, Springer.

Novak, M. and Guest, C. (1989). Caregiver response to Alzheimer's disease. *Int. J. Aging and Human Development*, **28**, 67–77.

Pearlin, L. L., Mullan, U. T., Semple, S. J. and Skaff, M. M. (1990). Caregiving and the stress process: An overview of concepts and their measures. *Gerontologist*, **30**, 583–593.

Poulshock, S. W. and Diemling, G. T. (1984). Families caring for elders in residence: Issues in the measurement of burden. *Gerontologist*, **39**(2), 230–239.

Pruchno, R. A. and Potashnik, S. L. (1989). Caregiving spouses. Physical and mental health in perspective. *J. Am. Geriatr. Soc.*, **37**(8), 697–705.

Rankin, E. D. (1990). Caregiver stress and the elderly: A familial perspective. *J. Gerontol. Soc. Work*, **15**, 57–72.

Sällström, C. (1994). Spouses' experiences of living with a partner with Alzheimer's disease. Umeå University Medical Dissertations, New Series No 39.

Thompson, E. H. and Doll, W. (1982). The burden of families coping with the mentally ill: An invisible crisis. *Family Relations*, **1**(31), 379–388.

Vitaliano, P. P., Young, H. M. and Russo, J. (1991a). Burden: A review of measures used among caregivers of individuals with dementia. *Gerontologist*, **31**, 67–75.

Vitaliano, P. P., Russo, J., Young, H. M., Becker, J. and Maiuro, R. D. (1991b). The screen for caregiver burden. *Gerontologist*, **31**, 76–83.

Zarit, S. H. and Zarit, J. M. (1987). The memory and behavior problems checklist— and the Burden interview. Gerontology Center, College of Health and Human Development, University Park, PA, Pennsylvania State University.

Zarit, S. H., Reever, K. E. and Bach-Peterson, J. (1980). Relatives of the impaired elderly: Correlates of feelings of burden. *Gerontologist*, **20**, 649–655.

4 Pharmacoeconomic Aspects

4.1 Drug Authorities' Policy on the Assessment of Drugs for Dementia

SUZANNE HILL and PATRICIA McGETTIGAN
University of Newcastle, New South Wales, Australia

THERAPEUTIC OPTIONS IN DEMENTIA

The development of drugs for the treatment of dementia remains in its infancy, although much consideration, particularly in relation to the socioeconomic aspects, has been given to this increasingly prevalent disorder. As dementia syndromes may have multiple aetiologies and pathophysiologies, it is unlikely that a single 'anti-dementia' drug will ever exist. It is more probable that a variety of drugs, affecting the symptoms of the disorder or modifying its aetiological or pathological processes, will eventually be developed. At present, tacrine and donepezil are targeted specifically at patients with Alzheimer's dementia, although neither affects the underlying process that causes loss of neurons and synapses and leads to functional and intellectual deterioration. Newer acetylcholinesterase inhibitors, such as ENA 713, are currently being investigated. Other therapeutic options, including antioxidants and mono-amine oxidase (B) inhibitors, have been assessed in the trial situation and found beneficial in delaying functional deterioration (Sano et al, 1997). It has recently been reported that a selective muscarinic M1-receptor partial agonist, SB-202026, appears to improve the cognitive performance of patients with probable Alzheimer's disease (Anon, 1997).

REGISTRATION AND REIMBURSEMENT ISSUES

In assessing new drugs, including those for the treatment of dementias, regulatory authorities consider their quality, safety and efficacy, as opposed to their costs or the economic consequences relating to their subsequent use. Social responsibility requires that society shares the cost of looking after its ill, and in many countries (in Europe, Canada and Australia), the state has

Health Economics of Dementia. Edited by Anders Wimo, Bengt Jönsson, Göran Karlsson and Bengt Winblad.
© 1998 John Wiley & Sons Ltd.

traditionally borne the brunt of the costs of health care provision. This has included medicines, the costs of which are reimbursed to the provider, in most cases, the pharmacist. While decisions about licensing/registration of drugs and the payment for them are usually considered separately, it has generally been the case in state-supported health care systems that, once registered, prescription drugs were reimbursed at, or close to, the prices requested by their manufacturers.

Increasingly, drug costs, and therefore reimbursement issues, are attracting attention from cash-strapped governments seeking to control spiralling health care expenditure. This has been particularly the case in Australia, where economic evaluation of new drugs for which reimbursement is sought has been a legal requirement since 1993 (Commonwealth of Australia, 1987). In Europe, Japan, Canada and the United States, the integration of economic evaluation throughout the clinical development process is encouraged, although to date, its inclusion in either registration or reimbursement submissions has not been required by law. While the registration process in the European Union (EU) has been centralised through the European Medicines Evaluation Agency (EMEA), drug companies may still opt to approach European regulatory authorities on a country-by-country basis. EU countries continue to negotiate drug prices individually with manufacturers and the levels of drug costs reimbursement vary between countries. The addition of the 'fourth hurdle' of economic data as a requirement for reimbursement has been considered to present a major challenge to both the methods of economic evaluation and the development of health care policy (Drummond, 1994).

We will now outline and discuss registration and reimbursement processes within the major pharmaceutical markets. We will consider in particular the issues that may influence the development of drug regulatory authorities' policy in relation to dementia.

DRUG REGISTRATION

Drug regulatory authorities undertake responsibility for the registration or licensing of new drugs for marketing within their own jurisdictions. Their aim in reviewing submissions from pharmaceutical manufacturers is to ensure that drugs approved for marketing are of adequate quality, safety and efficacy. In reaching a decision to license, data from laboratory studies, animal studies and Phase I–III studies in humans are considered.

In the evaluation of anti-dementia drugs, the assessment of data relating to quality and safety aspects is more straightforward than that concerning efficacy. Standards for pharmaceutical quality are well defined, although there may be difficulties when new drugs are not included in pharmacopoeias such as the British Pharmacopoeia or United States Pharmacopoeia. An estimate of safety is based on animal and human toxicology studies and adverse reaction reports from the Phase I–III trials. Given the relatively limited population exposed to a new drug during its development, pre-marketing data must be supplemented through post-marketing surveillance studies and voluntary adverse reaction reporting systems, although the limitations of both are well recognised. In common with other drugs, the issue in relation to anti-dementia drugs is balancing the possible risks with the benefits of therapy. This consideration leads inevitably to the questions of efficacy and effectiveness.

The evaluation of efficacy presents significant difficulties for regulatory authorities. This is due in no small part to the nature of dementia, in particular, Alzheimer's disease, characterised as it is by symptoms of dysmnesia, intellectual deterioration, changes in personality and behavioural abnormalities, which together result in social and occupational decline. There is no single symptom or feature of the disorder that can easily be translated into an outcome measure for a clinical trial—how, for example, may the impact of not pouring soup into the toaster be compared with that of being able to return to one's car in the parking lot?

In some respects, the problem of efficacy assessment in relation to anti-dementia drugs is similar to the difficulties encountered in assessing agents used for the treatment of other chronic illness. The impact of such conditions on the patient often owes more to effects on overall disability and quality of life than to change in a single, easily measured parameter. The case of interferon beta-1b in the treatment of multiple sclerosis is an example. Evidence for its efficacy is based on a single trial which suggested that it reduced the number of exacerbations of the relapsing-remitting form of the disease (The INF beta Multiple Sclerosis Group, 1995). Effects on disability and progression of the disease were not clearly established. However, the drug has been granted a product licence through the European Medicines Evaluation Agency (EMEA), a decision that may have been influenced by the demands of an active patient interest lobby and some enthusiastic clinicians (Richards, 1996). As a result, it may now be prescribed within the National Health Service (NHS) in the United Kingdom (UK) and considerable misgivings have been voiced, not only in relation to its effectiveness, but also concerning the lost opportunity costs it may generate (Richards, 1996; New et al, 1996). Some 38 000 patients in the UK are estimated to be eligible for treatment and the potential annual cost has been estimated at £380m, 10% of the current NHS drug bill (Walley and Barton, 1995). Prescribing guidelines have been issued (MacDonald et al, 1994), however, demand is widespread and usage may be considerable.

Riluzole (for the treatment of motor neuron disease) and dornase alfa (for cystic fibrosis) are further examples. In both cases, the diseases involved are chronic, progressive, disabling and eventually fatal, and it has been very difficult to interpret the value of these treatments in the absence of trials measuring the multiple outcomes that are of relevance to both patient and physician.

MEASUREMENT OF OUTCOMES: EFFICACY AND EFFECTIVENESS

The selection of outcomes with which to assess therapy is not straightforward. Trial outcomes can be considered as three types—'surrogate', 'clinical' and 'patient-relevant'. Some degree of overlap may occur between them and the relationship between them is not always well established (Herson, 1989; Temple, 1993; Fleming and DeMets, 1996). Clinical trials generally report either surrogate or clinical outcomes as these can usually be assessed over a relatively short period of time, a consideration that is obviously important in terms of rapid drug development.

Many of the problems in assessing efficacy relate to the use of surrogates when the effect of a potential treatment on clinically relevant outcomes cannot be assessed within the lifetime of a trial. For example, in the case of interferon for multiple sclerosis, reduction in the number of exacerbations was used as a surrogate for halting disease progression. Similarly, with respect to dornase alfa for the treatment of cystic fibrosis, improvement in pulmonary function (measured as the forced expiratory volume in one second) has been used as a surrogate for improved survival. In some cases, for example, the relationship between the fall in blood pressure and reduction in the risk of stroke, the relationship between surrogate and clinical outcome is well established. However, there have been other situations, such as the relationship between change in CD4 count and survival in patients with HIV, where the relationship has not been found to be consistent.

The selection and measurement of patient-/carer-relevant outcomes are recognised as being particularly difficult in anti-dementia drug trials. Any comprehensive measurement of the efficacy of an agent must measure and rate together additively several endpoints, the relevance to the patient or carer of which may be questionable. The main goals of treatment may be defined as symptomatic improvement, slowing or arrest of symptom progression and primary prevention (Committee for Proprietary Medicinal Products [CPMP], 1997). To date, drug therapy has addressed only symptomatic improvement, with efficacy being measured in terms of cognitive, functional and global endpoints. As the recently published CPMP document relating to the drug therapy of Alzheimer's disease acknowledges, however, there are difficulties in selecting patient-/carer-relevant outcomes, even within these domains.

In examining functional loss, as opposed to cognitive deterioration, the recently reported trial by Sano et al (1997), comparing selegiline and alpha-tocopherol, alone or in combination, with placebo, differed from previous trials involving patients with Alzheimer's disease. The primary outcome was the time to the occurrence of onset of any of the following endpoints: institutionalisation, loss of the ability to perform basic activities of daily living or severe dementia. Secondary outcomes included change in cognitive status. Treatment appeared to delay functional, but not cognitive, deterioration.

While there may be debate about the results of the trial because of the composite primary endpoint, and because statistical adjustments had to be made (Drachman and Leber, 1997), the selection of a functional endpoint represents recognition of an important reality in the treatment of Alzheimer's disease: patient function in daily life is the issue of clinical relevance. The results also illustrate the difficulty of reconciling a widely used surrogate outcome—cognitive score—with one that is patient-/carer-relevant.

AUTHORITIES' POLICIES ON THE REGISTRATION OF ANTI-DEMENTIA DRUGS

There has been considerable interest in harmonising regulatory requirements and establishing guidelines for drug development internationally. Under the aegis of the International Conference on Harmonisation of Regulatory Requirements (ICH), efforts to achieve this have been taking place over the past seven years, and have involved industry and regulatory authorities from the EU, Japan and the US. One of the driving forces in the process has been the industry's desire to speed up drug development, as well as moving towards a unified approval process. To date, the ICH has developed a Common Technical Document, harmonising some 45 topic areas relating to core safety, quality and efficacy aspects of the registration process. It is anticipated that final consensus will be achieved within the next three years.

In relation to the licensing of anti-dementia drugs specifically, common regulatory requirements do not yet exist in formal form. In practice, however, regulatory agencies in many countries employ some aspects of the Food and Drugs Administration (FDA) draft guidelines for anti-dementia drugs, issued in 1990 (Leber, 1990). The recently published EMEA guidelines, outlined below, are broadly similar (CPMP, 1997).

CURRENT GUIDELINES FOR THE CLINICAL EVALUATION OF ANTI-DEMENTIA DRUGS

(See Table 4.1.1)

Europe—the EMEA

In April 1997, the Committee for Proprietary Medicinal Products, the drugs evaluation division of the EMEA, issued a 'Note for guidance on medicinal products in the treatment of Alzheimer's disease'. While the principles are mainly applicable to evaluation of drugs for the treatment of Alzheimer's disease, they may be adapted for use for drug trials in other forms of dementia. The guidelines concentrate on assessment of efficacy in terms of symptomatic improvement in three specific areas: cognition (cognitive endpoint), activities of daily living (functional endpoint) and overall clinical response (global

Table 4.1.1. Summary of regulatory authorities' current requirements in relation to the licensing of anti-dementia drugs and the nature of existing guidelines (QOL = quality of life)

Authority/ Country	Registration requirements	Guidelines for the evaluation of anti-dementia drugs	Comments
EMEA: EU countries	Evidence of safety, quality and efficacy based on laboratory parameters, animal and human toxicology and Phase I–III studies in humans	Issued by the CPMP in draft form, July 1997. 3 Sections: 1: Diagnosis, grading of disease severity and selection of patients for trials 2: Assessment of therapeutic efficacy; cognitive, functional and global endpoints 3: Trial strategy: 6 month duration to demonstrate efficacy and one year extension to evaluate maintenance of efficacy	Assessment instruments not specified, but their development encouraged. QOL assessment not required as current instruments not validated Cost/economic considerations encouraged but not specifically required
FDA: United States	Investigational New Drug Application requirements (similar to EMEA) apply	Draft guidelines, 1990. Provide advice in relation to planning, design, conduct and interpretation of anti-dementia drug trials. Efficacy assessment includes a performance test of cognition and a clinical global assessment. Evaluation after 3 months therapy permitted. Information on maintenance of efficacy encouraged but no specific timespan advised	Assessment instruments not specified. QOL assessment not required as current measurement instruments not considered adequate No cost/economic considerations
Japan	Evidence of quality, safety and efficacy. Efficacy determined through comparison with the existing agent	Existing guidelines relate to 'cerebral circulation' and 'metabolism improvers'. Improvement, safety, usefulness assessment. Not obviously relevant to anti-dementia drug assessment	Assessment instruments not specified No cost/economic considerations

endpoint). Although not specifying the measurement instruments, the use of externally validated, pertinent and sensitive tools that 'may be calibrated in relation to various populations or sub-populations of different social, educational and cultural backgrounds' is encouraged.

While quality of life (QOL) is acknowledged as an important aspect of the treatment of dementia, due to the lack of validated methods for its measurement, there is no requirement at present for formal assessment of this dimension among either patients or caregivers.

In acknowledgement of the chronic, progressive nature of dementia, the guidelines specify that trials aimed at demonstrating short-term improvement should last six months and should include placebo and/or comparators where appropriate. It is suggested that studies of one year or more are necessary to evaluate the maintenance of efficacy.

The United States: the FDA

The FDA applies the general requirements of its Investigational New Drug Application (Department of Health and Human Services, 1991) to any company seeking to undertake Phase I–III studies of a new anti-dementia drug. In addition, specific guidelines have been published for the clinical evaluation of anti-dementia drugs (Leber, 1990). To gain an anti-dementia indication for a product, a sponsor must provide evidence that it 'has a clinically meaningful effect' and that it 'exerts its effect on the "core" manifestations of dementia'. It is suggested that these requirements may be met by demonstrating that the agent is superior to an appropriate control therapy, on the basis of a global assessment and a performance-based, objective assessment of cognitive function. A number of assessment instruments are suggested and their limitations are discussed. Reflecting the difficulty in assessing quality of life outcomes, there is no specific requirement for assessment of this parameter. In contrast to the CPMP draft requirements, the FDA will accept evidence of efficacy based on clinical assessment after three months of treatment. While encouraging the provision of information about the duration of a drug's efficacy in sustained use and the consequences of its withdrawal after chronic administration, no timespan for evaluation of the *maintenance* of efficacy is specified.

Japan

In Japan, the only guidelines so far developed regarding anti-dementia drugs relate to the evaluation of 'metabolism improvers' and cerebral vasodilators which are intended for the treatment of patients with cerebral infarction, haemorrhage or so-called vascular dementia (Sawada, 1995). Assessment is based on the evaluation of improvement rates, safety and 'usefulness'. Improvement rates are measured on 5–7-point scales in terms of general physical findings, subjective symptoms, psychiatric signs (behavioural abnormalities, cognitive function, memory disturbance and mood changes), neurological signs and activity of daily life. Overall final evaluation is based on global judgement of usefulness. Approval for new drugs generally is based on quality, safety and efficacy considerations. The efficacy of a new agent is compared with that of the 'standard drug' (i.e. the most commonly used drug) in current use for the indication and marketing approval is granted if the new agent produces the same or better results (Ikegami et al, 1994).

ISSUES

Obviously there are differences between the current guidelines, in particular with respect to duration of trials. Like multiple sclerosis and cystic fibrosis, Alzheimer's disease is progressive and, similarly, the rate of progression shows considerable individual variation. Trial duration may therefore impact significantly on the results. Our view would concur with that of the EMEA—that anti-dementia drug trials should be of at least six months' duration to demonstrate short-term improvement, and last for a year or more if the intention is to evaluate the maintenance of efficacy.

While both the EMEA and FDA guidelines require assessment of cognitive and global endpoints, the actual variables to be measured within each of these domains are not specified. This is not unreasonable however, given the cultural and social differences that may exist between populations of anti-dementia drug users. For example, in some countries care may be provided primarily in the home, while in others, the demented patient may be institutionalised at a relatively early stage of the disease. Clearly, outcomes considered advantageous in one milieu may differ from those of benefit in the other. The CPMP guidelines in their current form make specific reference to this, recognising that differing patient populations and backgrounds exist, and suggesting that measurement tools be calibrated for use in different languages and cultures. Reflecting the difficulties in assessing efficacy and/or effectiveness, neither guideline specifies the instruments to be used for the measurement of outcomes.

In catering for trials of anti-dementia drugs, guidelines must address the nature of any new drug—is it of marginal benefit, as has been suggested of tacrine, or does it fundamentally alter the course or clinical manifestations of the disease? Outcome parameters may be different depending on the type of drug. Is assessment of efficacy against placebo or active comparator the more relevant? As more anti-dementia drugs are developed and patients/carers become reluctant to risk placebo in the face of the inevitable and relentless progression of the disease, the latter option may dominate in trials. The design and interpretation of active comparator trials raises a number of important questions. The choice of comparator is important, but the determination of sample size is more important. Trials that are designed to show that two drugs are truly equivalent need significantly larger numbers of subjects than those designed to detect differences (Ware and Antman, 1997).

Is there a relationship between dose and clinical benefit?—in the case of tacrine, this is contentious. Studies reporting modest improvements in cognitive scale scores have attributed these to tacrine treatment and have suggested that higher doses had greater effect (Summers et al, 1986; Wilcock et al, 1993; Knapp et al, 1994). While some reviewers of the published literature concurred (Davis and Powchik, 1995), others were not convinced that a dose–benefit relationship existed (Wolfson et al, 1997; Qizilbash et al, 1997). Furthermore, the impact of duration of therapy on outcome remains unclear.

In contrast, a relationship appears to exist between tacrine dose and the frequency of adverse effects and withdrawal from trials. Tacrine has been associated with significant hepatotoxic and cholinergic adverse effects. In the trials overall, depending on the definition of 'adverse effects', 48–94% of patients experienced adverse drug reactions (ADRs) and 12% were 'severe' (Wolfson et al, 1997). Withdrawal rates from trials as a result of adverse events have been in the range of 18–25%, the higher rates occurring in the upper dose ranges. It is likely that in clinical practice, adverse drug reactions will have even more of a negative impact on compliance. The effect of poor adherence to therapy on effectiveness must be considered, as well as its contribution to lost opportunity costs.

In general clinical use, another relevant issue is the question of long-term therapy. The duration of treatment in the trials has varied from as short as three weeks to around forty weeks. It is unclear if the claimed beneficial effects of tacrine are maintained or if tolerance develops. In reality in clinical practice, it is likely that a timepoint exists for most patients beyond which further therapy achieves little benefit.

The fundamental issue of relevance in the assessment of anti-dementia drugs is their practical benefit to patients and carers, however outcomes are measured. Drug authorities' policies at the end of the day are driven by the need to assure availability of safe and effective drugs, yet at the same time to respond to community expectations of access to new drugs that may offer hope of effective treatment. In seeking to ameliorate this tragic disorder, the drugs registered for dementia to date have raised more questions than they have provided answers. This is reflected in their registration status worldwide, with some regulatory authorities, like those of the UK and Canada, either delaying licensing or failing to license them, while others, such as those of the US, Australia and Sweden, are granting early approval.

DRUG REIMBURSEMENT

Internationally, one of the common problems in the management of chronic diseases is the issue of rising drug costs. Most countries are facing increases in their total drug bill, and governments are therefore using or considering a number of cost-containment strategies in health care and pharmaceuticals. For example, in the Australian setting, drugs to treat chronic illnesses such as depression and hypertension account for significant proportions of the total expenditure on pharmaceuticals (Hill et al, 1997) and similar examples can be found in other countries. Whether drugs are purchased by individuals within the community, or through schemes which purchase drugs for the community as a whole at national, state or local level, choices must be made about which agents will be purchased and for which condition.

Like many populations affected by chronic illness, patients suffering from dementia are an 'at risk' population, and as such, in most countries with sophisticated social support structures, they receive significant amounts of support. This may take the form of subsidies for hospital or nursing care, subsidies for carer support, or subsidies for drugs. Many authorities have been forced to develop decision-making processes for deciding which health care interventions to purchase and these will vary extensively depending upon the structure of the health care sector.

In making decisions about which drugs to purchase, state-based and private purchasing organisations will consider similar questions about new products, and these are an extension of those asked by a Drug Regulatory Authority. The regulatory questions are: Does a drug work? How does it work? What is the right dose? Is it safe? and increasingly, How does it compare with the currently available treatment? The purchasing questions are: In whom does it work best? How does it compare to currently available therapy? Is it worth paying for? How much are the payers willing to pay?

There has been considerable debate about how best to answer these questions; what data should be used, how to collect the information, how to calculate the economic impact of new treatments. Decisions to buy or not to buy may be based on a number of additional factors, including the perceived value of treatment, the importance of the disease, the cost of the treatment, and the balance of concern in a national setting about industry viability versus public health.

ECONOMIC EVALUATION

The role of economic evaluation of pharmaceuticals in setting prices or making purchasing decisions has been controversial. In the UK, for example, the National Health Service (NHS) has covered the cost of all licensed medicines as long as they are not on the 'Selected List', a negative list established in 1985 that includes products (mostly, but not entirely, over-the-counter agents) which will not be reimbursed. To date, there has not been any use of economic evaluation techniques in deciding what to list or not list, as the pricing arrangements are conducted within a framework of overall profit control of the pharmaceutical industry. However, in light of the problems caused by the introduction of expensive products such as beta-interferon, consideration is being given to 'managed entry' of some drugs into the market, although it is not yet clear how this will occur.

ECONOMIC EVALUATION: CANADA

In Canada, a system has been developed where decisions about reimbursing drug costs are made at provincial level after licensing is handled at national level. The provinces have responded differently to the need to review pharmaceutical spending, with some implementing economic guidelines for decision making. The Canadian Co-ordinating Office for Health Technology Assessment (CCOHTA) is a non-profit organisation that is funded by federal, provincial and territorial governments, and was established to 'encourage the appropriate use of health technology by influencing decision makers through the scientific evaluation of medical procedures, devices and drugs'. It has developed guidelines for economic evaluation that have been used since 1994 and were revised in 1997.

The Canadian system has been developed on the basis that it is necessary to have an *independent* economic evaluation of drug products. Evaluations are commissioned and carried out by academic units or consultants, rather than being prepared by the pharmaceutical industry. The rationale for this approach is to have as unbiased a review as possible, but this creates its own difficulties. The major one to date has been that the resources needed to carry out reviews according to CCOHTA Guidelines are extensive and not readily available. However, a key advantage of an independent review is that the contents are in the public domain.

Tacrine has been reviewed for CCOHTA (Wolfson et al, 1997). The conclusion of the review was that 'the efficacy and effectiveness of tacrine in the treatment of Alzheimer's disease have not been convincingly established. For this reason an evaluation of the economic impact of tacrine is not warranted at this time.' This raises one of the methodological issues that has been at the centre of the debate about economic evaluation of pharmaceuticals—whether to base the evaluations on randomised controlled trials that assess efficacy or effectiveness with the economic evaluation 'piggy-backed' on to the RCT, or to use an approach that combines data from multiple sources, usually in a retrospective fashion, characterised by O'Brien (1996), as 'Frankenstein's monster'. In the case of tacrine, basing an analysis on the RCTs that were available was difficult, as, in the view of the reviewers, there was no convincing evidence of benefit and therefore nothing on which to 'piggy-back' an analysis.

Other economic analyses of the potential benefits of tacrine have been published (Lubeck et al, 1994; Henke and Burchmore, 1997; Wimo et al, 1997). In each of these, however, a key assumption is that a small change in the Mini-Mental State Examination score can be translated into a clinical benefit such as a decrease in nursing home use. It is unfortunate that this assumption is not yet well substantiated as it renders dependent cost-benefit and cost-effectiveness analyses extremely uncertain.

The Australian purchasing process has been established since 1992, and as a system probably has the most experience in using economic evaluation for making decisions about purchasing drugs. It is based around a nationalised reimbursement scheme for drugs used in the community (hospital drugs are covered under an alternative scheme) that has been in existence since the early 1950s (the Pharmaceutical Benefits Scheme, PBS). Australia was the first country to introduce a formal requirement for pharmacoeconomic data, and there has been considerable debate about the Guidelines that have been developed to describe the data requirements.

ECONOMIC EVALUATION: AUSTRALIA

The Australian system has been described in detail elsewhere (Henry and Johannesson, 1992; Glasziou and Mitchell, 1996; Sketris and Hill, in press). Briefly, once a drug is licensed, in order to have it listed on the PBS, companies must provide evidence to support its comparative efficacy, safety and cost-effectiveness. Data are reviewed in detail by the Department of Health and then considered by an independent expert advisory committee, the Pharmaceutical Benefits Advisory Committee. The Minister of Health makes the final decision about listing a drug, but cannot do so in the absence of a positive recommendation from the PBAC. If a drug is not listed, it can still be sold in Australia, but the market for non-PBS listed drugs is extremely limited.

The Guidelines are now in their second edition, with a third revision under way. Over 350 submissions have been reviewed by the Department and the PBAC. It is becoming clear that while there has been much debate about the Australian Guidelines' preference for cost-effectiveness analysis and the use of randomised controlled trials, these are not the only factors that influence the decision. Other considerations, such as the estimate of the incremental cost per quality-adjusted life-year (George et al, in press), may also be important, although the data at this stage are limited.

It is worth noting that no drug for dementia has yet been listed on the PBS. The secrecy provisions of the National Health Act, under which the Scheme operates, prevent any disclosure of whether drugs have been considered for listing but rejected, or whether a company has elected not to apply for listing. However, considering the similarity between other drugs for dementia and those for chronic disabling diseases, it is likely that such an application would require data about clinical- and patient-relevant outcomes, as well as an estimate of the value of these to society. One of the most difficult issues is how best to translate data from one setting to another to assist in this valuation (e.g. European trials or estimates of costs of care)—for this reason, many Australian subsidiaries of pharmaceutical companies are working with local experts to capture appropriate data before a drug is licensed.

In dementia, there is the key need to assess the impact of the disease on the quality of life *of carers* as well as patients, and then evaluating the impact. As this information is infrequently assessed in trials, it has been suggested that some of these issues can be addressed by the development of appropriate economic models. This may be particularly important where the clinical trials that have been conducted to support the application for a particular drug are relatively short in relation to the duration of the disease. This is not only an issue for assessment of the value of anti-dementia drugs; another example is drugs for osteoporosis where, in general, the trials have measured changes at relatively short-term treatment intervals, such as six to twelve months, and the changes have been measured in terms of bone density. Realistically, however, the burden of the disease will manifest primarily as fractures and their consequences that will not occur for at least 10 to 15 years after it is suggested that treatment be commenced. It is in this type of setting that careful economic modelling has the most potential to provide useful information to a decision-making body. However, the assumptions about effectiveness of therapy that are used in models are critical, and require careful assessment.

INDIRECT COSTS

The question of the inclusion of different types of costs is important in any assessment of the economic impact of a new drug, but particularly in drugs for dementia. The indirect costs of dementia are recognised to be substantial, but are difficult to measure in any given setting, and translate poorly from one health care system to another. The Australian guidelines currently tend to discourage the inclusion of indirect costs, though not to forbid it. However, time committed by a carer to looking after a patient with dementia is obviously of value, and will have monetary impact, and may change significantly if effective therapy for dementia is available. It may be in this type of setting that the methodology in economic evaluation of pharmaceuticals must develop most rapidly.

ANTI-DEMENTIA DRUGS: THE FUTURE

Within the global village, one may imagine the 'global' patient seeking access to medicines made available through the global marketplace. In practice, the desire of individual countries to retain autonomy with respect to drug supply has meant that common licensing requirements have been slow to evolve. This has been particularly the case in Europe, where what is potentially a single drug market remains, to a great extent, partitioned along national lines. The EMEA is intended to facilitate, through the principle of mutual recognition of national authorisations, the development of a unified market within the EU for medicinal products. It remains the case, however, that any member state may dispute registration authorisations granted within another state. The ICH aim of a single unified marketing approval process across American, Asian and European countries will clearly take some time to achieve.

While the development of a common licensing procedure would greatly facilitate the approval process, it would not remove the difficulties encountered *within* the process. All of these would remain, particularly in relation to the evaluation of efficacy. On the plus side, however, solutions developed might be accepted internationally. This would be of particular value in areas such as dementia, where drug evaluation is difficult. Key issues such as trial duration might be standardised, while social and cultural aspects of outcomes assessment could be tailored for specific populations or health care settings.

Medicine purchasing and reimbursement policies are highly variable internationally. However, rising drug costs have rendered the issue of economic assessment of pharmaceuticals internationally relevant as individual payers seek a mechanism to identify cost-effective drugs. The rationale for economic evaluation is that the assessment of health care interventions, including drug treatments, should extend beyond their clinical effects to their economic efficiency. In relating the outcomes of interventions to the consumption of resources in an explicit and quantitative fashion, economic analysis permits some measurement of the value for money of a drug. While numerous sets of guidelines have been developed, the existence of common elements in guidelines internationally is desirable to facilitate 'common readings' of worth. Ability to modify assessments to adjust for local conditions is also required. Finally, in relation to anti-dementia drugs, the thorny issue of quality of life, for both the patient and the primary carer, must be addressed.

REFERENCES

Anon. (1997). SB-202026 improves cognitive function in probable Alzheimers, *Inpharma*, **1103**, 7.

Committee for Proprietary Medical Products (CPMP) (1997). Note for guidance on medicinal products in the treatment of Alzheimer's disease. European Agency for the Evaluation of Medicinal Products, London.

Commonwealth of Australia, Hansard (1987). National Health Amendment Bill (No 2) Second Reading Speech. Canberra.

Davis, K. L. and Powchik, P. (1995). Tacrine, *Lancet*, **345**, 625–630.

Department of Health and Human Services. Title 21, Part 312, Code of Federal Regulations, Investigational New Drug Application (1991). Washington, DC, US Government Printing Office.

Drachman, D. A. and Leber, P. (1997). Treatment of Alzheimer's disease—searching for a breakthrough, settling for less, *N. Engl. J. Med.*, **336**, 1245–1247.

Drummond, M. F. (1994). Value for money assessments in Australia and beyond, *Spectrum Health Care Delivery and Economics*. Massachusetts, Decisions Resource Inc.

Fleming, T. R. and DeMets, D. L. (1996). Surrogate end-points in clinical trials: are we being misled? *Ann. Int. Med.*, **125**, 605–613.

George, B., Harris, A. and Mitchell, A. J. (in press). Reimbursement decisions and the implied value of life: cost-effectiveness analysis and decisions to reimburse pharmaceuticals in Australia, 1993–1996, in A. Harris (Ed.), *Proceedings of the Nineteenth Australian Conference of Health Economists*, Australian Studies in Health Service Administration, School of Health Services Management, University of New South Wales.

Glasziou, P. P. and Mitchell, A. S. (1996). Use of Pharmacoeconomic data by regulatory authorities, in *Quality of Life and Pharmacoeconomics in Clinical Trials*, 2nd edn, pp. 1141–1147 (Ed. B. Spilker), Philadelphia, PA, Lippincott-Raven Publishers.

Henke, C. J. and Burchmore, M. J. (1997). The economic impact of tacrine in the treatment of Alzheimer's disease, *Clinical Therapeutics*, **19**(2), 330–345.

Henry, D. A. and Johannesson, M. (1992). Economic analysis as an aid to subsidisation decisions, *PharmacoEconomics*, **1**, 54–67.

Herson J. (1989). The use of surrogate endpoints in clinical trials, *Stat. Med.*, **8**, 403–404.

Hill, S. R., Henry, D. A. and Smith, A. J. (1997). Rising prescription drug costs: whose responsibility? *Med. Journ. Aust.*, **167**, 6–7.

Ikegami, N., Mitchell, W. and Penner-Hahn, J. (1994). Pharmaceutical prices, quantities and innovation. Comparing Japan with the US, *PharmacoEconomics*, **6**(5), 424–433.

Knapp, M. J., Knopman, D. S., Solomon, P. R., Pendlebury, W. W., Davis, C. S. and Gracon, S. I. (1994). A 30-week randomised controlled trial of high-dose tacrine in patients with Alzheimer's disease, *JAMA*, **271**, 985–991.

Leber, P. (1990). Guidelines for the clinical evaluation of antidementia drugs, Washington, DC, Food and Drug Administration.

Lubeck, D. P., Mazonson, P. D. and Bowe, T. (1994). Potential effect of tacrine on expenditures for Alzheimer's disease, *Medical Interface*, October, 130–138.

MacDonald, W. I., for the Association of British Neurologists (1994). New treatment for multiple sclerosis. London.

New, B., on behalf of the Rationing Agenda Group (1996). The rationing agenda in the NHS, *Brit. Med. Journ.*, **31**, 1593–1601.

O'Brien, B. J. (1996). Economic evaluation of pharmaceuticals. Frankenstein's monster or Vampire of trials? *Medical Care*, **34**(12) suppl, DS99–DS108.

Qizilbash, N., Birks, J., Arrieta, J. L., Lewington, S. and Szeto, S. (1997). The efficacy of tacrine in Alzheimer's disease. In *Dementia and Cognitive Module of the Cochrane Database of Systematic Reviews* [updated June, 1997], The Cochrane Collaboration, Issue 3. Oxford, Update Software.

Richards, R. G. (1996). Interferon beta in multiple sclerosis: Clinical cost effectiveness falls at the first hurdle, *Brit. Med. Journ.*, **313**(7066), 1159–1160.

Sano, M., Ernesto, C., Thomas, R. G., Klauber, M., Schafer, K., Grundman, M., Woodbury, P., Growdon, J., Cotman, C. W., Pfeiffer, E., Schneider, L. S. and Thal, L. J. (1997). A controlled trial of selegiline, alpha tocopherol, or both as treatment for Alzheimer's disease, *New Eng. J. Med.*, **336**, 1216–1222.

Sawada (September 1995). Update on guidelines from Japan. Paper presented at the meeting of the International Working Group for the Harmonisation of Dementia Drug Guidelines. London, Royal Society of Medicine.

Sketris, I. and Hill, S. R. The Australian National publicly subsidized Pharmaceutical Benefits Scheme—any lessons for Canada? *Can. Journ. Clin. Pharmacol.*, in press.

Summers, W. K., Majoviski, L. V., Marsh, G. M., Tachiki, K. and Kling, A. (1986). Oral tetrahydroaminoacridine in long-term treatment of senile dementia, Alzheimer type, *New Eng. J. Med.*, **315**, 1241–1245.

Temple, R. (1993). Trends in pharmaceutical development, *Drug Information Journal*, **27**, 355–366.

The INF beta Multiple Sclerosis Study Group and the University of British Columbia MS/MRI analysis group (1995). Interferon beta-1b in the treatment of MS: Final outcome of the RCT, *Neurology*, **45**, 1277–1285.

Walley, T. and Barton, S. (1995). A purchaser perspective of managing new drugs: interferon beta as a case study, *Brit. Med. Journ.*, **311**, 796–799.

Ware, J. H. and Antman, E. M. (1997). Equivalence trials, *New. Eng. J. Med.*, **337**(16), 1159–1161.

Wilcock, G. K., Surmon, D. J., Scott, M., Boyle, M., Mulligan, K. and Neubauer, K. A. (1993). An evaluation of the efficacy and safety of tetrahydroaminoacridine (THA) without lecithin in the treatment of Alzheimer's disease, *Age and Ageing*, **22**, 316–324.

Wimo, A., Karlsson, G., Nordberg, A. and Winblad, B. (1997). Treatment of Alzheimer's disease with tacrine: a cost analysis model, *Alzheimer Disease and Associated Disorders*, **11**, 191–200.

Wolfson, C., Moride, Y., Perrault, A. and Vida, S. (June 1997). A study of the efficacy, effectiveness and economic impact of tacrine in Alzheimer's disease. Ontario, Canada, Canadian Coordinating Office for Health Technology Assessment (CCOHTA).

4.2 Designing Phase III Trials of Anti-dementia Drugs with a View towards Pharmacoeconomic Considerations

LON S. SCHNEIDER
University of Southern California, Los Angeles, USA

INTRODUCTION

This chapter will review the medication development process for anti-dementia drugs, and the current characteristics of Phase III trials in Alzheimer's disease. It will then proceed to discuss the limitations and issues involved in using Phase III data for pharmacoeconomic analyses. Although several approaches are possible, their validity is limited by the type of patients and data available in Phase III trials. The issues involved in cost-effectiveness analyses are also discussed.

THE MEDICATION DEVELOPMENT PROCESS

In order to consider the variations and designs of Phase III trials and how these designs impact on pharmacoeconomics it is important to understand the overall clinical drug development process. This process is traditionally divided into four phases (Table 4.2.1). Phase I represents the initial administration of a drug to humans. Objectives generally include the initial assessments of safety and tolerability and estimations of pharmacokinetics and pharmacodynamics in generally healthy volunteers (except for drugs with significant potential toxicity), and do not include estimations of efficacy. Phase II trials are intended to explore the circumstances of efficacy and safety in patients selected by clearly defined criteria for the illness, for example Alzheimer's disease defined by NINCDS–ADRDA workshop criteria (McKhann et al, 1984). Phase II is characterized by close monitoring, dose ranging and adjustments and evaluation of potential outcomes. The first evidence of efficacy is usually obtained in Phase II.

Health Economics of Dementia. Edited by Anders Wimo, Bengt Jönsson, Göran Karlsson and Bengt Winblad.
© 1998 John Wiley & Sons Ltd.

Table 4.2.1. Phases of clinical drug development

	Characteristics and goals	Typical study designs
Phase I	Initial administration to humans Initial safety tolerability Pharmacokinetics and pharmacodynamics Non-therapeutic objectives Conducted in healthy volunteers (except for drugs with significant potential toxicity) Early measurement of activity	Open within subject comparisons (randomization or blinding to enhance validity) Dose-tolerance studies Pharmacokinetic and pharmacodynamic studies
Phase II	Exploration of efficacy Patients selected by clearly defined criteria Close monitoring of trials Determine dosage and therapeutic regimen Evaluation of potential outcomes Evaluation of population subtypes	Randomized, placebo-controlled comparisons with baseline or between group comparisons Dose-response designs
Phase III	Confirmation of therapeutic efficacy and safety Further definition of dose response Exploration of use in wider populations or different disease stages Combinations with other drugs Extended exposure	Randomized, double-blind, parallel group, placebo-controlled, efficacy studies
Phase IV	After drug approval Extend prior demonstration of the drug's safety and efficacy, and dose Extended therapeutic use Studies related to approved indications Extension of an approved indication New dosage requiring routes of administration	Pharmacoeconomic studies Comparative efficacy studies Drug–drug interactions Dose-response Safety studies Mortality/morbidity studies

Sources: Federal Register 62(104): 29540–29546 (30 May 1997) International Conference on Harmonisation; Draft Guidelines on General Considerations for Clinical Trials.

Phase III trials typically follow on the completion of Phase II trials. They are intended to provide a confirmation of the therapeutic efficacy and safety observed in Phase II. Hypotheses of Phase III trials are rather specific. For example, in AD trials they usually address two or three primary outcomes, such as cognitive change or clinician's impression of improvement. In addition to being 'confirmatory,' Phase III trials are sometimes referred to as 'pivotal' because their results are often the basis upon which drugs are approved for clinical use by a governmental regulatory authority such as the United States Food and Drug Administration (FDA). Phase III trials that yield null results are unlikely to lead to a drug's marketing approval by the FDA. Usually two or more Phase III trials demonstrating efficacy and safety are required for marketing approval. In many countries 'marketing approval' means only that the drug may be offered for sale because basic efficacy has been established to a regulatory agency's satisfaction. But the agency does not comment on the overall effectiveness of the drug or whether insurers should pay for it. (As discussed elsewhere in this volume there are some differences in the approval process among countries that relate in part to health economic considerations).

Goals of Phase III trials may also include further defining dose response, the effects of extended exposure to a medication, and the exploration of a drug's efficacy and safety in more broadly defined populations or in different disease stages. As examples, a Phase III trial may compare two different dosages that were previously suggested to be effective in Phase II trials, or may assess efficacy over longer periods of time, or in more severe illness than a Phase II trial would. It is fair to say, however, that the goals of Phase III anti-dementia trials have been considerably more limited than in other therapeutic areas. Dose ranges are usually not fully explored; efficacy is usually assessed over the shortest allowable period of time (12 to 24 weeks); and only patients in a limited illness-severity range are assessed. Indeed, in anti-dementia clinical trials, Phase II trials often overlap or are allowed to be combined with Phase III, blurring the distinction between the two phases. Sometimes it is possible to combine Phases II and III, essentially by completing several efficacy and confirmation-of-efficacy trials.

Finally, Phase IV occurs (or the results are usually available) after a drug receives marketing approval. The objectives are to extend the prior demonstration of a drug's safety and efficacy, and appropriateness of dose. Studies are done that are related to the approved indication, including the extension of an approved indication. They may include further efficacy studies, assessments of comparative efficacy, safety studies, drug–drug interactions, morbidity and mortality studies and pharmacoeconomic studies.

It is in the context of the traditional Phase I to Phase IV medication development program that the role of pharmacoeconomics in Phase III studies needs to be considered. Although traditionally Phase IV is reserved for these types of studies, as drug development becomes more expensive, as national medical budgets place limits on medication prescribing, and (in the example of dementia) when drugs may have relatively modest effects, economic considerations need to be included throughout drug development. There is a prevailing opinion that merely demonstrating efficacy and safety compared to placebo in a controlled trial is not enough to justify the use of an anti-dementia drug in the community. Overall effectiveness, or how a drug works in the community with typical physicians and patients' needs to be demonstrated as well.

CURRENT CHARACTERISTICS OF PHASE III CLINICAL TRIALS IN ANTI-DEMENTIA MEDICATION DEVELOPMENT

Despite the descriptions of Phases I to IV and that they are meant as general guidelines, the current situation is that Alzheimer's disease Phase III trials are rather tightly defined and limited to the confirmation of efficacy and safety alone, and not to exploring various conditions of efficacy. Specifically, inclusion criteria for Phase III trials are often as limited as they are in Phase II; the same outcome instruments are used, and study designs are very similar. Current inclusion/exclusion criteria tend to create a fairly homogeneous group of patients with dementia of only mild to moderate severity, who are generally physically healthy, who usually do not have significant concomitant behavioral problems and are living as outpatients with caregivers. This, as will be discussed below, is hardly a typical group of AD patients.

Rather than exploring differing durations, these Phase III studies are of limited, fixed duration. Generally only one 3-month-long study and one 6-month-long clinical trial are offered to regulatory agencies as evidence of efficacy; and the experiences of about 2000 patients, including those from Phases I and II, are offered for evidence of safety.

The primary outcome criteria among the Phase III trials tend to be similar: the Alzheimer's Disease Assessment Scale–cognitive subscale (ADAS–cog), a Clinical Global Impression of Change Scale (CGIC), and an assessment of functional activities. The ADAS is taken as a test of cognitive function. A CGIC, essentially an experienced clinician's assessment, is taken as an index of clinically meaningful change. Finally, an assessment of activities of daily living is taken to determine whether or not medication treatment is associated with improved functioning compared to placebo. In addition to these three outcomes, other supplementary outcomes, including the Mini-Mental State Examination (MMSE, Folstein et al, 1975), cognitive tests that are speed-dependent, caregiver burden scales, behavior and mood assessments, as well as instruments designed to capture service utilization and costs, are used in these clinical trials. The purpose of the primary outcome ratings is to fulfill FDA's criteria, that an effective drug for the symptoms of dementia must show both cognitive improvement and clinically meaningful change. The European Agency for the Evaluation of Medicinal Products (EMEA) goes further, and requires also the demonstration of change in function or behavior for a medication to be deemed effective in dementia (http://www.eudra.org/emea.html).

Since currently the primary outcomes, at least the ADAS and the CGIC, are used nearly universally, the main area in which Phase III studies tend to vary both within and among proprietary medication development programs is in the use of secondary outcome measures. These assessments include a selection of additional and slightly differing functional or daily activities scales, quality of life scales, behavioral rating scales, caregiver symptoms or burden scales, or scales purporting to measure services consumed, or pharmacoeconomic outcomes. When the Phase II and Phase III clinical trials designs of the various cholinergic medications under development are compared, it is the range of drug dosage and the choice of secondary outcome scales that tend to differentiate their designs.

CURRENT ISSUES IN PHASE III CLINICAL TRIALS OF ANTI-DEMENTIA DRUGS

Three obvious concerns in designing Phase II and III clinical trials are that: excessive variability in the characteristics of patients selected for trials may mask potential drug effects; patients might be included who do not have AD; and extensive medical comorbidity may complicate the clinical presentation or affect outcome. Therefore, sponsors of clinical trials have attempted to reduce the clinical heterogeneity by using restrictive selection criteria for patients entering them.

The dementia population included in these trials generally consists of mildly to moderately impaired patients living at home with caregivers, with diagnoses of probable AD using NINCDS–ADRDA workshop criteria (McKhann et al, 1984). Study subjects, typically, are further required to be medically healthy without significant psychiatric symptoms, and with normal laboratory screening tests. Individual clinical trials vary, however, with respect to additional inclusion/exclusion criteria. For example, allowable MMSE ranges may be as broad as 10 to 26 points, or as narrow as 17 to 24 points (unpublished proprietary data). Similarly, age ranges vary, and may be as broad as 40 years or older, or as narrow as 65 to 80 years. There may be some variation, however, of allowable coexisting medical illness, electrocardiographic findings, and structural brain imaging features. For example, one study may insist that subjects have normal electrocardiograms while another may allow evidence of past myocardial infarction or certain conduction defects. Or the tolerance for T_2-enhanced subcortical lesions on magnetic resonance imaging may vary among trials.

Therefore, both the stringency and uniformity of certain selection criteria and the differences in other criteria among trials may lead to the enrollment of a group of subjects who are not representative of the overall clinical population of AD patients. Only a minority of AD patients in the community may fulfill the selection criteria for Phase III trials (see below). Moreover, placebo-treated patients in Phase III clinical trials are observed to decline cognitively at less than one-quarter the rate reported in clinic-based populations (e.g., approximately ½ to 3 MMSE points per year compared to 2.5 to 4 points per year reported in the clinics, e.g., Cory-Bloom et al, 1993). Some subgroups likely to be excluded from trials, such as those with delusions, extrapyramidal signs, or Lewy body variant of AD, may comprise 10 to 30% of the AD population and have a different natural history from other patients, possibly deteriorating more rapidly than others (Chui et al, 1994; Drevets et al, 1989).

Adverse effects are always of considerable importance in clinical practice but their frequency and severity are likely to be different under the highly controlled conditions of Phase III trial than in the community at large. This may be because patients in trials are healthier, and more likely to be compliant with medication. Speculatively, they may be more likely to report mild side-effects, and less likely to suffer from severe side-effects.

Finally, as a result of the selection criteria, clinical trials patients (both those who receive active medications and those who receive placebo) may be destined to have better outcomes than those ordinary patients in ordinary clinical practice.

COMPARISON OF A PHASE III CLINICAL TRIALS POPULATION WITH A CLINICAL POPULATION

With these considerations in mind, we tried to identify the percentage of patients with Alzheimer's disease in a general clinic population who would be provisionally eligible for randomized clinical trials, and the extent to which these patients represent the overall clinic-based population (Schneider et al, 1997). Patients diagnosed as probable or possible AD from the nine clinical sites of the State of California's Alzheimer's Disease Diagnostic and Treatment Centers were identified on the basis of their provisionally fulfilling the inclusion and exclusion criteria of two typical AD clinical trials (excluding ECG and brain imaging criteria). From a sample of 3470 subjects with possible or probable AD overall, we found only 4.4 or 7.9% would have been provisionally eligible based on the criteria from each of two Phase III trials.

Perhaps not surprisingly, provisionally eligible compared to ineligible patients were younger, *relatively* under-represented by women, better educated, wealthier, and more likely to be of European descent rather than Hispanic or African-American (Table 4.2.2). The major independent demographic predictors for eligibility were: income greater than $15 000 per year, male gender, and college education. Over 60% of probable AD patients would have been excluded because of significant behavioral problems; approximately one-quarter each would have been excluded because of significant medical or neurological problems, respectively. These results demonstrate that selection criteria for Phase III AD clinical trials result in a demographically and clinically constrained subgroup that is not representative of the overall clinic population. Quite significantly, any pharmacoeconomic modeling of this data would have to take these factors into account.

Table 4.2.2. Demographic characteristics for probable AD clinic patients compared to (a) those AD patients provisionally eligible for a typical Phase III AD clinical trial (Study 1) and to (b) patients actually enrolled in the trial (Knapp et al, 1994)

	Ineligible ADDTC sample	Provisionally eligible for Study 1	Tacrine clinical trial
N	1762	274	663
Age, yr (SD)	76.3 (7.9)	74.8 (8.9)	72.9 (8.0)
Gender, % female	71.0	*58.4*	*52.3*
Ethnicity			
% white	77.7	84.3	94.6
% black	7.6	*4.7*	*3.3*
% Hispanic	9.6	5.5	unknown
Education			
% college	35.5	*46.1*	*45.1*
% high school	*36.2*	33.2	43.9
% < high school	28.3	20.7	11.0
Living status, % alone			
	20.3	*0*	*0*
Yearly income, $ median	10 000–14 999	20 000–24 999	unknown
MMSE, mean (SD)	13.9 (7.6)	*18.4 (4.4)*	*18.5 (4.7)*

All differences were significant except for the italicized pairs in some rows.

Source: Adapted with permission from Schneider et al (1997).

APPROACHES TO PHARMACOECONOMICS USING PHASE III DATA

As discussed above, in general, and traditionally, health economic and pharmacoeconomic studies have been recommended to take place in Phase IV clinical drug development. Notably, however, this has not been the case with anti-dementia drugs. The first two cholinesterase inhibitors, tacrine and donepezil, were marketed without adequate Phase IV results. In the case of tacrine, the Phase IV studies that were undertaken (subsequent to marketing) focused only on the hepatotoxicity of the drug, while with donepezil the Phase IV studies that included pharmacoeconomic parameters were begun only after the medication was approved for marketing. In both instances, there were attempts to glean economic data from the Phase III trials (see below), and there has been substantial delay in the undertaking and publication of economic assessments.

In part because there are few published Phase III trials of viable, marketed medications for AD the main use of Phase III data for pharmacoeconomic modeling has been with the 6-month-long Phase III trial of tacrine (Knapp et al, 1994). Three examples of the use of this data to generalize pharmaco-economic impact are discussed below (Lubeck at al, 1994; Henke and Burchmore, 1997; Wimo et al, 1997).

The earliest study (Lubeck et al, 1994) included data only from the 30-week double-blind, randomized period of tacrine or placebo treatment. The authors calculated that tacrine use over this period could result in a 17% ($2243) reduction of the current costs of Alzheimer's disease per patient per year, assuming an MMSE decline of 4.6 pts/yr, life expectancy of 4.4 yrs, that 20% of a patient's lifespan with AD is spent in a nursing home, and that 50% of community care costs are avoided. When any of these parameters are varied cost savings vary from $3342 to an actual cost of $109. The basis for these estimates was made by comparing the 30-week data on the patients treated with tacrine to other external reports on the cost of Alzheimer's disease overall (e.g., Rice et al, 1991). The analysis was, in large part, predicated on the assumption that changes in the MMSE, a cognitive measure, could be correlated with changes in functional capacity and health care costs in a different group of subjects, although this correlation has been demonstrated to be rather weak (Galasko et al, 1991). As part of the analytic modeling, differing rates of MMSE change were associated with differing costs.

In the more recent study (Henke and Burchmore, 1997), data from the open-label follow-up study of the 663 patients enrolled in a 30-week Phase III placebo-controlled tacrine study were used as well (Knopman et al, 1994). In this study patients were followed until they died or required nursing home placement (or were lost to follow-up). Patients able to take higher doses were compared to those taking lower doses. The outcomes of interest in the economic model included mortality, longevity, time to nursing home placement, and estimates of the costs of community and nursing home care. These later estimates were taken from earlier reports on different populations at earlier times (e.g., Ernst and Hay, 1994). This model assumed that the loss of functional independence is associated with progression of the illness, and an increasing amount of home care until a patient is placed in a nursing home. Less emphasis was placed on cognitive or functional measures. The essential result of this analysis was that tacrine was associated with a cost savings of $9250 (7.5%) over the remaining lifetime that increased to $36 500 over five years in the patients who could take higher doses. Most of the cost saving in this model, however, was due to a delay in nursing home placement. Various sensitivity analyses provided a broad range of savings from approximately $600 to $24 000 depending on assumptions.

The authors of a cost-analysis study of tacrine (Wimo et al, 1997) also relied on changes in cognitive function on the MMSE, but in this case to estimate living situation (e.g., nursing home or home care) as a function of MMSE score in a subgroup of the Swedish AD population age 75 years or older and with MMSE scores ranging from 10 to 24. Assumptions included that tacrine's effect on MMSE could be projected as an effect on living situation, an annual rate of MMSE decline of 3 points, and survival of 5 years, were taken from other data. They estimated an overall 1.3% cost benefit (translating into about $320) and a hypothetical maximum of 11.3% under a highly unlikely set of conditions.

The models obviously differ from each other rather distinctly: relying either on the 30-week randomized period and cognitive change as a surrogate functional measure; or on data collected over the course of several years, and nursing home placement as a marker of functional loss and cost. The several limitations of these analyses involve the mapping of cognitive change to functional change, and the assumption that delay in institutionalization occurs without a change in length of stay in the nursing home, or in longevity, among others.

LIMITATIONS TO USING PHASE III DATA FOR PHARMACOECONOMIC ANALYSES

The magnitudes of the therapeutic differential effects in Phase III trials are certainly internally valid and unbiased measures of efficacy. As discussed above, even though a Phase III placebo-controlled trial can be subjected to contemporaneous, placebo-controlled cost analyses, or cost minimization, any differences observed between the treatment conditions, whether cognitive, functional, or economic, cannot be easily generalized to the population as a whole or to those likely to receive these medications. The Phase III trials as currently performed in Alzheimer's disease may lack externally valid or economically meaningful measures. The outcome measures used to define clinical effects such as the ADAS, the clinician's global impression of change, and the MMSE, do not necessarily translate into an accurate description of the patient in his or her community and may not convey overall economic impact. This is especially the case when one considers that unmeasured non-cognitive behavioral symptoms, changes in activities of daily living, dependency, living status, caregiver status, marital status, and other factors also contribute to the overall measurement of a treatment's effectiveness, and can be important and unmeasured factors for determining pharmacoeconomic effect.

The intensity of care that patients in Phase III clinical trials receive, whether randomized to drug or placebo, is incomparable to the care that ordinary patients would receive. For example, both drug and placebo patients are seen regularly and frequently by highly skilled multi-disciplinary treatment teams, laboratory tests are often extensive, and safety is carefully monitored. Considerable support and encouragement are given to caregivers and others who bring patients to the research clinic. The absolute costs of this clinical research care cannot be ignored when generalizing to the population. Patients in Phase II clinical trials not only are more carefully selected, but have less need for intensive care (i.e., they have few medical illnesses or behavioral management problems and have preserved basic activities of living). Yet they receive more intensive (and arguably better) care. This includes the placebo-treated patients who gain considerable non-specific benefits from enrolling in Phase III trials. For example, as discussed above, it is frequently observed that placebo-treated patients in 6-month-long clinical trials usually do not deteriorate on the

MMSE or ADAS to as great an extent as patients observed in other clinical samples and community-based samples.

Even when patients with co-morbid medical and behavioral conditions are included in a Phase III clinical trial, and are evenly distributed between both the drug and the placebo groups, the effect of these medical or psychiatric conditions on outcome are not likely to be analyzable. Firstly, there is the low statistical power of performing sub-group analyses in studies designed to demonstrate only a primary outcome effect; and, secondly, the purpose of a generalizable pharmacoeconomic assessment is to assess total net costs of dementia and its treatment and not merely a differential cost between two intensive treatments. In any event, the likelihood of both finding a statistically significant effect by chance (a type I error) and of not finding a significant differential effect when indeed there is one (a type II error) in this situation is high and the direction and magnitude of the error is likely to be considerable. Nevertheless, these patients would be more typical of ordinary community-dwelling patients and would make a better comparison group for cost-effectiveness studies.

COST-EFFECTIVENESS AND PHASE III TRIALS

The issue of pharmacoeconomic analysis in Phase III trials arises because the healthcare system is increasingly concerned with demonstrating that new products are not only efficacious, but also have meaningful practical value. These are societal issues as well as medical, 'do clinical benefits of medication justify their costs?', or, 'to what extent does medication use (or the costs associated with medication use) offset other medical or supportive care for dementia patients?'

Cost estimates are a way to demonstrate value to society. It may be helpful to think of a cost-effectiveness analysis as a demonstration of the relationship between the medical resources used ('costs') and the benefits obtained ('effects') for a medical or pharmaceutical intervention, compared with a specific alternative or standard approach. A cost-effectiveness ratio represents the *cost* difference between the intervention and a standard approach divided by the difference in *effectiveness* between the intervention and a standard approach. In theory, a cost-effectiveness analysis could be applied across a range of Phase III trials, involving several medications. But this would require that the differences in costs and effectiveness (perhaps the drug–placebo difference in outcome) are obtained using similar methods and reported in similar terms.

In pharmacoeconomics, a cost can be considered the value of the medical care and medication used, and can include both the estimated costs and any potential savings resulting from the intervention. In Phase III trials, the medical interventions can include the medications, physician services, nursing services, diagnostic testing, outcome assessments, nursing home care, complications of treatment, management of side-effects, monitoring of treatment, transportation to and from the clinic, and caregiver services. Indirect costs can be included, and include unpaid care by family members, or the time involved in obtaining care or receiving the medication. Indeed, it is well recognized that any treatment that reduces caregiver burden may have a substantial impact on the illness. A randomized clinical trial, focused on addressing the needs of caregivers, demonstrated that dementia patients lived longer in the community when their caregivers received specific intervention (Mittleman et al, 1996).

In order to do cost-effectiveness analyses in Phase III clinical trials, the total cost of the interventions must be calculated as well as the health effects. A particular concern in these trials is the standard health intervention to which the medication group is to be compared. On the one hand, the placebo group is an obvious comparison because the only essential difference between the treatments (i.e., drug vs placebo) is the administration of actual medication. This direct and contemporaneous analysis would give a differential estimate of the relationship between the resources used and the health effects achieved, that can be attributed almost entirely to the consequences of random medication assignment. The differential effect can be easily measured using the various outcome measures in the trial, and the cost of applying the medication, including the cost of managing side-effects, can be estimated in a fairly straightforward manner, limited only by the extent of measures obtained. Any cost-effectiveness observed in such a trial can be easily described and attributed to the medication. However, this would be essentially a differential treatment analysis in which the results are expressed as a cost-effectiveness ratio using the placebo group as the standard treatment group, and does not take into account the real costs or the real efficacy of treatment as compared to typical patients with Alzheimer's disease in the community. Although internally valid, the generalizability of this approach remains in question.

On the other hand, the overall costs associated with treatment in the drug and the placebo groups each can be compared to the cost of resources used as estimated from a standard and typical population of Alzheimer disease patients. This requires, however, the identification of such a relevant population and the feasibility of obtaining some estimate of overall health effects. This comparison, which was exemplified by the studies described above, has a disadvantage of being neither a contemporaneous nor a randomized comparison and is inherently subject to bias.

An interesting consideration is that the cost-effectiveness of placebo in the Phase III trial can be estimated and compared to the placebo and medication groups from other Phase III trials. If a standardized population of typical Alzheimer patients, receiving typical care, is used as the comparison group, then, in theory, different drugs and placebos from different Phase III trials could be compared with the standard group. (It would indeed be interesting if placebo in one trial was more cost-effective than placebo or medication from other virtually identically designed trials.) However, even here there would be a level of approximation and abstraction that would be difficult to interpret, since not all Phase III trials are conducted identically, and the current clinical effects of medications for Alzheimer's disease are modest. It is possible that the cost-effectiveness ratio calculated would actually be due to such methodological subtleties as slight differences in illness severity, frequency of assessments, unmeasured variables such as the possible use of estrogen replacement, or, finally, to unstable estimates or random-error variance because of the relatively small sample sizes of Phase III trials (even 700 patients constitute a 'small' clinical trial for these purposes).

A partial example of a cost-differential analysis is illustrated by results from a Phase III trial of a cholinesterase inhibitor similar to tacrine, velnacrine. In a six-month-long trial, velnacrine use was associated with 3.3 hours less of caregiving per day compared to placebo among other differences (Antouno, 1995). Even if it is determined by further analyses that this seemingly formidable (indirect) cost-saving is not offset by the costs of medication and side-effect management, the basic question still remains whether this caregiving effect would be seen in other, typical AD populations, or those with behavioral effects, and whether it occurred to a lesser extent in the placebo group.

SUMMARY

The strength of Phase III trials is their lean and efficient designs to demonstrate and confirm efficacy. Phase III of drug development was not intended to fully explore the utility of a treatment prescribed to typical patients under ordinary conditions. Phase III anti-dementia protocols currently include highly selected patients with only mildly severe dementia who are generally medically healthy and without behavioral problems. The trials require much more frequent visits, inter-disciplinary team contact, laboratory and diagnostic tests than are routinely used with ordinary patients. Therefore, the healthcare costs of patients in Phase III trials are very different from the costs of Alzheimer's disease patients not in clinical trials. One approach is to broaden the criteria for Phase III studies as part of the original drug development plan. An additional approach is to develop an identifiable comparison cohort of typical patients who did not enter the clinical trial and could be compared to the randomized patients, allowing for economic modeling. The final consideration is that Phase IV studies for economic benefit ought to be planned at the outset of a drug development program, and that Phase III should not be relied on to generate this important economic assessment.

STATEMENT

The author has received grants, contracts, and/or honoraria from Parke-Davis, Inc, Pfizer, Inc, Eisai, Inc, Novartis, Bayer, Janssen, SmithKline Beecham, as well as other developers of anti-dementia medications. No funding or other support was received expressly to support the research and writing of this chapter, however.

REFERENCES

Antuono, P. G., for the Mentane Study Group (1995). Effectiveness and safety of velnacrine for the treatment of Alzheimer's disease. *Arch. Intern. Med.*, **155**, 1766–1772.

Chui, H. C., Lyness, S., Sobel, E. and Schneider, L. S. (1994). Extrapyramidal signs and psychiatric symptoms predict faster rate of progression in Alzheimer's disease. *Arch. Neurology*, **51**, 676–681.

Corey-Bloom, J., Galasko, D., Hofstetter, C. R. et al (1993). Clinical features distinguishing large cohorts with possible AD, probable AD, and mixed dementia. *J. Am. Geriat. Soc.*, **41**, 31–37.

Dept. of Health and Human Services, Food and Drug Administration [Docket No. 97D-0188] (1997). International Conference on Harmonisation; Draft Guideline on General Considerations for Clinical Trials; Availability, p. 29540.

Drevets, W. C. and Rubins, E. H. (1989). Psychotic symptoms and the longitudinal course of senile dementia of Alzheimer type. *Biol. Psychiatry*, **25**, 39–48.

Ernst, R. L. and Hay, J. W. (1994). The U.S. economic and social costs of Alzheimer's disease revisited. *Am. J. Public Health*, **84**, 1261–1264.

Folstein, M. F., Folstein, S. E. and McHugh, P. R. (1975). 'Mini-mental state' a practical method for grading the cognitive state of patients for the clinician. *J. Psychiatr. Res.*, **12**, 189–198.

Galasko, D., Corey-Bloom, J. and Thal, L. J. (1991). Monitoring progression in Alzheimer's disease. *J. Amer. Geriat. Soc.*, **39**, 932–941.

Henke, C. J. and Burchmore, M. (1997). The economic impact of tacrine in the treatment of Alzheimer's disease. *Clinical Therapeutics*, **19**, 330–345.

Knapp, M. J., Knopman, D. S., Solomon, P. S., Pendlebury, W. W., Davis, C. S. and Gracon, S. I., for the Tacrine Study Group (1994). Controlled trials of high-dose tacrine in patients with Alzheimer's disease. *JAMA*, **271**, 985–991.

Knopman, D. and Gracon, S. (1994). Observations on the short-term 'natural history' of probable Alzheimer's disease in a controlled trial. *Neurology*, **44**, 260–265.

Knopman, D., Schneider, L., Davis, K. et al (1996). Long-term tacrine (Cognex®) treatment: Effects on nursing home placement and mortality. *Neurology*, **47**, 166–177.

Lubeck, D. P., Mazonson, P. D. and Bowe, T. (1994). Potential effect of tacrine on expenditures for Alzheimer's disease. *Med. Interface*, **7**, 130–138.

Mayeux, R., Stern, Y. and Sano, M. (1992). A comparison of clinical outcome and survival in various forms of Alzheimer's disease. In F. Boller, F. Forette, Z. Khachaturian, M. Poncet and Y. Christian (Eds), *Clinical Heterogeneity in Alzheimer's Disease*, pp. 4–11. New York, Springer-Verlag.

McKhann, G., Drachman, D., Folstein, M., Katzman, R., Price, D. and Stadlan, E. (1984). Clinical diagnosis of Alzheimer's disease: Report of the NINCDS-ADRDA Work Group under the auspices of Department of Health and Human Services Task Force on Alzheimer's disease. *Neurology*, **34**, 939–944.

Mittelman, M. S., Ferris, S. H., Shulman, E., Steinberg, G. and Levin, B. (1996). A family intervention to delay nursing home placement of patients with Alzheimer disease. A randomized controlled trial. *JAMA*, **276**(21), 1725–1731.

Peck, C. C., Barr, W. H., Benet, L. Z., Collins, J., Desjardins, R. E., Furst, D. E., Harter, J. G., Levy, G., Ludden, T., Rodman, J. H., Sanathanan, L., Schentag, J. J.,

Shah, V. P., Sheiner, L. B., Skelly, J. P., Stanski, D. R., Temple, R. J., Viswanathan, C. T., Weissinger, J. and Yacobi, A. (1992). Opportunities for integration of pharmacokinetics in rational drug development. *Clinical Pharmacol. Ther.*, **51**, 465–473.

Rice, D. P., Fox, P. J., Hauch, W. W. et al (1991). The burden of caring for Alzheimer's disease patients. US Department of Health and Human Services, *Proceedings of the 1991 Public Health Conference on Records and Statistics*, pp. 119–124.

Salmon, D. P., Thal, L. J., Butt, N. et al (1990). Longitudinal evaluation of dementia of the Alzheimer type: A comparison of 3 standardized mental status examinations. *Neurology*, **40**, 1225–1230.

Schneider, L. S., Olin, J. T., Lyness, S. A. and Chui, H. C. (1997). Eligibility of Alzheimer's disease clinic patients for clinical trials. *J. Am. Geriatr. Soc.*, **45**, 1–6.

Yesavage, J. A., Poulsen, S. L., Sheikh, J. et al (1988). Rates of change of common measures of impairment in senile dementia of the Alzheimer's type. *Psychopharmacology Bulletin*, **24**, 531–534.

Van Belle, G., Uhlmann, R. F., Hughes, J. P. et al (1990). Reliability of estimates of changes in mental status test performance in senile dementia of the Alzheimer type. *J. Clin. Epidemiol.*, **43**, 589–595.

Wimo, A., Karlsson, G., Nordberg, A. and Winblad, B. (1997). Treatment of Alzheimer disease with tacrine: a cost-analysis model. *Alzheimer Disease & Associated Disorders*, **11**(4), 191–200.

4.3 Evaluation of the Healthcare Resource Utilization and Caregiver Time in Anti-Dementia Drug Trials—A Quantitative Battery

A. WIMO, A.-L. WETTERHOLM
Umeå University, Umeå, Sweden, and Karolinska Institute, Huddinge, Sweden

V. MASTEY
Pfizer Pharmaceuticals Group, New York, USA

B. WINBLAD
Karolinska Institute, Huddinge Hospital, Huddinge, Sweden

INTRODUCTION

Alzheimer's disease (AD) is insidious in onset and results in a relentless and irreversible decline of function. It is characterized by symptoms of progressive memory loss, confusion and a variety of cognitive disabilities. Other symptoms including depression, agitation, psychosis and general deterioration in global intellectual abilities become so severe that they interfere with the person's customary occupational performance, often manifested by inappropriate social behavior. Thus, as the disease progresses, patients become unable to achieve even the simplest Activities of Daily Living (ADLs) without help. Eventually, this often leads to the patient requiring total care (Wimo et al, 1992). These characteristics make AD one of the most distressing and costly disorders among the elderly population (Huang et al, 1988; Østbye and Crosse, 1994; Gray and Fenn, 1993; Ernst and Hay, 1994; Wimo et al, 1997a).

Due to the increasing longevity of the general population, the prediction that the prevalence of AD will grow is now undisputed (Schneider and Guralnik, 1990; Manton et al, 1993; Rice et al, 1993; Wimo et al, 1992; Max, 1996). Indeed, AD is expected to reach epidemic proportions by the year 2020. As caregivers of patients with AD provide increasing levels of care as the disease progresses, they often experience difficulty dealing with the many cognitive and

Health Economics of Dementia. Edited by Anders Wimo, Bengt Jönsson, Göran Karlsson and Bengt Winblad.
© 1998 John Wiley & Sons Ltd.

behavioral problems experienced by the patient. Coping with these changes places the caregivers themselves in increasing jeopardy of health problems such as depression and anxiety (Schmall, 1996). For these reasons, the awareness of AD by families of patients, healthcare providers and society in general has grown, creating a major challenge for medicine and international economies (Yankner and Mesulam, 1991). Consequently, it is becoming increasingly important to assess not only the effects of treatment on healthcare utilization attributable to AD, but also the time spent by the caregivers caring for patients (Hepburn and Gates, 1988; Maletta, 1988). To calculate such variables, a questionnaire, designed to be used to estimate the potential benefits of therapies for AD in clinical trials, is presented. This questionnaire was used for the first time in a clinical trial on donepezil, a cholinesterase inhibitor (see Appendix).

THE NEED FOR ECONOMICALLY RELEVANT QUANTITATIVE DATA

Consumers expect and demand improvements in the quantity and quality of healthcare services provided. Previous healthcare reforms have concentrated on cost-containment measures and improved efficiency to ensure effective allocation of services. Restraining of increased management costs of AD by cost-containment strategies alone is unlikely. However, whilst only the prevention or cure of AD is likely to end the need for long-term care of AD patients completely, the symptomatic treatment of AD that is presently available may delay the time to the implementation of such care (Schneider and Guralnik, 1990).

Drugs constitute only a small proportion (1–2%) of the total costs of dementia care (Hay and Ernst, 1987; Østbye and Crosse, 1994), and the introduction of effective drug therapy for the care of dementia patients may benefit healthcare resource utilization (Mundell, 1993; Lubeck et al, 1994; Knopman et al, 1996; Max, 1996; Wimo et al, 1997b). With the many compounds in development for the treatment of AD, there is intensifying pressure on the pharmaceutical industry to collect economic data in Phase III studies that can be used by authorities to make decisions about the purchasing of drugs. Decision-makers, local drug purchasing groups or national authorities require cost comparisons of drug treatment to usual care to aid in the process of decision-making regarding healthcare resource allocation. For example, governments may consider reduced social security contributions as advantageous. These reductions may be obtained by maintaining patients with AD at a higher functional status with drug therapy. Indeed, in some countries, there are formal guidelines for the submission of economic evaluations: in France for reimbursement decisions for example, and Australia and Canada for drug pricing and reimbursement. Other interested groups include reimbursement/formulary committees, budget holders, physicians, advocacy groups and families.

ECONOMIC ASSESSMENT DESIGN DIFFICULTIES

Few prospective studies have been undertaken that investigate the impact of different treatment options for AD upon the patient, their caregivers and their utilization of healthcare resource. This is mainly due to a lack of specifically designed, reliable and quantitative tools to determine such variables. There are, however, a number of difficulties in the design of healthcare resource utilization assessments. For example, the symptoms, causes and the rate of progression of AD are heterogeneous, varying between individual patients and with age. Patients with severe dementia would be expected to receive more formal and informal care than patients with mild to moderately severe dementia who, depending upon their family situation, are more likely to be cared for at home (Rice et al, 1993). Consequently, the proportions of formal and informal care must be identified within a healthcare utilization assessment.

Other factors requiring consideration lie within varying sectors of the healthcare system which, as a consequence of budget-holding status, are the financial responsibility of different departments. This results in cost-shifting between various healthcare sectors, providing a complex scenario for cost assessment. Cross-cultural differences also exist in healthcare utilization, and these complicate comparative analysis. For example, the role of informal and formal caregiving differs reflecting the varying attitudes to the institutionalization of the elderly. As an alternative to the early institutionalization of the patient, some countries have intermediate care facilities providing outpatient and community care. In other countries, patient care is undertaken primarily within the family. Differences between countries due to financing, organizing and taxation levels also make comparisons of study results across countries difficult. Furthermore, there is a lack of consensus as to the value of treatment for AD. Provider, referral and treatment patterns differ between healthcare systems. Consequently, assessments are required that may be adapted for use across cultures.

To obtain basic data concerning the natural course of dementia, longitudinal, population-based studies are essential (Fratiglioni et al, 1992). Unfortunately, for practical and possibly ethical reasons, it is difficult to perform intervention studies over the whole survival period of the study groups, particularly as the major proportion of the total costs occur in the late stages of dementia. A reasonable solution is to apply models for costs and outcome measures. Alternatively, instruments may be designed that are sensitive to the characteristics of AD and that incorporate economically meaningful quantitative and qualitative assessments of the costs of caregiving and the total healthcare resource utilization of AD. This will aid the decision-making process regarding potential savings and cost comparisons of various therapeutic options and novel drugs for the treatment of AD that are beginning to emerge onto the market. This can only be achieved reliably by undertaking prospective, double-blind clinical studies of drug efficacy using specifically designed assessments of healthcare resource utilization.

THE RESOURCE UTILIZATION IN DEMENTIA (RUD) QUESTIONNAIRE

Total monetary costs resulting from a disease such as AD are normally calculated by a two-step process. Firstly, the utilization of the healthcare resource is estimated in terms of physical units, for example days or hours. These units of resource utilization are then converted into monetary costs. This Resource Utilization in Dementia (RUD) Questionnaire, described below, was designed to assess resource utilization. It assesses the healthcare resource utilization of the patient and caregiver and determines the level of formal and informal care attributable to AD.

The preferred method of measurement of healthcare utilization by AD patients and their caregivers is by structured interview. In order that all the information regarding healthcare resource use is obtained, this RUD Questionnaire may be administered by nurses, clinicians or specialists, or others. Patient participation in the evaluation of health surveys is difficult due to the decreases in cognition suffered by AD patients. In addition, other patient assessments (including cognitive functioning, ADLs, behavior, quality of life, etc.) are frequently administered during clinical trials, which may be a long and arduous experience for AD patients. Consequently, a proxy, that is, the caregiver, may be employed throughout the assessment to provide information about the patient. In addition, this problem may be solved by combining the administration of the RUD Questionnaire during home visits by a study nurse with visits to the physician's clinic. The RUD Questionnaire is summarized below in Table 4.3.1 and listed in full in the Appendix.

The RUD Questionnaire is divided into two parts. Part A constitutes the baseline assessments. Four sections include a general description of the primary caregiver and their relationship to the patient, the amount of time given up to assisting the patient with ADLs, their current employment status and work time lost through caring for the patient. The amount of hospitalization, physician time and medications consumed by the caregiver is also assessed. Two further sections determine the nature of the AD patients' living accommodation, home services and the amount of hospitalization, physician time and medications consumed by the patient.

Part B of the RUD Questionnaire is similar to the first, and is for use in all subsequent follow-up clinic visits at 3-month intervals up to one year. Questions regarding the characteristics of the primary caregiver are omitted, but more extensive questions are asked concerning alterations in the work status of the caregiver and the accommodation of the patient. The following assessment of healthcare utilization is described in more detail below.

Table 4.3.1. Structure of the Resource Utilization in Dementia (RUD) Questionnaire

Baseline assessment		Follow-up assessment	
Caregiver	Patient	Caregiver	Patient
Description of primary caregiver[a]	Accommodation	Caregiver time	Accommodation
Caregiver time	Healthcare resource utilization	Work status	Healthcare resource utilization
Work status		Healthcare resource utilization	
Healthcare resource utilization			

[a] It is assumed that the patient characteristics are described elsewhere with the Case Report Form of a clinical trial.

ACCOMMODATION AND HOME CARE

In addition to assistance with ADLs by professionals, family and friends in the community, the most significant component of the total cost of AD appears to be that of the quantity of long-term care in institutions (Welch et al, 1992). Previous studies have demonstrated that although the total figures for institutionalized and non-institutionalized patients may be similar, the cost breakdowns for the two settings are substantially different. The cost of formal care of non-institutionalized patients is mainly for social services (76%) and hospital care (13%) and other requirements including physician visits and medications. Alternatively, expenditure for institutionalized patients is largely accounted for by the institution itself (93%). For non-institutionalized patients, informal care accounts for approximately 75% of the total costs, whereas it is only approximately 12% of the costs for patients in nursing homes (Rice et al, 1993; Max et al, 1995). It is feasible that costs may be reduced by delaying the need for nursing home placement or decreasing utilization of emergency medical care and hospitalization (Odenheimer, 1989; Max, 1993; Max, 1996).

The decision to institutionalize an AD patient may be determined by the absence of a caregiver (a spouse, for example) or caregiver 'burden' that threatens caregivers' ability to continue to support the patient at home (Reisberg et al, 1987; Wimo et al, 1992; Donaldson et al, 1997). As caregivers of AD patients in the community spend more time managing behavioral and functional problems (e.g. hallucinations, wandering and incontinence) than any other activity (Max et al, 1995), patients are more likely to be institutionalized because of these symptoms than for cognitive decline.

The RUD Questionnaire determines the patient's living accommodation, including the patient's own home, intermediate forms of accommodation (e.g. 'service house' or 'home for the aged'), dementia-specific residential accommodation or other. Depending upon the design of a particular study, nursing home accommodation may also be included within this section of the RUD Questionnaire. For instance, if it is intended to include patients that move between nursing home and other types of accommodation in the study, then this alternative should be included in this section of the baseline and follow-up questionnaires. If, however, patients that are accommodated in nursing homes at the study baseline are to be excluded from the study, then this alternative should not be included in the baseline questionnaire.

As care terminology (nursing home, home for the aged, group living, meals-on-wheels, etc.) may differ between countries, the RUD Questionnaire may be modified and adapted accordingly. For multinational studies, each accommodation type is divided into the broad categories, described above. The time spent in each type of accommodation may be multiplied by the respective costs. The determination of the unit cost per day may be estimated from external sources reflecting the average cost for the different types of permanent and temporary living accommodation in different countries. For national studies, the categories of accommodation may be adapted to reflect the local terminology: for example, home care, residential care, service houses, group living, or nursing home care, and so on.

CAREGIVER TIME

In the majority of healthcare settings, a substantial proportion of the total costs of AD are absorbed by family members who generally become unpaid informal caregivers soon after diagnosis (Max, 1993; Weinberger et al, 1993; Stommel et al, 1994), particularly if they are elderly spouses (Grafström et al, 1992). As the cognitive and functional decline of the patient progresses and their dependency on assistance increases, the level of caregiver strain rises (Marchi-Jones et al, 1996). Many elements influence the extent of this caregiver 'burden', including the age and sex of the caregiver, the relationship to the patient, the overall health and the financial status of the patient and caregiver.

This RUD Questionnaire has been designed to capture the total time that the caregiver spends caring for the patient and essentially addresses two main issues. First is the time spent by the caregiver providing care to the patient (helping the patient with ADLs and supervision). Assisting the patient with ADLs is a key variable, particularly for cases where the primary caregivers are the adult children of the patient (Østbye and Crosse, 1994). It has been estimated that caregivers in the community spend 286 hours per month (almost 10 hours per day) supervising and assisting an AD patient with feeding, bathing, toileting and dressing, for example, while caregivers for patients in institutions spend 36 hours per month (Rice et al, 1993). Thus, a treatment that reduces caregiver time and burden might be expected to have a substantial impact on indirect costs.

The second issue of caregiver time involves more subtle changes in the health status of both the patient and the caregiver/family. For instance, the most common caregiver is likely to be a retired spouse who is unlikely to incur indirect costs from lost productivity. Alternatively, spouses and children of working age would be expected to incur indirect costs due to lost productivity. Consequently, this RUD Questionnaire also includes the time lost from work because of caregiving responsibilities, reduced income and loss of time to pursue hobbies, personal relationships, or recreational activities.

Principles for costing informal care are not the main focus for this chapter. Costing informal care is, however, difficult and includes a wide range of complex issues and approaches used include inconsistent and also controversial methods (Smith and Wright, 1994; see also Netten, 1990; and Chapter 2.8 in this book).

We have only some short notes on these issues. Total costs may be calculated by a number of methods. If time spent by the caregiver is work time, it may be valued at the average hourly rate for workers in a specific country plus any social insurance contributions. If the time spent by an employed caregiver is leisure time, it may be estimated from the average wage after tax. Lastly, the time spent by non-working caregivers and caregivers working over 50 hours per week may be valued as either of the following:

A. a zero value (assuming that the caregiver would normally have contributed to the person's care and well-being before disease onset), or
B. the value of the hourly rate equivalent to paid home help (the time replacement method).

Thus, an upper and a lower estimate for total caregiver time may be established. When comparing costs of caregiver time between different countries, an aggregate measure of formal and informal resource utilization should be used, as opposed to total annual costs.

Collecting resource utilization figures involves several obstacles. For example, if information regarding support in ADLs only is measured, informal care may be underestimated, while the inclusion of IADL and supervision needs make the figures of informal care more representative. However, informal care costs may be overestimated if an opportunity cost approach of the supervision and management of behavioral problems is not included. Although it is difficult to separate caregiver time from normal household activities, lost activity or earning opportunity costs due to caregiving activity may be calculated from the time used for independent household activities such as meal preparation, eating or sleeping. Activities that are given up due to caring for the patient (paid work or hobbies, for example) can also be estimated. However, if the caregiver did not work or partake in hobbies prior to the disease, then no benefit is forgone.

The age of the informal caregiver is obviously important because of the potential for work loss, as is the caregiver's occupation prior to and during the period of care. Hence, it is important to capture the characteristics of the caregiver at the study baseline, as in the *Description of the Primary Caregiver* in this Questionnaire.

HEALTHCARE RESOURCE UTILIZATION

Severe health consequences may arise through patients' inability to communicate discomfort or other symptoms and non-compliance with medications. These include increased frequency of physician and emergency visits and increased duration of hospital stays. Such factors may have a great economic impact as patients with AD have been reported to use the hospital more than normal age-matched controls of 45 years or older (Ernst and Hay, 1994). In addition, according to published studies, caregivers of cognitively-impaired patients are more likely to be hospitalized themselves, and are reported to visit the physician 46% more frequently for stress and depression, for example, than control subjects (George and Gwyther, 1986; Haley et al, 1987).

Apart from medication, the utilization of healthcare resource by both the patient and the caregiver may be divided into two categories: (1) hospitalization, and (2) ambulatory care.

Inpatient costs may be calculated by determining the number of days spent in different hospital wards (e.g. geriatric, psychiatric, surgical, emergency room, etc.), or by measurement of the number of hospital admissions and the cost per admission or Diagnosis Related Groups (DRG), if available. By the latter method, hospitalizations must be classified according to diagnosis and procedures undertaken.

In some countries, including Sweden, it is common practice for patients to be admitted and discharged from nursing homes on a regular basis. Costs for ambulatory care may be measured by multiplying the number of visits with the cost per visit. A list of unit costs for different types of visit (e.g. primary care physician, geriatrician, neurologist, psychiatrist, occupational therapist, psychologist, or others, such as emergency medicine) may be derived from external sources, depending upon the healthcare system in question. Information concerning the amount of time per visit may be used to classify visits into groups of different unit costs, and visits that have similar unit costs can be aggregated before they are costed. Other ambulatory costs that are considered in the RUD Questionnaire include patient services such as nursing visits, home help, food delivery, day care, transportation and others. The costs of such activities can be calculated by specifying the type of service, its frequency of use over a specified period (e.g. per week or month) and the average time spent per visit (Clipp and Moore, 1995).

MEDICATION

As AD generally affects elderly individuals, concurrent illnesses including depression, asthma, diabetes, hypertension, cerebrovascular disease (stroke), arthritis and congestive heart failure are commonly suffered by patients with AD. Although drugs constitute only a small proportion of the total costs of AD, this makes the cost differentiation between the treatment of separate conditions difficult. Furthermore, patient response to therapy is not the only measurement of treatment success when considering novel treatments for AD. The accumulation of emotional, psychological and practical problems relating to caregiving can overwhelm affected families. Caregivers often experience complaints associated with stress: gastrointestinal disturbances, headaches, depression, anxiety, and chronic fatigue (Anthony-Bergstone et al, 1988; Bergman-Evans, 1994; Hall et al, 1995; Schmall, 1996; George and Gwyther, 1986; Moritz et al, 1992). Indeed, more than 50% of caregivers are thought to be at risk from clinical depression (Drinka et al, 1987; Haley et al, 1987; Gallagher et al, 1989; Donaldson et al, 1997). As a consequence, some caregivers may use psychotropic drugs (Clipp and George, 1990). Caregivers of cognitively-impaired persons may use over 70% more prescribed drugs than control subjects (Ernst and Hay, 1994). This RUD Questionnaire is designed to gather information on the actual drugs used by the patients and their caregivers, the period of time of usage, and the dose prescribed. Hence, costs of daily medication can be calculated and the total drug costs may be determined.

DISCUSSION

The human and financial price of caring for patients with AD is immense and is predicted to escalate in future years. Although no cure or prevention exists for AD, treatment that improves or enhances cognitive function is a primary treatment goal in AD, as this may have significant economic, clinical and social ramifications. For example, since progressive cognitive impairment underlies the eventual functional disability in AD, maximizing cognition may prolong the autonomous life of the patient. It might be anticipated, therefore, that drug therapies that improve cognition in patients with AD may delay or postpone institutionalization (Knopman et al, 1996), the largest direct cost factor associated with AD (Welch et al, 1992). Alternatively, delaying institutionalization may transfer formal care responsibilities from nursing home staff to physicians and social service providers, and may shift direct cost payment to the patient and family, increasing the indirect cost of unpaid informal caregiving. However, this may be an acceptable alternative as families often consider that maintaining a patient at home is a desirable objective (Max, 1996).

On the other hand, improving the function of patients with AD could decrease unpaid informal caregiver time and improve patient and caregiver QOL. The stress associated with caring for an AD patient may also be reduced by enhancing cognitive function and delaying the loss of patients' ADLs, such as bathing, dressing or toileting. Finally, enhancing patients' cognitive function may also facilitate the timely diagnosis of concurrent diseases that are common in elderly patients. Moreover, improved compliance with existing treatments may reduce the costs associated with the management of co-morbidities (e.g. arthritis, diabetes or heart disease), thereby decreasing hospital and emergency department visits.

Cholinergic agents are currently the only approved drug treatment for the cognitive impairment of AD. This class of agent includes the cholinesterase inhibitors, muscarinic and nicotinic agonists, and indirect modifiers of acetylcholine release. Such drugs increase the cognitive and functional abilities of the patient by maintaining levels of acetylcholine neurotransmission, predominantly in the cortical and hippocampal brain regions, of AD patients (Schneider, 1996). Tacrine (Cognex^{TM}), a cholinesterase inhibitor, was the first such drug to become available for the symptomatic treatment of AD. Despite the added costs of the drug itself, treatment monitoring and withdrawals due to hepatotoxicity, it has been estimated that tacrine may generate significant savings in the current cost of untreated AD patients (Mundell, 1993; Lubeck et al, 1994; Henke et al, 1997; Wimo et al, 1997b) by delaying institutionalization for 9–12 months (Knopman et al, 1996). These data suggest that newer agents with equivalent or better risk–benefit profiles are likely to be at least, if not more, cost-effective than tacrine (Doraiswamy, 1996). However, as behavioral disturbances are probably better predictors of institutionalization than cognitive function, drugs that reduce such disturbances should be (and are) the focus of extensive research. Second-generation cholinesterase inhibitors that are long-acting, have predictable pharmacokinetics, and provide a high concentration of acetylcholine in the brain, are beginning to emerge into the marketplace (Schneider and Tariot, 1994). Donepezil (Aricept^{TM}) is the first of these second-generation cholinesterase inhibitors to receive marketing approval from the FDA and a central European filing for the treatment of mild to moderate AD. In contrast to tacrine, over 80% of patients in clinical trials who initiated treatment with once-daily donepezil completed treatment with an improvement or no further decline in cognitive function, without any evidence of hepatotoxicity (Rogers et al, 1996). Also, preliminary evidence from Phase III studies suggests that donepezil may delay the loss of ADLs by approximately 1 year (Friedhoff and Rogers, 1997). Furthermore, evidence from open-label studies suggests that the treatment effect of ChE inhibitors, including donepezil, is maintained for at least two years (Rogers et al, 1995). Thus, the treatment of AD with AChE inhibitors may translate into significant cost savings for the patient, caregiver and society in general.

Even if the economic evaluations referred to above indicate cost savings, they are not complete health economical evaluations. The demand for economic data on the costs of AD is increasingly requested by decision-makers. Currently, the potential of novel drug therapies to reduce the total costs of AD to society is uncertain. Drug therapies for AD cannot be evaluated using a conventional economic assessment in which the cost of therapy is compared with the savings in medical and other expenditures. Many of the benefits of the therapies under development affect indirect costs through reduced caregiver burden and improved QOL for both the patient and caregiver (Max, 1996). Instrumentation is required for use in longitudinal, prospective and comparative studies, to determine the benefits of specific drug therapy as compared with usual care. Any instruments used need to be sensitive to the unique circumstances of patients with AD and their caregivers and be applicable across cultures. The RUD Questionnaire described in this article was specifically designed for such purposes by investigating a number of different parameters of caregiver and patient healthcare utilization.

REFERENCES

Anthony-Bergstone, C. R., Zarit, S. H. and Gatz, M. (1988). Symptoms of psychological distress among caregivers of dementia patients. *Psychol. Aging*, 3, 245–248.

Bergman-Evans, B. (1994). A health profile of spousal Alzheimer's caregivers. Depression and physical health characteristics. *J. Psychosoc. Nurs. Ment. Health Serv.*, 32(9), 25–30.

Clipp, E. C. and George, L. K. (1990). Psychotropic drug use among caregivers of patients with dementia. *J. Am. Geriatr. Soc.*, 38(3), 227–235.

Clipp, E. C. and Moore, M. J. (1995). Caregiver time use: An outcome measure in clinical trial research on Alzheimer's disease. *Clin. Pharm. Ther.*, 58, 228–236.

Donaldson, C., Tarrier, N. and Burns, A. (1997). The impact of the symptoms of dementia on caregivers. *Brit. J. Psychiatry*, 170, 62–68.

Doraiswamy, P. M. (1996). Current cholinergic therapy for symptoms of Alzheimer's disease. *Primary Psychiatry*, 3(11), 56–68.

Drinka, T. J., Smith, J. C. and Drinka P. J. (1987). Correlates of depression and burden for informal caregivers of patients in a geriatrics referral clinic. *J. Am. Geriatr. Soc.*, 35(6), 522–525.

Drummond, M., Stoddart, G. L. and Torrance, G. E. W. (1987). *Methods for the Economic Evaluation of Health Care Programmes*, Oxford, UK, Oxford University Press.

Ernst, R. L. and Hay, J. W. (1994). The US economic and social costs of Alzheimer's disease revisited. *Am. J. Public Health*, 84, 1261–1264.

Fratiglioni, L., Viitanen, M., Backman, L., Sandman, P. O. and Winblad, B. (1992). Occurrence of dementia in advanced age: the study design of the Kungsholmen Project. *Neuroepidemiology*, 11 (suppl 1), 29–36.

Friedhoff, L. T. and Rogers, S. L. (1997). Donepezil lengthens time to loss of activities of daily living in patients with mild to moderate Alzheimer's disease—Results of a preliminary evaluation. *Neurology*, 48(3), A100(P02.026).

Gallagher, D., Rose, J., Rivera, P., Lovett, S. and Thompson, L. N. (1989). Prevalence of depression in family caregivers. *Gerontologist*, 29, 449–456.

George, L. and Gwyther, L. (1986). Caregiver well-being: a multidimensional examination of family caregivers of demented adults. *Gerontologist*, 26, 253–259.

Grafström, M., Fratiglioni, L., Sandman, P. O. and Winblad, B. (1992). Health and social consequences for relatives of demented and non-demented elderly. A population-based study. *J. Clin. Epidemiol.*, 45(8), 861–870.

Gray, A. and Fenn, P. (1993). Alzheimer's disease: the burden of the illness in England. *Health Trends*, **25**(1), 31–37.

Haley, W. E., Levine, E. G., Brown, S. L., Bartolucci, A. A., Berry, J. W. and Hughes, G. H. (1987). Stress, appraisal, coping, and social support as predictors of adaptational outcome among dementia caregivers. *Psychol. Aging*, **2**(4), 323–330.

Haley, W. E., Levine, E. G., Brown, S. L., Berry, J. W. and Hughes, G. H. (1987). Psychological, social, and health consequences of caring for a relative with senile dementia. *J. Am. Geriatr. Soc.*, **35**(5), 405–411.

Hall, G. R., Buckwalter, K. C., Stolley, J. M., Gerdner, L. A., Garand, L., Ridgeway, S. and Crump, S. (1995). Standardized care plan. Managing Alzheimer's patients at home. *J. Gerontol. Nurs.*, **21**(1), 37–47.

Hay, J. W. and Ernst, R. L. (1987). The economic costs of Alzheimer's disease. *Am. J. Public Health*, **77**(9), 1169–1175.

Henke, C. J. and Burchmore, M. J. (1997). The economic impact of tacrine in the treatment of Alzheimer's Disease. *Clinical Therapeutics*, **19**(2), 330–345.

Hepburn, K. W. and Gates, B. A. (1988). Family caregivers for non-Alzheimer's dementia patients. *Clin. Geriatr. Med.*, **4**(4), 925–940.

Huang, L., Cartwright, W. and Hu, T. (1988). The economic cost of senile dementia in the United States, 1985. *Public Health Rep.*, **103**, 3–7.

Knopman, D., Schneider, L., Davis, K. et al (1996). Long-term tacrine (Cognex) treatment: effects on nursing home placement and mortality. *Neurology*, **47**, 166–177.

Lubeck, D. P., Mazonson, P. D. and Bowe, T. (1994). Potential effect of tacrine on expenditure for Alzheimer's disease. *Medical Interface*, October, 132–138.

Maletta, G. J. (1988). Management of behavior problems in elderly patients with Alzheimer's disease and other dementias. *Clin. Geriatr. Med.*, **4**(4), 719–747.

Manton, K. G., Corder, L. S. and Stallard, E. (1993). Estimates of change in chronic disability and institutional incidence and prevalence rates in the U.S. elderly population from the 1982, 1984, and 1989 National Long Term Care Survey. *J. Gerontol.*, **48**(4), S153–166.

Marchi-Jones, S., Murphy, J. F. and Rousseau, P. (1996). Caring for the caregivers. *J. Gerontol. Nurs.*, **22**(8), 7–13.

Max, W. (1993). The economic impact of Alzheimer's disease. *Neurology*, **43** (suppl 4), S6–10.

Max, W. (1996). The cost of Alzheimer's disease. Will drug treatment ease the burden? *Pharmacoeconomics*, **9**(1), 5–10.

Max, W., Webber, P. A. and Fox, P. J. (1995). Alzheimer's disease: the unpaid burden of caring. *J. Aging Health*, **7**(2), 179–199.

Moritz, D. J., Kasl, S. V. and Ostfeld, A. M. (1992). The health impact of living with a cognitively impaired elderly spouse. *J. Aging Health*, **4**, 244–267.

Mundell, I. (1993). Is tacrine worth the price? *Inpharma*, **910**, 3–4.

Netten, A. (1990). An approach to costing informal care, Discussion paper 637, Personal Social Services Research Unit, University of Kent at Canterbury.

Nygaard, H. A. (1988). Strain on caregivers of demented elderly people living at home. *Scand. J. Prim. Health Care*, **6**(1), 33–37.

Odenheimer, G. L. (1989). Acquired cognitive disorders of the elderly. *Med. Clin. North Am.*, **73**(6), 1383–1441.

Østbye, T. and Crosse, E. (1994). Net economic costs of dementia in Canada. *Can. Med. Assoc. J.*, **151**(10), 1457–1464.

Reisberg, B., Borenstein, J., Salob, S. P., Ferris, S. H., Franssen, E. and Georgotas, A. (1987). Behavioural symptoms in Alzheimer's disease: phenomenology and treatment. *J. Clin. Psychiatry*, **48** (suppl 48), 9–15.

Rice, D. R., Fox, P. J., Max, W., Webber, P. A., Lindeman, D. A., Hauck, W. W. and

Segura, E. (1993). The economic burden of Alzheimer's disease care. *Health Aff. Millwood*, **12**, 165–176.

Rogers, S. L. and Freidhoff, L. T. and The Donepezil Study Group (1996). The efficacy and safety of donepezil in patients with Alzheimer's disease: results of a US multicentre, randomized, double-blind, placebo-controlled trial. *Dementia*, **7**, 293–303.

Rogers, S. L., Perdomo, C. and Friedhoff, L. T. (1995). Clinical benefits are maintained during long-term treatment of Alzheimer's disease with the acetylcholinesterase inhibitor, E2020. *Eur. Neuropsychopharmacol.*, **5**(3), 386(P-8-21).

Rogers, S. L., Yamanishi, Y. and Yamatsu, K. (1991). E2020: the pharmacology of a piperidine cholinesterase inhibitor. In R. Becker and E. Giacobini (Eds), *Cholinergic Basis for Alzheimer Therapy*, pp. 314–320. Boston, Birkhäuser.

Schmall, V. L. (1996). Dealing with Alzheimer's disease: Caregiver issues. *Consult. Pharm.*, **11** (suppl E), 25–31.

Schneider, E. L. and Guralnik, J. M. (1990). The aging of America. Impact on health care costs. *JAMA*, **263**(17), 2335–2340.

Schneider, E. L. and Tariot, P. N. (1994). Emerging drugs for Alzheimer's disease: mechanisms of action and prospects for cognitive enhancing medications. *Med. Clin. North Am.*, **78**, 911–934.

Schneider, L. S. (1996). New therapeutic approaches to Alzheimer's disease. *J. Clin. Psychiatry*, **57** (suppl 14), 30–36.

Smith, K. and Wright, K. (1994). Informal care and economic appraisal: a discussion of possible methodological approaches. *Health Econ.*, **3**, 137–148.

Snow, C. (1996). Medicare HMOs develop plan for future of Alzheimer's programming. *Modern Healthcare*, 23 September, 66–70.

Stommel, M., Collins, C. E. and Given, B. A. (1994). The costs of family contributions to the care of persons with dementia. *Gerontologist*, **34**(2), 199–205.

Weinberger, M., Gold, D. T., Divine, G. W., Cowper, P. A., Hodgson, L. G., Schreiner, P. J. and George, L. K. (1993). Expenditures in caring for patients with dementia who live at home. *Am. J. Public Health*, **83**, 338–341.

Welch, H. G., Walsh, J. S. and Larson, E. B. (1992). The cost of institutional care in Alzheimer's disease: nursing home and hospital use in a prospective cohort. *J. Am. Geriatr. Soc.*, **40**, 221–224.

Wimo, A., Gustafsson, L. and Mattson, B. (1992). Predictive validity of factors influencing the institutionalization of elderly people with psychogeriatric disorders. *Scand. J. Prim. Health Care*, **10**(3), 185–191.

Wimo, A., Karlsson, G., Sandman, P. O., Corder, L. and Winblad, B. (1997a). Cost of illness due to dementia in Sweden. *Int. J. Geriatr. Psychiatry*, **12**, 857–861.

Wimo, A., Karlsson, G., Nordberg, A. and Winblad, B. (1997b). Treatment of Alzheimer's disease with tacrine, a cost analysis model. *Alzheimer Dis. Assoc. Disord.*, **11**, 39–45.

Winblad, B., Hill, S., Beermann, B. and Wimo, A. (1997). Issues in the economic evaluation of treatment for dementia. *Alzheimer Dis. Assoc. Disord.*, **11** (suppl 3), 39–45.

Yankner, B. A. and Mesulam, M.-M. (1991). Seminars in medicine of the Beth Israel Hospital, Boston. β-Amyloid and the pathogenesis of Alzheimer's disease. *N. Engl. J. Med.*, **325**(26), 1849–1857.

Appendix: The Resource Utilization in Dementia (RUD) Questionnaire

THE RESOURCE UTILIZATION IN DEMENTIA (RUD) QUESTIONNAIRE GUIDELINES AND QUESTIONNAIRE

A. Wimo, A.-L. Wetterholm, V. Mastey, and B. Winblad

A   **BASELINE QUESTIONNAIRES**

A1   **Caregiver**

A1.1   Description of primary caregiver
A1.2   Caregiver time
A1.3   Work status
A1.4   Health care resource utilization

A2   **Patient**

A2.1   Accommodation
A2.2   Health care resource utilization

B   **FOLLOW-UP QUESTIONNAIRES**

B1   **Caregiver**

B1.1   Caregiver time
B1.2   Work status
B1.3   Health care resource utilization

B2   **Patient**

B2.1   Accommodation
B2.2   Health care resource utilization

GUIDELINES FOR THE RUD

A-SECTION: BASELINE

A1.1.4 Staff are not accepted as informative caregivers (but of course they are accepted to care for the patient). If the first caregiver for some reason during the study period (disease, death, moving, etc.) does not fulfill the criteria any longer, a new caregiver according to the defined criteria can be included. The date and the type of new caregiver must be noted.

A1.2 Caregiver time

The first questions refer to how much time has been spent on care during this typical care episode while the B questions refer to the number of days that support was given during the period. Example: if a daughter makes 16 visits during the period (here one month) to her demented mother and supports her in ADL, and the daughter at every visit spends 2 hours there, then the first answer is '2' and the second is '16'. If part of the total time is IADL and supervision activities, then the total time should be divided into relevant parts (ADL, IADL and supervision). The number of days/month for the activities may also vary (example: there may be support in ADL at 4 occasions/week, supervision every day but IADL-support only once a week.

A1.2.1 This question covers ADL (Activities of Daily Life).

A1.2.2 This question covers IADL (Instrumental ADL).

A1.2.3 Supervision (or surveillance) is related to the risk for dangerous events, such as risks of fire, walking into a road alone, walking outside without sufficient clothes if weather cold, etc. Help questions: can the patient be left alone for part of day? If so, for how many hours? Can the patient be left alone at nights?

A1.3 Caregiver Work Status

A1.3.1 Caregivers sick-listed ≤ 1 month (1 month = 30 days) are regarded as working for pay (option 1) while sick listed > 1 month = option 2).

A1.3.2 Early retirement: pension insurance, part pension, contract pension, that is not related to disease.

Own health problems: Early pension due to disease, sick-listed > 1 month.

The sick-listing may change at follow-up visits. To care for subject: includes both if the caregiver has stopped work and is paid for the care or is not paid for it.

A1.3.4 Caregiving responsibilities: All kinds of caregiving of the patient; not only because of the patient's dementia.

A1.4 Caregiver Health Care Resource Utilization

A1.4.3 DRG = Diagnose Related Groups, a remuneration system in health care. If you are not familiar with it: leave it, but always note the major diagnosis/reason for hospitalization.

A1.4.4 If there are more hospitalization events than 4 and other specialities than those noted, please write them down near the specified columns.

A1.4.5 Emergency room: episode at the Emergency Department at a hospital, irrespective of whether the caregiver meets a doctor or a nurse. The episode must be related to a caregiver disease, if the caregiver is accompanying someone else it should not be registered. Planned visits to specialists or GPs or emergency visits to GPs at public health centers should be registered at **A1.4.6**.

A2.1 Patient Living Accommodation

Care organization and types of accommodation for the elderly vary between countries and the following 'definitions' are supposed to serve as a guide for classification of the accommodation. Even if there are gray areas (see Chapter 2.8 in this book), you should classify the subject's accommodation.

Own home

'Usual living', that is a flat (apartment) or a house or similar which was not originally designed for care or social support. However, in their own home, some adjustments for care may be done to accommodate the needs of a patient. If the subject lives in the same house as for instance his/her son, and the house is owned by the son, the living place of the subject is still classified as 'own home'.

Intermediate forms of accommodation (not dementia-specific)
Service house: A permanent habitation where the residents live in their own apartments in a particular building. The apartment fulfills quality criteria for private living in
physical terms. Home service is available from staff when needed. Day Center activities
(see below) are mostly available in the building. Staff density is lower than in homes for
the aged.
Home for the aged/Old people's home: A permanent habitation where the residents live
in their own room in a particular building where home service is regularly available
from staff in the house. Little or no medical-technical equipment is available. Generally
there are staff also available during the night even if their number is limited.

Dementia-specific residential accommodation
Group Living (Group Homes, Group Dwellings, Collective Living and similar):   A
permanent habitation for 4–10 demented where the residents live in their own room or
a small apartment and where facilities/rooms for mutual activities such as meals and
other forms of social life are available. Staff are trained in dementia care and are
available around the clock. The demented receive community and care under staff
supervision, according to specified goals for dementia care. The specified goals may
vary but are mostly based on a nursing theory of dementia care (such as managing
behavioral disturbances, apraxia, agnosia, memory impairment). Staff may be nurses,
licenced practical nurses (assistant nurses), home aids or special dementia carers.

Long-term institutional care
A care unit with care wards where nursing care is provided around the clock to those
who are chronically ill and unable to perform daily activities. Staff are nurses, licenced
practical nurses (assistant nurses) and orderlies. Staff are available around the clock.
Medical–technical equipment is available.
    Nursing home care may sometimes not be allowed at baseline (depends on inclusion/
exclusion criteria).

A2.2 Patient Health Care Resource Utilization
A2.2.7   District nurse option: all types of visits by registered nurses even if they are
called something different.
Home health aid/orderly option: also register visits by licenced practical nurses/assistant
nurses here.
Meals on wheels: register just public-paid delivered meals.

Day care
Day care units are usually defined as 'day care' (the namings may vary) in administrative terms. All the following types of day care should be noted as 'day care'. Note
that visits to, for instance, physiotherapists or occupational therapists which are not
part of day care should just be registered above (A2.2.6). Do not double-register those
visits.
Day care for demented: Demented receive, under staff supervision, community and
care according to specified goals for dementia care, at a particular place, generally for
5–7 hours/day. The specified goals may vary but are mainly based on a nursing theory
of dementia care (such as managing behavioral disturbances, apraxia, agnosia, memory
impairment) and the staff are trained in dementia care. Staff may be nurses, licenced
practical nurses (assistant nurses), home aids or special dementia carers. The patients
mostly come from their own homes but may also come from service houses and homes
for the aged. Generally 2–3 staff serve 7–12 demented persons.

Day Center: Elderly persons, not necessarily ill, receive activation, occupational therapy and social support during part of the day at a particular place. Staff are often occupational therapists with assistants. If no registered staff (such as occupational therapists or physiotherapists) are available, do not register. The patients mostly come from own homes, service houses or homes for the aged.

Somatic Day Care: Patients receive care at a particular place, generally for 5–7 hours/day according to specified goals, focused mainly on rehabilitation and physical training. Staff may be nurses, physiotherapists, occupational therapists, psychologists. Assistants to these staff categories are often available. Somatic day care may be located at hospitals ('day hospitals') or as independent units. The patients mostly come from own homes but may also come from service houses, homes for the aged or nursing homes.

Transportation: Just register public-paid transport, not transport by spouses, children, etc.

Other: If volunteer organizations' work is registered here, note that it is this type of support.

B-SECTION: FOLLOW-UP VISIT

B1.2 Caregiver Work Status
Since changes from baseline (and between the follow-ups) are of interest it is important for the investigator to look at the previous registration. Regarding caregivers, the focus is on the changes of work time and work situation due to care responsibilities.

The most common alternative for caregiver-spouses will be: did not work at baseline and did not do it at follow-up(s) either.

For caregiver-children it will probably be: worked at baseline and no change at follow-ups. However, other scenarios will also be possible and a specific 'scenario schedule' has been produced (not given here) which may be of use (but try to register the questionnaire first).

B1.2.1   Note that the questions focus on paid work during part of or the whole period. If the caregiver has changed job or working time or gets paid for care, all this is considered as paid work. Also note that if the caregiver was 'short time' sicklisted at baseline or last visit (< 1 month), then he/she was registered as working at baseline.

B1.2.2   Stopped working: Caregivers sick-listed ≤ 1 month at the visit are regarded as working for pay (option 2), while sick-listed > 1 month and still is sick-listed at visit, register option 1. If caregiver was sick-listed > 1 month during period but has started to work again, register option 2.

B1.2.3   'Changed your job or working situation' includes new jobs but also changes in working time. If a caregiver has started to get paid for the care of the demented, it also means a changed working situation.

B1.2.4   Note that if the caregiver has started to get paid for the care of the demented, this number of hours (in the example 2 hours/day = 14 hour/week) is a part of the work for pay (see 4a–b). Example: if the caregiver reduces working time in their regular job from 40 hours to 20 hours per week but gets paid for care 2 hours/day, the total new work time is 20 + (2 × 7) = 34 hours per week. If there is no pay for the care but the work time is reduced to 20 hours/week, then the work time is 20 hours per week.

B1.2.5a   'Regular job' means the work that was registered at baseline.

B1.2.6   This question focuses on occasional episodes which do not influence the regular working time, for instance when the caregiver must leave work because the demented has lost her/his way. If there have been both occasional events (question 6) *and* a change in regular work time because of caregiving responsibilities (question 5), then register at both, otherwise do not double-register.

B2.1   Patient Living Accommodation

B2.1.4   The first four options deal with deterioration of the patient while options 5–8 describe improvement. There is a risk of overlap between these alternatives, but try to choose the most relevant and just one alternative.

B2.1.5   This question deals with short-time accommodation (not emergency hospital care). If there are problems in distinguishing between for instance nursing home care and short-time care at nursing homes organized by geriatric clinics, just register at one place, preferably at **B2.2.4** (see next section) but make a note in the margin about these problems.

THE RESOURCE UTILIZATION IN DEMENTIA (RUD) QUESTIONNAIRE BASELINE QUESTIONNAIRE

A1 CAREGIVER

A1.1 Description of Primary Caregiver

1. Date of birth __ / __ / __
   dd/mm/yy

2. Age ____ years

3. Sex:

   1. Male ☐
   2. Female _____ ☐

4. Relationship to patient

   1. Husband ☐
   2. Wife ☐
   3. Child ☐
   4. Friend ☐
   5. Other _____ ☐
   (Staff not allowed)

5. Marital status

   1. Married/Cohabiting ☐
   2. Never married ☐
   3. Divorced/Separated ☐
   4. Widowed _____ ☐

6. Number of children currently living with you
   ____ child(ren)

7. Do you live with the patient?

   1. Yes ☐
   2. No ☐

A1.2 Caregiver Time

1. On a typical care day during the last month, how much time per day did you spend assisting the patient with tasks such as toilet visits, eating, dressing, grooming, walking and bathing?

    |___|___| hours per day

    1(b).   During the last month, how many days did you spend providing these services to the patient? _____ days

2. On a typical care day during the last month, how much time per day did you spend assisting the patient with tasks such as shopping, food preparation, housekeeping, laundry, transportation, taking medication, and managing financial matters?

    |___|___| hours per day

    2(b).   During the last month, how many days did you spend providing these services to the patients? _____ days

3. On a typical care day during the last month, how much time per day did you spend supervising (that is, preventing dangerous events) the patient?

    |___|___| hours per day

    3(b).   During the last month, how many days did you spend providing these services to the patient? _____ days

A1.3 Caregiver Work Status

1. Do you currently work for pay?

    1. Yes ☐ If **yes**, answer questions 3 to 5
    2. No ☐ If **no**, answer question 2 **only**

2. Why did you stop/reduce working?

    1. Never worked ☐
    2. Reached retirement age ☐
    3. Early retirement ☐
       (not disease-related) ☐
    4. Laid off ☐
    5. Own health problems ☐
    6. To care for patient ☐
    7. Other _____ ☐

3. How many hours do you work in total for pay per week?

    |_|_| hours/week

    3(a). Of this number of hours, are you for some part paid to care for the patient?

        1. Yes ☐
        2. No ☐

    3(b). If **yes**, how many hours per week?

    |_|_| hours/week

4. During the last month, have you needed to cut down the number of hours that you usually work each week because of your caregiving responsibilities?

    1. Yes ☐
    2. No ☐

    4(a). If **yes**, how many hours did you cut down?

    |_|_| hours/week

5. During the last month, please specify the number of times that your caregiver responsibilities affected your work in the following ways.

    1. Missed a whole day of work

    |_|_| Number of times

    2. Missed a part of a day of work

    |_|_| Number of times

A1.4 Caregiver Health Care Resource Utilization

1. During the last month, were you admitted to a hospital (for more than 24 hours)?

   1. Yes ☐ If **yes**, go to question 2
   2. No ☐ If **no**, go to question 5

2. During the last month, how many times were you hospitalized?

   | | | times

3. For each hospitalization (during the last month), please provide the diagnosis or reason for hospitalization.

Hospitalization number	Major diagnosis or reason for hospitalization	DRG code (if possible)
1		
2		
3		
4		

4. Please specify the **total** number of nights spent in each type of ward (for all hospitalizations during the last month).

Ward	Number of nights
Geriatric	
Psychiatric	
Internal medicine	
Surgery	
Other (please specify)	

5. During the last month, did you receive care in a hospital emergency room (for less than 24 hours)?

   1. Yes ☐
   2. No ☐

   5(a). If **yes**, how many times?

   | | | times

6. During the last month, did you receive care from a doctor, physical therapist, psychologist, or other health care professional?

1. Yes ☐
2. No ☐

6(a). If **yes**, please specify the number of visits for each type of care received.

Type of care	Number of visits during last month
General practitioner	
Geriatrician	
Neurologist	
Psychiatrist	
Physiotherapist	
Occupational therapist	
Social worker	
Psychologist	
Other (e.g. specialist; please specify)	

7. Are you currently taking any medication (prescription or over-the-counter)?

1. Yes ☐
2. No ☐

7(a). If **yes**, please complete the following table.

Name of medication	Strength (mg)	Number of times per day	Number of days taken in the last month

A2. PATIENT

A2.1 Patient Living Accommodation

1. Please specify the patient's current living accommodation.

    1. Own home ☐
    2. Intermediate forms of accommodation (not dementia-specific) ☐
    3. Dementia-specific residential accommodation ☐
    4. Long-term institutional care* ☐
    5. Other _____ ☐

* If nursing home accommodation is permitted at baseline, if not this alternative should be deleted

   1(a). If the patient lives in her/his own home, who does the patient live together with?

   1. Alone ☐
   2. Spouse ☐
   3. Other ☐
   4. Not applicable _____ ☐

A2.2 Patient Health Care Resource Utilization

1. During the last month, was the patient admitted to a hospital (for more than 24 hours)?

    1. Yes ☐   If **yes**, go to question 2
    2. No ☐   If **no**, go to question 5

2. During the last month, how many times was the patient hospitalized?

    | | | times

3. For each hospitalization (during the last month), please provide the diagnosis or reason for hospitalization.

Hospitalization number	Major diagnosis or reason for hospitalization	DRG code (if possible)
1		
2		
3		
4		

4. Please specify the **total** number of nights spent in each type of ward (for all hospitalization during the last month).

Ward	Number of nights
Geriatric	
Psychiatric	
Internal medicine	
Surgery	
Other (please specify)	

5. During the last month, did the patient receive care in a hospital emergency room (for less than 24 hours)?

    1. Yes ☐
    2. No ☐

5(a). If **yes**, how many times?

    | | | times

6. During the last month, did the patient receive care from a doctor, physical therapist, psychologist or other health care professional?

1. Yes ☐
2. No   ☐

6(a). If **yes**, please specify the number of visits for each type of care received.

Type of care	Number of visits during last month
General practitioner	
Geriatrician	
Neurologist	
Psychiatrist	
Physiotherapist	
Occupational therapist	
Social worker	
Psychologist	
Other (e.g. specialist; please specify)	

7. For each service listed below, please specify the number of times the service was received during the last month and the average number of hours per visit.

Service	Number of visits during last month	Number of hours per visit
District nurse		
Home aid/orderly		
Food delivery		
Day care		
Transportation (public-paid)		
Other (e.g. please specify)		

FOLLOW-UP QUESTIONNAIRES

B1 CAREGIVER

B1.1 Caregiver Time

1. On a typical care day since the last visit, how much time per day did you spend assisting the patient with tasks such as toilet visits, eating, dressing, grooming, walking and bathing?

   | | | hours per day

   1(b). Since the last visit, how many days did you spend providing these services to the patient? _____ days

2. On a typical care day since the last visit, how much time per day did you spend assisting the patient with tasks such as shopping, food preparation, housekeeping, laundry, transportation, taking medication, and managing financial matters?

   | | | hours per day

   2(b). Since the last visit, how many days did you spend providing these services to the patient? _____ days

3. On a typical care day since the last visit, how much time per day have you spent supervising (that is, preventing dangerous events) the patient?

   | | | hours per day

   3(b). Since the last visit, how many days have you spent providing these services to the patient? _____ days

B1.2 Caregiver Work Status

1. Since the last visit, have you been working for pay (part or the whole period)?

    1. Yes ☐ If **yes**, answer question 2
    2. No   ☐ If **no**, go to section B1.3

2. Since the last visit, have you stopped working completely?

    1. Yes ☐ If **yes**, answer question 7 **only**
    2. No   ☐ If **no**, go to question 3

3. Since the last visit, have you changed your job or working situation?

    1. Yes ☐ If **yes**, answer questions 4 to 7
    2. No   ☐ If **no**, answer question 6

4. How many hours in total do you work for pay per week?

    |___|___| hours/week

    4(a). Of this number of hours, are you for some part paid to care for the patient?

       1. Yes ☐
       2. No   ☐

    4(b). If **yes**, how many hours per week?

       |___|___| hours/week

5. Since the last visit, have you needed to cut down the number of hours that you work in your regular job because of your caregiving responsibilities?

    1. Yes ☐
    2. No   ☐

    5(a). If **yes**, how many hours did you cut down?

       |___|___| hours/week

6. Since the last visit, please specify the number of times that your caregiver responsibilities affected your work in the following ways.

    1. Missed a whole day of work

       |___|___| number of times

    2. Missed a part of a day of work

       |___|___| number of times

7. Why did you stop/reduce working?

    1. Reached retirement age ☐
    2. Early retirement ☐
       (not disease-related)
    3. Laid off ☐
    4. Own health problems ☐
    5. To care for the patient ☐
    6. Other ☐
    7. Not applicable _____ ☐

B1.3 Caregiver Health Care Resource Utilization

1. Since the last visit, have you been admitted to a hospital (for more than 24 hours)?

   1. Yes ☐ If **yes**, go to question 2
   2. No   ☐ If **no**, go to question 5

2. Since the last visit, how many times have you been hospitalized?

   |___|___| times

3. For each hospitalization (since the last visit), please provide the diagnosis or reason for hospitalization.

Hospitalization number	Major diagnosis or reason for hospitalization	DRG code (if possible)
1		
2		
3		
4		

4. Please specify the **total** number of nights spent in each type of ward (for all hospitalizations since the last visit)

Ward	Number of nights
Geriatric	
Psychiatric	
Internal medicine	
Surgery	
Other (please specify)	

5. Since the last visit, have you received care in a hospital emergency room (for less than 24 hours)?

   1. Yes ☐
   2. No   ☐

   5(a). If **yes**, how many times?

   |___|___| times

6. Since the last visit, have you received care from a doctor, physical therapist, psychologist or other health care professional?

1. Yes ☐
2. No ☐

6(a). If **yes**, please specify the number of visits for each type of care received.

Type of care	Number of visits since the last visit
General practitioner	
Geriatrician	
Neurologist	
Psychiatrist	
Physiotherapist	
Occupational therapist	
Social worker	
Psychologist	
Other (e.g. specialist; please specify)	

7. Are you currently taking any medication (prescription or over-the-counter)?

1. Yes ☐
2. No ☐

7(a). If **yes**, please complete the following table.

Name of medication	Strength (mg)	Number of times per day	Number of days taken since the last visit

B2.1 Patient Living Accommodation

1. Since the last visit, has the patient **permanently** changed his/her living accommodation (i.e. moved to another location and is currently living in this new location)?

    1. Yes ☐ If **yes**, answer questions 2 to 4
    2. No   ☐ If **no**, answer question 5

2. Please specify the patient's current living accommodation.

    1. Own home ☐
    2. Intermediate forms of accommodation (not dementia-specific) ☐
    3. Dementia-specific residential accommodation ☐
    4. Long-term institutional care ☐
    5. Other _____ ☐

3. Please specify the date at which the change occurred.

    __ / __ / __
    dd/mm/yy

4. Please specify the principal reason for this change in living accommodation.

    1. Worsening of patient's cognitive function ☐
    2. Worsening of patient's ability to perform daily tasks (e.g., feeding, dressing, housekeeping, etc.) ☐
    3. Increase in patient's behavior problems ☐
    4. Poor caregiver health ☐
    5. Improvement of patient's cognitive function ☐
    6. Improvement of patient's ability to perform daily tasks (e.g., feeding, dressing, housekeeping, etc.) ☐
    7. Improvement of patient's behavior ☐
    8. Improved caregiver health ☐
    9. Other _____ ☐

5. Since the last visit, has the patient **temporarily** changed living accommodation (i.e. moved to a new location for more than 24 hours and then back to the original location)?

    1. Yes ☐
    2. No   ☐

    5(a). If **yes**, please specify where the subject temporarily moved to. Please specify the patient's current living accommodation.

        1. Own home ☐
        2. Intermediate forms of accommodation (not dementia-specific) ☐
        3. Dementia-specific residential accommodation ☐
        4. Long-term institutional care ☐
        5. Other _____ ☐

5(b). Please specify the number of nights spent in this temporary living accommodation.

		Number of nights
1.	Own home	⎵⎵⎵
2.	Intermediate forms of accommodation (not dementia-specific)	⎵⎵⎵
3.	Dementia-specific residential accommodation	⎵⎵⎵
4.	Long-term institutional care	⎵⎵⎵
5.	Other _____	⎵⎵⎵

B2.2 Patient Health Care Resource Utilization

1. Since the last visit, has the patient been admitted to a hospital (for more than 24 hours)?

   1. Yes ☐   If **yes**, go to question 2
   2. No ☐   If **no**, go to question 5

2. Since the last visit, how many times has the patient been hospitalized?

   ☐☐ times

3. For each hospitalization (since the last visit), please provide the diagnosis or reason for hospitalization.

Hospitalization number	Major diagnosis or reason for hospitalization	DRG code (if possible)
1		
2		
3		
4		

4. Please specify the **total** number of nights spent in each type of ward (for all hospitalization since the last visit).

Ward	Number of nights
Geriatric	
Psychiatric	
Internal medicine	
Surgery	
Other (please specify)	

5. Since the last visit, has the patient received care in a hospital emergency room (for less than 24 hours)?

   1. Yes ☐
   2. No ☐

   5(a). If **yes**, how many times?

   ☐☐ times

6. Since the last visit, has the patient received care from a doctor, physical therapist, psychologist or other health care professional?

1. Yes ☐
2. No ☐

6(a). If **yes**, please specify the number of visits for each type of care received.

Type of care	Number of visits since the last visit
General practitioner	
Geriatrician	
Neurologist	
Psychiatrist	
Physiotherapist	
Occupational therapist	
Social worker	
Psychologist	
Other (e.g. specialist; please specify)	

7. For each service listed below, please specify the number of times the service has been received since the last visit and the average number of hours per visit.

Service	Number of visits since last visit	Number of hours per visit
District nurse		
Home aid/orderly		
Food delivery		
Day care		
Transportation (public-paid)		
Other (e.g. please specify)		

4.4 Clinical and Economic Considerations of Anti-dementia Drug Treatment

HOWARD FELDMAN
University of British Columbia, Vancouver, Canada

BERNARD PRIGENT
Pfizer Canada Inc., Kirkland, Canada

INTRODUCTION

The development and approval process for novel anti-dementia pharmacologic therapies has been driven by the efforts of academics, government regulators and the pharmaceutical industry. The first milestone for anti-dementia drug development has been and will continue to be the demonstration of clinical efficacy. For a drug to be approved for the indication of treatment of dementia most regulatory authorities have issued either draft or completed guidelines which address minimal efficacy criteria (Mohr et al, 1995; Leber, 1990; CPMP, 1992). Such efficacy criteria in most countries currently include the demonstration of statistically significant differences between drug and placebo-treated subjects both on objective cognitive tests as well as on clinical global assessments in randomized clinical trials. In the European guidelines (CPMP, 1992), particular attention is paid to activities of daily living in addition to the usual 'dual criteria'. More recently there has been appropriate emphasis in the clinical dementia research literature on the non-cognitive aspects of dementia, especially on behavioral changes and how they influence outcome and care costs in dementia and Alzheimer's disease (AD) in particular. Such recognition seems likely to add new efficacy domains over time for the approval of anti-dementia drugs.

Beyond the demonstration of efficacy there comes a need to address issues of effectiveness and efficiency to allow the optimal approach to treatment within the usual community setting. This assessment is both clinically and economically imperative as government resources shrink in the face of continually escalating health care costs and novel therapeutics. Thus beyond clinical trial

Health Economics of Dementia. Edited by Anders Wimo, Bengt Jönsson, Göran Karlsson and Bengt Winblad.
© 1998 John Wiley & Sons Ltd.

efficacy, 'effectiveness' can be thought of as the clinical benefit that should be measurable with the novel therapeutic/intervention in a broader cross-section of AD patients in the environment of usual clinical practice and usual care. This consideration of effectiveness will also include a consideration of risk/benefit. Further to effectiveness there is a need to then show that there is 'efficiency' for a novel therapeutic/intervention, that is cost-benefit and/or cost-effectiveness. Following the demonstration of statistically significant differences in efficacy outcome measures from large Phase III clinical trials, such proof of clinical effectiveness and efficiency will be demanded by formularies, health maintenance providers (HMOs) or governments. To address questions of the effectiveness and efficiency of therapy the information that has been gathered from large community-based epidemiological studies which have included costing of care with attention to both direct and indirect costs will be very useful, particularly from the standpoint of modeling. Both actual data as well as modeling will likely be needed to demonstrate effectiveness and efficiency, given the particularly long course and temporal dispersion of clinical milestones in both AD and related neurodegenerative dementias.

This chapter will use the example of the cholinesterase inhibitors tacrine and donepezil that have met the regulatory requirements in many countries to address specific points about efficacy, effectiveness and efficiency. The limitations of current information and the direction that will be required to advance the studies of effectiveness and efficiency will be discussed.

EFFICACY

Definition: Refers to the clinical benefits of the drug being established under the ideal and restrictive experimental conditions of a clinical trial in Phases II and III of drug development.

Background: Alzheimer's disease typically affects the domains of cognition, behavior and function along its course. To make a claim for an anti-dementia drug clinical efficacy has been specified by most regulatory authorities to include both positive effects on objective measures of cognitive function as well as on clinical global assessments. To date, there has not been a specification of efficacy in the FDA guidelines (Leber, 1990) concerning functional and behavioral outcomes of the emerging AD treatments. However, the draft European guidelines (CPMP, 1992) propose that there should be benefits in 'behavior closely connected with function' to make a drug claim. The acetyl-cholinesterase (AchE) inhibitors, donepezil and tacrine, stand alone at present, as having met these regulatory hurdles and having been approved in the United States and many other countries for the symptomatic treatment indication of mild to moderate severity Alzheimer's disease. A number of AchE inhibitors which are in development are also anticipated to be approved over the next 1–2 years (Anand et al, 1996; Cummings et al, 1997). It is instructive to review some of the bases of efficacy assessments which have led to their approval in order to understand their limitations when extrapolated to assess effectiveness and efficiency.

The regulatory emphasis on cognitive benefits in objective psychometric test measures has directed trial clinicians to refine measurement instruments to those that can adequately detect significant changes during the short Phase II–III trial periods of 12–24 weeks. Though a number of instruments have been developed (Rosen et al, 1984; Randolph, 1998; Wesnes, 1985), it has been the Alzheimer Disease Assessment Scale-Cognitive Subscales (ADAS-cog) (Rosen et al, 1984) that has had the widest acceptance over the past several years. Mean differences between placebo and drug treated groups have been taken to be the yardstick of efficacy for this primary outcome measure in clinical trials. In presenting clinical trial efficacy results there are a variety of approaches taken. The intention to treat (ITT) analysis will usually include all subjects who have been randomized following their baseline visit and who will have been exposed to the study drug prior to dropping out/prior to completion of the study. Their last observed efficacy-evaluable visit data would generally be carried forward to the study termination. Such an ITT analysis is generally accepted to be a conservative approach for AD. The fully evaluable or observed cases will usually include those subjects who have completed the study protocol while meeting the criteria for being efficacy-evaluable by virtue of their compliance to the study drug and study protocol. With both tacrine and donepezil the treatment effect sizes have been uniformly larger in fully evaluable or observed cases. Where pharmacoeconomic studies are undertaken as add-on studies to efficacy clinical trials it is imperative that data be captured on all subjects with recognition that non-completers are potentially a more severely affected and declining group of patients (Feldman et al, 1997).

Table 4.4.1 illustrates some of the ITT data from selected Phase III pivotal trials of tacrine and donepezil for the ADAS-cog (Knapp et al, 1994; Rogers et al, 1998).

It is particularly difficult to actually compare the ADAS-cog efficacy between these two drugs even within randomized double-blind placebo-controlled trials. Tacrine had a high drop-out rate in its pivotal trials, which created a large efficacy difference in comparing ITT to fully evaluable cases. Donepezil, with a relatively lower drop-out rate, had much less difference between its ITT group and its fully evaluable cases. In the Knapp study (Knapp et al, 1994) subjects from the ITT group were offered the opportunity to receive open label tacrine following their drop out and then were included in the analysis at week 30. This approach likely attenuated the treatment differences, particularly as the placebo group had 10% of patients receiving tacrine at week 30, and only 76% of the 160 mg tacrine randomized group were receiving tacrine at any dose at week 30. In assessing the comparative efficacy of these two drugs as well as the other emerging AchE inhibitors it should be noted that to date there have been no head-to-head comparative trials reported.

Table 4.4.1.

ADAS-Cog results	Tacrine Knapp, M. J. et al, JAMA (1994)				Donepezil Rogers, S. L. et al, Neurology (1998)		
	Placebo	80 mg	120 mg	160 mg	Placebo	5 mg	10 mg
Mean drug-placebo differences (ITT)		−1.4	−2.0	−2.2		−2.49	−2.88
95% CI		−3.5 to 0.7	−3.5 to −0.5	−3.5 to −0.8			
p value		0.20	0.008	0.002		<0.0001	<0.0001
Mean change from baseline (ITT) ± SEM	2.5			0.5	1.82 ±0.49	−0.67 ±0.51	−1.05 ±0.51
95% CI	1.5 to 3.5			−0.5 to 1.5			
Percentage fully evaluable subjects	68	48	32	27	80	85	68

Table 4.4.2.

Clinical global assessment results	Tacrine Knapp, M. J. et al, JAMA (1994)				Donepezil Rogers, S. L. et al, Neurology (1998)		
	Placebo	80 mg	120 mg	160 mg	Placebo	5 mg	10 mg
Mean drug-placebo differences (ITT)		−0.1	−0.2	−0.2		−0.36	−0.44
95% CI		−0.04 to 0.1	−0.04 to −0.006	−0.04 to −0.01			
p value		0.33	0.04	0.04		<0.0047	<0.0001
Percentage pts completing study	68	48	32	27	80	85	68

Furthermore it is desirable when comparing efficacy results to consider a variance term to allow for the determination of a treatment effect size. Cohen has recommended that the standard deviation of either the mean of the baseline scores or the mean of the change scores be utilized as the variance term to be used in the calculation of the treatment effect sizes (Cohen, 1988). This approach will not compensate, however, for differences in inclusion criteria, center effects, or differences in testing instruments and approaches.

Given that the mean ADAS-cog changes have been measured in double-blind placebo-controlled conditions for only 12–26 weeks generally there is only limited information available to assess longer term efficacy which is the necessary endpoint for effectiveness and efficiency analyses. Open label studies provide some data points beyond the double-blind placebo study period but the lack of placebo controls and retrieved drop outs limits conclusions about efficacy (Knopman et al, 1996; Rogers and Friedhoff, 1998). Naturalistic projected rates of decline are used as the comparator group for such open label studies though the comparability of the study populations is not clear. Only 24% of those subjects who enrolled in a Phase II double-blind placebo-controlled donepezil study were still participating in the open label continuation study at 3.5 years (Rogers and Friedhoff, 1998). Prior studies have reported a mean 6–9 point annual ADAS decline in untreated AD patients of mild to moderate severity with a mean difference score of four points taken to be the rough equivalent of six months of decline (Stern et al, 1994; Mohs et al, 1995).

The second measure of specified clinical efficacy for an anti-dementia drug has been the clinical global impression. This has been assigned importance in determining that the drug under investigation has a clinically meaningful effect, which can be identified by a skilled clinician. This scale has been prescribed by the FDA (Leber, 1990) to determine that the psychometric test score improvements are accompanied by an independent measure of global clinical efficacy. It has not been the intention that small changes, which are of uncertain clinical significance, are picked up but rather that those which are clinically meaningful be identified. In the original unstructured Clinical Global Impression of Change (CGIC) there was little sensitivity to treatment effects with considerable variance. Current clinical global measures such as the Alzheimer's Disease Cooperative Study-Clinical Global Impression of Change (ADCS-CGIC) (Schneider et al, 1997a) have been derived using multidimensional probes of behavior, cognition and function interviewing both caregivers and patients with a semi-structured approach. The seven-point global impression scale provides an intermediate score of 4 which indicates no change, 3 minimal improvement, 2 moderate improvement, and 1 marked improvement with mirror image anchor points below 4 through 7 for worsening.

Table 4.4.2 presents some of the results of the clinical global assessments from selected pivotal studies of tacrine and donepezil (ITT) (Knapp et al, 1994; Rogers et al, 1998).

It can be seen from these figures that the impact of current treatments as judged by the clinical global assessment is modest, with the anticipated difficulties this will present to the clinician in a usual care setting. Further to this mean change assessment of clinical global assessments there is the additional issue of responders and how these can be defined. During the validation studies of the Alzheimer's Disease Cooperative Study-Clinical Global Impression of Change (ADCS-CGIC) (Schneider et al, 1997a) it was noted that at six months 38% of untreated AD patients outside of a clinical trial remain unchanged. This number corresponds quite closely to the % of placebo and treated subjects who do not change on the clinical global assessment during the 6-month clinical trial period (Schneider et al, 1997a). Beyond the 12–26 week double-blind placebo-controlled study periods there is again difficulty in assessing clinical global efficacy absent a control group. Longer-term benefits of tacrine and donepezil on clinical global assessments remain consequently difficult to evaluate. In a long-term open label donepezil study (Rogers and Friedhoff, 1998) a comparison of slopes on a disease staging instrument (CDR-sum of the boxes) (Berg et al, 1992) showed an attenuation of donepezil-treated patients compared to untreated patients. However, consideration of such long-term open label studies should take into account those subjects who fail to complete the study period as there is some evidence that their baseline characteristics and course may not be the same as completers (Feldman et al, 1997).

The dual criteria of the FDA have limited the attention given to the assessment of the non-cognitive domains in Alzheimer's disease and other dementia-related disorders. Recently the development of dementia-specific scales for behavior and function (Cummings et al, 1994; Gauthier et al, 1993; Teunisse and Derix, 1991) has facilitated the measurement of these key domains to both patients and caregivers. Information about efficacy in these key domains in the tacrine and donepezil data bases is significantly lacking despite their clear importance in predicting costs of care and caregiver burden (Østbye and Crosse, 1994; Canadian Study of Health and Aging, 1994a). In fact these are clearly the domains where practitioners will undoubtedly be looking for efficacy despite the clear indications for use that will be provided to clinicians in the product monographs. Much of the information related to behavioral changes has been acquired with tacrine beyond the Phase III trials in uncontrolled or limitedly controlled settings with much smaller than desirable sample sizes (Kaufer et al, 1996). Larger scale prospective studies with primary behavioral outcome measures are currently ongoing with donepezil.

EFFECTIVENESS

Definition: Refers to the clinical benefit that can be demonstrated with a drug/intervention in a broad cross-section of AD patients in the environment of usual clinical practice (usual care). This will include consideration of risk/benefit.

Background: To move from efficacy trials to assessment of effectiveness the process must involve removing the bias of the more tightly controlled Phase II and III clinical trials. There are a variety of limitations in the generalizability of data from the Phase II and III trials in AD that are developed to demonstrate efficacy and meet the regulatory requirements. The first is the research setting and the environment where such clinical trials take place. This setting rarely resembles usual clinical care, particularly in dementia trials where there are extensive questionnaires and instruments administered by highly specialized research teams. Most clinical trial sites for Phase II and III efficacy trials have supported infrastructure allowing staff that would not otherwise be part of usual dementia care. Such additional staff and patient attention has been shown to influence long-term dementia milestones (Albert et al, 1997). Second are the actual participants in the pivotal AD clinical trials. Subjects to date have been selected with diagnosed 'clinically probable' Alzheimer's disease by NINCDS-ADRDA criteria (McKhan et al, 1984) without significant comorbidity. This precludes the participation of a large number of AD subjects who will ultimately be treated when regulatory approval is received. In fact it has been estimated that ten AD subjects need to be reviewed to find one suitable candidate for a Phase II–III clinical trial (Schneider et al, 1997b).

Thirdly, a major problem in the geriatric population is the concurrent use of polypharmacy. As with comorbidity the use of polypharmacy, particularly those medications such as antidepressants, neuroleptics and anxiolytics, will most often exclude subjects from participating in an AD clinical trial yet they are very widely used in the care of patients with Alzheimer's disease. Again, once a novel AD medication is approved its use with multiple medications will occur yet there will be little clinical trials experience to fall back on from the controlled setting of a clinical trial. Fourthly, it has been estimated that 50% of AD subjects live in institutions (Canadian Study of Health and Aging, 1994b), yet in efficacy trials, living in an institution will preclude participation as will lacking a caregiver. A narrow segment of mild to moderate severity AD subjects are permitted to participate in pivotal trials, leaving large segments of the actual disease population unstudied for efficacy in a randomized double-blind placebo-controlled trial. At the level of compliance in the donepezil Phase III 302 study (Rogers et al, 1998), subjects had to demonstrate greater than 80% compliance, or be precluded from participating in the trial. It is important to note that compliance greater than 80% will not be the norm once a drug is approved for AD treatment. Efficacy studies thus do not address the issue of partial compliance as most relevant to a real life setting.

In contrast to such efficacy studies, effectiveness studies will address how a treatment performs in a more real life setting. The generalizability of results from clinical trials of efficacy cannot be assumed for the reasons outlined above. Thus to demonstrate effectiveness requires an evaluation of the new medication/intervention in the usual care setting. Such studies and their methodologies have yet to be fully worked out but are evolving in the face of demand. Amongst the challenges in designing effectiveness studies is the relative absence of measurement instruments used in usual care settings. Apart from the MMSE (Folstein et al, 1975) there are no scales used from clinical trials that are particularly well suited to usual care or currently in use. In conceptual terms there is the potential and need for the clinical global assessment to be extrapolated to the usual care setting, perhaps with the linkage of goal attainment or defined target symptoms assessment (Rockwood et al, 1993, 1996). Shortened cognitive, functional and behavioral scales will all need to be developed and validated before they can be adopted to usual care settings where they could become part of the effectiveness evaluation. Additionally, issues of quality of life of both caregivers and patients will need to be addressed in determining the effectiveness of a drug/treatment intervention. The issue of how an AD patient's quality of life can be measured remains to be defined and operationalized (Whitehouse et al, 1997).

In addressing effectiveness there is a need as well to consider the risk/benefit ratio. Assessing the risk side of this ratio involves the consideration of dropout rates related to adverse events, the nature of the adverse events and the frequency with which they occur. The need to monitor for side-effects becomes one of the cost drivers on the risk side. Whereas the tables above on tacrine and donepezil demonstrate that the cognitive efficacy at the higher doses of both is of the same order the risk/benefit ratio favors donepezil for reasons of fewer adverse events, the lack of required laboratory monitoring and the increased compliance with the most effective doses. The benefits of this ratio are not easily measured in pivotal clinical trials for reasons of the non-representativeness of the study sample, the timelines used, and the lack of generalizability of the study sample.

To demonstrate effectiveness in a clinical study would likely require a long-term (>2 years) observational study of treated patients in their community with usual care from their primary care physician. At present it is not possible to reach this level of effectiveness assessment as the methodological issues above remain to be reconciled. The measurement of effectiveness may be facilitated by emerging electronic technologies for the office such as computer-based disease guidance systems. These diagnostic systems would allow the usual care of community physicians to be captured and logged into a central database. Such a process for development and evaluation of treatment responses could allow a more uniform approach to issues of assessment, diagnosis, and management, which in turn could aid effectiveness assessment.

One emerging study approach to longer-term effectiveness could be the use of survival analysis of the major disease milestones comparing usual care to a specific intervention. The demonstration in the study of Sano et al (1997) that vitamin E could delay selected disease outcomes such as functional milestones, nursing home placement, CDR staging and death has raised the potential of this approach in measuring effectiveness; however the lack of concurrent differences in cognitive measures has raised concern.

It should be clear, based on the above discussion, that seeking evidence of effectiveness prematurely in drug development could compromise the necessary demonstration of efficacy. The current approach of keeping these program developments sequential and separated would seem justified. That is, efficacy trials for Phase II and III and effectiveness trials in Phase III-B and IV following regulatory approval.

EFFICIENCY

Definition: Refers to the demonstration of potential cost-benefits resulting from the use of a therapeutic agent/intervention in clinical practice. An evaluation of efficiency will allow for the comparative analysis of alternative therapies in terms of both their cost and their consequences (Drummond, 1997).

Background: As new therapies become available, the economic implications of their clinical benefits need to be formally assessed to demonstrate efficiency. Such economic evaluation must be based on the conduct of pharmacoeconomic studies, comparing the costs and consequences of the new treatment with the relevant alternatives (Canadian Coordinating Office, 1994).

The four main types of pharmacoeconomic analysis include cost-minimization analysis, cost-effectiveness analysis, cost-utility analysis and cost-benefits analysis (Bookman et al, 1996).

COST-MINIMIZATION ANALYSIS

In cost-minimization analysis the consequences of the two interventions being compared are identical. Therefore, the analysis reduces to a comparison of cost alone. For two drugs of similar efficacy and side-effects the economic analysis would compare the costs of the drugs plus the cost of any associated medical intervention. To date this has no immediate applicability to tacrine or donepezil or to any of the upcoming drugs in development. It seems unlikely that, given the complexity and heterogeneity of cost drivers in this illness, such an approach will be applicable.

COST-EFFECTIVENESS ANALYSIS

In cost-effectiveness analysis the consequences of treatment interventions are being assessed in the most appropriate physical units. Physical units could range from clinical measures, such as MMSE/ADAS-cog points to time to institutionalization through lives saved/life-years gained (Canadian Coordinating Office, 1994). Cost-effectiveness analysis results in the choice of intervention which minimizes cost for a given measure of effectiveness.

COST-UTILITY ANALYSIS

In cost-utility analysis the consequences of treatment intervention are measured in terms of quality-adjusted life-years based on information on preferences of individuals toward the interventions being studied. The preferences of individuals reflect the gains in welfare or satisfaction (often called 'utilities') arising from the treatment. The inherent problems of measuring quality of life in patients with AD have been recognized (Whitehouse et al, 1997). The potential to use the caregiver's quality of life as a surrogate is being explored through the demonstration of benefit of pharmacological interventions and remains to be demonstrated.

COST-BENEFITS ANALYSIS

In cost-benefits analysis all of the costs and consequences of treatment interventions are measured in the same unit: money, usually using the willingness to pay approach (O'Brien et al, 1995).

APPROACHES

All pharmacoeconomic studies must be comparative. Applying pharmacoeconomics to the present generation of AchE drug therapies thus is indeed difficult. It requires a comparison of a new drug intervention with 'usual care' where there is no other disease-specific treatment available as a comparator (Drummond, 1997). In all studies, costs and consequences are measured as increments, that is, as differences between two alternatives. With the very recent approval of donepezil there have not yet been any direct comparative trials with tacrine, which has been limiting, though formularies will likely insist on such data where limited budgets exist. The available references on pharmacoeconomic AD trials are still very limited. There have been two recently published review papers (Molnar and Dalziel, 1997; Max, 1996).

Each of the first pharmacoeconomic studies reported on AchE inhibitors has relied on economic modeling rather than actual longitudinal data to perform their cost analysis (Lubeck et al, 1994; Henke and Burchmore, 1997; Wimo et al, 1997).

This modeling involves a transformation of efficacy data from clinical trials to effectiveness data; a fundamental step toward projecting associated costs over the remaining lifetime of both a treated and untreated group of patients. Both Lubeck et al (1994) and Wimo et al (1997) chose to model on the MMSE efficacy benefits from tacrine to placebo-treated subjects from the 30 week placebo-controlled study (Knapp et al, 1994). A model was subsequently constructed which projected over the remaining lifetime of a treated and untreated group of patients.

In the key point of translating efficacy into effectiveness data the authors endorsed the assumption that the MMSE score is directly linked to placement in institution (Lubeck et al, 1994; Wimo et al, 1997) and/or the use of community care (Lubeck et al, 1994). The limitations of this assumption must be considered. The decision to institutionalize an AD patient is driven by a variety of factors, most of which are not cognitive (Cohen et al, 1993; Gold et al, 1995; Aneshensel et al, 1993). These include the family's economic and social resources, the health and age of the caregiver as well as their level of burden, the patient's ability to perform activities of daily living, and the presence of behavioral disturbances. Though there are generally relationships between cognitive decline and the above factors such relationships are not invariable. Feldman recently reported on a pharmacoeconomic study where it was the functional scale Disability Assessment for Dementia scores (DAD) (Gauthier et al, 1993) rather than ADAS-cog scores that determined community service utilization (Feldman et al, 1997).

A further limitation of such a modeling exercise is the short period of efficacy assessment that then serves as the basis of a much longer projected time for cost estimates where compliance to study medication can only be very roughly estimated. Where actual longer-term open label study data are available there is a significant rate of drop out that needs to be considered. In the long-term open-label extension of donepezil study 201, 65% participating had dropped out by 3.5 years (Rogers and Friedhoff, 1998). Such corrections to models will be needed as fuller long-term data sets emerge, particularly from more usual care settings.

From the economic side the actual cost estimates of AD care in models are derived from different published sources and populations potentially dissimilar to those participating in clinical trials. It is known for example that clinical trial participants will have delayed institutionalization compared to non-participants in trials (Albert et al, 1997).

An alternative modeling approach was taken by Henke and Burchmore (1997). Data on the effectiveness of tacrine were derived from the published results of a two year open-label follow-up study of patients originally enrolled in a placebo-controlled trial (Knopman et al, 1996). The economic analysis was based on a model of the lifetime costs of care for someone newly diagnosed with mild to moderate Alzheimer's disease with the same assumptions for the calculations of cost and disease progression. Although the use of long-term data, and the study endpoints chosen, are closer to a naturalistic setting major limitations still remain as patients recruited in the long-term study with tacrine can only be considered to represent a very small percentage of highly selected AD patients able to tolerate the medication.

These three studies represent a first attempt to evaluate the economic impact of tacrine by adopting an analytic horizon extending far enough into the future to capture important clinical outcomes. Findings from the three independent published studies with modeling from clinical trials data indicate that it is possible to identify either substantial (Lubeck et al, 1994; Henke and Burchmore, 1997) or at least modest beneficial effects on the Alzheimer's disease costs through the use of a cholinesterase inhibitor. To more fully examine the efficiency of this class and other emerging treatments for AD there will be a need for effectiveness data and longer-term studies of treated patients.

Thus beyond recognizing the shortcomings of modeling, clinical trial methodology in AD should evolve to allow economic analysis to be conducted alongside clinical trials. Although such analysis could be conducted at any stage of the drug clinical development process, the stronger candidates for economic analysis have to be medium- to long-term (1–3 years) effectiveness data. Such trials looking both at cost-effectiveness and cost utility have already been successfully conducted to asses non-pharmacological intervention and are certainly feasible, though they will likely need to be conducted in usual care settings rather than as add-on studies to Phase III double-blind placebo-controlled clinical trials (Wimo et al, 1994, 1995; Brodaty and Peters, 1991).

CONCLUSIONS

In the development of Alzheimer's disease treatment the first milestone of demonstrating efficacy for the acetylcholinesterase inhibitors has been taken. The challenge for this class of medications and those that will emerge will be to demonstrate their effectiveness and ultimately their efficiency in the context of usual clinical practice.

ACKNOWLEDGEMENTS

The authors wish to gratefully acknowledge the helpful contribution of Ms Agnes H. Sauter in the preparation of this manuscript.

REFERENCES

Albert, S. M., Sano, M., Marder, K. et al (1997). Participation in clinical trials and long-term outcomes in Alzheimer's disease. *Neurology*, **49**, 38–43.

Anand, R. and Gharabawi, M. (1996). An overview of the development of SDZ ENA 713, a brain selective cholinesterase inhibitor. In R. Becker and E. Giacobini (Eds), *Alzheimer Disease: From Molecular Biology to Therapy*, pp. 239–243, Boston, Birkhauser.

Aneshensel, C. S., Pearlin, L. I. and Schuler, R. H. (1993). Stress, role captivity, and the cessation of caregiving. *J. Health Soc. Behav.*, **34**, 54–70.

Berg, L., Miller, J. P., Baty, J., Rubin, E. H., Morris, J. C. and Figiel, G. (1992). Mild senile dementia of the Alzheimer type. 4. Evaluation of intervention. *Ann. Neurol.*, **31**, 242–249.

Bookman, J. L., Townsend, J. T. and McGhan, W. F. (1996). *Principles of Pharmacoeconomics*. Cincinnati, OH, Harvey Whitney.

Brodaty, H. and Peters, K. E. (1991). Cost-effectiveness of a training program for dementia carers. *International Psychogeriatrics*, **3**, 11–22.

Canadian Coordinating Office for Health Technology Assessment (1994). *Guidelines for Economic Evaluation of Pharmaceuticals*. Canada.

Canadian Study of Health and Aging Working Group (1994a). Patterns of caring for people with dementia in Canada. *Canadian Journal on Aging*, **13**, 470–487.

Canadian Study of Health and Aging Working Group (1994b). Canadian Study of Health and Aging: study methods and prevalence of dementia. *J. Can. Med. Assoc.*, **150**, 899–913.

Cohen, C. A., Gold, D. P., Shulman, K. I., Wortley, J. T., McDonald, G. and Wargon, M. (1993). Factors determining the decision to institutionalize dementing individuals: a prospective study. *Gerontologist*, **33**, 714–720.

Cohen, J. (1988). *Statistical Power Analysis for the Behavioral Sciences*, 2nd edn, Hillsdale, NJ, Lawrence Erlbaum.

CPMP Working Party on Efficacy of Medicinal Products (1992). Anti-dementia Medicinal Products. Note for guidance (Draft 5). Commission of the European Communities; November: 111/3705-91-EN.

Cummings, J. L., Mega, M., Gray, K., Rosenberg-Thompson, S., Carusi, D. A. and Gornbein, J. (1994). The Neuropsychiatric Inventory. *Neurology*, **44**, 2308–2314.

Cummings, J., Bieber, F., Mas, J., Orazem, J. and Gulanski, B. (1997). Metrifonate in Alzheimer's disease: results of a dose-finding study. In K. Iqbal, B. Winblad, T. Nishimura et al (Eds), *Alzheimer's Disease: Biology, Diagnosis and Therapeutics*, pp. 665–669, Chichester, John Wiley.

Drummond, M. (1997). *Methods for the Economic Evaluation of Health Care Programmes*. Oxford, Oxford University Press.

Feldman, H., Donald, A., Sauter, A. and Parys, W. (1997). A protocol to evaluate pharmacoeconomics in a clinical trial. 13th International Conference and 7th Annual European Meeting. Helsinki: Alzheimer's Disease International, Alzheimer Europe, Alzheimer Society of Finland.

Folstein, M. F., Folstein, S. and McHugh, P. R. (1975). Mini-mental state: A practical method for grading the cognitive state of patients for the clinician. *J. Psychiatr. Res.*, **12**, 189–198.

Gauthier, L., Gauthier, S., Gelinas, I., McIntyre, M. and Wood-Dauphinee, S. (1993). Assessment of functioning and ADL, 6th Congress of the International Psychogeriatric Association, Berlin: 9 (Abstract).

Gold, D. P., Reis, M. F., Markiewicz, D. and Andres, D. (1995). When home caregiving ends: a longitudinal study of outcomes for caregivers of relatives with dementia. *J. Am. Geriatr. Soc.*, **43**, 10–16.

Henke, J. C. and Burchmore, M. J. (1997). The economic impact of Tacrine in the treatment of Alzheimer's disease. *Clinical Therapeut.*, **19**(2), 330–345.

Kaufer, D. I., Cummings, J. L. and Christine, D. (1996). Effect of tacrine on behavioral symptoms in Alzheimer's disease: an open label study. *J. Geriatr. Psychiatry Neurol.*, **9**, 1–6.

Knapp, M. J., Knopman, D. S., Solomon, P. R., Pendlebury, W. W., Davis, C. S. and Gracon, S. I. (1994). A 30-week randomized controlled trial of high-dose tacrine in patients with Alzheimer's disease. The Tacrine Study Group. *JAMA*, **271**, 985–991.

Knopman, D. S., Schneider, L. S., Davis, K. L. et al (1996). Long-term tacrine (Cognex) treatment: Effects on nursing home placement and mortality. *Neurology*, **47**, 166–177.

Leber, P. (1990). Guidelines for the Clinical Evaluation of Anti-dementia Drugs. First draft. Rockville, MD.

Lubeck, D. P., Mazonson, P. D. and Bowe, T. (1994). Potential effects of Tacrine on expenditures for Alzheimer's disease. *Medical Interface*, October, 132–138.

Max, W. (1996). The cost of Alzheimer's disease: Will drug treatment ease the burden? *PharmacoEconomics*, **9**(1), 5–10.

McKhann, G., Drachman, D. A., Folstein, M., Katzman, R., Price, D. L. and Stadlan, E. M. (1984). Clinical diagnosis of Alzheimer's disease—Report of the NINCDS-ADRDA Work Group under the auspices of Department of Health and Human Services Task Force on Alzheimer's disease. *Neurology*, **34**, 939–944.

Mohr, E., Feldman, H. and Gauthier, S. (1995). Canadian guidelines for the development of anti-dementia therapies: A conceptual summary. *Can. J. Neurol. Sci.*, **22**(1), 62–71.

Mohs, R. C., Marin, D. B., Green, C. R. and Davis, K. L. (1995). Instruments for measuring the efficacy of treatments for Alzheimer's Disease. In E. Giacobini and R. Becker (Eds), *Alzheimer Disease: Therapeutic Strategies. Neurology.*

Molnar, F. J. and Dalziel, W. B. (1997). The pharmacoeconomics of dementia therapies. Bringing the clinical, research and economic perspectives together. [Review]. *Drugs & Aging*, **10**, 219–233.

O'Brien, B. J., Novosel, S., Torrance, G. and Streiner, D. (1995). Assessing the economic value of a new antidepressant: A willingness to pay approach. *PharmacoEconomics*, **8**(1), 34–45.

Østbye, T. and Crosse, E. (1994). Net economic costs of dementia in Canada. *Can. Med. Assoc. J.*, **151**, 1457–1464.

Randolph, C. (1998). Repeatable battery for the assessment of dementia (RBAD). *Psychological Corporation*, in press.

Rockwood, K., Stolee, P. and Fox, R. A. (1993). Use of goal attainment scaling in measuring clinically important change in the frail elderly. *J. Clin. Epidemiol.*, **46**, 1113–1118.

Rockwood, K., Stolee, P., Howard, K. and Mallery, L. (1996). Use of goal attainment scaling to measure treatment effects in an anti-dementia drug trial. *Neuroepidemiology*, **15**(6), 330–338.

Rogers, S. L. and Friedhoff, L. T. (1998). Long-term efficacy and safety of donepezil in the treatment of Alzheimer's disease: an interim analysis of the results of a US multicenter open label extension study. *European Neuropsychopharmacology*, **8**, 67–75.

Rogers, S. L., Farlow, M. R., Mohs, R., Freidhoff, L. T. and Donepezil Study Group (1998). A 24-week, double-blind, placebo-controlled trial of donepezil in patients with Alzheimer's disease. *Neurology*, **50**, 136–145.

Rosen, W. G., Mohs, R. C. and Davis, K. L. (1984). A new rating scale for Alzheimer's disease. *Am. J. Psychiatry*, **141**, 1356–1364.

Sano, M., Ernesto, C., Thomas, R. G. et al (1997). A controlled trial of selegeline, alpha-tocopherol, or both as treatment for Alzheimer's disease. *N. Engl. J. Med.*, **336**, 1216–1222.

Schneider, L. S., Olin, J. T., Doody, R. S. et al (1997a). Validity and reliability of the Alzheimer's Disease Cooperative Study—Clinical global impression of change. *Alzheimer Dis. Assoc. Disord.*, **11**, S22–S32.

Schneider, L. S., Olin, J. T., Lyness, S. A. and Chui, H. C. (1997b). Eligibility of Alzheimer's disease clinic patients for clinical trials. *J. Am. Geriatr. Soc.*, **45**, 923–928.

Stern, R. G., Mohs, R. C., Davidson, M. et al (1994). A longitudinal study of Alzheimer's disease: Measurement, rate and predictors of cognitive deterioration. *Am. J. Psychiatry*, **151**, 390–396.

Teunisse, S. and Derix, M. M. (1991). Measurement of activities of daily living in patients with dementia living at home: Development of a questionnaire. [Dutch]. *Tijdschrift voor Gerontologie en Geriatrie*, **22**, 53–59.

Wesnes, K. (1985). A fully automated psychometric test battery for human psychopharmacology. In *Abstracts of the IVth World Congress of Biological Psychiatry*, p. 153, Philadelphia.

Whitehouse, P. J., Orgogozo, J.-M., Becker, R. E. et al (1997). Quality-of-life assessment in dementia drug development. *Alzheimer Dis. Assoc. Disord.*, **11** (Supp 3), 56–60.

Wimo, A., Karlsson, G., Nordberg, A. and Winblad, B. (1997). Treatment of Alzheimer's disease with Tacrine—A cost-analysis model. *Alzheimer Dis. Assoc. Disord.*, **11**, 191–200.

Wimo, A., Mattson, B., Krakau, I., Eriksson, T., Nelvig, A. and Karlsson, G. (1995). Cost-utility analysis of group living in dementia care. *Int. J. Technol. Assess. Health Care*, **11**(1), 49–65.

Wimo, A., Mattsson, B., Krakau, I., Eriksson, T. and Nelvig, A. (1994). Cost-effectiveness analysis of day care for patients with dementia disorders. *Health Economics*, **3**, 395–404.

4.5 Ethical Considerations in Pharmacoeconomic Trials in Dementia

STEPHEN G. POST

Case Western Reserve University, Cleveland, OH, USA

The introduction of cholinesterase inhibitors for treatment of mild to moderate Alzheimer disease (AD) is on the one hand promising. Nursing Home Placements (NHP) may be somewhat delayed, and patients who retain greater independence and functional capacity may be able to remain employed longer or require less expensive caregiving later in the course of the disease. The ideal economic outcome would occur if anti-dementia compounds could delay the onset of symptoms of AD, allowing the potentially affected 'old-old' to die of other causes before manifesting the disease. But there are no anti-dementia compounds as of yet that are profoundly enhancing of quality of life, or highly effective. They are all at best modest in their effects (Rogers et al, 1996), and therefore contrast sharply with the use of a highly effective compound such as insulin in response to diabetes.

DELAY IN NURSING HOME PLACEMENT: AN AMBIGUOUS GOAL?

The pharmacoeconomic aspect of anti-dementia drug research focuses for the most part on the goal of delayed NHP. This is an understandable goal in that NHP does impose significant financial burdens on either families or the taxpayer. In the United States, for example, families must pay for nursing home care directly until their private resources are more or less exhausted, at which point public entitlements can become available. In contrast to the United States, Canadian public entitlements cover all nursing home care, but create a significant added tax burden. Whatever the balance between family and public financial duties, NHP is a costly proposition. Thus, one major study of a cholinesterase inhibitor indicated that NHP is considerably delayed for patients maintained on high dose throughout the course of AD to the point of placement (Knopman et al, 1996).

Health Economics of Dementia. Edited by Anders Wimo, Bengt Jönsson, Göran Karlsson and Bengt Winblad.
© 1998 John Wiley & Sons Ltd.

But ethically, delay in NHP is an ambiguous goal. It means that even more burden will be shifted to family caregivers, who will also assume more costs in most countries.

As an alternative to making delay in NHP a goal, might we develop better long-term care facilities to help relieve caregivers who have reached their limits? Indeed, by asserting that delay is such an especially worthwhile goal, we convey to caregivers that even when they are exhausted and beyond their capacities for caring, there is something wrong with placing a loved one in a nursing home. Yet there are many cases where NHP would be the best thing for patient and caregiver.

Perhaps the most disturbing aspect of defining delay in NHP as a goal is that it implies application of these various compounds throughout the course of AD, or at least until the time of NHP. This amounts to a permanent or near permanent application, contrary to what may be of benefit to either the demented patient or the caregiver.

As many new anti-dementia compounds are approved in future years, families and society will face a remarkably complex ethical issue of their proper application, consistent with the principles of autonomy, beneficence, and justice. It is somewhat premature to address this issue without much more extensive outcome data. No doubt the pharmacoeconomic analysis will prove significant, but it should not submerge the larger ethical questions nor set aside the rights of families to determine whether the application of anti-dementia compounds is for the patient's good in the individual case. Because these questions can be submerged, I now turn to them in some depth.

ENHANCING THE QUALITY OF LIFE FOR INDIVIDUALS WITH AD

The most important impact of anti-dementia compounds is not economic; rather, the essential question is whether or not their application is consistent on a case-by-case basis with the well-being of the patient. The art of medicine begins with the moral principles of the minimization of harm and the maximization of benefit in the case of the individual patient; economic considerations remain central matters in just allocation, but these should not overpower patient beneficence.

The use of an anti-dementia compound may or may not enhance the quality of life of the AD-affected individual. Some patients may for a period regain their sense of self-identity, or feel a brief liberation from the isolation of speech limitations. Improved functioning and quality of life can be evident by global clinical assessment as well as through statistical analysis of cognition. Any anti-dementia compound can provide a ray of hope for a patient, and hope is recognized as good.

In patients who begin treatment with anti-dementia compounds at or near diagnosis, there is much benefit in helping them to retain their capacities for as long as possible. But in sharp contrast, for patients already significantly demented, the application of an anti-dementia compound may be a very mixed blessing. For these patients, temporary partial 'awakenings' with anti-dementia compounds in the context of an irreversible progressive dementing condition such as AD create enormous ethical issues. In such cases, patients who have already navigated the difficult crises of cognitive decline and adjustment to the demented condition may have to go through adjustment a second time. For example, the individual who has lost insight into his or her loss of capacity may be awakened into renewed awareness and therefore into renewed anxiety; or the individual who has experienced aggressive behavioral problems that have since been successfully treated may, under the influence of an anti-dementia compound, revisit these problems. Thus, for AD patients who have negotiated significant AD decline, the sudden intrusion of a temporary awakening may or may not enhance quality of life; for caregivers, some of the most taxing phases of care may need to be virtually repeated.

This first case account came over my e-mail system (23 June 1997) through the Cleveland Area Chapter of the Alzheimer's Association:

At last night's Shaker Heights–Mt. Pleasant support group, the subject of anti-dementia drugs came up. One caregiver (Dorothy A, daughter) brought the Dr's prescription for the drug to the meeting and said she wasn't sure if she wanted to give it to her mom. Through the beautiful group process, they helped her decide what to do! You could see the relief on her face, and the decision ended up being no. Fortunately she had already discussed the pros and cons of the drug with her brother, and was ready to come to a decision once more input had been received. (I had handouts with me too.) But one family's story was especially moving, and is one that you might want to include in your study . . . Katie S. (wife) shared with Dorothy how much the new drug has changed the situation with her husband. He is once again obsessing about finances, whereas before Aricept, he had finally gotten to the point where he wasn't aware anymore—which was a relief for the family. He was very frustrated and suspicious about the financial situation earlier in the disease.

Also, Katie shared that the children can no longer come over and talk openly about their problems and issues at home and with their own families, because he is now aware enough to be concerned and start worrying again. You might want to follow up with her and get the whole story, and hear the good aspects too.

The above case indicates how complex the decisions to place an already seriously demented patient on an anti-dementia compound can be. Positively considered, symptoms are temporarily mitigated and a degree of insight is regained. On the other hand, intense anxiety is also regained. Are these limited but significant awakenings beneficent? As I have argued in a recent book, if there is one kind point in the progression of AD, it may be when the patient comes to the point of forgetting that he or she forgets, because it is precisely at this point that the anxiety of insight in self-loss subsides (Post, 1995).

Amid the ravages of AD, families and clinicians are easily enchanted and awed by newly approved compounds. For family members there is the potential of regaining the presence of a loved one able to recognize them again and to function better for at least some period of time. For physicians, there is the sense of at least some limited medicinal power over a progressive and incurable disease.

However, new anti-dementia compounds should not be prescribed routinely. Each patient's response must be carefully monitored with regard to quality of life. Every caregiver should know that the application of a compound is a deeply personal and value-laden decision requiring the careful exercise of compassion and good judgment. Caregivers should know that there is nothing wrong with withdrawing an anti-dementia treatment that does not seem to be enhancing quality of life.

My concern is that pharmacoeconomic analysis with delayed NHP as endpoint may well overlook these important issues of quality of life in the patient's experience. As I was revising this chapter, the following lines arrived at my desk over e-mail:

> Cecilia's mom was started on the new drug and it did push her back into a difficult stage of wandering and 'wanting to go home' to the point that Cecilia stopped it after finding her mom actually leaving the house.

ENDPOINTS FOR DISCONTINUING TREATMENT

How long into the progression of AD should clinically important functional deterioration be delayed? The underlying loss of neurons is not slowed, but cognitive symptoms may be ameliorated until the neuronal loss can no longer support synaptic activity. At some threshold of cognitive decline, however, the level of fragmentation reaches a point where the application of an anti-dementia compound has nothing of benefit to offer (unless the compound contributes, in ways that existing psychiatric medications do not, to the management of behavioral problems). These compounds are recommended for mild and moderate stages of AD, after which they could be withdrawn. Yet many patients involved in the drug trials have continued to take compounds with no defined endpoint.

Compounds such as selegiline and vitamin E, in contrast to the cholinesterase inhibitors, may act by reducing neuronal damage (Sano et al, 1997). Data suggest no cognitive benefits, but some functional benefits (e.g., eating, using the toilet, grooming), leading to somewhat lower levels of dependence on caregivers. These compounds may in some cases delay death. Thus, while caregiver burden may be slightly ameliorated, the patient's lifespan may be somewhat enlarged, resulting in extended caregiving.

Pharmacoeconomic analysis tends to presuppose the long-term use of anti-dementia compounds, leading to the possible expansion of the lifespan in the context of progressive dementing diseases that many people would prefer to escape by an earlier death.

CONCLUDING ENVOI: INFORMED CONSENT IN TRIALS OF ANTI-DEMENTIA COMPOUNDS

The doctrine of informed consent in human subjects research is vitally important. Competent subjects must always be allowed the opportunity to make comprehending choices to participate in research programs. People with a diagnosis of AD *must* be told of their diagnosis in order to consent to either therapeutic or non-therapeutic research. However, many people, by the time of diagnosis, are no longer competent to consent.

In the United States and in many other countries, incompetent people with AD are enrolled in therapeutic and nontherapeutic research based on the consent of the responsible family member who acts as a proxy. There is renewed controversy in the United States regarding proxy consent for non-therapeutic research, even when the research is AD-related. Increasingly, it appears in the United States that a considerable amount of AD research that will not benefit the incompetent research subject may no longer be allowed to proceed based on proxy consent. Thus, researchers must depend much more than ever before on involving people immediately upon diagnosis in discussion of nontherapeutic research programs.

This development in the United States is unfortunate. AD is a dreadful disease that requires our concerted research efforts. Nontherapeutic research, *so long as it is AD-specific*, involving incompetent patients based on proxy consent, is a necessity. Subjects should of course always be treated with respect and dignity, and harm should in all possible instances be avoided.

Having stated the above, I immediately assert that research on anti-dementia drugs is categorically therapeutic, since all current ethics guidelines allow for any compound 'with the potential' of direct benefit to be designated as therapeutic. It would be unethical for the doctrine of informed consent to be carried to the extreme of denying demented patients the potential benefits of experimental compounds.

REFERENCES

Knopman, D. S., Schneider, L. S., Davis, K. L. et al (1996). Long-term tacrine (Cognex) treatment: Effects on nursing home placement and mortality. *Neurology*, **47**, 166–177.

Post, S. G. (1995). *The Moral Challenge of Alzheimer Disease*, Baltimore, MD, Johns Hopkins University Press.

Rogers, S. L., Friedhoff, L. T. and the Donepezil Study Group (1996). The efficacy and safety of Donepezil in patients with Alzheimer's disease: results of a US multicentre, randomized, double-blind, placebo-controlled trial. *Dementia*, **7**, 293–303.

Sano, M., Ernesto, C., Thomas, R. G., Klauber, M. R., Schafer, K., Grundman, M., Woodbury, P., Growdon, J., Cotman, C. W., Pfeiffer, E., Schneider, L. S. and Thal, L. J. (1997). A controlled trial of selegiline, alpha-tocopherol, or both as treatment for Alzheimer's disease. *New Eng. J. Med.*, **336**, 1217–1222.

4.6 Issues in Cross-Cultural Assessment of Economic Outcomes in Dementia

ELKE WITTHAUS

Department of Clinical Development, Hoechst Marion Roussel, Frankfurt, Germany

INTRODUCTION

A 20% reduction in the number of people requiring assistance for personal care was one of the US health care goals formulated for the elderly population in 1990. It has been suggested that this goal can only be achieved by recognizing Alzheimer's disease as a major cause of impaired function in the elderly, and devising more effective treatments (Mayeux, 1996).

Dementia, and primarily Alzheimer's disease, has become an important area of drug research and development. New compounds are currently entering the market and more will enter it in future. The medical need is already huge and, according to population forecasts (e.g. Evans et al, 1991; Dinkel, 1996), will grow constantly over the next few decades. From a health economic perspective the expected increase in demented subjects translates into a growing need for various types of ambulatory and institutional care services, which present the predominant cost components in the management of this condition. Yet while health care planners find themselves confronted with escalating requirements for care services, they also face growing budgetary constraints. In a situation of this kind, which is typical for many countries at present, drugs for the treatment of dementia are frequently expected to offer twin benefits: on the one hand, they are expected to improve or stabilize the patients' condition and, on the other, to yield economic savings as a result of improved patient health (Rice et al, 1993; Lubeck et al, 1994; Henke and Burchmore, 1997). The link between these two outcomes has, however, not been very well established.

Health Economics of Dementia. Edited by Anders Wimo, Bengt Jönsson, Göran Karlsson and Bengt Winblad.
© 1998 John Wiley & Sons Ltd.

WHEN DO EFFECTIVE TREATMENTS REDUCE COSTS?

Generally, health gains resulting from a treatment do not necessarily reduce overall health care costs at the same time. For example, a concurrent cost saving effect is questionable if the health gain prolongs survival in an otherwise fatal disease, without curing or significantly alleviating the condition. In chronic non-life-threatening diseases, however, the situation may be different and depends in large part on the treatment effect on disease-related disability or daily functioning. Dementia is usually perceived as belonging to this latter disease category, despite the fact that a number of studies have shown increased mortality in the demented (e.g. Evans et al, 1991; Skoog et al, 1993). Since disability and loss of independence increase as the disease progresses (at least in the most prevalent type of dementia, Alzheimer's disease), the need for care increases as well. It is, therefore, possible to specify circumstances under which savings would theoretically occur following the introduction of a new treatment for dementia.

The prerequisites which permit a reasonable forecast of potential savings can be summarized as follows: First, the health care system should provide a catalogue of services characterized by diversity and hierarchy. Diversity means distinction between services useful for different levels of need. Hierarchy means that higher efforts and costs are dedicated to the more demanding disease stages. Secondly, the corresponding health policy should follow a decision rule that allocates the more expensive services to the more severely ill. Finally, the range of services should be accessible to the majority of the population of interest. Figure 4.6.1 illustrates a system which fulfills these criteria.

This policy model does not yet reflect the organization of care for the demented in the majority of countries, although in some countries a comparable model has indeed evolved. For instance, Sweden, where a relatively large proportion of the health care budget is spent on the demented, has a somewhat similar cost structure (Wimo et al, 1997a). However, potential savings are small where health care budgets for the elderly with mental health problems, or for mental health care in general, are small. Potential savings are similarly small where care decisions are primarily taken on the basis of social factors. It has been shown that variations in the cost of health care provision for dementia are not systematically related to level of need in the target population of dementia care (e.g. Philips, 1995).

PREDICTING THE COSTS OF CARE FROM DISEASE SEVERITY

There is some evidence of a severity-dependent gradient in health care consumption by demented subjects (e.g. Wimo et al, 1992; Severson et al, 1994; Heyman et al, 1997). As yet, however, there is a lack of databased

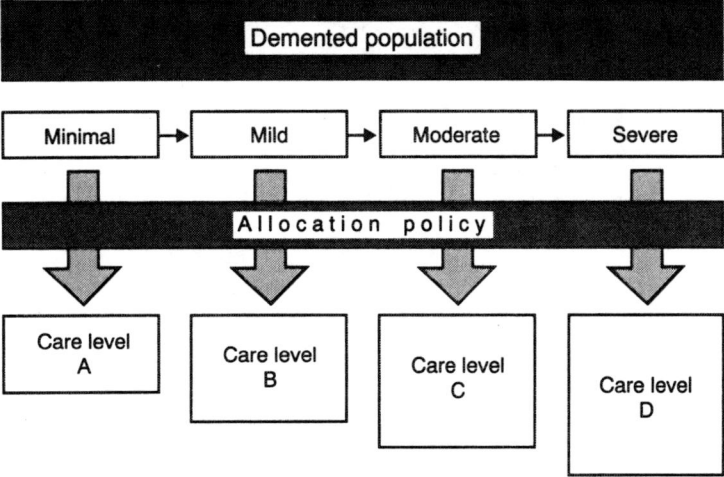

Figure 4.6.1. Health policy model of severity-dependent allocation of care

models capable of predicting the costs of care on the basis of disease severity or other characteristics which determine the level of care needed.

One of the few databases providing a direct link between disease severity and health care consumption is the Kungsholmen Project (Fratiglioni et al, 1994). This database has provided an empirical basis for modeling economic outcomes of new anti-dementia drugs in Sweden (Wimo et al, 1997b). However, the model based on the Kungsholmen database reflects the situation in Sweden and is not applicable to other countries unless the cost structure and decision rules are similar. There are, indeed, only a few countries with decision rules in place which would allow a comparable modeling exercise. One example is Germany where the long-term care insurance scheme (Pflegeversicherung) distinguishes between three levels of need. Each level is recompensated either with a volume of service or with money. However, the levels of need are only very roughly defined and it has been argued that the dementia-specific disabilities are not adequately reflected in the underlying classification system (Zerfass et al, 1997).

A lack of empirical data on disease-stage-driven costs has been an important problem with the few economic evaluations of new anti-dementia treatments which have been carried out to date (Lubeck et al, 1994; Henke and Burchmore, 1997). Due to the relatively speculative nature of some of the assumptions made, the savings projected by these studies are open to question. Efforts are therefore required to generate an empirical link between cost data and patient outcome data. Large multicentre multinational clinical trials are increasingly being used as a data source for this purpose. A number of issues occur in the context of planning and evaluating such studies.

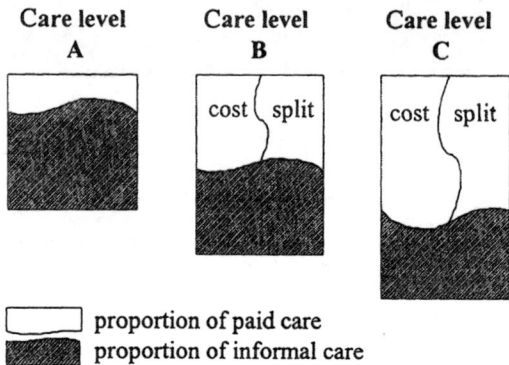

proportion of paid care
proportion of informal care

Figure 4.6.2. Illustration of fragmentation of care providers/purchasers

PROVIDERS AND PURCHASERS OF DEMENTIA CARE

Regional differences in the organization and funding of health care present a general problem for cross-cultural economic evaluation. Providers and purchasers of dementia care are characterized by diversity and fragmentation between and often even within individual countries. There are also variations in the volumes of money and care provided for demented populations. For example, community-based services such as home care, day care or visiting nurse services are available to different extents, are organized in different ways, and vary in the extent to which they are reimbursed.

The mix of purchasers presents a substantial difficulty for the economic evaluation of dementia care even within a single country or region. Figure 4.6.2 illustrates the issue. For example, in France, patients staying in long-term care institutions may 'choose' between psychiatric hospitals, nursing homes or other long-stay hospitals. For some of these institutions, there is a cost split between public and private purchasers. While psychiatric hospitals are funded by the social security system, nursing homes are usually paid for by the residents unless their financial means are insufficient. In the UK, there are more levels of residential care, including a range of residential homes, nursing homes, psychiatric hospitals (fewer now due to the UK's deinstitutionalization policy) and sheltered housing. Except for NHS hospitals, most alternatives are paid for privately. Care in other long-term care institutions is reimbursed by public purchasers in cases where the patient has no financial means. A similar cost split exists for care facilities in the ambulatory sector.

The availability and financing of formal services influences in turn the fraction of care which needs to be provided by informal caregivers. Usually, informal carers represent a major, albeit unofficial, part of the health care system since they provide large volumes of care. Their contribution is partially reimbursed by specific allowances in a few countries only. Among these countries are Germany, Sweden and Italy.

In Germany the long-term care insurance which was established in 1995 as part of the social insurance system follows a policy of spending according to disability, not income. However, within the different care levels spending on ambulatory care differs according to the provider in that the expenditure for a patient receiving informal care is 50% lower than for a similarly disabled patient receiving formal care. Thus, the economic impact of any intervention would be difficult to predict and would vary according to the proportion of formal and informal care.

To add to the complexity of the purchaser/provider problem, health care organization in many countries is continually changing. Mental health care has been targeted for a switch from institutional to community care in countries where until recently long-term care institutions were common, such as Germany, Sweden and the UK. These switches present difficulties in assessing the economic impact of any intervention.

Economic evaluation of dementia care in any particular country ultimately requires a detailed health policy analysis, thoroughly characterizing the organization and funding of care. Most of the cost-of-illness studies currently available from the literature do not provide a sufficient level of detail. As stated above, the health policy analysis should include an assessment of the decision criteria for placing patients into long-term care institutions. It is critically important to analyze to which extent (if at all) volumes of care are determined by disease severity.

THE IMPORTANCE OF A SOCIETAL PERSPECTIVE

Clearly, the evolving mix of funding for dementia care, involving patients, their families and different public purchasers, is also likely to involve different levels of interest in and perception of economic arguments. The perspective of the target audience is critical in deciding on the range of costs and benefits to be considered in economic evaluations of new treatments for dementia. New pharmacological treatments will lead to increases in drug budgets for dementia, but these increases may be matched or outweighed by savings within other budgets. Decision-making from a societal perspective will take into account the total cost impact of the new drug, including not only the cost of purchasing the drug but the impact of its use on the costs of other services. However, whether the purchaser of the drug will appreciate savings elsewhere is a matter of uncertainty.

Due to the diversity of components of care for the demented the societal perspective is an even more theoretical construct here than it is in other disease areas. As with other serious mental health problems, care for the demented comprises medical care, community care, social services, and voluntary care (including informal care). The fragmentation of budgets and the restricted perspectives of different purchasers presents a challenge for researchers in and outside the pharmaceutical industry who wish to establish the economic impact of an intervention. Cost shifting between different forms of health care provision may be obscured if costs are examined from a limited purchaser's perspective alone.

ESTIMATING THE ECONOMIC IMPACT OF NEW TREATMENTS

The collection of resource-use data in intervention studies, most of which are multinational, is a relatively new approach to estimating the economic impact of new treatments. As yet, this approach is exploratory in nature. Depending on the size of the study populations and on the variation in costs between different regions within the study, typical patterns of care and costs may be identified. Once identified, these patterns need to be correlated with effectiveness outcomes. Changes in clinical outcomes may not, however, be directly accompanied by changes in resource use, and indeed the impact on resource use may not be observable within the time horizon of the clinical trial. The choice of the right range of measures and of suitable instruments is therefore critical.

The assessment of the economic impact of a new treatment involves a comparative evaluation of the balance between costs and effects of the new treatment and a relevant alternative. Clinical studies in dementia have so far used placebo as the comparator treatment. From an economic perspective placebo does not represent a do-nothing alternative, but a 'true' comparator: the organization and provision of care (in a given country) to which the new drug is a supplement. So far, there are no published comparisons between different drugs. This is not surprising since no drug has yet sufficiently diffused into common practice patterns to be called a standard approach. This is probably still true although new drugs are attracting substantial clinical interest.

Cost consequences have not yet been prospectively established for any anti-dementia drug. The analyses presented for tacrine (Lubeck et al, 1994; Henke and Burchmore, 1997) used effects on cognition and other clinical outcomes from randomized clinical trials, conducted in the US, and assumed effects on a range of costs. It is not sufficient, however, to project cost estimates from clinical outcomes. Effectiveness outcomes need to be considered too and this requires a critical review of current clinical outcome measures.

NEW TREATMENTS: EFFECT ON MORBIDITY

Efficacy in dementia studies is usually assessed on the basis of a number of scales and tools, most of which reflect specific aspects of the disease. Some are acknowledged as primary outcome measures. Even these are subject to current debate and improvement, as reflected by the ongoing Instrument Development Project conducted by the Alzheimer's Disease Cooperative Study (summarized by Mackell et al, 1997). To what extent these clinical instruments are useful for economic evaluation is much less clear.

For economic purposes more holistic measures are in fact desirable, which reflect the multidimensional nature of the disease on the one hand, and describe clearly distinguishable health states in the population of interest on the other. The efficacy measures required for regulatory approval such as the Alzheimer's Disease Assessment Scale (ADAS) are only of limited value. Cognitive performance is given a high weight in clinical trials. However, outcomes reflecting the patient's degree of dependence or need for care should be more broadly defined and may include prevention of disease progression, extension of disability-free life expectancy, delay of institutionalization, decrease in caregiver burden, or increase in quality of life of patients and caregivers. The inclusion of this type of outcomes in clinical studies evaluating new anti-dementia treatments (e.g. Sano et al, 1997) is still rare.

Global measures of disease severity, for example the Clinical Dementia Rating scale (CDR; Hughes et al, 1982) or the Global Deterioration Scale (GDS; Reisberg, 1988), do, however, fulfill some of the above criteria. They are staging instruments and cover a broad spectrum of domains. Moreover, they have been used in a number of important studies such as the Rotterdam study (Hofman et al, 1991), the Kungsholmen study (Fratiglioni et al, 1994) and the Consortium to Establish a Registry for Alzheimer's Disease (CERAD; Morris et al, 1993), all of which have provided population-based estimates of severity distribution or progression. However, the CDR and GDS are both to some extent subjective measures and the validity of the scores depends on training and experience. Their use in a study requires additional training of the raters to ensure sufficient reliability of the scores generated.

The CDR and the GDS are nevertheless useful instruments for the assessment of disease progression. Prevention or delay of progression are clinically meaningful outcomes of anti-dementia drug treatment; avoiding the more severe disease states should be beneficial for demented individuals and their families. These outcomes are also economically meaningful since the more severe disease stages are the more costly ones.

Despite the fact that the CDR and GDS scales measure disease progression, it is not yet clear whether drugs which are effective according to CDR and GDS criteria achieve a genuine delay in disease progression or are merely symptomatic. Drugs which do achieve a genuine effect on disease progression will modify the disease history in the individual patient and, if used by significant populations, will change the distribution of disease severity. This type of effect has not been shown for cholinesterase inhibitors (Aricept Package Insert, 1997), although recent evidence indicates that the neuroprotective agent propentofylline does delay the progression of dementia (Karlsson et al, 1998).

Generating evidence on disease progression is challenging due to the long observation periods required to observe progression and variability in the course of disease. Many studies are conducted for 6 months only, and relatively few for 12 months. However, only a fraction of a demented population has marked disease progression within this time frame.

A patient's level of dependency represents an economically meaningful outcome since it reflects the need for assistance and care. The importance of this domain has been strengthened by the European Agency for the Evaluation of Medicinal Products (EMEA). The Agency requires that new anti-dementia drugs be evaluated for changes in cognition, global performance *and* activities of daily living. The Agency does not, however, specify how daily functionality should be assessed and, in fact, daily functioning is still considered an understudied area in dementia studies. A number of new dementia-specific measures are under development (e.g. Gauthier et al, 1993; Stern et al, 1994; Galasko et al, 1997). The problems with current instruments are that many were developed for general geriatric assessment, focus on a limited set of basic activities and are therefore insufficiently sensitive to change in demented populations.

NEW TREATMENTS: EFFECT ON QUALITY OF LIFE

In dementia, measurement of patients' perceived quality of life is not usually undertaken since the subjective world of the demented is not directly accessible and their impaired judgment does not seem to allow self-assessment. Proxy assessment has been explored to some extent (e.g. Albert et al, 1996). However, little research has been conducted in this field. Likewise, utility measures which allow the calculation of quality-adjusted life-years are not straightforwardly applicable in the demented and, again, little research has been done to date to evaluate the usefulness of proxy assessments.

NEW TREATMENTS: EFFECT ON INFORMAL CAREGIVERS

Informal care is an essential part of dementia care and potentially more sensitive to changes in the patients' condition and treatment effects than formal paid care (e.g. Clipp and Moore, 1995; Haley, 1997; Max, 1996). Informal carers are frequently the primary providers of community care and the shift from institutional to community care which is ongoing in many countries increases their burden. Since informal caregivers not only sacrifice time and money but also suffer physical and emotional stress, social isolation and poor health, the burden they face is multidimensional. A number of instruments have been designed to assess both the objective and subjective burdens of caregiving (e.g. reviewed by Vitaliano et al, 1991). Most of these have only been used in limited settings and are not available for multinational use. There

Unpaid care by family or friends		
☐ None		
Type of care provided (check all that apply)	Time spent in a typical day	
	Hours	Minutes
☐ Feeding	⎿⊥⏌	⎿⊥⏌
☐ Toileting	⎿⊥⏌	⎿⊥⏌
☐ Bathing	⎿⊥⏌	⎿⊥⏌
☐ Dressing	⎿⊥⏌	⎿⊥⏌
☐ Administering medication	⎿⊥⏌	⎿⊥⏌
☐ Supervision	⎿⊥⏌	⎿⊥⏌
☐ Housekeeping	⎿⊥⏌	⎿⊥⏌
☐ Transportation	⎿⊥⏌	⎿⊥⏌
☐ Other	⎿⊥⏌	⎿⊥⏌

Figure 4.6.3. Quantification of informal care in Caregiver Activities Time Survey (CATS)

is a need for comprehensive but easy-to-use instruments with multinational applicability, and additional research is needed to improve and validate current tools.

Estimates of time spent by informal caregivers indicate volumes as large as 60 to 70 hours per week, determined by stage of disease, the availability and use of support services and the contribution of other caregivers (Rice et al, 1993). Precision of measurement is probably an important issue in reaching a reliable estimate of informal caregiver care time, as is the need to distinguish between usual household tasks and the additional workload due to illness. One instrument capable of assessing time spent by paid and unpaid caregivers as well as a number of baseline characteristics (age, sex, relationship with the patient, social network) is the Caregiver Activities Time Survey (CATS, Figure 4.6.3) which was first described by Clipp and Moore (1995). A significant positive relationship was shown between unpaid caregiver time and cognitive and non-cognitive impairment. The instrument has since been subject to continuous improvements and has been used in a number of studies, including multinational studies.

Another consideration which needs attention is the direct financial burden of dementia for patients and their families. Since full financial provision for comprehensive care is rare, a proportion of the professional care is often paid for privately. A comprehensive assessment of the financial burden of dementia should therefore include out of pocket expenses. Whether these are sensitive to treatment effects is an open question.

NEW TREATMENTS: EFFECT ON MORTALITY

There is substantial evidence showing increased mortality rates in demented as compared with non-demented subjects (Barcley et al, 1985; Diesfeldt et al, 1986; Knopman et al, 1988; Martin et al, 1987; Sulkava et al, 1992; Walsh et al, 1990; Evans et al, 1991; Heeren et al, 1992; Skoog et al, 1993). There is also some evidence indicating that the increase in mortality is dependent on disease severity (Barcley et al, 1985; Martin et al, 1987; Cooper et al, 1996; Witthaus et al, submitted). It is therefore theoretically possible that effective treatments for dementia would in turn prolong survival. In patients treated with tacrine there was a trend towards prolonged survival in the cohort with the best clinical response (Knopman et al, 1996).

Concerns about the economic implications of an effect of anti-dementia drugs on longevity have already been expressed (*BMJ* editorial, **314**, March 1997). The long-term economic impact of any treatment will depend in part on whether or not survival is affected. This does not necessarily mean, however, that initial savings will be offset by downstream expenditure in the lifetime gained. For example, patients may live longer in milder disease stages and die from competing causes of death before reaching a high level of dependency. Although the long observation periods required will make it difficult to observe any effect of treatment on mortality, the possibility of extended survival needs to be considered in economic evaluation.

NEW TREATMENTS: EFFECT ON THE COSTS OF CARE

The expected effect of treatment on the cost of dementia care involves a shift of costs within the forms of care provided for individuals with dementia (Figure 4.6.4). As explained above, the assumption underlying this expected effect is that the allocation and provision of care is sensitive to patient performance at all levels. It is, however, unknown how sensitive the organization of dementia care is to changes in the patient's condition.

As discussed above, the monetary value of shifts between different forms of dementia care depends on the total volume of (paid) care for the demented and

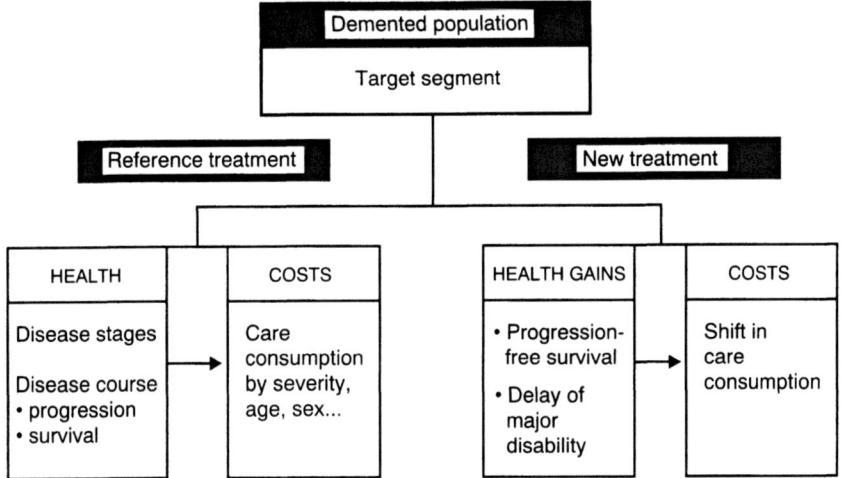

Figure 4.6.4. Conceptual model of treatment effects

the rules for the allocation of patients to the different care components. The target population for anti-dementia drugs is usually patients with mild or moderate disease who may not consume significant paid resources. Therefore, it may not be possible to observe any economically significant transitions in the distribution of care within any clinical trial although the lifetime economic advantages of treating these patients may be important. Modeling over many years may therefore be necessary to show any true economic impact.

In terms of measurement this means that all relevant cost elements need to be covered, including volumes of informal care. It will be important in this regard to determine whether avoiding institutional and paid community care as a result of treatment does, in turn, affect the burden for informal caregivers. A further issue of relevance here is that, as explained above, considerable methodological uncertainties exist as to how time and efforts of informal caregivers should be valued.

NEW TREATMENTS: EFFECT MODIFIERS

Pharmacological treatment of dementia is not the only factor influencing outcome. As in other psychiatric disorders, the social environment, including social network and family relationships, will have an effect on the disease course and therefore modify any pharmacological treatment effect. Consequently, the social environment needs to be assessed in studies aiming at establishing treatment effects. This will allow more meaningful analysis, but add to the complexity of studies.

CONCLUDING REMARKS

The assessment of the economic impact of new anti-dementia treatments is a challenging task. It requires the collection of a broad range of data which must then be used in models to predict the long-term consequences of treatment. The decision on the range and type of data that should be gathered and the instruments that should be used for their collection is part of the challenge. Despite the potentially limited perspectives of major decision makers, a broad spectrum of benefits and costs needs to be assessed and a societal perspective taken.

The design of multinational, combined clinical-economic studies in dementia therefore requires very careful consideration. It necessarily involves some risk, not least because it will take a few years until some of the outcome measures and scales currently under development will be sufficiently validated and acknowledged. However, since health care decision makers at all levels are likely to require evidence-based justification for the additional costs of new drugs there is probably no better alternative.

REFERENCES

Albert, S. M., Del Castillo-Castaneda, C., Sano, M. et al (1996). Quality of Life in patients with Alzheimer's disease as reported by patient proxies, *J. Am. Geriatr. Soc.*, **44**, 1342–1347.

Barcley, L. L., Zemcov, A., Blass, J. P. et al (1985). Survival in Alzheimer's disease and vascular dementias, *Neurology*, **35**, 834–840.

Clipp, E. C. and Moore, M. J. (1995). Caregiver time use: An outcome measure in clinical trial research on Alzheimer's disease, *Clin. Pharmacol. Ther.*, **58**, 228–236.

Cooper, B., Bickel, H. and Schaufele, M. (1996). Early development and progression of dementing illness in the elderly: a general-practice based study, *Psychol. Med.*, **26**, 411–419.

Diesfeldt, H. F. A., Van Honte, L. R. and Moerkens, R. M. (1986). Duration of survival in senile dementia, *Acta. Psychiatr. Scand.*, **73**, 366–371.

Dinkel, R. H. (1996). Development of dementia to the year 2050, *Gesundheitswesen*, **58**, 50–55.

Evans, D. A., Smith, L. A., Scherr, P. A., Albert, M. S., Funkenstein, H. H. and Hebert, L. E. (1991). Risk of death from Alzheimer's disease in a community population of older persons, *Am. J. Epidemiol.*, **134**, 403–412.

Fratiglioni, L., Forsell, Y., Torres, H. A. and Winblad, B. (1994). Severity of dementia and institutionalization in the elderly: prevalence data from an urban area in Sweden, *Neuroepidemiology*, **13**, 79–88.

Galasko, D., Bennett, D., Sano, M. et al (1997). An Inventory to Assess Activities of Daily Living for Clinical Trials in Alzheimer's Disease, *Alzheim. Disea. Assoc. Disord.*, **11**, S33–S39.

Gauthier, L., Gauthier, S., Gélinas, I., McIntyre, M. and Wood-Dauphinee, S. (1993). Functional assessment in Alzheimer's disease. *Abstract of the 16th Annual meeting of the Canadian College of Neuropsychopharmacology and the British Association of Psychopharmacology*, June, Montreal, Canada.

Haley, W. E. (1997). The family caregiver's role in Alzheimer's disease, *Neurology*, **48**, 25–29.

Heeren, T. J., Van Hemert, A. M. and Rooymans, H. G. M. (1992). A community-based study of survival in dementia, *Acta. Psychiatr. Scand.*, **85**, 415–418.

Henke, C. J. and Burchmore, M. J. (1997). The economic impact of tacrine in the treatment of Alzheimer's disease, *Clinical Therapeutics*, **19**, 330–345.

Heyman, A., Peterson, B., Fillenbaum, G. and Pieper, C. (1997). Predictors of time to institutionalization of patients with Alzheimer's disease: the CERAD experience, part XVII, *Neurology*, **48**, 1304–1309.

Hofman, A., Rocca, W. A., Brayne, C. et al (1991). The prevalence of dementia in Europe: a collaborative study of 1980–1990 findings, *International Journal of Epidemiology*, **20**, 736–748.

Hughes, C. P., Berg, L., Danziger, W. L., Coben, L. A. and Martin, R. L. (1982). A new clinical scale for the staging of dementia, *Brit. J. Psychiat.*, **140**, 566–572.

Karlsson, I., Kittner, B., Rother, M. et al (1998). A double-blind, placebo-controlled study of the effects of withdrawing propentofylline therapy (submitted).

Knopman, D. S., Kitto, J., Deinard, S. and Heiring, J. (1988). Longitutional study of death and institutionalization in patients with primary degenerative dementia, *J. Am. Geriatr. Soc.*, **36**, 108–122.

Knopman, D., Schneider, M. D., Davis, K., Talwalker, S., Smith, F., Hoover, T. et al (1996). Long-term tacrine (Cognex) treatment: Effects on nursing home placement and mortality, *Neurology*, **47**, 166–177.

Lubeck, D. P., Mazonson, P. D. and Bowe, T. (1994). Potential effect of tacrine on expenditures for Alzheimer's disease, *Med. Interface*, **7**, 130–138.

Mackell, J. A., Ferris, S. H., Mohs, R., Schneider, L., Galasko, D., Whitehouse, P. et al (1997). Multicenter evaluation of new instruments for Alzheimer's disease clinical trials: summary of results, *Alzheim. Disea. Assoc. Disord.*, **11**, S65–S69.

Martin, D. C., Miller, J. K., Kapoor, W., Arena, V. C. and Boller, F. (1987). A controlled study of survival with dementia, *Arch. Neurol.*, **44**, 1122–1126.

Mayeux, R. (1996). Development of a national prospective study of Alzheimer's disease, *Alzheim. Disea. Assoc. Disord.*, **10**, 38–44.

Max, W. (1996). The cost of Alzheimer's disease. Will drug treatment ease the burden? *PharmacoEconomics*, **9**, 5–10.

Morris, J. C., Edland, S., Clark, C., Galasko, D., Koss, E., Mohs, R. et al (1993). The Consortium to Establish a Registry for Alzheimer's Disease (CERAD), *Neurology*, **43**, 2457 2465.

Philips, V. L. (1995). Community care for severely disabled people on low incomes, *BMJ*, **311**, 1121–1123.

Reisberg, B., Ferris, S. H., de Leon, M. J. and Crook, T. (1988). Global deterioration scale (GDS), *Psychopharmacology Bulletin*, **24**, 661–663.

Rice, D. P., Fox, P. J., Max, W., Webber, P. A., Lindeman, D. A., Hauck, W. W. et al (1993). The economic burden of Alzheimer's disease care, *Datawatch*, 164–176.

Sano, M., Ernesto, Ch., Thomas, R. G., Klauber, M. R., Schafer, K., Grundman, M. et al (1997). A controlled trial of selegiline, alpha-tocopherol, or both as treatment for Alzheimer's disease, *N. Engl. J. Med.*, **336**, 1216–1222.

Severson, M. A., Smith, G. E., Tangalos, E. G., Peterson, R. C., Kokmen, E., Ivnik, R. J. et al (1994). Patterns and predictors of institutionalization in community-based dementia patients, *J. Am. Geriatr. Soc.*, **42**, 181–185.

Skoog, I., Nilsson, L., Palmertz, B., Andreasson, L. A. and Svanborg, A. (1993). A population based study of dementia in 85-year-olds, *N. Engl. J. Med.*, **328**, 153–158.

Stern, Y., Albert, S. M., Sano, M. et al (1994). Assessing patient dependence in Alzheimer's disease, *J. Gerontol.*, **49**(5), M216–M222.

Sulkava, R., Vaden, J. and Erkinjuntti, T. (1992). Survival in Alzheimer's disease (AD) and multi-infarct dementia (MID) in the 1980s, *Neurology*, **42**, 143.

Vitaliano, P. P., Young, H. M. and Russo, J. (1991). Burden: A review of measures used among caregivers of individuals with dementia, *The Gerontologist Society of America*, **31**, 67–75.

Walsh, J. S., Welch, H. G. and Larson, E. B. (1990). Survival of outpatients with Alzheimer-type dementia, *Ann. Intern. Med.*, **113**, 429–434.

Wimo, A., Mattsson, B. and Gustafson, L. (1992). Predictive validity of factors influencing the institutionalization of elderly people with psycho-geriatric disorder, *Scand. J. Prim. Health Care*, **10**, 185–191.

Wimo, A., Karlsson, G., Sandman, P. O., Corder, L. and Winblad, B. (1997a). The cost of illness due to dementia in Sweden, *Int. J. Geriatr. Psychiatr.*, **12**, 857–861.

Wimo, A., Karlsson, G., Nordberg, A. and Winblad, B. (1997b). Treatment of Alzheimer's disease with tacrine—a cost analysis model, *Alzheim. Disea. Assoc. Disord.*, **11**, 191–200.

Witthaus, E., Ott, A., Barendregt, J. J., Breteler, M. and Bonneux, L. (submitted). The burden of mortality and morbidity from dementia.

Zerfass, R., Daniel, S., Sattel, H. et al (1997). Degree of disability of demented patients as judged by relatives and experts (disability insurance), *Psychiatr. Prax.*, **24**, 84–87.

4.7 Nursing Home Placement and Mortality as Outcomes in Clinical Trials of Anti-dementia Drugs: Methodological Issues

S. GRACON and F. SMITH

Parke-Davis Pharmaceutical Research, Ann Arbor, MI, USA

INTRODUCTION

In this chapter we hope to provide a practical approach to the collection of data which can be used to document reduced burden of care and support cost-effectiveness of new therapies for patients with Alzheimer's disease (AD). The approach is based upon re-examination of our experience in patients treated with tacrine (Cognex[R]) where the focus was on nursing home placement and mortality.

THE TACRINE EXPERIENCE

Tacrine, a cholinesterase inhibitor, was approved in the United States in 1993 for the symptomatic treatment of mild to moderate dementia of the Alzheimer's type. Approval was based upon the results of two, randomized, double-blind, placebo-controlled clinical trials of 12- (Farlow et al, 1992) and 30- (Knapp et al, 1994) weeks duration. Statistically significant differences versus placebo were demonstrated on the Alzheimer's Disease Assessment Scale cognitive subscale (ADAS Cognitive), the Mini-Mental State Examination (MMSE), the Clinician Interview-Based Impression of Change (CIBIC) as well as on a caregiver-rated global assessment and assessments of patients on activities of daily living. Data supportive of efficacy were derived from two additional cross-over studies (Eagger et al, 1991; Wilcock et al, 1993) and three studies that employed enrichment designs (Davis et al, 1992; Forrette et al, 1995; Foster et al, 1996).

Health Economics of Dementia. Edited by Anders Wimo, Bengt Jönsson, Göran Karlsson and Bengt Winblad.
© 1998 John Wiley & Sons Ltd.

The clinical development of tacrine was complicated by a high dropout rate from controlled trials. The forced dose escalation and ensuing dose-related cholinergic side-effects caused many patients to discontinue treatment. The mandatory withdrawal of patients if liver transaminase levels (specifically alanine aminotransferase; ALT) exceeded three times the upper limit of normal resulted in approximately 25% of patients stopping treatment, at least temporarily. Patients who had to stop tacrine treatment were doing at least as well on average as patients who continued. Stopping tacrine treatment was associated with a measurable decline in cognitive performance (Knapp et al, 1994; Davis et al, 1992). Despite these difficulties the efficacy data were compelling and tacrine is now approved in more than 25 countries worldwide and has proven safe in use in clinical practice (Gracon et al, in press).

The CIBIC was one of two primary outcome measures. It was used to ensure that the magnitude of the treatment effect was clinically meaningful and recognizable to an experienced clinician (Knopman et al, 1994; Leber, 1990; CPMP, 1997). Unfortunately, the magnitude of the treatment effect was judged more by the mean treatment difference for drug versus placebo comparisons on the ADAS cognitive, a 70 point scale on which untreated patients worsen 6–12 points per year. The estimated difference between drug and placebo on the ADAS cognitive was in the order of 2–5 points. A difference described as small by some experts, trivial by others and modest at best by still others.

Although tacrine was approved, these opinions created uncertainty about the value of tacrine treatment in Alzheimer's disease. Because only an estimated 10–40% of patients improved in response to tacrine treatment, questions arose as to the ability to predict, prior to treatment, which patients were likely to improve. Possibly a more puzzling issue was the entrenched nihilistic attitude towards the diagnosis and treatment of patients with AD. The persistence of this attitude is surprising given that tacrine was the first drug to demonstrate significant beneficial effects in a previously untreated, fatal illness.

Speculation arose as to numbers of patients who would be started on tacrine treatment and the numbers who would respond and could be maintained on treatment. The long-term benefit of treatment also came into question and, specifically, whether the effects observed over 3 to 6 months in controlled clinical trials would persist and translate into long-term effects on major disease milestones such as a delay in nursing home placement, a positive economic outcome and delayed mortality, a potential negative economic outcome.

The regulatory approval of new drugs as safe and effective is separated from the reimbursement process and the process of adding new drugs to formularies (Johnson and Bootman, 1994). In this age of cost containment, the high cost of new drugs, especially in a new therapeutic category, raises concerns about diagnostic accuracy, use patterns and cost-effectiveness. The approval of new drugs can result in a significant increase in health care expenditures. For example, if all AD patients in the US were treated with tacrine the cost would be \$4.7 billion, based upon an annual cost of \$1620 per patient (Gunderson, 1995). Assuming that about one third of patients actually improve in response to tacrine treatment and non-responders are taken off medication then the cost would be closer to \$1.5 billion. On the other hand, if patients with mild memory loss associated with aging were treated, the cost could rise dramatically. Obviously, insurers want to reduce such uncertainty about cost-effectiveness and see cost-benefit assessment become an integral part of new drug evaluation. Requiring experts to make the diagnosis of AD, either through a hospital based restricted drug distribution system as occurred with tacrine in France or through specific labelling requirements, is a first step to ensuring new treatments are used only in the intended patient population.

It is because of complex issues that some payers did not reimburse for tacrine treatment and Parke-Davis sought new data to support long-term benefit and cost-effectiveness.

THE NATURAL HISTORY OF ALZHEIMER'S DISEASE

Figure 4.7.1 depicts the natural history of the clinical phase of AD from initial symptoms to death (Jost and Grossberg, 1995; Seversen et al, 1994; Piccini et al, 1995). MMSE score (Folstein et al, 1975) is displayed on the vertical axis as a surrogate of disease severity, and time in years from first symptom is shown on the horizontal axis. The 'clinical course' of AD can last a decade or longer, while the underlying neurochemical, biochemical, and neuropathological changes begin years and perhaps decades before symptoms appear (Jost and Grossberg, 1995; Heyman et al, 1987). The time from initial symptoms to diagnosis can exceed 3 years. Eventually, cognitive decline leads to loss of functional independence (Drachman et al, 1990). Depression and anxiety are common symptoms early in the disease course in more mildly impaired patients, who may be aware of their cognitive loss (Levy et al, 1996). More troublesome neuropsychiatric symptoms such as delusions, hallucinations, agitation, and aggression generally occur later and in more severely impaired patients (Heyman et al, 1987; Levy et al, 1996). These symptoms are unpredictable and can wax and wane during the disease course (Levy et al, 1996).

In the United States and Australia, an estimated three of every four patients with AD will enter a nursing home with an average stay of 3 years until death (Welch et al, 1992; Brodaty et al, 1993). The total cost of AD in the US is estimated at \$90 billion (US National Institute of Health); the cost of nursing home care alone is more than \$40 000 per patient per year (US National Institute of Health; Ernst and Hay, 1994). For many families, the decision to institutionalize the patient is more traumatic than the patient's death. Nursing home placement, although an imprecise measure of disease severity, is a major disease milestone and a major determinant of cost of illness.

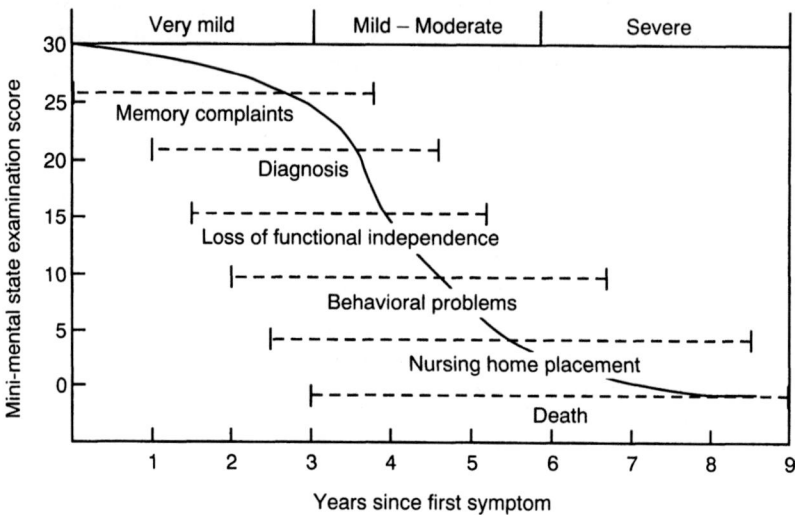

Figure 4.7.1. Natural history of Alzheimer's disease

Early diagnosis and treatment of AD is critical to maximizing benefit both to the patient and to the caregiver. It is important to intervene early in the illness, before the quality of life of both the patient and the caregiver has deteriorated to a point where treatment only prolongs an already difficult situation. If effective treatment begins early enough in the disease course, milestones such as loss of functional independence and nursing home placement can be delayed. When to stop treatment can be a more troublesome dilemma which raises ethical concerns (Post and Whitehouse, 1992).

Nursing home placement is not the outcome of interest in many countries. The economics of disease management vary from country to country, and it is important to collect data that allow modeling based upon the country of interest. It is not enough to simply determine that nursing home placement is delayed and that life is not prolonged. Concurrent assessment of the level of dependency of the patient on others for cognitive support, behavior and basic activities of daily living as they relate to the burden of care are of greater concern. The assumption has been that a delay in nursing home placement is a function of the patient being more functionally independent in the home. This assumption must be proven.

Numerous studies have shown significant, albeit modest, correlations between changes in cognitive function, global severity of illness, functional abilities and behavior (Stern et al, 1994; Heyman et al, 1997; Kramer-Ginsberg et al, 1988). There are also significant correlations between severity of illness (How far?; Drachman et al, 1990) in each of these domains and the need for nursing home care (Stern et al, 1990; Uhlmann et al, 1987). However,

Table 4.7.1. Logistic regression analysis of nursing home placement or mortality at week 30

Comparison	Odds ratio	95% CI	Difference favors	p-value
80 mg/day vs placebo[a]	1.1	[0.3, 3.8]	80 mg/day	0.833
120 mg/day vs placebo	1.6	[0.6, 4.1]	120 mg/day	0.338
160 mg/day vs placebo	2.8	[1.0, 7.8]	160 mg/day	0.046*

[a] The sample size for the 80-mg/day treatment group was considerably smaller, approximately one-third that of the placebo group.
* $p < 0.05$

treatment effects on quantitative measures of severity of illness have not been accepted as surrogates for outcomes such as nursing home placement. Perhaps that is because the magnitude of the treatment effect in absolute terms on measures like the ADAS cognitive is considered too small. It is also the tremendous heterogeneity in this patient population which makes reliably predicting outcome for individual patients impossible.

THE 30-WEEK TACRINE STUDY

The effects of tacrine on quantitative measures in cognitive, global, functional and behavioral domains as well as on mortality and nursing home placement were assessed in the 30-week, randomized, double-blind, placebo-controlled study (Knapp et al, 1994; Knopman et al, 1996). Using logistic regression, patients randomized to tacrine 160 mg/day were significantly more likely to remain alive or at home than patients on placebo (Odds Ratio = 2.8; p = 0.046) with a dose response effect (see Table 4.7.1). Similar results were obtained by Smith et al using a Cox regression analysis (Smith et al, 1996). However, 30 weeks is a short period of time relative to the natural history of AD and too few events occurred to provide convincing evidence of a beneficial effect of tacrine.

LONG-TERM TREATMENT EFFECTS: NURSING HOME PLACEMENT AND MORTALITY

Two years after the 30-week study was completed, attempts were made to contact the families of all patients originally randomized. The purpose was to determine whether patients were alive and, if so, whether they were still living at home. Subsequently 90% of the original sample were included in analyses of nursing home placement and all patients were included in analyses of mortality (Knopman et al, 1996). In order to avoid the criticism that only caregivers who were dedicated maintained patients on tacrine long term we examined the cohort of patients who remained on tacrine treatment up to the time of nursing

Table 4.7.2. Logistic regression analyses of NHP and mortality at follow-up, by tacrine dose (mg/day) for patients who were on tacrine

Comparison	Odds ratio	95% CI	Difference favors	p-value
NHP				
>80 to 120 vs 20 to 80	2.7	[1.4, 5.2]	>80 to 120	0.003
>120 to 160 vs 20 to 80	2.8	[1.5, 5.2]	>120 to 160	0.001
Mortality				
>80 to 120 vs 20 to 80	1.3	[0.5, 3.3]	>80 to 120	0.602
>120 to 160 vs 20 to 80	2.6	[0.9, 7.1]	>120 to 160	0.063

home placement. We used patients taking tacrine 80 mg/day or less as the comparative group for logistic regression analyses.

The probability of nursing home placement was significantly reduced for patients taking doses >80 to 120 mg/day (OR = 2.7; p = 0.003) and >120 mg/ day to 160 mg/day (OR = 2.8; p = 0.001) compared with patients receiving doses <80 mg/day (Table 4.7.2). After 300 days, 25% of patients in the low-dose group had entered a nursing home compared with 5% of patients who received higher doses. An additional 400 plus days elapsed before 25% of patients in the higher-dose groups had entered a nursing home (Figure 4.7.2). No statistically significant effects on mortality were seen.

One criticism of this approach was the fact that the dose-titration was not accounted for in the logistic regression. Analyses were repeated using Cox proportional hazards model with time dependent covariates, which gave a more conservative result that remained statistically significant (Smith et al, in press). Unfortunately, this portion of the study was neither randomized nor blinded and the potential for selection bias clearly existed so that these data, although being consistent with expectations, were not readily accepted.

LONG-TERM TREATMENT EFFECTS: QUANTITATIVE MEASURES

In order to determine if long-term effects generalized to quantitative measures, patients still living at home were invited to return to the clinic for assessments on the MMSE, Global Deterioration Scale (GDS; Reisberg et al, 1982), Instrumental Activities of Daily Living (IADL), and Physical Self Maintenance Scale (PSMS; Lawton and Brody, 1969). Patients who continued to receive tacrine were compared with patients who had stopped tacrine treatment (Knopman et al, 1998). All comparisons favored the on-tacrine cohort. Statistically significant or near significant results were seen for the PSMS and IADL, respectively, indicating that patients who continued treatment were performing basic activities of daily living to a greater degree than patients who stopped (Table 4.7.3). Again, treatment assignment was not random nor blinded, and attrition could have influenced the final results in either direction.

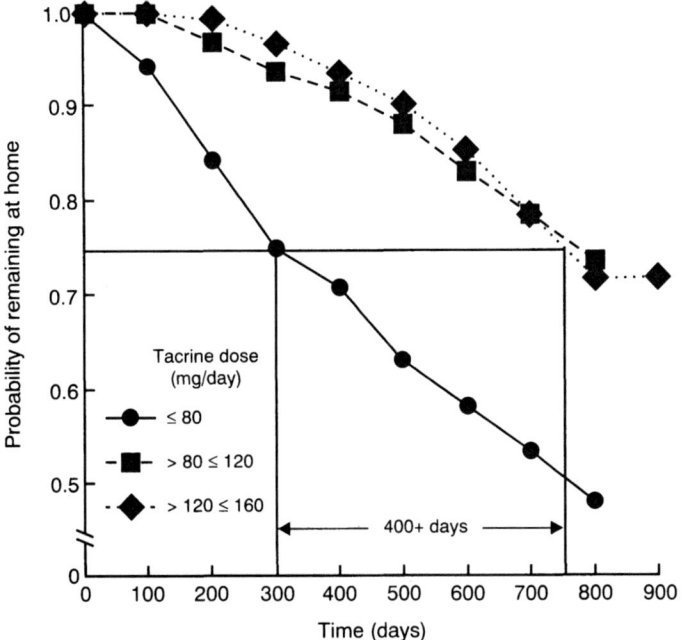

Figure 4.7.2. Impact of tacrine on nursing home placement

Table 4.7.3. Analysis of MMSE, GDS, IADL, and PSMS: patients on versus off tacrine

	MMSE	GDS	IADL	PSMS
Sample Sizes[a]				
On tacrine	185	197	194	196
Off tacrine	75	92	97	96
Total N	260	289	291	292
On vs Off Cognex				
Treatment difference	1.807	−0.113	−1.665	−1.917
95% CI	(−0.6, 4.2)	(−0.4, 0.2)	(−3.6, 0.2)	(−3.4, −0.5)
Difference favors	On tacrine	On tacrine	On tacrine	On tacrine
p-value	0.146	0.505	0.086	0.010*

[a] The number of patients with data varies among efficacy parameters because some patients lacked either a baseline or follow-up assessment.
* $p < 0.05$

More patients who were off tacrine were already in nursing homes and unavailable for assessment. This could result in an underestimate of the magnitude and significance level for the treatment effect.

The impact of tacrine on the economics of AD has been modeled using both quantitative measures from the 30-week study (Lubeck et al, 1994; Gray, 1995) and data from long-term follow-up using outcomes of nursing home placement and mortality (Henke and Burchmore, 1997). Sensitivity analyses have also been conducted and only the most conservative analyses failed to provide evidence of a cost benefit.

Although these results are provocative and useful for hypothesis generation, it is clear that the burden of proof required for studies showing cost-effectiveness is no less rigorous than that to support regulatory approval for safety and efficacy. Appropriately designed and controlled prospective studies are necessary to provide definitive data.

METHODOLOGICAL CONSIDERATIONS FOR PROSPECTIVE STUDIES

STUDY DESIGN

There are no alternatives to prospective, randomized, double-blind, controlled trials (Noseworthy, 1988). Comparisons with historical controls cannot be accepted because of potential selection bias, and contemporaneous controls, although seemingly more appropriate, are acceptable only if there was random assignment to treatment and control groups. Attrition from the study is a major issue and all patients randomized must be followed as long as possible. It would be difficult, if not unethical, to argue for a placebo-controlled, long-term study in AD. It may be possible to extend a Phase II dose-response study or to study an approved treatment or a widely available agent with reported beneficial effects (e.g. vitamin E; Sano et al, 1997) to provide direct comparative data.

It is direct comparative data, against which costs can be applied on a country by country basis, that are important. Although 75% of patients may enter a nursing home in the US, this is clearly not the case in many other cultures where only a small fraction of patients enter nursing homes or have nursing home placement as an option. Data must be collected to capture all aspects of the natural history of disease progression. If the treatment is effective and the effects are robust, one would expect to find internal consistency across multiple domains and outcomes.

STUDY DURATION

In a population of patients with mild to moderate AD (MMSE 10–28 with a mean of 20) the time for 50% of the control patients to enter a nursing home would be in the order of 3 years (Knopman et al, 1996). Over this same period, our experience suggests only about 10% of the sample would have died. In order to capture a significant number of deaths, a study lasting up to 5 years would be required. A more severely impaired population could be studied and therefore more patients would reach these endpoints in a shorter time, but this would limit the generalizability of results to only severe patients and studying only severe patients may in fact bias against finding a treatment effect if severe patients are no longer responsive to treatment.

PATIENT POPULATION

Payers are concerned about the generalizability of results of cost-effectiveness studies. To the extent possible, the patient and caregiver populations studied should be comparable to the population that would receive the drug post-approval. For example, exclusion of patients with concurrent illnesses or those receiving concurrent medications should be kept to a minimum.

The patient population should be broadly defined by the severity of cognitive decline that one would include in a standard trial for efficacy, for example MMSE scores ranging from 8 or 10 through 26 or 28. A separate study of more severely impaired patients may also be worthwhile. In both cases the sample size, by necessity, will be large, in the order of 150–200 patients per treatment group because of the marked heterogeneity of the disease, as well as the patient and caregiver population (Mayeux et al, 1985). Assessments and data collection should be as simple as possible but adequate to capture all elements of the natural history (cognitive, activities of daily living, global severity of illness, and behavior) to be applied to models of disease management and cost as they exist in different countries. It would be of benefit to harmonize assessments and data collection for these studies and therefore make external comparisons more relevant.

RANDOMIZATION

The number of study sites should be limited to those which can recruit adequate numbers of patients. The objective is to use the minimum number of sites necessary and to encourage sites to fill the treatment blocks multiple times. This helps to control for different levels of caregiver and patient support, which can differ substantially between centers. Effective caregiver training alone has been shown to delay nursing home placement (Brodaty et al, 1993; Mittelman, 1990). Consideration should be given to stratifying on one and at most two key factors such as severity of illness, age, familial versus sporadic cases, as well as presence or absence of an apolipoprotein E4 allele which may themselves influence time to nursing home placement.

For Phase II placebo-controlled, dose-response studies of 6 months' duration, it is highly desirable to retain patients on their randomized doses in a blinded fashion beyond the end of the placebo-controlled period. This could provide a low-dose, randomized, controlled trial over a long period of time. Patients on placebo could transition to the highest dose and the delay in starting drug treatment could be used in analysis strategies to determine if the treatment delays disease progression. This is similar in concept to the randomized 'on design' proposed by Paul Leber, M.D. of the FDA.

CONCURRENT MEDICATIONS

Patients enrolled in the study should not be taking other central nervous system medications such as anxiolytics, antidepressants or antipsychotics at the time of enrollment. However, these agents may be used in the course of the trial if they are medically necessary and helpful to the caregiver in maintaining the patient at home or in managing the patient in a nursing home. This helps to retain patients in the study, adds to the value of economic analyses and helps to generalize the results to a broader patient sample. The ability to avoid other prescription medications associated with disease progression is in fact another index of effectiveness. All medications being taken at the time of study entry and all medications taken during the course of the study should be captured.

OUTCOMES

The outcomes selected should capture as many domains of the natural history of the disease as possible and should be simple, understandable, and applicable in a variety of cultures where burden of care may be far more important than nursing home placement. Systematic assessment of all patients randomized up to the point of death is essential to providing data where sources of potential bias through attrition can be addressed. The assessments should be completed routinely at least every 4 months and, if possible, assessments should be made at the time of nursing home placement.

QUANTITATIVE MEASURES

Cognitive: The Mini-Mental State Examination is a simple, brief, widely used cognitive assessment. It has been shown to be sensitive longitudinally to change (Folstein et al, 1975). It correlates significantly with both functional and behavioral measures, and is predictive of the major endpoints of interest relating to health care requirements, nursing home placement, and death (Tombaugh and McIntyre, 1992).

Global: In the absence of a demonstrably better instrument, the Global Deterioration Scale of Reisberg (1982) is adequate to capture severity of illness and has appropriate anchors, which can be readily applied in many cultures.

Behavioral: None of the behavioral measures currently available have been adequately validated in long-term controlled trials. Behavioral symptoms are highly variable and largely unpredictable. The value of the Neuropsychiatric Inventory as an outcome measure is the inclusion of an assessment of caregiver distress, which provides an index of caregiver emotional burden (Cummings et al, 1994). This instrument does require time to complete and training for administration but is likely to gain acceptance because of the assessment of caregiver distress.

Functional: The PSMS consists of six items (toiletting, feeding, dressing, grooming, physical dependency and bathing), each of which is clearly anchored and rated on a scale of 1 through 5 with a rating of 1 indicating complete independence, and 5 total dependence (Green et al, 1993). This scale is simple to administer, even by phone, and it has been used to determine placement requirements. The items are clearly a reflection of the burden placed upon the caregiver in caring for the patient's basic needs.

ENDPOINT OUTCOMES

Nursing Home Placement: All of the patients randomized to treatment must by definition be living at home and not in an assisted living situation. The inclusion of patients and families already in assisted living situations complicates the analysis unnecessarily. The nature of each new care situation needs to be defined in enough detail to allow accurate cost assignment. The alternatives for patient care continue to grow and defining the limits of assisted living versus skilled care versus custodial care is important. Analyses should allow provision for hospitalizations, collection of discharge diagnoses and flexibility for temporary placements, for example, hospitalization due to a fracture, followed by discharge to a care facility, followed by return to the home after rehabilitation.

Patients with dementia are more likely to enter a hospital than normal age-matched elderly, and their length of stay is likely to be influenced by the severity of the dementing illness (Johnston et al, 1987; Binder and Robins, 1990). Collecting dates of hospitalization and discharge diagnoses is critical for determining cost assignment.

Death: The issue of whether treatment may reduce mortality is non-ignorable. If patients are delayed in the time it takes for them to enter a nursing home and their life expectancy is prolonged then there may have been no cost saving and there may in fact be incremental costs associated with treatment.

ATTRITION/DROPOUTS

All patients who are randomized should be followed on all measures until death, even if consent to continue taking study medication is withdrawn. This allows examination of data to identify potential sources of bias which can take place if the dropout rate in one group is different from another. Patients who enter a nursing home should continue to have quantitative measures completed. Nursing home placement is only a surrogate for severe disability and the decision to place the patient in a nursing home may, in some cases, be independent of disease severity. This approach allows the use of survival methods using various levels of dependency as the endpoint with a consistent definition of equivalent to nursing home placement (Stern et al, 1997).

If in fact therapy is effective, attrition from the study is most likely to occur from the low-dose or control group; this could bias against showing a treatment effect if all patients are not followed to the endpoint of death.

STATISTICAL CONSIDERATIONS

If our assumptions about effective therapies are met, the data on cognitive function, activities of daily living, behavior and global severity should be internally consistent with analyses of nursing home placement. Application of costs can be modeled and adjusted to reflect the appropriate setting. Sensitivity parameters can be applied to estimate best case and worst case scenarios.

CONCLUSION

The challenge is to make clinical drug evaluation more sensitive to the economic realities of health care. The most reliable data can be generated within the context of well designed studies which also provide proof of efficacy. In each culture, an accurate determination of direct and indirect costs of AD against the natural history of the disease is needed. It must include quantitative measures of cognitive function, global severity of illness, activities of daily living, and behavior, in addition to nursing home placement and death. Harmonization of assessments and outcomes in economic studies would increase the reliability of decisions based upon clinical trial data.

REFERENCES

Berg, L., Miller, J. P., Storandt, M., Duchek, J., Morris, J. C., Rubin, E. H. et al (1988). Mild senile dementia of the Alzheimer type, 2: longitudinal assessment, *Ann. Neurol.*, **23**, 477–484.

Binder, E. F. and Robins, L. N. (1990). Cognitive impairment and length of hospital stay in older persons, *J. Am. Geriatr. Soc.*, **38**, 759–766.

Brodaty, H., McGilchrist, C., Harris, L. and Peters, K. E. (1993). Time until institutionalization and death in patients with dementia. Role of caregiver training and risk factors, *Arch. Neurol.*, **50**, 643–650.

Committee for Proprietary Medicinal Products (CPMP) (1997). Note for Guidance on Medicinal Products in the Treatment of Alzheimer's Disease, 24 July, London, UK.

Cummings, J. L., Mega, M., Gray, K., Rosenberg-Thompson, S., Carusi, D. A. and Gornbein, J. (1994). The neuropsychiatric inventory: comprehensive assessment of psychopathology in dementia, *Neurology*, **44**, 2308–2314.

Davis, K. L., Thal, L. J., Gamzu, E. R., Davis, C. S., Woolson, R. F., Gracon, S. I. et al (1992). A double-blind, placebo-controlled multicenter study of tacrine for Alzheimer's Disease, *N. Engl. J. Med.*, **327**, 1253–1259.

Drachman, D. A., O'Donnell, B. F., Lew, R. A. and Swearer, J. M. (1990). The prognosis in Alzheimer's disease. 'How far' rather than 'how fast' best predicts the course, *Arch. Neurol.*, **47**, 851–856.

Eagger, S. A., Levy, R. and Sahakian, B. (1991). Tacrine in Alzheimer's Disease, *Lancet*, **337**, 989–992.

Ernst, R. L. and Hay, J. W. (1994). The US economic and social costs of Alzheimer's disease revisited, *Am. J. Public Health*, **84**, 1261–1264.

Farlow, M., Gracon, S. I., Hershey, L. A., Lewis, K. W., Sadowsky, C. H. and Dolan-Ureno, J. (1992). A controlled trial of tacrine in Alzheimer's disease, *JAMA*, **268**, 2523–2529.

Folstein, M. F., Folstein, S. E. and McHugh, P. R. (1975). Mini-mental state, *J. Psychiatr. Res.*, **12**, 189–198.

Forrette, F., Hoover, T., Gracon, S., de Rotrou, J., Hervy, M. P., Lechevalier, B. et al (1995). A double-blind, placebo-controlled, enriched population study of tacrine in patients with Alzheimer's disease, *Eur. J. Neurol.*, **2**, 229–238.

Foster, N. L., Petersen, R. C., Gracon, S. I. and Lewis, K. (1996). An enriched-population, double-blind, placebo-controlled, crossover study of tacrine and lecithin in Alzheimer's disease, *Dementia*, **7**, 260–266.

Gracon, S. I., Knapp, M. J., Berghoff, W. G., Pierce, M., DeJong, R., Lobbestael, S. J. et al (in press). Safety of tacrine: clinical trials, treatment IND and postmarketing experience, *Alzheimer Dis. Assoc. Disord.*

Gray, A. M. (1995). The economic impact of Alzheimer's disease, *Rev. Contemp. Pharmacother.*, **6**, 327–334.

Green, C. R., Mohs, R. C., Schmeidler, R., Aryan, M. and Davis, K. L. (1993). Functional decline in Alzheimer's disease: a longitudinal study, *J. Am. Geriatr. Soc.*, **41**, 654–661.

Gunderson, C. H. (1995). The impact of new pharmaceutical agents on the cost of neurologic care, *Neurology*, **45**, 569–572.

Henke, C. J. and Burchmore, M. J. (1997). The economic impact of tacrine in the treatment of Alzheimer's disease, *Clinical Therapeutics*, **19**, 330–345.

Heyman, A., Peterson, B., Fillenbaum, G. and Pieper, C. (1997). Predictors of time to institutionalization of patients with Alzheimer's disease. The CERAD experience, Part XVII. *Neurology*, **48**, 1304–1309.

Heyman, A., Wilkinson, W. E., Hurwitz, B. J., Helms, M. J, Haynes, C. S., Utley, C. M. and Gwyther, L. P. (1987). Early-onset Alzheimer's disease: clinical predictors of institutionalization and death, *Neurology*, **37**, 980–984.

Johnson, J. A. and Bootman, J. L. (1994). Pharmacoeconomic analysis in formulary decisions: an international perspective, *Am. J. Hosp. Pharm.*, **51**, 2593–2598.

Johnston, M., Wakeling, A., Graham, N. and Stokes, F. (1987). Cognitive impairment, emotional disorder and length of stay of elderly patients in a district general hospital, *B. J. Med. Psychol.*, **60**, 133–139.

Jost, B. C. and Grossberg, G. T. (1995). The natural history of Alzheimer's disease: a brain bank study, *J. Am. Geriatr. Soc.*, **43**, 1248–1255.

Knapp, M. J., Knopman, D. S., Solomon, P. R., Pendlebury, W. W., Davis, C. S. and Gracon, S. I. (1994). A 30-week randomized controlled trial of high-dose tacrine in patients with Alzheimer's disease, *JAMA*, **271**, 985–991.

Knopman, D. S., Knapp, M. J., Gracon, S. I. and Davis, C. S. (1994). The clinician interview-based impression of change (CIBIC): a clinician's global change rating scale in Alzheimer's disease, *Neurology*, **44**, 2315–2321.

Knopman, D., Schneider, L., Davis, K., Talwalker, S., Smith, F., Hoover, T. and

Gracon, S. (1996). Long-term tacrine (Cognex) treatment: effects on nursing home placement and mortality, *Neurology*, **47**, 166–177.

Knopman, D., Schneider, L., Davis, K., Gracon, S. and Smith, F. (1998). Long-term tacrine treatment effects, *Neurology*, **50**, 567–568.

Kramer-Ginsberg, E., Mohs, R. C., Aryan, M., Lobel, D., Silverman, J., Davidson M. and Davis, K. L. (1988). Clinical predictors of course for Alzheimer patients in a longitudinal study: a preliminary report, *Psychopharmacol Bull.*, **24**.

Lawton, M. P. and Brody, E. M. (1969). Assessment of older people: self-maintaining and instrumental activities of daily living, *Gerontology*, **9**, 179–186.

Leber, P. (1990). Guidelines for the evaluation of antidementia drugs: first draft, 8 November. US Food and Drug Administration, Division of Neuropharmacology.

Levy, M. L., Cummings, J. L., Fairbanks, L. A., Bravi, D., Calvani, M. and Carta, A. (1996). Longitudinal assessment of symptoms of depression, agitation and psychosis in 181 patients with Alzheimer's disease, *Am. J. Psychiatry*, **153**, 1438–1443.

Lubeck, D. P., Mazonson, P. D. and Bowe, T. (1994). Potential effect of tacrine on expenditures for Alzheimer's disease, *Med. Interface*, **7**, 130–138.

Mayeux, R., Stern, Y. and Spanton, S. (1985). Heterogeneity in dementia of the Alzheimer type: evidence of subgroups, *Neurology*, **35**, 453–461.

Mittleman, M. S. (1990). A randomized trial of family caregiver support in the home management of dementia, *J. Am. Geriatr. Soc.*, **38**, 446–454.

Noseworthy, J. H. (1988). There are no alternatives to double-blind, controlled trials, *Neurology*, **38** (suppl 2), 76–79.

Piccini, C., Bracco, L., Falcini, M., Pracucci, G. and Amaducci, L. (1995). Natural history of Alzheimer's disease: prognostic value of plateau, *Journal of the Neurological Sciences*, **131**, 177–182.

Post, S. G. and Whitehouse, P. J. (1992). Ethics and dementia: current issues dementia and the life prolonging technologies used: an ethical question, *Alzheimer Dis. Assoc. Disord.*, **6**, 3–6.

Reisberg, B., Ferris, S. H., de Leon, M. J. and Crook, T. (1982). The global deterioration scale for assessment of primary degenerative dementia, *Am. J. Psychiatry*, **139**, 1136–1139.

Sano, M., Ernesto, C., Thomas, R., Klauber, M. R., Schaffer, K., Grundman, M. et al (1997). A controlled trial of selegeline, alpha-tochopherol, or both as treatment for Alzheimer's disease, *N. Engl. J. Med.*, **336**, 1216–1222.

Seversen, M. A., Smith, G. E., Tangelos, E. G., Petersen, R. C., Kokmen, E., Ivnik R. J. et al (1994). Patterns and predictors of institutionalization in community-based dementia patients, *J. Am. Geriatr. Soc.*, **42**, 181–185.

Smith, F., Gracon, S., Knopman, D. and Schneider, L. (in press). Tacrine treatment and nursing home placement: application of the Cox proportional hazards model with time-dependent covariates, *Drug Inf. J.*, **32**.

Source: US National Institutes of Health, National Institute on Aging.

Stern, Y., Albert, M., Brandt, J., Jacobs, D. M., Tang, M-X., Marder, K. et al (1994). Utility of extrapyramidal signs and psychosis as predictors of cognitive and functional decline, nursing home admission and death in Alzheimer's disease: prospective analyses from the predictors study, *Neurology*, **44**, 2300–2307.

Stern, Y., Hesdorffer, D., Sano, M. and Mayeux, R. (1990). Measurement and prediction of functional capacity in Alzheimer's disease, *Neurology*, **40**, 8–14.

Stern, Y., Tang, M., Albert, M. S., Brandt, J., Jacobs, D. M., Bell, K. et al (1997). Predicting time to nursing home care and death in individuals with Alzheimer's disease, *JAMA*, **277**, 806–812.

Tombaugh, T. N. and McIntyre, N. J. (1992). The mini-mental state examination: a comprehensive review, *J. Am. Geriatr. Soc.*, **40**, 922–935.

Uhlmann, R. F., Larson, E. B. and Buchner, D. M. (1987). Correlations of mini-mental state and modified dementia rating scale to measures of transitional health status in dementia, *J. of Gerontology*, **42**(1), 33–36.

Welch, H. G., Walsh, J. S. and Larson, E. B. (1992). The cost of institutional care in Alzheimer's disease: nursing home and hospital use in a prospective cohort, *J. Am. Geriatr. Soc.*, **40**, 221–224.

Wilcock, G. K., Surmon, D. J., Scott, M., Boyle, M., Mulligan, K., Neubauer, K. A., O'Neill, D. and Royston, V. H. (1993). An evaluation of the efficacy and safety of tetrahydroaminoacridine (THA) without lecithin in the treatment of Alzheimer's disease, *Age Ageing*, **22**, 316–324.

4.8 Outcomes Research and Alzheimer's Disease: A Pharmaceutical Industry Perspective

VERA MASTEY

Pfizer Pharmaceuticals Group, New York, USA

INTRODUCTION

Over the last 20–30 years, not only has health care expenditure expanded rapidly in absolute terms but—as a percentage of gross national product—it has surpassed other categories of expenditure (OECD, 1995). The universal reaction has been that decisions regarding allocation of health care resources now involve many payers, including governments, formulary committees, insurance companies and managed care organizations, as they all look for ways to contain this growth (Sloan and Grabowski, 1997).

This is no easy task because the drivers of health care costs are powerful and increasingly fueled by a growing number of elderly people in many countries, with increasing needs for treatment and management of long-term medical conditions and age-related disorders, among them Alzheimer's disease.

International policies to contain health care costs have often focused on drugs, since these are a visible and seemingly easily managed element of health care costs. Such policies have been flawed not simply because drugs represent only about 10% of total health care expenditure, but also because efforts to curtail costs have on occasion provided evidence at a later date of actually reducing efficiency at the same time (Soumerai et al, 1994).

Interventions and policies to control drug expenditures have been introduced to depress both demand and supply. These include limiting reimbursement, introducing patient co-payments (Bloor and Freemantle, 1996a) and budgetary restrictions, providing information and feedback to physicians and establishing prescribing guidelines (Bloor and Freemantle, 1996b). In addition, there have been demands on the pharmaceutical industry by governments and payers to provide them with information about the 'cost-effectiveness' of newly

Health Economics of Dementia. Edited by Anders Wimo, Bengt Jönsson, Göran Karlsson and Bengt Winblad.
© 1998 John Wiley & Sons Ltd.

introduced therapies, to help them make informed resource allocation decisions. Whereas traditionally physicians have been the pharmaceutical industry's primary customers for information relating to new drug therapies, it must now also direct its efforts towards many new customers, including governments, private payers, formularies, and so on (Andersson, 1995).

Outcomes research is the systematic study of the impact of disease on society and individuals and how medicines affect the quality of life, resource utilization and cost of treating these diseases. Outcomes research provides a means for assessing the costs and effectiveness of a specific health care intervention and supplies payers with key information needed to make decisions about pricing, reimbursement and formulary inclusion. In addition, outcomes research provides pharmaceutical companies with valuable information that can be used to promote a new drug or to help establish relationships with opinion leaders and customers (physicians, patients, governments) through communication of study results.

OUTCOMES RESEARCH GOALS IN ALZHEIMER'S DISEASE

Alzheimer's disease is an insidious, progressive neurodegenerative disorder, marked by memory loss, confusion, impaired judgment and speech, and other cognitive disabilities. In time, other symptoms including agitation, depression, psychosis and general impaired functioning may become so severe that patients often require total care (Wimo et al, 1992).

Alzheimer's disease is the most common cause of dementia in the elderly, affecting 3% of men and women aged 65 to 74, and increasing in prevalence with age (Alzheimer's Education and Referral Center). Studies have estimated that the prevalence rates double approximately every five years up to the age of around 95 (Jorm et al, 1987). It is estimated that some 4 million people in the US have Alzheimer's disease, 5 to 6 million people in Western Europe and almost 2 million people in Japan (Evers, 1997). The aging of the population will cause a dramatic increase in the number of individuals with Alzheimer's disease; it is estimated that by the year 2040, there will be more than 10 million people in the US with Alzheimer's disease (Evans, 1990; US Congress OTA, 1987).

The impact of Alzheimer's disease is enormous, not just on the patient but on the caregiver at home and on society in general. In its early phases, much of the burden of care falls to the immediate family, with particular impact on both the sufferers' and caregivers' quality of life. In advanced stages, patients often require institutionalization, with all its implications and costs. Estimates of the overall economic burden in the US alone range from $80 billion to $100 billion in annual total treatment costs (Snow, 1996).

There is currently no cure for Alzheimer's disease patients but, in some countries, new therapies are now available for those patients with mild to moderate Alzheimer's disease which are designed to improve cognitive and global function (Aricept™, Cognex™, Exelon™).

From a pharmaceutical industry perspective, the successful introduction of a new therapy for the treatment of Alzheimer's disease will include clinical, marketing and outcomes research strategies and initiatives aimed at addressing the many challenges specific to this illness and the particular needs of all relevant customers. Outcomes research is especially important in Alzheimer's disease because standard measures of clinical efficacy, such as improvements in cognitive function measured on the Alzheimer's Disease Assessment Scale—cognitive subscale (ADAS-Cog) or Mini-Mental State Examination (MMSE), may not be relevant to all customers. Outcomes research studies help us to communicate these clinical benefits in a more meaningful way: patient function and behavior, caregiver burden and quality of life, health care resource utilization and cost savings.

USING OUTCOMES RESEARCH TO ADDRESS PHARMACEUTICAL INDUSTRY CHALLENGES

Outcomes research can be used effectively to address the political, clinical and economic challenges specific to Alzheimer's disease. Examples of these are given below.

- The introduction of therapies for the treatment of Alzheimer's disease will increase drug expenditures in a disease area where these have traditionally been relatively low. In parallel, the aging of the population common to all Western countries will result in a large increase in the number of individuals with Alzheimer's disease, and a corresponding increase in the number of elderly patients requiring long-term and acute care. The social and fiscal effects of these factors will pose a major challenge for health care decision-makers and put more pressures on the need to restrain the rise in costs imposed by new drug therapies.

  Challenge—To develop 'value for money' arguments to support reimbursement and formulary inclusion of new drug therapies.

  Outcomes Research response—To demonstrate that positive effects on cognitive and global function reduce Alzheimer's disease costs and ease patient and caregiver burden.

The use of health economic arguments during pricing and reimbursement negotiations relies upon decision-makers focusing not only on the price of the medicine, but to a greater extent on the outcomes achieved. In the case of

Alzheimer's disease, these customer groups will need to be convinced that if new therapies can delay the onset of more severe symptoms, cost savings can be identified within the health care system. For example, the patients may not require high-dependency care so early and the net cost of treating these patients might be reduced.

For chronic diseases such as Alzheimer's disease, health economic models can be used to predict the benefits of interventions by extrapolating the short-term effects and outcomes benefits demonstrated in clinical trials to the longer-term scenario. The utility of these models depends upon the quality of input data (clinical and economic), and upon the robustness of the extrapolation method (e.g. Markov model). Properly constructed models are becoming more widely accepted by a variety of key customers.

Including measures of patient function and behavior, caregiver quality of life, caregiver burden and patient and caregiver health care resource utilization in appropriate clinical studies can also help to describe the benefits of therapy.

- There are considerable differences between countries in the level and type of care provided for patients and caregivers. Many countries have not appropriately budgeted for Alzheimer's disease, and financial support and health care services are not readily available to patients and caregivers.

  Challenge—To improve the level of care provided to patients and caregivers.

  Outcomes Research response—To communicate information to policy-makers about the economic and social burden of Alzheimer's disease for patients, caregivers and society, the need for better disease management and the role of drug therapy in effective patient management.

Governments and policy-makers have an elected responsibility to direct health care resource utilization to those areas of greatest practical need. These customers are important decision-makers in the management of Alzheimer's disease, as the burden of this particular disease can impact on the budgets of different departments in many countries (such as health and social services).

Outcomes research can help them understand how new therapies could alter the pattern of service provision and reduce the overall burden of care to society. For example, if new therapies enable patients to be maintained at home for longer than is currently the case, social services may be required to provide flexible and responsive home care resources for longer periods of time. On the health services side, this may mean that the patient requires less inpatient care in local mental health units for treatment or for respite.

These programs are important for educating decision-makers about the true burden of Alzheimer's disease, emphasizing the need for better therapeutic management and placing the role and cost of drug treatment in its true perspective. The skill lies in understanding the dynamics of the health care system in each country such that critical data can be provided to raise awareness regarding the economic and social consequences of this disease and to show that the cost of drug treatment is just a small component of the overall burden of Alzheimer's disease.

Examples of these initiatives include health policy round-table meetings, in which a cross-section of participants from all areas of the health care services meet to develop a consensus on the support that is needed for Alzheimer's disease patients and their caregivers, the roles of primary and secondary care and the appropriate role of drug therapy. The publication of the outcomes of these meetings in the form of health policy papers and research findings in specialized Alzheimer's disease journals is valuable.

Cost-of-illness studies that estimate the economic burden of Alzheimer's disease in specific countries address these issues as well by determining principal cost drivers, identifying research priorities and, thus, influencing social, health and economic policies for this illness (Østbye and Crosse, 1994).

- Awareness of Alzheimer's disease is low in most countries and the symptoms tend to be regarded by patients and their families as part of the natural aging process. Sufferers and carers often do not seek help from their physicians until 'things have begun to go wrong' and patients are in the later stages of the disease, when problems have become severe. Patients living alone may only come to the attention of primary care physicians if they have been admitted to hospitals as an emergency. At these later stages medical treatments are less beneficial.

Challenge—To raise awareness of Alzheimer's disease among potential patients and their families and to increase early consultations when patients are in the mild stages and treatments are available.

Outcomes Research response—To sensitize patients and caregivers to the potential economic and quality-of-life benefits of early diagnosis and treatment of Alzheimer's disease.

Patients value their independence, as do their caregivers, and outcomes research programs can provide evidence of quality-of-life improvements attributable to drug therapy for certain patient groups. Again, including measures of patient function and behavior in appropriate clinical studies can assess these benefits. In those countries where a patient co-payment for medicines is made, patients and caregivers will need to understand such value-for-money arguments.

- The diagnosis of Alzheimer's disease appears to be almost exclusively provided by specialists rather than by primary care physicians. The diagnosis often takes place later in Europe than in the US, and the reasons for this are thought to be lack of simple, specific diagnostic criteria, the previous lack of effective therapy for cognitive defects in Alzheimer's disease, and the adverse effect on patient and family of the diagnosis of a disease that is perceived as incurable and progressive (Breteler, 1992).

Challenge—To improve diagnosis at the primary care level.

Outcomes Research response—To collaborate in the development of disease management tools and diagnostic guidelines.

The responsibility of primary care physicians to use cost-effective medicines has been reinforced by many policies, including such reforms as them taking budgetary responsibility (as in the UK and Germany).

Our goal is to sensitize them to the ways in which the management process of Alzheimer's disease can be re-engineered to produce improved outcomes through the appropriate usage of new therapies and their inclusion in disease management guidelines; for example, evidence of improvements in patient quality of life and cost savings attributable to delays in nursing home admissions.

- Alzheimer's disease intensely influences and affects the lives of relatives and caregivers. Without the contribution of carers, both social and health care providers may face increased costs, should higher levels of intervention become necessary earlier in the progression of the disease. Caregiver burden is not widely understood, and must be addressed through research and communication of the findings.

  Challenge—To understand fully the needs of caregivers and to provide support.

  Outcomes Research response—To measure the effect of drug therapy in easing caregiver burden and to communicate the benefits of therapy to policymakers, physicians and caregivers.

There are significant social, psychological and financial impacts on the informal carers of Alzheimer's disease patients. Caregivers suffer from stress, lack of sleep, fatigue, somatic complaints, anxiety and depression, which may result in their own need for medication and support (Clipp and George, 1990; Jones and Peters, 1992).

Our responsibility is to help caregivers to 'see' how the appropriate usage of new therapies might improve the cognitive and global functioning of some patients, and thereby reduce some of the burden on themselves. Outcomes research can provide this evidence of improved quality of life for these carers.

In order to demonstrate this, appropriate measurements are included in clinical studies to provide relatively hard data on the impacts that drug therapy will have on selected outcomes; for example, specific measurements of caregiver quality of life, psychological, social and physical burden, time spent providing care to a patient and time missed from work. The findings of these studies should be communicated to payers, providers, prescribers, patients and caregivers through quality journals.

FUTURE NEEDS

The major challenge facing everyone today is to increase efficiency and productivity within our health care systems. This will require a change in the way health care provision is viewed and a move away from cost-containment towards efficiency, value and optimum patient outcomes. More knowledge is needed about the range of care that should be provided for different diseases and patient groups, and of the financial implications. Many different programs now exist for payers and providers to improve clinical, patient and economic outcomes through better disease management. All these initiatives will require the ability to measure the outcomes of treatments so as to assess their effectiveness.

Drug companies have a specific role and responsibility in this area to assist in the development of reliable, valid methodologies for economic analysis and to communicate with decision-makers such that levels of knowledge and expertise are raised. This will involve increased collaboration among health care decision-makers in the development of studies, disease management programs, treatment protocols and guidelines.

Alzheimer's disease is currently the third most expensive disease to treat in the US following cancer and heart disease (Snow, 1996). Prevalence rates are expected to continue to increase because of the dramatic aging of the population in many Western countries, and this medical need is currently underserved. Current acetylcholinesterase inhibitors represent advances in the treatment of the symptoms of Alzheimer's disease, and these therapies may bring not just quality-of-life improvements for both sufferers and carers, but also improvements in health care utilization in the whole system.

Pharmacoeconomic analyses will have an increasingly significant influence on health care decisions affecting people with dementia. In future, outcomes research collaborations between pricing and reimbursement authorities, prescribers, payers, patients, carers, researchers, economists and drug companies are essential to ensure that decision-makers are provided with information that will enable them to make the most effective use of limited resources.

REFERENCES

Alzheimer's Disease Education & Referral Center (1996). National Institute on Aging. *Alzheimer's Disease: Fact Sheet.*
Andersson, F. (1995). Why is the pharmaceutical industry investing increasing amounts in health economic evaluations? *Int. J. Technol. Assess. Health Care*, **11**(4), 750–761.

Bloor, K. and Freemantle, N. (1996a). Lessons from international experience in controlling pharmaceutical expenditure. I influencing patients. *BMJ*, **312**, 1469–1471.

Bloor, K. and Freemantle, N. (1996b). Lessons from international experience in controlling pharmaceutical expenditure. II influencing doctors. *BMJ*, **312**, 1525–1527.

Breteler, M. M. B., Cluas, J. J., van Duijin, C. M. et al (1992). Epidemiology of Alzheimer's disease. *Epidemiol. Rev.*, **14**, 59–82.

Clipp, E. C. and George, L. K. (1990). Psychotropic drug use among caregivers of patients with dementia. *J. Amer. Geriatr. Soc.*, **38**, 227–235.

Evans, D. (1990). Estimated prevalence of Alzheimer's disease in the United States. *Milbank Q.*, **68**, 267–289.

Evers, P. (1997). *Diseases of the Elderly: Markets and Developments*, p. 34. Financial Times Pharmaceuticals and Health Care Publishing. London, Pearson Professional.

Jones, D. A. and Peters, T. J. (1992). Caring for elderly dependants: effects on the quality of life. *Age Ageing*, **21**, 421–428.

Jorm, A. F., Korten, A. E. and Henderson, A. S. (1987). The prevalence of dementia: A quantitative integration of the literature. *Acta. Psychiatr. Scan.*, **76**, 465–479.

Organization for Economic Cooperation and Development (1995). New directions in health care policy. *Health Policy Studies, No. 7*.

Østbye, T. and Crosse, E. (1994). Net economic costs of dementia in Canada. *Can. Med. Assoc. J.*, **151**, 1457–1464.

Sloan, F. A. and Grabowski, G. H. (1997). The impact of cost-effectiveness on public and private policies in health care. An international perspective. Introduction and overview. *Soc. Sci. Med.*, **45**(4), 505–510.

Snow, C. (1996). Medicare HMOs develop plan for future of Alzheimer's programming. *Modern Healthcare*, 23 September, 66–70.

Soumerai, S. B., McLaughline, T. J., Ross-Degnan, D., Casteris, C. S. and Bollini, P. (1994). Effects of limiting Medicaid drug-reimbursement benefits on the use of psychotropic agents and acute mental health services by patients with schizophrenia. *N. Engl. J. Med.*, **331**, 650–655.

US Congress Office of Technology Assessment (1987). *Losing a Million Minds: Confronting the Tragedy of Alzheimer's Disease and other Dementias*. Washington, DC, US Government Printing Office.

Wimo, A., Gustafsson, L. and Mattson B. (1992). Predictive validity of factors influencing the institutionalization of elderly people with psychogeriatric disorders. *Scand. J. Prim. Health Care*, **10**(3), 185–191.

5 Final Remarks

5.1 A Proposed Health Economics Research Agenda for Dementia

BENGT WINBLAD
Karolinska Institute, Stockholm, Sweden

GÖRAN KARLSSON, BENGT JÖNSSON
Stockholm School of Economics, Stockholm, Sweden

ANDERS WIMO
Karolinska Institute, Stockholm, Sweden

Our main conclusion from working with this book is that the health economics of dementia is in its infancy. The database is small, although expanding, and the methodological problems are obvious. The social and economic consequences of dementia are enormous and there are reasons to believe that new drugs and other care strategies could have a positive influence on the situation of patients and caregivers. However, the present research mostly includes short-term studies on patients with mild and moderate dementia, mainly focusing on cognitive function, ADL and, from the economic point of view, on the effects of institutionalisation. Based on the discussions in this book and other research contacts, it is obvious that the research field must be broadened and a research agenda focusing on the social impact and health economics aspects of dementia could, *inter alia*, include the following studies:

- Research on outcome measures relevant for the patient. This research should have a wide approach: not just cognitive and functional capacity, but also behaviour, mood, psychiatric symptoms and quality of life. Endpoints used in clinical trials are not obviously appropriate in a health economic study.
- There should also be a focus on the caregiver's situation, including burden, coping, depression, quality of life and resource use, but also on principles for costing informal care. This involves both methodological and empirical issues. What should be measured, how should it be measured, and how should the measure be incorporated in a health economics study?
- Research which increases the understanding of the course of the disease, from onset to death. There are several important issues that should be

Health Economics of Dementia. Edited by Anders Wimo, Bengt Jönsson, Göran Karlsson and Bengt Winblad.
© 1998 John Wiley & Sons Ltd.

taken into account when the course of the disease is analysed. This requires epidemiological, individual, longitudinal data of good quality, but also some kind of modelling in order to structure the data. In order to perform health economics analyses it is important to understand how the disease progresses from mild, through moderate, to severe dementia. Much of the course of dementia occurs in severe dementia, causing great suffering, and considerable resource utilisation and costs. In spite of this, little is known about treatment effects in this stage.

- Study periods for drug interventions have so far been short, mostly one year or less. The long-term effects can be analysed with various approaches such as the use of modelling techniques, for instance Markov models, and open follow-up studies. An interesting approach regarding progression and survival would be the establishment of a link between longitudinal population-based studies and clinical trials. Hitherto, pharmaceutical interventions with anti-dementia drugs studies have mostly been single drug studies, with only modest results. Combination studies including drugs with different ways of acting should also be performed, as well as studies focusing on combined treatment strategies such as drugs and non-pharmacological treatment strategies (e.g. drugs combined with day care and support to family members).

- The relationship between the progression of the disease, place of living and cost is complex. How these factors interact depends on the organisation of care. The organisation of care is differentiated between many countries, with various care alternatives between the patient's own home and nursing homes. We also need improved methods of describing different care alternatives in such a way as to facilitate international comparisons.

- Many demented patients suffer from other disorders as well. It is essential to know to what extent comorbidity affects cost and outcome, but this is rarely analysed.

- In many studies, costs of dementia care are based on the general costs of different care alternatives. However, this may be misleading since demented patients probably have other care needs in, for instance, a ward or at home, such as constant necessity of surveillance. Different degrees of severity of dementia also demand different forms of care support. Therefore, dementia-specific per item costs should be calculated and compared with general per item costs.

- Discussions regarding efficacy vs effectiveness are essential when the results of clinical trials are evaluated. A study population's representativeness in terms of type and degree of dementia (is severe dementia excluded?), age, sex, and family situation, and also its representativeness regarding distribution of care organisation are both factors of importance. Potential intervention effects in terms of savings are therefore linked to effects of the type of care/accommodation. If a study period, for example, lasts a year and there are changes in the organisation of care during this period (such as closing down institutions), the effect of this may surpass potential intervention effects.

Dementia is one of the most devastating and costly groups of diseases and its impact on the care systems in different countries will increase. Given the present literature, the need for a great expansion of health economics research on dementia is obvious and we hope that this book will be a contribution to this field.

Index

INDEX

Index compiled by Geoffrey C. Jones

Lightning Source UK Ltd.
Milton Keynes UK
UKOW05n2119210514

232067UK00001B/16/A